Nutraceutical and Functional Foods in Disease Prevention

Raj K. Keservani
Chhatrapati Shahu Ji Maharaj Group of Institutions, India

Anil K. Sharma
Delhi Institute of Pharmaceutical Sciences and Research, India

Rajesh K. Kesharwani
Nims University Rajasthan, India

A volume in the Advances in
Human Services and Public Health
(AHSPH) Book Series

IGI Global
DISSEMINATOR OF KNOWLEDGE

Published in the United States of America by
IGI Global
Medical Information Science Reference (an imprint of IGI Global)
701 E. Chocolate Avenue
Hershey PA, USA 17033
Tel: 717-533-8845
Fax: 717-533-8661
E-mail: cust@igi-global.com
Web site: http://www.igi-global.com

Library of Congress Cataloging-in-Publication Data

Names: Keservani, Raj K., 1981- editor | Sharma, Anil K., 1980- editor | Kesharwani, Rajesh K., 1978- editor
Title: Nutraceutical and functional foods in disease prevention / Raj K. Keservani, Anil K. Sharma, and Rajesh K. Kesharwani, Editors.
Description: Hershey PA : Medical Information Science Reference, [2018]
Identifiers: LCCN 2017018636| ISBN 9781522532675 (hardcover) | ISBN 9781522532682 (ebook)
Subjects: | MESH: Dietary Supplements | Functional Food | Primary Prevention
Classification: LCC RA784 | NLM QU 145.5 | DDC 613.2--dc23 LC record available at https://lccn.loc.gov/2017018636

This book is published in the IGI Global book series Advances in Human Services and Public Health (AHSPH) (ISSN: 2475-6571; eISSN: 2475-658X)

British Cataloguing in Publication Data
A Cataloguing in Publication record for this book is available from the British Library.

Advances in Human Services and Public Health (AHSPH) Book Series

ISSN:2475-6571
EISSN:2475-658X

Editor-in-Chief: Jennifer Martin, RMIT University, Australia

MISSION

The well-being of the general public should be a primary concern for any modern civilization. Ongoing research in the field of human services and public healthcare is necessary to evaluate, manage, and respond to the health and social needs of the global population.

The **Advances in Human Services and Public Health (AHSPH)** book series aims to publish high-quality reference publications focused on the latest methodologies, tools, issues, and strategies for managing the health and social welfare of the public. The AHSPH book series will be especially relevant for healthcare professionals, policy makers, government officials, and students seeking the latest research in this field.

COVERAGE

- Poverty
- Health policy
- Healthcare Reform
- Social Welfare Policy
- Access to Healthcare Services
- Public Welfare
- Public Funding
- Medicare and Medicaid
- Assistance Programs
- Social Work

IGI Global is currently accepting manuscripts for publication within this series. To submit a proposal for a volume in this series, please contact our Acquisition Editors at Acquisitions@igi-global.com or visit: http://www.igi-global.com/publish/.

The Advances in Human Services and Public Health (AHSPH) Book Series (ISSN 2475-6571) is published by IGI Global, 701 E. Chocolate Avenue, Hershey, PA 17033-1240, USA, www.igi-global.com. This series is composed of titles available for purchase individually; each title is edited to be contextually exclusive from any other title within the series. For pricing and ordering information please visit http://www.igi-global.com/book-series/advances-human-services-public-health/102256. Postmaster: Send all address changes to above address.

Titles in this Series

For a list of additional titles in this series, please visit:
https://www.igi-global.com/book-series/advances-human-services-public-health/102256

Ethical Issues in Social Work Practice
Antonio Sandu (Ştefan cel Mare University of Suceava, Romania) and Ana Frunza (LUMEN Research Center in Social and Humanistic Sciences, Rmania)
Information Science Reference • ©2018 • 328pp • H/C (ISBN: 9781522530909) • US $195.00

Global Perspectives on Human Migration, Asylum, and Security
Christina M. Akrivopoulou (Hellenic Open University, reece)
Information Science Reference • ©2018 • 268pp • H/C (ISBN: 9781522528173) • US $185.00

Nutraceuticals and Innovative Food Products for Healthy Living and Preventive Care
Amit Verma (SDAU, India) Kajal Srivastava (GBPUAT, India) Shivom Singh (ITM University, India) and Hukum Singh (Forest Research Institute, India)
Medical Information Science Reference • ©2018 • 462pp • H/C (ISBN: 9781522529705) • US $245.00

Health Information Systems and the Advancement of Medical Practice in Developing Countries
Kgomotso H. Moahi (University of Botswana, Botswana) Kelvin Joseph Bwalya (University of Johannesburg, South Africa) and Peter Mazebe II Sebina (University of Botswana, Botswana)
Medical Information Science Reference • ©2017 • 350pp • H/C (ISBN: 9781522522621) • US $200.00

Examining the Role of Environmental Change on Emerging Infectious Diseases and Pandemics
Maha Bouzid (University of East Anglia, UK)
Information Science Reference • ©2017 • 327pp • H/C (ISBN: 9781522505532) • US $200.00

Sexual Misconduct in the Education and Human Services Sector
Christopher Schwilk (Shippensburg University, USA) Rachel Stevenson (Shippensburg University, USA) and David Bateman (Shippensburg University, USA)
Information Science Reference • ©2017 • 291pp • H/C (ISBN: 9781522506577) • US $190.00

For an entire list of titles in this series, please visit:
https://www.igi-global.com/book-series/advances-human-services-public-health/102256

IGI Global
DISSEMINATOR OF KNOWLEDGE

701 East Chocolate Avenue, Hershey, PA 17033, USA
Tel: 717-533-8845 x100 • Fax: 717-533-8661
E-Mail: cust@igi-global.com • www.igi-global.com

Table of Contents

Detailed Table of Contents

The human body harbors ten times more bacterial cells than human cells. These bacterial cells form the human microbiome that plays a vital role in human health. An imbalance in the gut microbiome (i.e., dysbiosis) can result in various pathological conditions. This dysbiosis can be refurbished with the supplement of "probiotics." Probiotics have thus been defined as non-pathogenic micro-organisms that, when ingested, exert a positive influence on host health or physiology. The most commonly used probiotic bacteria comes from two genera: Lactobacillus and Bifidobacterium. Various research findings have proposed a correlation between the alteration of microbiota (composition/activity/density) with disorders like infectious diarrhea, inflammatory bowel diseases, obesity, to name a few. The ultimate effect of administration of probiotics on health or physiology is either direct or indirect. This chapter summarizes the concept of probiotics, their therapeutic aspect along with possible mechanism of action.

Probiotics have become the major breakthrough in therapeutic applications due to their various health promoting effects in humans by maintaining the homeostasis of the intestine and prevent microbial imbalance (dysbiosis) without any side effects. Dysbiosis in the microbial population is the major cause for several diseases in humans. Treatment of diseases using antibiotics is not recommended due to high cost, side effects, and the loss of intestinal friendly bacteria. Probiotics work in symbiotic association with the intestine and produce several metabolites which not only regulate the growth of pathogenic bacteria but also provide vital nutrients which contribute to human health. The present chapter highlights about the role of probiotics in treatment and prevention of different human diseases.

Obesity is a medical condition caused by the accumulation of excess fat in the body. The main causes of obesity are lifestyle, less physical activity, and increased health problems. Overweight and obesity have increased over the past 20 years in many regions of the world, particularly the prevalence of obesity in childhood. It is not only a problem of developed countries but also becoming a growing burden for the developing countries. Functional foods might play important role in prevention or treatment of overweight. Functional foods for obesity influences the energy balance equation regulated by the control of energy intake or of energy dissipated as heat (thermogenesis).

Obesity has now become an epidemic affecting wide variety of population across the world. It is associated with a cluster of cardiovascular diseases and other related metabolic disorders such as diabetes, hypertension, and cancer which is mainly caused due to the dysbiosis in the energy intake and expenditure. Researchers have found a wide variety of functional foods from different sources which help in combating and prevention of obesity and its related diseases. Recent advancement in nutritional science has led to the development of several functional foods with low glycemic index. The present chapter highlights about the problems related to obesity and the importance of various functional foods which have great potential to be incorporated in our daily diet to curb the menace of obesity.

Hypertension is the major cause of mortality amongst many cardiovascular risk factors causing 7.5 million deaths annually. Macronutrient and micronutrient deficiencies are very common in general population and have broad-ranging physiological effects in-vivo which lessen inflammatory cascades and vascular reactivity. A recent trend is to perform nutritional epidemiological studies linking overall diet pattern to the lifestyle, examining the link between food and nutrients of diet to risk of chronic diseases. This chapter would deal with pharmacological and pathological basis of hypertension, utilization of dietary fibers, functional foods, nutraceuticals for hypertensive populations as well as to those with increased cardiovascular risks.

Diets rich in fats and cholesterol are mainly responsible for the production of free radicals which contribute to the incidence of hyperlipidemia and hypercholesterolemia. Both of these are the major factors responsible for CVDs. Hyperlipidemia is characterized by elevated level of total cholesterol (TC), low-density lipoprotein (LDL) and very low-density lipoprotein (VLDL), and reduced level of high-density lipoprotein (HDL) in serum. The main role of diet is to provide ample amount of nutrients to meet the nutritional requirements of an individual. However, there are increasing scientific approaches helping the hypothesis that some food ingredients have beneficial effects over and above the provision of the basic nutrients. So in this chapter, the main focus is food categorized under nutraceutical and functional food and their various protective roles in the case of hyperlipidemia.

Section 5
Brain and Neurodegenerative Disorders

This chapter presents an overview of various complementary nutritional approaches for the management of brain disorders. Numerous epidemiological studies emphasize the growing burden of brain disorders worldwide. Due to the complex pathophysiology, lack of precise diagnostic and therapeutic options, there is growing need to have alternative approaches. One important strategy for the prevention and treatment of brain impairment is based on dietary supplements, functional foods, and nutraceuticals. The current chapter illustrates various aspects of available nutritional products for the brain disorder. Considering the recent surge in the nutritional products and as it destined to play an important role in future, existing regulatory framework is explained here which ensures purity, safety, and efficacy of the marketed products.

Nutraceuticals and functional foods have attracted considerable interest recently because of their well-known safety and potential nutritional and therapeutic effects. Nutraceuticals include food supplements, dietary supplements, value-added processed foods, as well as non-food supplements such as tablets, soft gels, and capsules etc. which are packed with bioactive components. Life expectancy continues to rise and along with a rise in the lifestyle diseases (i.e., obesity, diabetes, hypertension, cardiovascular diseases, and neurodegenerative disorders). Functional foods and nutraceuticals constitute a great promise to improve health, neurodegenerative disorders, and aging-related chronic diseases. A collective effort by the academia, industry, government, and research organization must keep on promoting nutraceutical and functional food to contain the menace of lifestyle diseases.

Section 6
Anemia

WHO database mentions that the global anemia-affected population is 24.8%. To name a few conditions in which compromisation of the red blood corpuscles and hemoglobin occurs are iron deficiency anemia, gestational anemia, anemia due to malaria and parasitism, hemolytic anemia, sickle cell anemia. The line of treatment in case of anemia involves administration of iron supplements, plasmapheresis, steroids, blood transfusion at regular intervals, and lifestyle changes. The systematic approach applied for the pharmaceutical molecules should be equally inculcated in the case of nutraceuticals. The traditional system when woven carefully with the novel drug delivery system will give effective nutrient delivery. Functional foods have inherent nutritional value. Nutraceuticals and functional food cannot cure the anemic condition, but help the patient lead life almost like a normal individual.

Section 7
Cancer

Cancer is an insidious disease affecting mankind in every country. The progression of cancer cells from one part of the body to another (metastasis) is one of the biggest problems in curing cancer. The present study brings new hope of future therapies to fight cancer. Designing an appropriate food to maintain proper health has become a necessity worldwide. Due to this, the food industries in many countries are modifying their products as a response to consumer demands. In recent years, many of the natural products are gaining popularity as nutraceuticals.

Preface

Science will never be a finished book. Any development over time reveals more and deeper difficulties. – Albert Einstein

Science is a way of thinking much more than it is a body of knowledge. – Carl Sagan

This book, *Nutraceutical and Functional Foods in Disease Prevention*, was motivated by the desire we and others have had to further the evolution of the core course in Nutraceuticals Science. This book ensembles the therapeutics of different food materials and covers maximum burning life style oriented health issues which can be solved or prevented, to bestow the dispersed valuable information huddled in a compact form. This book encircles the different views of nutraceuticals against obesity, cardiovascular disease, brain disorder, neurological diseases, hypertension, hyperlipidemia, ageing and cancer etc. The essence of each chapter is written by expert, experienced and renowned scientists, researchers across the world with updated knowledge to provide valuable information of nutraceuticals role in life style diseases to readers, researchers, academician, scientists and industrialists around the globe.

CHAPTER COMPOSITION

This book has 15 chapters and divided into nine sections. Section 1, "Probiotic," includes two chapters. Chapter 1, "An Overview of the Therapeutic Aspect of Living Drugs Probiotics," by Vandana Bharat Patravale and Amita Keertimaan Joshi, from India provides an overview of probiotics and its role in current scenario to boost our body system. The authors also given concreate idea about the living probiotics and its positive influence on host health or physiology. The living probiotics of human or gut microbiota is a hugely diverse, largely unexplored ecosystem that is closely related to various diseases conditions. These bacterial cells form the human microbiome that plays a vital role in human health. An imbalance in the gut microbiome, i.e., dysbiosis, can result in various pathological conditions. This dysbiosis can be refurbished with the supplement of "Probiotics". The ultimate effect of administration of probiotics on health or physiology is either direct or indirect. This chapter summarizes the concept of probiotics, their therapeutic aspect along with possible mechanism of action.

Chapter 2, "Impact of Probiotics in Human Health and Disease Treatment," is by Jagan Mohan Rao Tingirikari from South Korea, and Muthu Vijaya Sarathy and Ashok Kumar Karthigarani from India. In this chapter authors express their idea about the Probiotics has become the major breakthrough in therapeutic applications due to their various health promoting effects in humans by maintaining the homeostasis of the intestine and prevent microbial imbalance (dysbiosis) without any side effects. The present chapter highlights about the role of probiotics in treatment and prevention of different human diseases.

Section 2, "Obesity," includes Chapters 3 and 4. The Chapter 3, "Recent Trends in Functional Foods for Obesity Management," by Amrita Poonia from India, revealed their idea that the Obesity is a medical condition caused by the accumulation of excess fat in the body. The main causes of obesity are sedentary life style, less physical activity and increased health problems. It is not only a problem of developed countries but also becoming a growing burden for the developing countries. This chapter throws light on the problem of obesity among various age groups of the society and further described the prevalent trends and future prospects of functional foods for obesity management. It also discusses how functional foods play important role in prevention and treatment of overweight. Functional foods for obesity influences the energy balance equation regulated by the control of energy intake or of energy expenditure dissipated as heat (thermogenesis). In this section the Chapter 4, "Functional Foods for Treatment and Prevention of Obesity and Its Associated Disorders," very well described by Jagan Mohan Rao from South Korea about the obesity, has now become an epidemic affecting wide variety of population across the world. Researchers have found a wide variety of functional foods from different sources which helps in combating and prevention of obesity and its related diseases. Recent advancement in nutritional science has led to the development of several functional foods with low glycemic index. The present chapter highlights about the problems related to obesity and the importance of various functional foods which has great potential to be incorporated in our daily diet to curb the menace of obesity.

Section 3, "Cardiovascular," contains Chapters 5 and 6. Chapter 5 is titled "Roles of Nutraceuticals and Functional Food in Prevention of Cardiovascular Disease: Sustaining Health" by Shahrul Bariyah Hamid, and Auni Fatin Abd Hamid from Malaysia. The chapter provides an overview of cardiovascular disease, a major cause of mortality worldwide. It relates economic and social impacts to the disease, especially in developing countries. One of the approaches to addressing this challenge is increasing awareness within society, through implementation of education programs. It is important for society to understand the types and roles of the risk factors leading to cardiovascular disease. Emphasis is on the role of functional food and nutraceuticals as dietary sources that could prevent development of cardiovascular disease. The chapter highlights roles of nutraceuticals and functional food sources from medical plants, seeds, berries, and tropical fruits in lowering risk factors. Key findings from trials conducted in Asia, China, Europe, and America provide supporting evidence for the importance of functional food to health, and its potential for modifying the level of risk factors related to cardiovascular diseases.

Chapter 6, "Nutraceutical Intervention of Phytosterols in Cardiovascular Aging," well portrayed by Charu Gupta, Dhan Prakash and Sneh Gupta from India, the role of Phytosterols and phytostanols in cardiovascular diseases. Phytosterols and phytostanols are structurally and functionally related to cholesterol but differ from cholesterol in the structure of the side chain. Phytosterols lower total and low density lipoprotein (LDL) blood cholesterol by preventing cholesterol absorption from the intestine, so they have been known as blood cholesterol-lowering agents. Phytosterols are naturally found in fruits, vegetables, nuts and mainly oils. Dietary phytosterol intakes normally range from 160-400 mg/day with variations depending on food culture and major food sources. Dairy foods remain a food of choice for use as delivery vehicle for many functional ingredients including phytosterols and there are many dairy products available in the global markets which are enriched with phytosterols. The use of phytosterols in commonly consumed dairy products may soon provide an effective tool against CVD and its introduction to our food products is worth anticipating in the near future as nutraceuticals for healthy ageing.

Section 4 mainly deals with Hypertension and Hyperlipidemia and well described in Chapter 7 and 8 in detail. Chapter 7 titled "Dietary Fibers and Nutraceuticals in Prevention of Hypertension," authored by John Intru Disouza, Kiran Shivaji Patil, Pratik Shailendra Kakade, Vandana Bharat Patravale, India is about role of dietary food in hypertension and, described that hypertension is the major cause of mortality amongst many cardiovascular risk factors causing 7.5 million deaths annually. Macronutrient and micronutrient deficiencies are very common in general population and have broad-ranging physiological effects in-vivo which lessen inflammatory cascades and vascular reactivity. A recent trend is to perform nutritional epidemiological studies linking overall diet pattern to the lifestyle, examining the link between food & nutrients of diet to risk of chronic diseases. This chapter would deal with pharmacological and pathological basis of hypertension, utilization of dietary fibers, functional foods, nutraceuticals for hypertensive populations as well as to those with increased cardiovascular risks. Chapter 8, "The Protective Role of

Nutraceuticals and Functional Food in Hyperlipidemia" by Raushan Kumar and Syed Ibrahim Rizvi, India outlined about the role of nutraceuticals and functional food as protective against hyperlipidemia. Diets rich in fats and cholesterol are mainly responsible for the production of free radicals which mainly contributes to the incidence of hyperlipidemia and hypercholesterolemia. Both of these are the major factors responsible for CVDs. Hyperlipidemia is characterized by elevated level of total cholesterol (TC), low-density lipoprotein (LDL) and very low-density lipoprotein (VLDL), and reduced level of high-density lipoprotein (HDL) in serum. The main role of diet is to provide ample amount of nutrients to meet the nutritional requirements of an individual, however, there are increasing scientific approaches helping the hypothesis that some food ingredients have beneficial effects over and above the provision of the basic nutrients. So in this chapter, our main focus is food i.e. categorized under Nutraceutical and functional food and there various protective role in the case of hyperlipidemia.

Section 5, "Brain and Neurodegenerative Disorders," contains Chapters 9 and 10, titled "Role of Diet, Functional Foods, and Nutraceuticals in Brain Disorders," by Vandana Bharat Patravale, Shivraj Vasantrao Naik and Shrikant Ninaji Dhage, India, and "Nutraceuticals Role in Stress, Aging, and Neurodegenerative Disorders," by Manisha Choudhary, Sandeep Tripathi, and Rajesh Kumar Kesharwani, India, respectively. Chapter 9 presents an overview of various complementary nutritional approaches for the management of brain disorders. Numerous epidemiological studies emphasize the growing burden of brain disorders worldwide. Considering the recent surge in the nutritional products and as it destined to play an important role in future, existing regulatory framework is explained here which ensures purity, safety, and efficacy of the marketed products.

Chapter 10, "Nutraceuticals Role in Stress, Aging, and Neurodegenerative Disorders," explained nutraceuticals and functional foods have attracted considerable interest recently because of their well-known safety and potential nutritional and therapeutic effects. Nutraceuticals include food supplements, dietary supplements, value-added processed foods as well as non-food supplements such as tablets, soft gels, and capsules etc. which are packed with bioactive components. Life expectancy continues to rise and along with a rise in the lifestyle diseases i.e. obesity, diabetes, hypertension, cardiovascular diseases and neurodegenerative disorders. Functional foods and nutraceuticals constitute a great promise to improve health, neurodegenerative disorders, and aging-related chronic diseases.

Section 6, "Anemia," deals with Chapter 11, "Nutraceutical and Functional Foods in Treatment of Anemia," is written by Vandana B. Patravale, Namrata A. Kadwadkar, Shalaka R. Patki, John Intru DiSouza, from India. The definition of anemia in clearly states that it is 'a condition in which there is a deficiency of red cells or of hemoglobin in the blood, resulting in pallor and weariness.' WHO database mentions globally anemia affected population is 24.8%. To name a few conditions in which compromisation of the Red Blood corpuscles and Hemoglobin occurs are Iron Deficiency Anemia, Gestational Anemia, Anemia Due to Malaria And Parasitism, Hemolytic Anemia, Sickle Cell Anemia. The line of treatment in case of anemia involves administration of Iron supplements, plasmapheresis, steroids, blood transfusion at regular intervals, and lifestyle changes. The systematic approach applied for the pharmaceutical molecules should be equally inculcated in the case of nutraceuticals. The traditional system when woven carefully with the Novel Drug Delivery System will give effective nutrient delivery. Functional Foods have inherent nutritional value. Nutraceuticals and functional food cannot cure the anemic condition, but help provide patient to lead day to day life almost like a normal individual.

Section 7, "Cancer," contains one chapter, Chapter 12, "Nutraceutical and Functional Foods in Cancer Management and Therapy" written by Sakshi Bajaj, Satish Manchanda, of India. Authors specified that Cancer is an insidious disease affecting mankind in every country. Current cancer treatments, such as chemotherapy, radiotherapy and surgery, may induce unwanted side effects compromising health and also well-being of patients. Now days, consumers are considering food not only for basic nutrition but for other health benefits also. Fruits and vegetables containing phytoconstituents are gaining popularity as potent anticarcinogenic agents such as allicin in garlic, isoflavones in soybeans, lycopene in tomato, alpha carotene in carrot, sulforaphane in broccoli and other glucosinolates in cruciferous plants. Their ability to reduce cancer incidence in these studies is likely related to apoptosis. Cancer is one of the major deadly diseases and complexities of all diseases are such that no single available anticancer agent can satisfactory combat the multiple disorders of the disease. In this context, nutraceuticals are promising candidates to treat cancer. Therefore, this chapter attempts to focus on promising therapeutic potential of nutraceuticals and highlight their chemical constituents in deadly disease like cancer.

In Section 8, "Antioxidant," Chapter 13, "Clinical Role of Antioxidants in Treatment of Diseases" from India gives clear picture about the antioxidants role in clinical. Antioxidants are our first line of defense system against free radical damage and are critical for maintaining optimum health care. Although, most of the present day research is focused on the potential benefits of antioxidant nutrients or supplements. It has become clear that the best protection against oxidative stress involve a wide assortment of interrelated antioxidants and antioxidant cofactors. Additionally, the combination of several suboptimal concentrations of these kinds of detoxifying supplements may have an additive or even synergistic role to decrease the risk of some of diseases which caused due to aging. Adequate intake of antioxidants, such as B-carotene and vitamin C or some of fruit and vegetables which have essential antioxidants are especially found to decrease the risk of cancer and coronary heart disease (CHD).

Section 9, "Biochemic and Lactoserum," begins with Chapter 14, "Biochemic System of Medicine: Oldest form of Nutraceutical Therapy," by Srijan Goswami, Sagarika Mitra, Piyasee Paul, Dipjyoti Dey, and Sankalan Das, India. In this chapter authors illustrated that the Biochemic System of Medicine also known as the Inorganic Cell Salt Therapy, pioneered by Dr. Wilhelm Heinrich Schuessler, following the footsteps of Dr. Samuel Hahnemann, is the oldest form of Nutraceutical Therapy, approved and recognized by the World Health Organization as one of the Complementary Therapy. The chapter presents the fundamental ideology and concepts that underlies the promising system of Biochemic Medicine in a concise, simple and to the point as possible. The chapter begins with a brief introduction to Biochemic system, nutrition science and concepts of Nutraceuticals, followed by a brief history and literature review. It covers Biochemic System of Medicine and its relevant concepts finally closing the chapter with conclusion.

Chapter 15, "Lactoserum: A Complete Nutraceutical," by Charu Gupta, Dhan Prakash from India, and Consuelo Pacheco from Argentina, clearly illustrated that lactoserum as complete nutraceuticals. The whole chapters summarized as Lactoserum, a byproduct of cheese industry, is rich in nutrients but still it is discharged directly into the environment. It has many human applications that promise to be a complete nutraceutical for the future generations. It is of high nutritive value and its products can be used as functional ingredients in food and pharmaceutical applications and as nutrients in dietary and health foods. They contain full spectrum of amino acids including essential and branched-chain amino acids which are important in tissue growth and repair. The other biological activities of lactoserum are antibiotic, anti-cancer, anti-toxin, immune-enhancer, and prebiotic (growth enhancement of gut microflora such as bifidobacteria). Lactoserum can thus be used as nutraceutical in various products like infant formulas, food supplements, cheese spreads, sports bars and beverages to meet a variety of health goals for people of all ages including animal feed.

This book is constructed in such a form that it covers the burning life style induced diseases and role of nutraceuticals to cure or prevent it, and future prospective highlighted in pharmaceutical and medical application. A collective effort by the academia, industry, government and research organization must keep on promoting nutraceutical and functional food to contain the menace of lifestyle diseases. We are quite hopeful that this particular compilation would receive the interest of its target audience. The editors are an email a way to accept any suggestion, comment or critics. In last section book contains compilation of references, list of contributors and subject index.

Imagination is more important than knowledge. For knowledge is limited, whereas imagination embraces the entire world, stimulating progress, giving birth to evolution. – Albert Einstein

Raj K. Keservani
Chhatrapati Shahu Ji Maharaj Group of Institutions, India

Anil K. Sharma
Delhi Institute of Pharmaceutical Sciences and Research, India

Rajesh K. Kesharwani
Nims University Rajasthan, India

Section 1
Probiotic

Chapter 1
An Overview of the Therapeutic Aspect of Living Drugs Probiotics

Vandana Bharat Patravale
Institute of Chemical Technology, India

Amita Keertimaan Joshi
B. V. Patel PERD Centre, India

ABSTRACT

The human body harbors ten times more bacterial cells than human cells. These bacterial cells form the human microbiome that plays a vital role in human health. An imbalance in the gut microbiome (i.e., dysbiosis) can result in various pathological conditions. This dysbiosis can be refurbished with the supplement of "probiotics." Probiotics have thus been defined as non-pathogenic micro-organisms that, when ingested, exert a positive influence on host health or physiology. The most commonly used probiotic bacteria comes from two genera: Lactobacillus and Bifidobacterium. Various research findings have proposed a correlation between the alteration of microbiota (composition/activity/density) with disorders like infectious diarrhea, inflammatory bowel diseases, obesity, to name a few. The ultimate effect of administration of probiotics on health or physiology is either direct or indirect. This chapter summarizes the concept of probiotics, their therapeutic aspect along with possible mechanism of action.

DOI: 10.4018/978-1-5225-3267-5.ch001

INTRODUCTION

Probiotics are non-pathogenic micro-organisms that, when ingested, exert a positive influence on host health or physiology by inhabiting in the gut microbiota. Various fermented food in our diet provide probiotics to human body. Interestingly, the useful microbial flora of the gut has been described as "Jataragni" (fire in the stomach) as the sustaining force of all living beings, while, "Takra," *i.e.*, fermented milk, as "Amrita" or elixir in, CHARAKA SAMHITA. Much later, in 1907, Elie Metchnikoff, proposed the first scientific rationale for the role of *Lactobacilli* in maintaining health and longevity. WHO defines "Probiotics" as live microorganisms which, when administered in adequate amounts, have a beneficial effect on the health of the host (FAO/WHO, 2002). Lactic acid bacteria (LAB) and *bifidobacteria* were the first identified probiotics (Ouwehand, Salminen, & Isolauri, 2002). The impact of modulation in gut microbiota has been implicated in a variety of diseases conditions. Due to the involvement of gut microbiota in regulation of numerous physiological pathways, it can be presumed to be a full-fledged organ. Various research findings have proposed a correlation between the alteration of microbiota (composition/activity/density) with disorders like., infectious diarrhea, inflammatory bowel diseases, obesity, oral health, hypertension, hypercholesterolemia, to name a few. The ultimate effect of administration of pharmaceutical formulations containing live health-beneficial bacteria (probiotics) on health or physiology is either direct or indirect, via, alteration of the immune response. This chapter summarizes the concept of probiotics in conjunction with therapeutic aspect of probiotics in different disease conditions along with possible mechanism of action.

GUT MICROBIOTA

Human gut microbiota is a fascinating, unexplored ecosystem. Gut microbiome is a'mini-ecosystem' created by a collection of microbes inhabiting the human gastrointestinal (GI) tract. The intestinal lumen harbors 500 to 1000 different species of living microbes. By an estimate, there are 10 times higher number of microbes than the cells in human body and collectively the genome of these microbes is 50 times larger than the human genome. The predominant bacterial phyla in the human gut, *Bacteroides* and *Firmicutes,* are obligate anaerobes. Bacteroides phylum include *B. fragilis* and *B. vulgates*. Bacteroides are involved in the digestion of carbohydrate resulting in lowering of intestinal pH that inhibit the growth of harmful bacteria.

While, the phylum *Firmicutes* (strong wall) includes the genera of Lactobacillus, Clostridium, and Bacillus.

The intestinal microbiota is not homogeneous; the density of bacterial cells varies throughout the GI tract depending upon the physiological condition of the GI tract viz., intestinal pH gradient, intestinal oxygen gradient, bile acids etc. The gut microbiota is a continuously evolving ecosystem, depending upon various exogenous and endogenous factors (Flint, Scott, Louis, & Duncan, 2012). The evolution of the microbiota takes in three stages of the human life (Figure 1):

From Birth to Weaning

Interestingly, the newborn human gut is a sterile GI tract, which is quickly inhabited by microbes during birthing process. The type of delivery (vaginal birth versus caesarean section) and the type of diet (breast feeding versus formula feeding) are few of the factors that affect the colonization patterns. The initial colonizing microbes are facultative anaerobes which establish the conditions for the eventual obligate anaerobes. The initial bacteria that colonize gut are *Bifidobacterium spp.* and *Bacteroids spp.* Vaginally born babies have predominant population of *Bifidobacterium* as compared to the babies born via caesarean section, wherein the majority population is from *Staphylococcus spp.* and *Propionibacterium spp.* Eventually, delivery process significantly determines the immune system development via gut microbiome. Babies delivered via caesarean section have been found to have lower fecal bacterial cell count as compared to babies born vaginally.

The early microbiome in infants evolves and adapts for the lactose utilization from the milk (breast milk as well as formula milk). However, solely breastfed babies have a highly stable and less variable bacterial microbiome, with *Bifidobacterium* being the predominant bacteria colonizing the gut, as compared to bottle fed babies (Flint, Scott, Louis, & Duncan, 2012; Duncan, 2013).

From Weaning to Normal Diet

After weaning, once the solid food intake is established, the microbiota becomes more diverse and by the age of 3, attains resemblance to the adult microbiome. At this stage, the population of *Firmicutes* bacteria increases significantly. Interestingly, by the age of 2 years, the microbiota of a breast fed baby and formula fed babies becomes indistinguishable. By the age of 3 years, the microbiota acquires relative stability, although some compositional evolution of microbiota continues in later years of life (Flint, Scott, Louis, & Duncan, 2012; Wang, Du, Xu, Cheng, & Liu, 2017).

Old Age

The microbiota becomes less diverse with the old age and *Firmicutes and Bifidobacterium* bacteria population decreases significantly. Predominantly, the microbes population has *Bacteroidetes* (Flint, Scott, Louis, & Duncan, 2012).

Overall the microbiota composition is depended upon the factors, viz., diet (calories, processed food vs vegetable and fruit based, composition etc.), antibiotic usage, acid suppression, cultural factors, geographic factors, age, etc. The host (human GI tract) and GI inhabiting bacteria (Probiotics) share a symbiotic relationship. These colonized microbes determine the physiological, immune, metabolic and behavioral development and also future disease susceptibility. An intact microbiome is essential for the development and function of the mucosa- or, gut-associated immune system (mucosa-associated lymphoid tissue or gut-associated lymphoid tissue), immunologic tolerance, epithelial and barrier function, motility, and vascularity (Quigley 2016). The commensal microbiota also preserves the primary homeostatic functions of life as, pathogen exclusion, immunomodulation, upregulation of cytoprotective genes, prevention and regulation of apoptosis, and maintenance of barrier function (O'Hara & Shanahan, 2006; Turnbaugh & Gordon, 2009; Sekirov, Russell, Antunes, & Finlay, 2010).The microbiome, not only, actively and significantly contribute to the metabolic functions of the body, but are seemingly capable of influencing the development and function of the central nervous system, leading to a new conceptual dimension of the microbiota-gut-brain axis (Yarandi, Peterson, Treisman, Moran, & Pasricha, 2016). Overall, healthy microbiome offers beneficial effects via (Duncan, 2013):

Figure 1. Transformation of sterile gut microbiome to a well-established, stable gut microbiota, at various stages of life

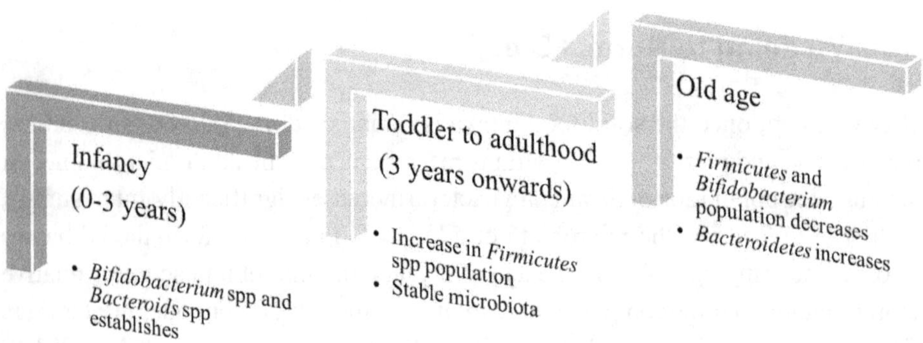

1. Gut bacteria ferment the non-digestible carbohydrates resulting in the production of short chain fatty acids. This results in lowering of the gut pH that enhances absorption of the minerals calcium, magnesium, zinc, and iron.
2. Acidic gut environment results in conditions which are less conducive for the invading pathogenic bacteria to inhabit.
3. Gut bacteria control the proliferation and differentiation of the gut epithelium especially goblet cells. This results in a thicker epithelium for the protection and enlarged surface area for the absorption of the nutrients.
4. Gut bacteria also induces regulatory T cells in gut lymphatic follicles thereby enabling the host to tolerate a large number of antigens.

Thus, a compositional alteration of the microbiota, wherein, harmful bacteria exceed the beneficial bacteria results in dysbiosis (Arnold, Roach, & Azcarate-Peril, 2016). Consequently, dysbiosis increases the host's disease susceptibility. An imbalance or dysfunctionality in the microbiota, leads to infection, inflammation, allergy, chronic GI diseases, colorectal cancer, and obesity (Wang, Du, Xu, Cheng, & Liu, 2017). Restoring this imbalance by supplementing the microbiota with probiotics and prebiotics has proven to be a valuable tool in the treatment of some of the diseases (Figure 2).

Figure 2. Various disease conditions arising due to imbalanced gut microbiota viz., dysbiosis

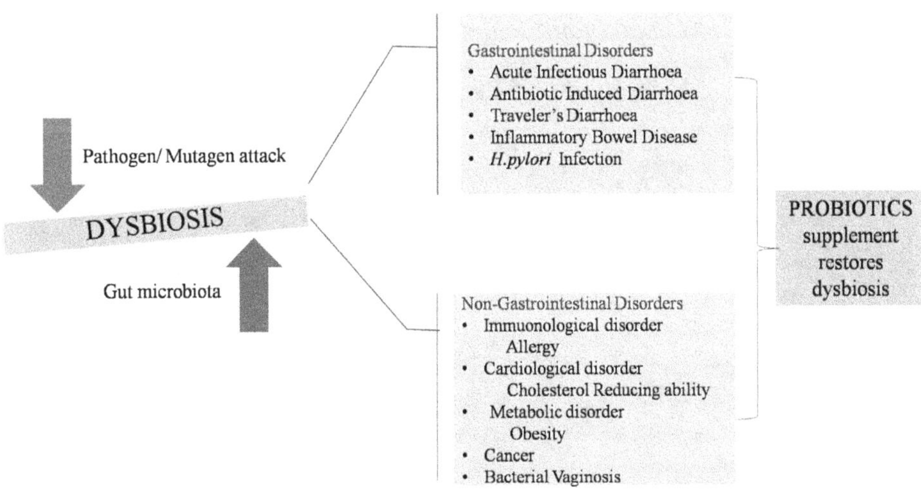

MECHANISM OF ACTION OF PROBIOTICS

Probiotics have been found to be effective in the treatment of wide array of diseases ranging from infectious, allergic and inflammatory to cancer. This itself suggests multiple pathways of action of probiotics. Different probiotic bacterial strains exert their effect through diverse mechanisms (Figure 3). Although the exact mechanism of probiotic bacteria action is not well understood, various potential mechanism of probiotic action has been postulated (Marteau, 2003; Fedorak & Madsen, 2004):

1. Modulation of epithelial barrier function
2. Competitive exclusion of pathogen
3. Increased Adhesion to Intestinal Mucosa
4. Production of Antimicrobial Substances
5. Immunomodulatory effect of probiotic

Enhancement of Barrier Function

Intestinal epithelium functions as one of the important defensive barrier mechanism of the body against the external/pathogenic microorganism. The defensive tools in the arsenal of the intestinal epithelium are mucous layer, antimicrobial peptides, secretory IgA and the epithelial junction adhesion complex (Ohland & Macnaughton, 2010). On disruption of this defensive barrier, the pathogenic bacteria can enter the intestinal

Figure 3. Mechanisms of probiotic action

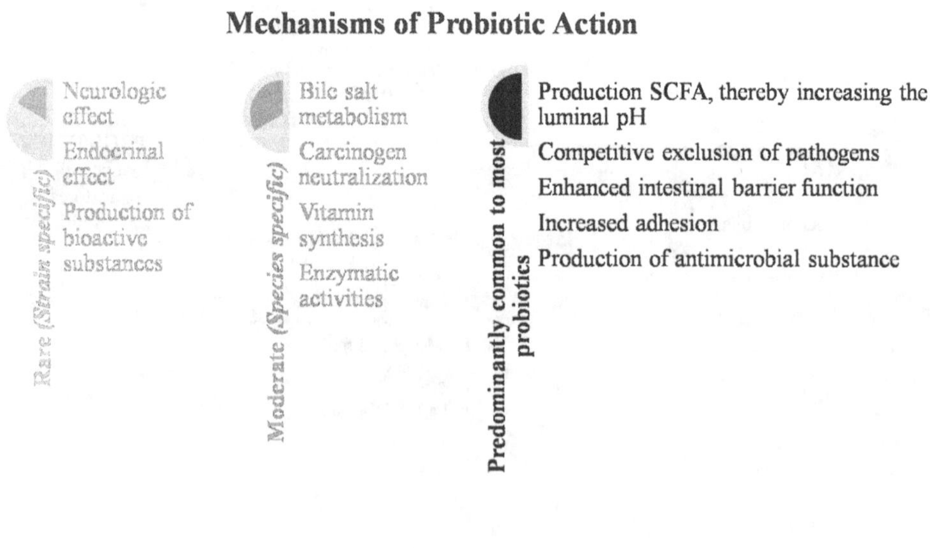

submucosa and result in inflammatory intestinal diseases like, inflammatory bowel diseases. Use of probiotic can enhance the barrier function of the intestine through various mechanisms, viz., increase in mucus secretion (Mack, 2003), enhancing the expression of genes coding for tight junction proteins (Anderson 2010), preventing the pro-inflammatory cytokines induced intestinal damage. Probiotics have also been reported to enhance the repair of the intestinal damage.

Competitive Exclusion of Pathogen

Competition for available nutrients and for mucosal adhesion sites results in Bacterium-to-bacterium competitive interaction or exclusion. Different probiotic bacteria uses different strategies to eliminate pathogenic bacteria. In order to win the battle, the bacterium can create hostile intestinal microenvironment for the pathogenic bacteria by releasing antimicrobial substances, such as lactic and acetic acid (Schiffrin & Blum, 2002). To exclude or reduce the pathogenic bacteria, probiotic bacteria can also create steric hindrance at the pathogen receptor site or competitive depletion of essential nutrients (Bermudez-Brito, Plaza-Diaz, Munoz-Quezada, & Gomez-Llorente, 2012).

Increased Adhesion to Intestinal Mucosa

Prerequisite for colonization of bacteria is their adhesion to the intestinal mucosa, which thereby modulates the human immune system. Probiotic bacteria interact with Intestinal Epithelial Cells (IECs) and mucus, through surface determinants. These IECs secrete glycoprotein mucin, which is the main component of the mucus. Increased mucus production, along with binding to microbial binding sites in the intestinal epithelium, by probiotic bacteria results in protection from the pathogenic bacteria (Hirano, Yoshida, Sugiyama, Koide, Mori, & Yokochi, 2003; Buck, Altermann, Svingerud, & Klaenhammer, 2005; Sanchez, Darimont, Drapeau, Emady-Azar, Lepage, Rezzonico,…Tremblay, 2010). To strengthen gut barrier function, probiotic bacteria have also been found to induce the release of small peptides and proteins, defensins, from the intestinal epitheial cells. Defensins are the peptides that are active against bacteria, fungi and virus. Defensins are the bacterial cell membrane disrupting peptides. Most of these proteins destroy pathogenic bacteria by disrupting the cell wall enzymatically or cell membrane non-enzymatically. These peptides bind electrostatically to anionic phospholipid groups of the cell membrane to create pores in the membrane; consequently, this results in bacterial cell lysis (Furrie, Macfarlane, Kennedy, Cummings, Walsh, O'neil, & Macfarlane, 2005; Ayabe, Satchell, Wilson, Parks, Selsted, & Ouellette, 2000; Ganz, 2003; Gallo & Hooper, 2012).

Production of Antimicrobial Substances

Probiotic bacteria produce a diverse array of substances, viz., low molecular weight (<1000 KDa) compounds such as lactic acid, acetic acid, and antibacterial substances (>1000 KDa), bacteriocins. Organic acids, like lactic acid, acetic acid, have strong inhibitory action on Gram negative bacteria. Undissociated form of acid is taken up by the pathogenic bacteria, which eventually gets dissociated in the cytoplasm of the bacteria. The resultant acidic cyotoplasmic pH and accumulation of the ionic organic acid causes pathogenic bacterial cell death. On the other hand, probiotic bacteria, like Lactic acid producing bacteria (LAB) produce small peptides, known as bacteriocins, having antimicrobial property against Gram-positive bacteria. Bacteriocins, destroy the pathogenic bacteria via, pore formation or by inhibiting the cell wall synthesis (Hassan, Kjos, Nes, Diep, & Lotfipour, 2012; Bierbaum & Sahl, 2009). Apart from these substances, probiotics have been found to produce health promoting fatty acids and de-conjugated bile acids. Some strains of *bifidobacteria* and *lactobacilli* have been found to produce a potent anti-carcinogenic compound, conjugated linoleic acid (CLA), while CLA produced by *L. plantarum* have been found to have anti-obesity activity in mouse model. While, de-conjugated bile acids have been found to have strong anti-microbial activity. Interestingly, probiotics protect themselves, via unknown mechanism, from de-conjugated bile acids (Oelschlaeger, 2010).

Immunomodulatory Effect of Probiotic

Probiotics interact with epithelial and dendritic cells (DCs), monocytes/macrophages and lymphocytes to exert immunomodulatory effect. Probiotics downregulate Toll-like receptor (TLR) expression and secretion of metabolites that inhibit entry of TNFα in mononuclear cells. Cell wall components of probiotics like, *lactobacilli* bind and stimulate TLR-2 and TLR-6. Activation of TLR-2 results in increase in transepithelial resistance to pathogenic bacteria (Vizoso Pinto, 2009; Gómez-Llorente, Muñoz, & Gil, 2010). *Bifidobacterium* also activates TLR-2 that results in increased production of IL-10 and prolonged survival of dendritic cells (Hoarau, 2006). Another set of membrane bound receptors located in cytoplasm, NOD like Receptors (NLRs), play a crucial immunomodulatory role wherein TLR are expressed in low levels. Amongst 20 different NLRs, two, NOD1 and NOD2, have been characterized in detail. NLRs are involved in the formation of inflammasomes, that activates caspase-I. NLRs also upregulate the transcription and production of inflammatory mediators like, cytokines, COX-2 (Chen, Shaw, Kim, & Nuñez, 2009; Hakansson & Molin, 2011).

PROBIOTICS: *THE LIVING DRUGS*

The concept of well-maintained gut barrier and a balanced microbiota forms the basis of use of probiotics in the treatment of various disease conditions (Figure 3). Probiotics have been proven to be effective therapeutically or prophylactically in various gastrointestinal as well as non-gastrointestinal disorders.

- Probiotics in non-gastrointestinal disorders
- Probiotics in gastrointestinal disorders

PROBIOTICS IN NON-GASTROINTESTINAL DISORDERS

Acute Infectious Diarrhea

One of the most widely documented use of probiotics is in the treatment of acute infectious diarrhea. *L. rhamnosus* GG, *L. reuteri, L casei Shirota, L plantarum, Bifidobacterium Bb12, Streptococcus thermophilus, VSL#3 (*a mixture of four strains of *lactobacilli: L. acidophilus, L. paracasei, L. bulgaricus, L. plantarum,* three strains of *bifidobacteria: B. breve, B. infantis, B. longum, one strain of S. thermophilus)* are some of the commonly used probiotics for the treatment of acute infectious diarrhea. The probable mechanism of action of probiotics in acute infectious diarrhea include: competitive exclusion of pathogens, lowering of luminal pH and production of bacteriocins, and promotion of the production of mucus. Effect of probiotics in rotavirus induced diarrhea has been widely studied and probiotics have been found to significantly shorten the duration of diarrhea. Guandalini et al., (2000) carried out a multicentered clinical trial in Europe to evaluate the effectiveness of *Lactobacillus* GG in rotavirus induced diarrhea. *Lactobacillus* GG was found to significantly reduce the duration of diarrhea in children as compared to placebo group. In another double blind placebo-controlled randomized clinical trial, wherein 75% of the enrolled subjects were infected with rotavirus infection, administration of *L. reuteri*SD2222 strain for five days, significantly reduced the duration of diarrhea in subjects as compared to placebo group (Shornikova, Casas, Isolauri, Mykkanen, & Vesikari, 1997). Three different strains of *L. rhamnosus* strains, 573L/1, 573L/2, and 573L/3, were also found to be significantly shorten the duration of rotavirus induced diarrhea in Poland (Szyman´ski, Pejcz, Jawien, Chmielarczyk, Strus, & Heczko, 2006). *Bifidobacterium* Bb12-supplemented powdered milk was found to increase the antibody titer by 30.4% in 175 school children in Thailand. While, administration of *Bifidobacterium* Bb12 alone and co-administration of *Bifidobacterium* Bb12 and *S. thermophilus* didn't result in an increase in antibody titer (Saavedra, Bauman, Oung, Perman, & Yolken, 1994). Various studies have shown that different probiotics have variation in therapeutic outcome. In one of the randomized clinical trial, 571 of the enrolled rotavirus infected children were given different species and strains of probiotics viz., *L. casei, L. delbrueckii, L. acidophilus, S. thermophilus* and *Bifidobacterium bifidum, S. boulardii, Bacillus clausii or Enterococcus faecium.* Surprisingly, the diarrheal duration was reduced only in groups receiving *L. casei, L. delbrueckii, L. acidophilus, S.thermophilus* and *Bifidobacteriumbifidum* (Canani, Cirillo, Terrin, Cesarano, Spagnuolo, De Vicenzo, Albano, Passariello, De Marco, Manguso, & Guarino, 2007). A combination of four strains of probiotics, *VSL#3*, has been reported to hasten the patient recovery from rotavirus induced diarrhea (Dubey, Rajeshwari, Chakravarty, & Famularo, 2008). There have been few meta-analysis reports for evaluating the therapeutic potential of probiotics in acute infectious diarrhea (Szajewska & Mrukowicz, 2001). Szajewska and Mrukowicz concluded that probiotics reduce the duration of diarrhea to less than 3 days. Amongst various probiotics reported to be effective in acute diarrhea, *Lactobacillus* GG exhibit the most consistent outcome. Niel et al., (2002) reported a linear relation between dose of the therapeutic outcome and dose of *Lactobacillus* and *Lactobacillus* has a therapeutic potential in acute infectious diarrhea. Various studies have reported the therapeutic potential of *Lactobacillus* GG in acute infectious diarrhea, however, the prophylactic benefits have not been yet proven (Mastretta 2002; Szajewska, Kotowska, Mrukowicz, Armańska, & Mikołajczyk, 2001).

On the contrary, colitis by *C. difficile* is difficult to treat and recurrence is often reported. The treatment of choice includes oral metronidazole or oral vancomycin. Potential of probiotics to reduce the chances of recurrence has been studied in few small scale randomized trials (Surawicz McFarland, Greenberg, Rubin, Fekety, Mulligan, Garcia, Brandmarker, Bowen, Borjal, & Elmer, 2003; Wullt, Hagslätt, & Odenholt, 2003). The subjects recruited in these study had at least suffered one episode of *C. difficile* infection. In one of the study, subjects were administered *S. boulardii* b.i.d for 28 days (Surawicz McFarland, Greenberg, Rubin, Fekety, Mulligan, Garcia, Brandmarker, Bowen, Borjal, & Elmer, 2003), while in the other the subjects received the *L. plantarum* 299V for 38 days (Wullt, Hagslätt, & Odenholt, 2003). Surawicz et al (2003) reported recurrence episode in 17% of the subjects that were receiving *S. boulardii* as against the placebo group. While, Wullt et al, (2003) reported 4 cases of recurrence out of 12 recruited subjects being administered *L. plantarum* in comparison to 6 cases of recurrence out of 9 recruited subjects on placebo treatment.

Antibiotic-Induced Diarrhea

Perturbation of normal intestinal flora by antibiotics results in imbalance of the gut microbiome. As a result, opportunistic bacteria, like *C. difficle*, may over grow resulting in diarrhea. This gut microbiome imbalance also results in reduction of short chain fatty acid production, which is an essential nutrient for enterocyte and water and electrolyte absorption. Concurrently, there is also a reduction in the population of carbohydrate digesting bacteria in the gut. Cumulatively, all this consequently results in diarrhea (Firmansyah, Penn, & Lebenthal, 1989; Clausen, Bonnen, Tvede, & Mortensen, 1991). *C. difficle*, *Klebsiella oxytoca*, multidrug resistant *Salmonella*, *C. albicans*, and *C. tropicalis* are the most commonly implicated bacterial agents in antibiotic induced diarrhea. Conventionally, in an attempt to normalize the gut microbiome, probiotics have been supplemented with antibiotic treatment. *S. boulardii*, *L. rhamnosus, Bifidobacterium longum, L. acidophilus, Bifidobacterium lactis* are few of the commercially available probiotic preparations, commonly available as freeze dried powder, for the treatment of antibiotic induced diarrhea (Kotzampassia & Giamarellos-Bourboulis, 2012). Several studies have been carried out to evaluate the potential of probiotics, co-administered with antibiotics, in diarrhea induced by antibiotics. A meta-analysis of 63 randomized clinical trials concluded that there is a strong correlation in probiotic administration and reduction in diarrhea induced by antibiotics (Hempel, Newberry, Maher, Wang, Miles, Shanman, Johnsen, & Shekelle, 2012). Another meta-analysis concluded that co-administration of *S. boulardii* significantly reduces the incidence of antibiotic induced diarrhea in adults (McFarland, 2007). In case of *C. difficle* associated diarrhea, only *S. boulardii* have been proven to be effective (Tung, Dolovich, & Lee, 2009). *S. boulardii* neutralizes the toxins produced by *C. difficle* by releasing proteases, increasing the concentration of intestinal polyamines and modulating the levels of inflammatory cytokines (Vandenplasetal, 2009). Therapeutic effect of probiotics has also been reported in a large meta-analysis of 16 clinical studies carried out since 1990 in pediatric patients. Despite the heterogeneity in all these 16 clinical studies, probiotics were found to have significant preventive role in diarrhea (Johnston, Goldenberg, Vandvik, Sun, & Guyatt, 2011).

Traveler's Diarrhea

Traveler's diarrhea is one of the most common form of diarrhea caused by the consumption of contaminated food, water or beverages. The most common causative pathogens include, enteropathogenic *E. coli*, enteroaggregative *E. coli*, *Salmonella* species, *Shigella* species, *Campylobacter jejuni*, *Yersinia enterocolitica*, *Plesiomonas shigelloides*, *Vibrio parahemolyticus*, *Aeromonashydrophila*, and *Vibrio cholerae*.

Probiotics have been evaluated both prophylactically as well as therapeutically in traveler's diarrhea. There has been mixed reports on the efficacy of probiotics in traveler's diarrhea. Different trials with *L. acidophilus* and *L. rhamnosus* GG have reported them to be ineffective in the treatment of Traveler's diarrhea while, a small trial with *S. boulardii* have reported it to be potentially effective in traveler's diarrhea (Katelaris, Salam, & Farthing, 1995; Hilton, Kolakowski, Singer, & Smith, 1997; Oksanen, Salminen, Saxelin, Hämäläinen, Ihantola-Vormisto… Salminen, 1990; Kollaritsch, 1989). However, geographical variation in the efficacy of *S. boulardii* has been suggested by Kollaritsch, (1989). In a meta-analysis, Macfarl and concluded that, *L. rhamnosus* GG, *L. casei* DN-114001, and *S. boulardii* are evidently effective in the treatment of traveler's diarrhea while, *L. acidophilus* is ineffective (McFarland, 2010).

Inflammatory Bowel Disease (IBD)

Crohn's disease (CD), Ulcerative colitis (UC), and nonspecific colitis are collectively termed as IBD characterized by inflammation of the GI tract accompanied by pain, diarrhea and bleeding. UC is confined to the colonic mucosal lining while, CD can affect any segment of the GI tract. Reduction in the population of *Bifidobacteria* and *Lactobacilli* bacteria has been observed in patients with UC (Mylonaki, Rayment, Rampton, Hudspith, & Brostoff, 2005; Bullock, Booth, & Gibson, 2004). Regardless of the underlying genetic predisposition or immunologic effector mechanism defect, role of enteric flora has been implicated in many studies (Fedorak & Madsen, 2004). Anti-TNFα drugs, immunomodulators and selective adhesion inhibitors are used for the treatment of UC and CD, however, approximately one-fifth of the patients suffer from remission within a year of the treatment. Remission of IBD with the usage of certain antibiotics such as metranidazole, ciprofloxacin etc. suggest a potential role of gut microbiota (Damaskos & Kolios, 2008; Fedorak, 2008; Geier, Butler, & Howarth, 2007). Hence, restoring dysbiosis by supplementing with probiotics seems to be a rational approach in the treatment of IBD. The potential of VSL#3 have been evaluated in patients with UC. VSL#3 were found to modulate cytokine levels similar to corticosteroid treatment in patients with UC. VSL#3 down regulate IL-1240p level and induce the production of IL-10 (Ng, Plamondon, Al-Hassi, Kamm, Knight, & Stagg, 2008a; 2008b). A randomized double blind trial have proven a comparable efficacy and remission rate of *E.coli Nissele* to that of mesalamine treatment (Rembacken, Snelling, & Hawkey, 1999). A similar outcome was reported in a double blind trial, wherein comparison of S. *boulardii* and mesalamine resulted in an equivalent therapeutic outcome (Kruis, Schutz, Fric, Fixa, Judmaier, & Stolte, 1997). While, in an open label trial, 53% of UC patient, being treated with a combination of VSL#3 and mesalamine or corticosteroid, exhibited remission

(Bibiloni, Fedorak, Tannock, Madsen, Gionchetti, Campieri, De Simone, & Sartor, 2005). A combination of VSL#3 and balsalazide was found to be effective in mild to moderate UC patients in comparison of VSL#3 or balasalazide alone (Tursi, Brandimarte, Giorgetti, Forti, Modeo, & Gigliobianco, 2004).

Lactobacillus johnsonii LA1 and *LGG* were found to be ineffective in controlling CD (Penneret, 2005; Marteau, Lemann, & Seksik, 2005). *Lactobacillus rhamnosus* GG was not found to have any superiority over placebo in patients with active CD as well as in remission, in a double-blind, randomized, placebo-control trials (Schultz, Timmer, Herfarth, Sartor, Vanderhoof, & Rath, 2004; Bousvaros, Guandalini, Baldassano, Botelho, Evans, Ferry… Hibberd, 2005). For establishing the routine use of probiotics in the treatment of IBD, large scale clinical trials are needed.

H. pylori Infection

H. pylori is a microaerophilic causative rod for gastritis, peptic ulcer and risk factor for gastric malignancies. Complete eradication using antibiotic therapy is often not achieved. Unsuccessful antibiotic therapy often leads to side effects viz., antibiotic resistance, augmented bacterial virulence, adverse drug reactions, to name a few (Boltin, 2016). Gastric microbiota undergoes considerable changes during *H. pylori* colonization, hence use of probiotics to restore the normal gastric microbiota seems to be a potential approach for the treatment of *H. pylori* infection (Andersson, Lindberg, Jakobsson, Backhed, Nyren, & Engstrand, 2008). Certain lactic acid bacterial strains and *Bifidobacterium* strains have been found to reduce proliferation and urease activity of *H. pylori, in vitro* and are reported to thwart *H. pylori* infection *in vivo* in animals (Sgouras, Maragkoudakis, Petraki, Martinez-Gonzalez, Eriotou…Mentis, 2004). Bacteriocins produced by probiotics and their anti-inflammatory property reduce the proliferation and colonization of *H. pylori. L. johnsonii*ncc533 was found to reduce the *H. pylori* colonization in children after 4 weeks of oral administration in a double blind controlled trial (Cruchet, Obregon, Salazar, Diaz, & Gottenland, 2003). Same strain, in another trial, when administered in combination with cranberry juice eradicated *H. pylori* by 22.9% (Gotteland, Andrews, Toledo, Muñoz, Caceres, Anziani…Salazar, 2008). Similar results have been reported with *S. boulardii* (Gotteland, Poliak, Cruchet, & Brunser, 2005). On the other hand, although *L. Gasseri*OLL 2716 (LG21) have been found to reduce the *H.pylori* induced inflammation, it didn't affect the colonization density of *H. pylori*. Efficacy of co-administered probiotics and antibiotic treatment has also been evaluated in various clinical trials. In a randomized, double blind controlled clinical trial, antibiotic and omeprazole treatment, with (fermented milk containing *L. casei*dn-114001) and without probiotic was administered to *H. pylori* infected children. In probiotic supplemented children, eradication rate was increased to

84.6% in comparison to the group without probiotic treatment that exhibited 57.5% eradication (Sýkora, Valecková, & Amlerová, 2005). On the contrary, in another study, treatment with yogurt containing *B. animalis* and *L. casei* for 3 months didn't improved the eradication rate of *H. pylori* (Goldman, Barrado, Balcarce, Rua, Oshiro, & Calcagno, 2006). Overall, it can be concluded that probiotics cannot eradicate the *H. pylori*, however, colonization density of *H. pylori* can be decreased and eradication rate can be increased upon their usage. Also, the efficacy of probiotics in *H. pylori* infection is strain dependent (Vandenplas, Huys, & Daube, 2015).

PROBIOTICS IN NON-GASTROINTESTINAL DISORDER

Allergy and Immune Response

According to hygiene hypothesis, an inverse relation exists between exposure and incidence of infections in early life and developing atopy/allergy later in life (Strachan, 2000). A number of studies have suggested altered gut microbiota composition during allergic condition. *Bifidobacterium* population in the microbiota has been found to reduce significantly in allergic subjects especially, in atopic eczema condition. *Bifidobacterium bifidum* population, in particular, is significantly reduced while a higher count of *B. adolescentis* and *B. longum* have been found in allergic patients as compared to normal healthy human gut flora. Simultaneously, an increase in *Clostridium*, *Bacteroides* and *Staphylococcus* population has also been reported in allergic individuals (Grönlund, Arvilommi, Kero, Lehtonen, & Isolauri, 2000). During infancy, the successful maturation of gut mucosal immune system requires constant stimulation by the developing gut microbiota. The mode of delivery during birth contributes significantly to the composition of the gut microbiota. Gut microbiota rich in *B. adolescentis*, *Clostridium*, *Bacteroides* and *Staphylococcus* population has higher amount of immunoglobulin (Ig) E-levels (He, Ouwehand, Isolauri, Hashimoto, Benno, & Salminen, 2001). An elevated level of IgE in the serum is a characteristic feature of Atopic sensitization (allergy) (Simpson, Tan, Winn, Svensén, Bishop, & Heckerman, 2010). Gut microbiota tune the infant immune system for Th-1 mediated Th-2 expression through TGF-ß and IgA secretion. A healthy microbiota has a balanced Th-1/Th-2 and food tolerance. Limited microbial exposure in infants results in a skewed Th-1 and Th-2 balance, towards Th-2, a characteristic of allergy (Kalliomaki & Isolauri, 2002). Probiotics can modulate the gut microbiota to restore Th-1/Th-2 balance, thereby alleviating risk and symptoms of allergy. Probiotics interact with intestinal mucosa and stimulate T- cells to differentiate into Th-1 via., IFN-α, IL-2, and IL-12; while, Th-2 is down regulated via IL-4. Consequently,

Ig-E production is reduced and Ig-A level is increased. This reduces the allergic response (Sanfilippo, Li, Seth, Balwin, Menozzi, & Mahida, 2000). Preventive co-administration of pre- and pro-biotics in pregnant women for two to four weeks prior to delivery significantly reduced the occurrence of IgE mediated atopic allergy in the initial two years of life of such kids. However, for the same duration, there was no difference in the occurrence of cumulative incidences of allergy in comparison to placebo treatment (Kukkonen, Savilahti, Haahtela, Juntunen-Backman, Korpela, & Poussa, 2008). Prenatal and 6 months post birth, infants were administered *Lactobacillus rhamnosus GG* (*LGG*) resulted in reduction of occurrence of atopic dermatitis by half in comparison to that of control group (Kalliomäki, Salminen, Arvilommi, Kero, Koskinen, & Isolauri, 2001). While, the other study concluded that prenatal administration of *LGG* reduced the incidence of atopic allergy by half, however, *LGG* does not have any preventive effect in atopic allergies (Kalliomäki, Salminen, Poussa, & Isolauri, 2007).*Lactobacillus acidophilus* strain inefficiency towards atopic allergies signifies the probiotic strain specificity towards atopic allergies (Taylor, Hale, Wiltschut, Lehmann, Dunstan, & Prescott, 2006). Prenatal co-administered *Lactobacillus GG* and *B. lactis* reduced the risk of atopic eczema and sensitivity towards allergens (Huurre, Laitinen, Rautava, Korkeamäki, & Isolauri, 2008). On the other hand, a mixture of *Lactobacillus GG*, *L. rhamnosus* LC705, *B. breve*, and *Propioniobacterium freudenreichii* ssp. *Shermanii* JS didn't showed any affect in reducing atopic eczema (Viljanen, Savilahti, Haahtela, Juntunen-Backman, Korpela, Poussa…Kuitunen, 2005). Evidently, probiotics have the ability to modulate the immune response. Hence, potential of *LGG* has been under investigation as a vaccine adjuvant. In one such randomized, double-blind, placebo-controlled study, *LGG* was administered 28 days after administration of live- attenuated influenza vaccine. An increase in protective hemagglutinin inhibition titers against the virus with no side effect were observed, suggesting the potential of *LGG* as a potential vaccine adjuvant (Davidson, Fiorino, Snydman, & Hibberd, 2011).

Regardless of probiotic strain variation, certain probiotics have been found to be effective in atopic eczema, however, utility and efficacy of probiotics in other allergic conditions still needs to be evaluated. Overall, large scale clinical trials and meta-analysis are still needed for establishing the role of probiotics in allergic conditions.

Cholesterol Reducing Ability

In a recent study, probiotics have been reported to have cholesterol reducing capability. Various doctrines have been proposed viz., binding of cholesterol to probiotic bacterial cell surface and its incorporation in the probiotic cellular membrane, short-chain fatty acids production from oligosaccharides, co-precipitation of cholesterol with deconjugated bile (Kumar, Nagpal, Kumar, Hemalatha, Verma, Kumar…Yadav, 2012), conversion of cholesterol to coprostanolin (Philippe, 2014), and bile salt hydrolase mediated bile deconjugation (Lye, Rahmat-Ali, & Liong, 2010). However, the most widely accepted theory is the hydrolysis of amide bond of bile salts conjugate. Bile salts conjugate with glycine or taurine to form bile salt conjugates. These highly soluble conjugates enter the blood circulation wherein, they get accumulated. *Lactobacillus* and *Bifidobacterium* release hydralase, which cleaves amide bond in the bile salt conjugates. The free bile acid is then eliminated from the body. Bile salts produced by liver hepatocytes increases the cholesterol and fat transport across intestinal epithelium. *L. acidophilus* and few other species of *Lactobacilus*, have been reported to bind the exogenous cholesterol in their cell membrane (Kumar, Nagpal, Kumar, Hemalatha, Verma, Kumar…Yadav, 2012). *Sterolibacterium denitrificans* produces cholesterol dehydrogenase that converts cholesterol to cholest-4-en-3-one which is converted into coprostanol and excreted from the body (Ooi, & Liong, 2010). However, all the probiotic strains don't possess cholesterol reducing ability. The search for probiotics with excellent cholesterol reducing ability is still underway (Ishimwe, Daliri, Lee, Fang, & Du, 2015).

Obesity

The core cause of obesity has been an imbalance in energy intake and energy expenditure. However, recent studies suggest a significant role played by gut microbiota in obesity. Obese subjects have a altered gut microbiota composition, with reduced population of *Bacteroidetes* and a corresponding increase in *Firmicutes* (Ley, Turnbaugh, Klein, & Gordon, 2006). Although few studies suggest an increase of *Actinobacteria* coupled with reduction of *Bacteroidetes* (Turnbaugh & Gordon, 2009). In either condition, *Bacteroidetes* population is reduced. This bacterial composition shift results in increased energy harvesting capacity of gut from food and induction of low level of inflammation. The altered obese microbiota generates Short Chain Fatty Acids (SCFA) from the indigestible portion of food eg., resistant starch. Carbohydrates are the substrate for SCFAs. SCFAs generate additional 10% caloric intake and moreover, SCFAs augment the process of *de novo* lipid synthesis (Schwiertz, Taras, Schäfer, Beijer, Bos, Donus, & Hardt, 2010; Macfarlane & Macfarlane, 2011). Pro- and anti-inflammatory cytokines from certain bacteria have also been linked to increased risks of obesity (Hotamisligil, 2006). Loss of mucosal integrity due to gut dysbiosis seems to be the major cause of inflammation in obesity (Cani, Possemiers, Van de Wiele, Guiot, Everard, Rottier… Delzenne, 2009). *L. rhamnosus*PL60 administered for 8 weeks in high-fat diet-induced obese mice resulted in weight loss, presumably, due to production of anti-obesity agent, conjugated linoleic acid (Lee, Park, Seok, Baek, Kim, Lee... Park, 2006). In another study in high-fat diet-induced obese mice, 4 weeks administration of VSL#3, reduced the serum and liver triglycerides level (Esposito, Iacono, Bianco, Autore, Cuzzocrea, Vajro... Meli, 2009). While, administration of *Lactobacillus salivarius* UCC118 Bac (+) increased the population of *Bacteroidetes* and *Proteobacteria*, along with reduction in *Actinobacteria*, although, *Firmicutes* poplutaion count remained unchanged in mice (Murphy, Cotter, Hogan, O'Sullivan, Joyce, Fouhy... Shanahan, 2013). *Lactobacillus acidophilus* NCDC 13, also increased the Bifidobacterium in mice, without altering the body weight (Arora, Anastasovska, Gibson, Tuohy, Sharma, & Bell, 2012). Co administered *Lactobacillus curvatus* HY7601 and *Lactobacillus plantarum* KY1032 reduced fat accumulation, weight gain and pro-inflammatory cytokine levels while it upregulated the fatty acid oxidation genes (Park, Ahn, Park, Huh, Yoo, Yu, Sung, McGregor, & Choi, 2013). In humans, early postnatal microbiota development seems to influence the body weight phenotype and predisposition to adult obesity via., microbial metabolite like, SCFAs (Mischke & Plosch, 2013) . The effect of probiotic in obesity and weight loss seems to be strain and species specific. *L. rhamnosus* GGMCC is the only probiotic to have positive affect in weight loss in humans. *L. rhamnosus* CGMCC also reduces the leptin level (Sanchez, Darimont, Drapeau, Emady-Azar, Lepage, Rezzonico... Tremblay, 2014).While, *L.plantarum* LG42, *L. gasseri* SBT2055and L. *plantarum* co-therapy with KY103 and *L. curvatus*HY7601 seems to be effective in weight loss in animals (Rouxinol-Dias, Pinto, Janeiro, Rodrigues, Moreira, Dias, & Pereira, 2016). Evidently, although limited, an interplay of diet and microbiota seems to play a critical role in inducing obesity. However, further studies and meta-analysis in this area needs to carried out to establish the significance of restoring microbiota balance in reducing obesity.

Cancer

Cancer of large intestine is one the most common forms of cancer with high mortality and morbidity. Epidemiological studies have suggested an interlink between colon cancer and diet (Geier, Butler, & Howarth, 2006). Reversible reduction in fecal ß-glucuronidase, nitroreductase and azoreductase in healthy individuals suggest that consumption of fermented milk products containing lactobacilli and *bifidobacteria* may play a role in preventing cancer of the colon and rectum (Geier, Butler, & Howarth, 2006). The exact mechanisms responsible for this effect are not fully understood and may be linked to different factors. Various mechanisms have been proposed that include: Physicochemical alteration viz., pH and redox potential, of luminal environment, host immune activation resulting in activation of anti-tumerogenic factors that either neutralize or block mutagens, production of butyric acid that induces apoptosis in enterocytes (Lan, Lagadic-Gossmann, Lemaire, & Jan, 2007). However, the efficacy of probiotics is strain specific. *L. casei*Shirota is reported to be efficacious in cancer (Morotomi, 1996). *B. adolescentis* SPM0212 was found to inhibit cell proliferation in a dose dependent manner of a colon cancer cell line: HT-29, SW 480,and CaCo-2, *in vitro* (Kim, Lee, Kim, Cho, Yang, Chung, Kim, & Ha, 2008).*Enterococcus faecium* CRL 183 when administered for 24 weeks exhibited 40% reduction in adenocarcinoma in rats (Sivieri, Spinardi-Barbusan, Barbisan, Bedani, Pauly, Carlos, Benzatti,Vendramini, & Rossi, 2008).

Bacterial Vaginosis

Vaginosis is a disease condition characterized by alteration of vaginal microbial ecology. The normal vaginal flora comprises of *Lactobacillus* predominantly. In vaginosis, *Lactobacillus* population is replaced by anaerobes and *Gardnerella vaginalis.* This results in increased vaginal pH over 4.5, which causes burning sensation or discomfort during urination (McGroarty, 1993). Bacterial vaginosis is one of the most prevalent pathological condition in women worldwide. Vaginal or oral administration of antibiotics like, metranidazole or clindamycin is usual treatment course in bacterial vaginosis. However, relapse is usually reported with antibiotic treatment. Hence, probiotics are being explored as an alternative treatment for bacterial vaginosis. A Cochrane database systematic review reported that vaginal administration of *Lactobacillus* was more effective than oral administration of metronidazole (Oduyebo, Anorlu, & Ogunsola, 2009). Oral administration of *L. acidophilus,* or intra-vaginal administration of *L. acidophilus* or *L. rhamnosus GR*-1 and *L. fermentum* RC-14, have been found to increase the vaginal lactobacilli numbers and restore the vaginal microbiota to normal, and cure women of bacterial vaginosis (Reid, Beuerman, Heinemann, & Bruce, 2001). However, contradictory reports on the efficacy of intravaginal instillation of lactobacilli for the treatment of bacterial vaginosis suggest the need for large scale, multicenter trials (Falagas, Betsi, & Athanasiou, 2007).

SAFETY OF PROBIOTIC THERAPY

Safety of probiotics is one of the major concerns of the probiotic therapy. There has been a rapid surge in the usage of probiotics in recent years, sometimes, in completely new therapeutic areas without much evidence. This has increased the probability of potential infection by probiotic bacteria itself. Although, most of these bacteria harbor in the gastrointestinal tract, the probability of manifestation of natural infection cannot be ruled out. Few cases of bacteremia, sepsis, endocarditis by *L. rhamnosus* GG or *L. casei* has been reported. *S. boulardii* has been reported to cause fungal sepsis. Although, all such cases have been reported in patients with severe disease condition like, diabetes, ICU patients, bowel syndrome, cancer (Boyle, Robins-Browne, & Tang, 2006). It, therefore, becomes essential to be cautious while opting for the probiotic therapy. Different probiotics have different safety profile which needs to be considered vigilantly while selecting the probiotic supplement (Olveira, & González-Molero, 2016). *Lactococcus* and *Lactobacillus* are classified under GRAS status, while the members of the *Streptococcus* and *Enterococcus* genera and some other genera of lactic acid bacteria have been classified as opportunistic pathogens. Absence of pathogenicity and infectivity, platelet-aggregating activity, mucus-degradation activity, production of harmful metabolites and antibiotic resistance are few of the criteria that need to be assessed for probiotics intended for therapeutic use (Ishibashi & Yamazaki, 2010).

FUTURE PERSPECTIVE

Imbalance in the microbiota or dysbiosis has been linked to various disease conditions. Restoring this imbalance has proven to be an effective approach to treat many disease conditions. Transplantation of a foreign gut microbiota to restore the dysbiosis is one such approach under intensive research (Bakken, 2009). Khoruts et al. (2010) transplanted the microbial population from a healthy donor in a *Clostridium difficile* associated disease (CDAD) patient. The microbial composition changed from *Firmicutes*- and *Bacteroidetes*-deficient to *Bacteroidetes* dominated along with the disappearance of the CDAD symptoms. However, further studies are underway to determine the conditions leading or promoting the successful transplantation of healthy microbiota. Gut microbiota exhibit interpersonal diversity depending upon the conditions like, diet, age etc. Majority of the studies are based on the gut microbiota of subjects under western diet. There is a growing need to establish global microbiota composition (Blaser, 2011). Also, impact of various environmental, diet shift, usage of antibiotics, surgery, drugs, on the composition of microbiota needs to be studied. Another important aspect of probiotic research is the need for technological advancement for the in-depth understanding the gut microbiome. Use of high- throughput sequencing technology in gut microbiome research has opened up the gate for compositional and functional analysis of gut microbiome. Engineered organoids derived from human stem cells, high-throughput culturing, and microfluidics assays are few of the emerging technologies being explored for comprehensive gut microbiome research (Arnold, Roach, & Azcarate-Peril, 2016).

CONCLUSION

Gut microbiota is a hugely diverse, largely unexplored ecosystem that is closely related to various diseases conditions. Host microbiota is being implicated and correlated in an increasing variety of disease states and disorders, viz., influenza, retrovirus transmission, autoimmune demyelination, behavioral disorders, Alzheimer's etc. (Daliri, & Lee, 2016). There is a mounting need to transform these findings for successful use in humans. However, the role of gut microbiota in all such disorders needs to be studied in depth using novel techniques like, sequencing followed by large scale, multi-centered, clinical trials across different population groups. Probiotics have huge potential in numerous therapeutic applications; however, their safety must be established prior to large scale human usage. The outcome of such study may provide enough evidence to establish alteration in gut microbiome composition as an early predictor of diseases states.

REFERENCES

Anadón, A., Martínez-Larrañaga, M. R., Arés, I., & Martínez, M. A. (2016). Prebiotics and Probiotics: An Assessment of Their Safety and Health Benefits. In Probiotics, Prebiotics, and Synbiotic. Elsevier Inc. doi:10.1016/B978-0-12-802189-7.00001-0

Anderson, R. C., Cookson, A. L., McNabb, W. C., Park, Z., McCann, M. J., Kelly, W. J., & Roy, N. C. (2010). Lactobacillus plantarum MB452 enhances the function of the intestinal barrier by increasing the expression levels of genes involved in tight junction formation. *BMC Microbiology*, *10*(1), 316. doi:10.1186/1471-2180-10-316 PMID:21143932

Andersson, A. F., Lindberg, M., Jakobsson, H., Backhed, F., Nyren, P., & Engstrand, L. (2008). Comparative analysis of human gut microbiota by barcoded pyrosequencing. *PLoS One*, *3*(7), e2836. doi:10.1371/journal.pone.0002836 PMID:18665274

Arnold, J. W., Roach, J., & Azcarate-Peril, M. A. (2016). Emerging Technologies for Gut Microbiome Research. *Trends in Microbiology*, *24*(11), 887–901. doi:10.1016/j.tim.2016.06.008 PMID:27426971

Arora, T., Anastasovska, J., Gibson, G., Tuohy, K., Sharma, R. K., Bell, J., & Frost, G. (2012). Effect of Lactobacillus acidophilus NCDC 13 supplementation on the progression of obesity in diet-induced obese mice. *British Journal of Nutrition*, *108*(08), 1382–1389. doi:10.1017/S0007114511006957 PMID:22289627

Ayabe, T., Satchell, D. P., Wilson, C. L., Parks, W. C., Selsted, M. E., & Ouellette, A. J. (2000). Secretion of microbicidal alpha defensins by intestinal Paneth cells in response to bacteria. *Nature Immunology*, *1*(2), 113–118. doi:10.1038/77783 PMID:11248802

Bakken, J. S. (2009). Fecal bacteriotherapy for recurrent Clostridium difficile infection. *Anaerobe*, *15*(6), 285–289. doi:10.1016/j.anaerobe.2009.09.007 PMID:19778623

Bermudez-Brito, M., Plaza-Díaz, J., Muñoz-Quezada, S., Gómez-Llorente, C., & Gil, A. (2012). Probiotic Mechanisms of Action. *Annals of Nutrition & Metabolism*, *61*(2), 160–174. doi:10.1159/000342079 PMID:23037511

Bibiloni, R., Fedorak, R. N., Tannock, G. W., Madsen, K. L., Gionchetti, P., Campieri, M., ... Sartor, R. B. (2005). VSL#3 probiotic-mixture induces remission in patients with active ulcerative colitis. *The American Journal of Gastroenterology*, *100*(7), 1539–1546. doi:10.1111/j.1572-0241.2005.41794.x PMID:15984978

Bierbaum, G., & Sahl, H. G. (2009). Lantibiotics: Mode of action, biosynthesis and bioengineering. *Current Pharmaceutical Biotechnology*, *10*(1), 2–18. doi:10.2174/138920109787048616 PMID:19149587

Bischoff, S., & Crowe, S. E. (2004). Food allergy and the gastrointestinal tract. *Current Opinion in Gastroenterology*, *20*(2), 156–161. doi:10.1097/00001574-200403000-00018 PMID:15703638

Blaser, M. (2011). Antibiotic overuse: Stop the killing of beneficial bacteria. *Nature*, *476*(7361), 393–394. doi:10.1038/476393a PMID:21866137

Boltin, D. (in press). Probiotics in Helicobacter *pylori*-induced peptic ulcer disease. *Best Practice & Research. Clinical Gastroenterology*. doi:10.1016/j.bpg.2015.12.003 PMID:27048901

Bousvaros, A., Guandalini, S., Baldassano, R. N., Botelho, C., Evans, J., Ferry, G. D., ... Hibberd, P. L. (2005). A randomized, double-blind trial of *Lactobacillus GG* versus placebo in addition to standard maintenance therapy for children with Crohn's disease. *Inflammatory Bowel Diseases*, *11*(9), 833–839. doi:10.1097/01.MIB.0000175905.00212.2c PMID:16116318

Boyle, R. J., Robins-Browne, R. M., & Tang, M. L. K. (2006). Probiotic use in clinical practice: What are the risks? *The American Journal of Clinical Nutrition*, *83*(6), 1256–1264. doi:10.1093/ajcn/83.6.1256 PMID:16762934

Buck, B. L., Altermann, E., Svingerud, T., & Klaenhammer, T. R. (2005). Functional analysis of putative adhesion factors in *Lactobacillus acidophilus* NCNCFM. *Applied and Environmental Microbiology*, *71*(12), 8344–8351. doi:10.1128/AEM.71.12.8344-8351.2005 PMID:16332821

Bullock, N. R., Booth, J. C., & Gibson, G. R. (2004). Comparative composition of bacteria in the human intestinal microflora during remission and active ulcerative colitis. *Current Issues in Intestinal Microbiology*, *5*, 59–64. PMID:15460067

Canani, R. B., Cirillo, P., Terrin, G., Cesarano, L., Spagnuolo, M. I., De Vicenzo, A., ... Guarino, A. (2007). Probiotics for treatment of acute diarrhoea in children: Randomised clinical trial of five different preparations. *British Medical Journal*, *335*(7615), 340. doi:10.1136/bmj.39272.581736.55 PMID:17690340

Cani, P. D., Possemiers, S., Van de Wiele, T., Guiot, Y., Everard, A., Rottier, O., ... Delzenne, N. M. (2009). Changes in gut microbiota control inflammation in obese mice through a mechanism involving GLP-2-driven improvement of gut permeability. *Gut*, *58*(8), 1091–1103. doi:10.1136/gut.2008.165886 PMID:19240062

Chen, G., Shaw, M. H., Kim, Y. G., & Nuñez, G. (2009). NOD-like receptors: Role in innate immunity and inflammatory disease. *Annual Review of Pathology*, *4*(1), 365–398. doi:10.1146/annurev.pathol.4.110807.092239 PMID:18928408

Clausen, M. R., Bonnen, H., Tvede, M., & Mortensen, P. B. (1991). Colonic fermentation to short-chain fatty acids is decreased in antibiotic-associated diarrhea. *Gastroenterology*, *101*(6), 1497–1504. doi:10.1016/0016-5085(91)90384-W PMID:1955116

Cruchet, S., Obregon, M. C., Salazar, G., Diaz, E., & Gottenland, M. (2003). Effect of the ingestion of a dietary product containing *Lactobacillus johnsonii* La1 on *Helicobacter pylori* colonization in children. *Nutrition (Burbank, Los Angeles County, Calif.)*, *19*(9), 716–721. doi:10.1016/S0899-9007(03)00109-6 PMID:12921879

Daliri, E.B.M., Lee, B. H. (in press). New perspectives on probiotics in health and disease. *Food Science and Human Wellness*. .10.1016/j.fshw.2015.06.002

Damaskos, D., & Kolios, G. (2008). Probiotics and prebiotics in inflammatory bowel disease: Microflora 'on the scope'. *British Journal of Clinical Pharmacology*, *65*(4), 453–467. doi:10.1111/j.1365-2125.2008.03096.x PMID:18279467

Davidson, L. E., Fiorino, A. M., Snydman, D. R., & Hibberd, P. L. (2011). *Lactobacillus GG* as an immune adjuvant for live-attenuated influenza vaccine in healthy adults: A randomized double-blind placebo-controlled trial. *European Journal of Clinical Nutrition*, *65*(4), 501–507. doi:10.1038/ejcn.2010.289 PMID:21285968

Dubey, A. P., Rajeshwari, K., Chakravarty, A., & Famularo, G. (2008). Use of VSL#3 in the treatment of rotavirus diarrhea in children: Preliminary results. *Journal of Clinical Gastroenterology*, *42*(Suppl. 3 Pt. 1), S126–S129. doi:10.1097/MCG.0b013e31816fc2f6 PMID:18806703

Duncan, B. (2013). Prebiotics, Probiotics, and Health Promotion: An Overview. In *Bioactive Food as Dietary Interventions for Liver and Gastrointestinal Disease* (pp. 449–463). Elsevier Inc. doi:10.1016/B978-0-12-397154-8.00005-1

Esposito, E., Iacono, A., Bianco, G., Autore, G., Cuzzocrea, S., Vajro, P., ... Meli, R. (2009). Probiotics reduce the inflammatory response induced by a highfatdiet in the liver of young rats. *The Journal of Nutrition*, *139*(5), 905–911. doi:10.3945/jn.108.101808 PMID:19321579

Falagas, M. E., Betsi, G. I., & Athanasiou, S. (2007). Probiotics for the treatment of women with bacterial vaginosis. *Clinical Microbiology and Infection*, *13*(7), 657–664. doi:10.1111/j.1469-0691.2007.01688.x PMID:17633390

FAO/WHO. (2002). *Joint FAO/WHO Working Group on Drafting Guidelines for the Evaluation of Probiotics in Food. Guidelines for the evaluation of probiotics in food: report of a Joint FAO/WHO Working Group on Drafting Guidelines for the Evaluation of Probiotics in Food.* London, ON, Canada: FAO/WHO.

Fedorak, R. N. (2008). Understanding why probiotic therapies can be effective in treating IBD. *Journal of Clinical Gastroenterology*, *42*(Suppl 3 Pt 1), S111–S115. doi:10.1097/MCG.0b013e31816d922c PMID:18806699

Fedorak, R. N., & Madsen, K. L. (2004). Probiotics and the Management of Inflammatory Bowel Disease. *Inflammatory Bowel Diseases*, *10*(3), 286–299. doi:10.1097/00054725-200405000-00018 PMID:15290926

Firmansyah, A., Penn, D., & Lebenthal, E. (1989). Isolated colonocyte metabolism of glucose, glutamine, n-butyrate, and beta-hydroxy-butyrate in malnutrition. *Gastroenterology*, *97*(3), 622–629. doi:10.1016/0016-5085(89)90633-1 PMID:2753323

Flint, H. J., Scott, K. P., Louis, P., & Duncan, S. H. (2012). The role of the gut microbiota in nutrition and health. *Nature Reviews. Gastroenterology & Hepatology*, *9*(10), 577–589. doi:10.1038/nrgastro.2012.156 PMID:22945443

Furrie, E., Macfarlane, S., Kennedy, A., Cummings, J. H., Walsh, S. V., O'neil, D. A., & Macfarlane, G. T. (2005). Synbiotic therapy *(Bifidobacteriumlongum*/Synergy 1) initiates resolution of inflammation in patients with active ulcerative colitis: A randomised controlled pilot trial. *Gut*, *54*(2), 242–249. doi:10.1136/gut.2004.044834 PMID:15647189

Gallo, R. L., & Hooper, L. V. (2012). Epithelial antimicrobial defence of the skin and intestine. *Nature Reviews. Immunology*, *12*(7), 503–516. doi:10.1038/nri3228 PMID:22728527

Ganz, T. (2003). Defensins: Antimicrobial peptides of innate immunity. *Nature Reviews. Immunology*, *3*(9), 710–720. doi:10.1038/nri1180 PMID:12949495

Geier, M. S., Butler, R. N., & Howarth, G. S. (2006). Probiotics, prebiotics and synbiotics: A role in chemoprevention for colorectal cancer? *Cancer Biology & Therapy*, *5*(10), 1265–1269. doi:10.4161/cbt.5.10.3296 PMID:16969130

Geier, M. S., Butler, R. N., & Howarth, G. S. (2007). Inflammatory bowel disease: Current insights into pathogenesis and new therapeutic options; probiotics, prebiotics and synbiotics. *International Journal of Food Microbiology*, *115*(1), 1–11. doi:10.1016/j.ijfoodmicro.2006.10.006 PMID:17137666

Goldman, C. G., Barrado, D. A., Balcarce, N., Rua, E. C., Oshiro, M., Calcagno, M. L., ... Boccio, J. R. (2006). Effect of a probiotic food as an adjuvant to triple therapy for eradication of *Helicobacter pylori* infection in children. *Nutrition (Burbank, Los Angeles County, Calif.)*, *22*(10), 984–988. doi:10.1016/j.nut.2006.06.008 PMID:16978844

Gómez-Llorente, C., Muñoz, S., & Gil, A. (2010). Role of Toll-like receptors in the development of immune tolerance mediated by probiotics. *The Proceedings of the Nutrition Society*, *69*(03), 381–389. doi:10.1017/S0029665110001527 PMID:20416121

Gotteland, M., Andrews, M., Toledo, M., Muñoz, L., Caceres, P., Anziani, A., ... Salazar, G. (2008). Modulation of *Helicobacter pylori* colonization with cranberry juice and *Lactobacillus johnsonii*La1 in children. *Nutrition (Burbank, Los Angeles County, Calif.)*, *24*(5), 421–426. doi:10.1016/j.nut.2008.01.007 PMID:18343637

Gotteland, M., Poliak, L., Cruchet, S., & Brunser, O. (2005). Effect of regular ingestion of *Saccharomyces boulardii*plus inulin or *Lactobacillus acidophilus* LB in children colonized by *Helicobacter pylori. Acta Paediatrica (Oslo, Norway)*, *94*(12), 1747–1751. doi:10.1111/j.1651-2227.2005.tb01848.x PMID:16421034

Grönlund, M. M., Arvilommi, H., Kero, P., Lehtonen, O. P., & Isolauri, E. (2000). Importance of intestinal colonisation in the maturation of humoral immunity in early infancy: A prospective follow up study of healthy infants aged 0-6 months. *Archives of Disease in Childhood. Fetal and Neonatal Edition*, *83*(3), F186–F192. doi:10.1136/fn.83.3.F186 PMID:11040166

Guandalini, S., Pensabene, L., Zikri, M. A., Dias, J. A., Casali, L. G., Hoekstra, H., ... Weizman, Z. (2000). *Lactobacillus* GG administered in oral rehydration solution to children with acute diarrhea: A multicenter European study. *Journal of Pediatric Gastroenterology and Nutrition*, *30*(1), 54–60. doi:10.1097/00005176-200001000-00018 PMID:10630440

Hakansson, A., & Molin, G. (2011). Gut microbiota and inflammation. *Nutrients*, *3*(6), 637–682. doi:10.3390/nu3060637 PMID:22254115

Hassan, M., Kjos, M., Nes, I. F., Diep, D. B., & Lotfipour, F. (2012). Natural antimicrobial peptides from bacteria: Characteristics and potential applications to fight against antibiotic resistance. *Journal of Applied Microbiology*, *113*(4), 723–736. doi:10.1111/j.1365-2672.2012.05338.x PMID:22583565

He, F., Ouwehand, A. C., Isolauri, E., Hashimoto, H., Benno, Y., & Salminen, S. (2001). Comparison of mucosal adhesion and species identification of bifidobacteria isolated from healthy and allergic infants. *FEMS Immunology and Medical Microbiology*, *30*(1), 43–47. doi:10.1111/j.1574-695X.2001.tb01548.x PMID:11172990

Hempel, S., Newberry, S. J., Maher, A. R., Wang, Z., Miles, J. N., Shanman, R., ... Shekelle, P. G. (2012). Probiotics for the prevention and treatment ofantibiotic-associated diarrhea: A systematic review and meta-analysis. *Journal of the American Medical Association*, *307*, 1959–1969. doi:10.1001/jama.2012.3507 PMID:22570464

Hilton, E., Kolakowski, P., Singer, C., & Smith, M. (1997). Efficacy of *Lacto-bacillus* GG as a diarrheal preventive in travelers. *Journal of Travel Medicine*, *4*(1), 41–92. doi:10.1111/j.1708-8305.1997.tb00772.x PMID:9815476

Hirano, J., Yoshida, T., Sugiyama, T., Koide, N., Mori, I., & Yokochi, T. (2003). The effect of *Lactobacillus rhamnosus*on enterohemorrhagic*Escherichia coli* infection of human intestinal cells in vitro. *Microbiology and Immunology*, *47*(6), 405–409. doi:10.1111/j.1348-0421.2003.tb03377.x PMID:12906100

Hoarau, C., Lagaraine, C., Martin, I., Velge-Roussel, F., & Lecranchu, Y. (2006). Supernatant of Bifidobacterium breve induces dendritic cell maturation, activation, and survival through a Toll-like receptor pathway. *The Journal of Allergy and Clinical Immunology*, *117*(3), 696–702. doi:10.1016/j.jaci.2005.10.043 PMID:16522473

Hotamisligil, G. S. (2006). Inflammation and metabolic disorders. *Nature*, *444*(7121), 860–867. doi:10.1038/nature05485 PMID:17167474

Huurre, A., Laitinen, K., Rautava, S., Korkeamäki, M., & Isolauri, E. (2008). Impact of maternal atopy and probiotic supplementation during pregnancy on infant sensitization. *Clinical and Experimental Allergy*, *38*(8), 1342–1348. doi:10.1111/j.1365-2222.2008.03008.x PMID:18477013

Ishibashi, N., & Yamazaki, S. (2001). Probiotics and safety. *The American Journal of Clinical Nutrition*, *73*(2Suppl.), 465S–470S. doi:10.1093/ajcn/73.2.465s PMID:11157359

Ishimwe, N., Daliri, E., Lee, B., Fang, F., & Du, G. (2015). The perspective on cholesterol-lowering mechanisms of probiotics. *Molecular Nutrition & Food Research*, *59*(1), 94–105. doi:10.1002/mnfr.201400548 PMID:25403164

J. C., Ursell, L.K., Parfrey, L. W., Knight, R. (2012). The Impact of the Gut Microbiota on Human Health: An Integrative View. *Cell*, *148*(16), 1258–1270. PMID:22424233

Johnston, B. C., Goldenberg, J. C., Vandvik, P. O., Sun, X., & Guyatt, G. H. (2011). Probiotics for the prevention of pediatric-associated diarrhea. *Cochrane Database of Systematic Reviews*, CD004827. PMID:22071814

Kalliomaki, M., & Isolauri, E. (2002). Pandemic of atopic diseases—a lack of microbial exposure in early infancy? *Current Drug Targets. Infectious Disorders*, *2*(3), 193–199. doi:10.2174/1568005023342452 PMID:12462124

Kalliomäki, M., Salminen, S., Arvilommi, H., Kero, P., Koskinen, P., & Isolauri, E. (2001). Probiotics in primary prevention of atopic 392 disease: A randomised placebo-controlled trial. *Lancet*, *357*(9262), 1076–1079. doi:10.1016/S0140-6736(00)04259-8 PMID:11297958

Kalliomäki, M., Salminen, S., Poussa, T., & Isolauri, E. (2007). Probiotics during the first 7 years of life: A cumulative risk reduction of 388 eczema in randomized, placebo-controlled trial. *The Journal of Allergy and Clinical Immunology*, *119*(4), 1019–1021. doi:10.1016/j.jaci.2006.12.608 PMID:17289135

Katelaris, P. H., Salam, I., & Farthing, M. J. (1995). *Lactobacilli* to preventtraveler's diarrhea? *The New England Journal of Medicine*, *333*(20), 1360–1391. doi:10.1056/NEJM199511163332016 PMID:7566045

Khoruts, A., Dicksved, J., Jansson, J. K., & Sadowsky, M. J. (2010). Changes in the composition of the human fecal microbiome after bacteriotherapy for recurrent Clostridium difficile-associated diarrhea. *Journal of Clinical Gastroenterology*, *44*, 354–360. PMID:20048681

Kim, Y., Lee, D., Kim, D., Cho, J., Yang, J., Chung, M., Kim, K., & Ha, N. (2008). Inhibition of proliferation in colon cancer cell lines and harmful enzyme activity of colon bacteria by Bifidobacteriumadolescentis SPM0212. *Archives of Pharmcal Research,* 468–473.

Kollaritsch, H. (1989). Traveller's diarrhea among Austrian touriststowarm climate countries: II Clinical features. *European Journal of Epidemiology*, *5*(3), 355–362. doi:10.1007/BF00144838 PMID:2792310

Kotzampassia, K., & Giamarellos-Bourboulis, E. J. (2012). Probiotics for infectious diseases: More drugs, less dietary supplementation. *International Journal of Antimicrobial Agents*, *40*(4), 288–296. doi:10.1016/j.ijantimicag.2012.06.006 PMID:22858373

Kruis, W., Schutz, E., Fric, P., Fixa, B., Judmaier, G., & Stolte, M. (1997). Double-blind comparison of an oral *E. coli* preparation and mesalazine in maintaining remission of ulcerative colitis. *Aliment Pharmacology & Theraputics*, *11*(5), 853–858. doi:10.1046/j.1365-2036.1997.00225.x PMID:9354192

Kukkonen, K., Savilahti, E., Haahtela, T., Juntunen-Backman, K., Korpela, R., Poussa, T., ... Kuitunen, M. (2008). Long-term safety and impacton infection rates of postnatal probiotic and prebiotic(synbiotic) treatment: Randomized, double-blind, placebo-controlled trial. *Pediatrics*, *122*(1), 8–12. doi:10.1542/peds.2007-1192 PMID:18595980

Kumar, M., Nagpal, R., Kumar, R., Hemalatha, R., Verma, V., Kumar, A., ... Yadav, H. (2012). Cholesterol-lowering probiotics as potential biotherapeutics for metabolic diseases. *Experimental Diabetes Research*, *2012*, 902917. doi:10.1155/2012/902917 PMID:22611376

Lan, A., Lagadic-Gossmann, D., Lemaire, C., & Jan, G. (2007). Acidic extracellular pH shifts colorectal cancer cell death from apoptosis to necrosis upon exposure to propionate and acetate, major end-products of the human probiotic propionibacteria. *Apoptosis*, *12*(3), 573–591. doi:10.100710495-006-0010-3 PMID:17195096

Lee, H. Y., Park, J. H., Seok, S. H., Baek, M. W., Kim, D. J., Lee, K. E., ... Park, J. H. (2006). Human originated bacteria, Lactobacillus rhamnosus PL60, produce conjugated linoleic acid and show anti-obesity effects in diet induced obese mice. *Biochimica et Biophysica Acta*, *1761*(7), 736–744. doi:10.1016/j.bbalip.2006.05.007 PMID:16807088

Ley, R. E., Turnbaugh, P. J., Klein, S., & Gordon, J. I. (2006). Microbial ecology: Human gut microbes associated with obesity. *Nature*, *444*(7122), 1022–1023. doi:10.1038/4441022a PMID:17183309

Lye, H. S., Rahmat-Ali, G. R., & Liong, M. T. (2010). Mechanisms of cholesterol removal by lactobacilli under conditions that mimic the human gastrointestinal tract. *International Dairy Journal*, *20*(3), 169–175. doi:10.1016/j.idairyj.2009.10.003

Macfarlane, G. T., & Macfarlane, S. (2011). Fermentation in the human large intestine its physiologic consequences and the potential contribution of prebiotics. *Journal of Clinical Gastroenterology*, *45*(Suppl.), S120–S127. doi:10.1097/MCG.0b013e31822fecfe PMID:21992950

Mack, D. R., Ahrne, S., Hyde, L., Wei, S., & Hollingsworth, M. A. (2003). Extracellular MUC3 mucin secretion follows adherence of *Lactobacillus* strains to intestinal epithelial cells in vitro. *Gut*, *52*(6), 827–833. doi:10.1136/gut.52.6.827 PMID:12740338

Marteau, P., Lemann, M., & Seksik, P. (2005). Ineffectiveness of *Lactobacillus johnsonii*la1 for prophylaxis of postoperative recurrence in Crohn's disease: A randomised, double-blind, placebo-controlled getaid trial. *Gut*, *23*, 443–454.

Marteau, P., & Shanahan, F. (2003). Basic aspects and pharmacology of probiotics: An overview of pharmacokinetics, mechanisms of action and side-effects. *Best Practice & Research. Clinical Gastroenterology*, *17*(5), 725–740. doi:10.1016/S1521-6918(03)00055-6 PMID:14507584

Mastretta, E., Longo, P., Laccisaglia, A., & Gianino, P. (2002). Effect of *Lactobacillus* GG and breast-feeding in the prevention of rotavirus nosocomial infection. *Journal of Pediatric Gastroenterology and Nutrition*, *35*(4), 527–531. doi:10.1097/00005176-200210000-00013 PMID:12394379

McFarland, L. V. (2010). Probiotics and diarrhea. *Annals of Nutrition & Metabolism*, *57*(1), 10–11. doi:10.1159/000309016 PMID:20829585

McFarland, L. V. (2010). Systematic review and meta-analysis of *Saccharomyces boulardii*in adult patients. *World Journal of Gastroenterology*, *16*(18), 2202–2222. doi:10.3748/wjg.v16.i18.2202 PMID:20458757

McGroarty, J. A. (1993). Probiotic use of lactobacilli in the human female urogenital tract. *FEMS Immunology and Medical Microbiology*, *6*(4), 251–264. doi:10.1111/j.1574-695X.1993.tb00337.x PMID:8499891

Mischke, M., & Plosch, T. (2013). More than just a gut instinct—The potential interplay between a baby's nutrition, its gut microbiome and the epigenome. *American Journal of Physiology. Regulatory, Integrative and Comparative Physiology*, *304*(12), R1065–R1069. doi:10.1152/ajpregu.00551.2012 PMID:23594611

Morotomi, M. (1996). Properties of *Lactobacillus casei*Shirota strain as probiotics. *Asia Pacific Journal of Clinical Nutrition*, *5*, 29–30. PMID:24394462

Murphy, E. F., Cotter, P. D., Hogan, A., O'Sullivan, O., Joyce, A., Fouhy, F., ... Shanahan, F. (2013). Divergent metabolic outcomes arising from targeted manipulation of the gut microbiota in diet induced obesity. *Gut*, *62*(2), 220–226. doi:10.1136/gutjnl-2011-300705 PMID:22345653

Mylonaki, M., Rayment, N. B., Rampton, D. S., Hudspith, B. N., & Brostoff, J. (2005). Molecular characterization of rectal mucosa-associated bacterial flora in inflammatory bowel disease. *Inflammatory Bowel Diseases*, *11*(5), 481–487. doi:10.1097/01.MIB.0000159663.62651.4f PMID:15867588

Ng, S. C., Plamondon, S., Al-Hassi, H. O., Kamm, M. A., Knight, S. C., & Stagg, A. J. (2008a). M1202 Effective probiotic treatment (VSL#3), but not placebo, in acute ulcerative colitis is associated with downregulation of inflammatory intestinal dendritic cells. *Gastroenterology*, *134*(4), A3610. doi:10.1016/S0016-5085(08)61677-7

Ng, S. C., Plamondon, S., Al-Hassi, H. O., Kamm, M. A., Knight, S. C., & Stagg, A. J. (2008b). Corticosteroids increase interleukin-10 and inhibit interleukin-12p40 production by intestinal dendritic cells in acute ulcerative colitis: Novel mechanisms of therapy. *Gastroenterology*, *134*(4), A646. doi:10.1016/S0016-5085(08)63015-2

O'Hara, A. M., & Shanahan, F. (2006). The gut flora as a forgotten organ. *EMBO Reports*, *7*(7), 688–693. doi:10.1038j.embor.7400731 PMID:16819463

Oduyebo, O. O., Anorlu, R. I., & Ogunsola, F. T. (2009). The effects of antimicrobial therapy on bacterial vaginosis in non-pregnant women. *Cochrane Database of Systematic Reviews*, *3*, CD006055. PMID:19588379

Oelschlaeger, T. A. (2010). Mechanisms of probiotic actions – a review. *International Journal of Medical Microbiology*, *300*(1), 57–62. doi:10.1016/j.ijmm.2009.08.005 PMID:19783474

Ohland, C. L., & Macnaughton, W. K. (2010). Probiotic bacteria and intestinal epithelial barrier function. *American Journal of Gastrointestinal and Liver Physiology*, *298*(6), G807–G819. doi:10.1152/ajpgi.00243.2009 PMID:20299599

Oksanen, P. J., Salminen, S., Saxelin, M., Hämäläinen, P., Ihantola-Vormisto, A., Muurasniemi-Isoviita, L., ... Vapaatalo, H. (1990). Prevention of travellers' diarrhoea by *Lactobacillus* GG. *Annals of Medicine*, *22*(1), 53–93. doi:10.3109/07853899009147242 PMID:2184847

Olveira, G., & González-Molero, I. (*In-press*). Actualización de probióticos, prebióticos y simbióticos en nutrición clínica. *Endocrinología y Nutrición*. doi:10.1016/j.endonu.2016.07.006

Ooi, L. G., & Liong, M. T. (2010). Cholesterol-lowering effects of probiotics and prebiotics: A reviewof in vivo and in vitro findings. *International Journal of Molecular Sciences*, *11*(6), 2499–2522. doi:10.3390/ijms11062499 PMID:20640165

Ouwehand, A. C., Salminen, S., & Isolauri, E. (2002). Probiotics: An overview of beneficial effects. *Antonie van Leeuwenhoek*, *82*(1/4), 279–289. doi:10.1023/A:1020620607611 PMID:12369194

Park, D. Y., Ahn, Y. T., Park, S. H., Huh, C. S., Yoo, S. R., Yu, R., ... Choi, M. S. (2013). Supplementation of Lactobacillus curvatus HY7601 and Lactobacillus plantarum KY1032 in diet-induced obese mice is associated with gut microbial changes and reduction in obesity. *PLoS One*, *8*(3), e59470. doi:10.1371/journal.pone.0059470 PMID:23555678

Penner, R. M., Madsen, K. L., & Fedorak, R. N. (2005). Postoperative Crohn's disease. *Inflammatory Bowel Diseases*, *11*(8), 765–777. doi:10.1097/01.MIB.0000171273.09757.f2 PMID:16043993

Philippe, G. (2014). Metabolism of cholesterol and bile acids by the gut microbiota. *Pathogens (Basel, Switzerland)*, *3*, 14–24. PMID:25437605

Quigley, E. M. M. (2016). Basic Definitions and Concepts: Organization of the Gut Microbiome. *Gastroenterology Clinics of North America*, 1–8. PMID:28164844

Reid, G., Beuerman, D., Heinemann, C., & Bruce, A. (2001). Probiotic Lactobacillus dose required to restore and maintain a normal vaginal flora. *FEMS Immunology and Medical Microbiology*, *32*(1), 37–41. doi:10.1111/j.1574-695X.2001.tb00531.x PMID:11750220

Rembacken, B. J., Snelling, A. M., Hawkey, P. M., Chalmers, D. M., & Axon, A. T. R. (1999). Chalmers DM, Axon AT Non-pathogenic *Escherichia coli* versus mesalazine for the treatment of ulcerative colitis: A randomised trial. *Lancet, 354*(9179), 635–639. doi:10.1016/S0140-6736(98)06343-0 PMID:10466665

Rouxinol-Dias, A. L., Pinto, A. R., Janeiro, C., Rodrigues, D., Moreira, M., Dias, J., & Pereira, P. (2016). Probiotics for the control of obesity – Its effect on weight change. *Porto Biomedical Journal, 1*(1), 12–24. doi:10.1016/j.pbj.2016.03.005

Saavedra, J. M., Bauman, A., Oung, I., Perman, J. A., & Yolken, R. H. (1994). Feeding of *Bifidobacteriumbifidum*and *Streptococcus thermophilus*to infants in hospital for prevention of diarrhea and shedding of rotavirus. *Lancet, 344*(8929), 1046–1049. doi:10.1016/S0140-6736(94)91708-6 PMID:7934445

Sánchez, B., Urdaci, M. C., & Margolles, A. (2010). Extracellular proteins secreted by probiotic bacteriaas mediators of effects that promote mucosa- bacteria interactions. *Microbiology, 156*(11), 3232–3242. doi:10.1099/mic.0.044057-0 PMID:20864471

Sanchez, M., Darimont, C., Drapeau, V., Emady-Azar, S., Lepage, M., Rezzonico, E., ... Tremblay, A. (2014). Effect of Lactobacillus rhamnosus CGMCC1.3724 supplementation on weight loss and maintenance in obese men and women. *British Journal of Nutrition, 111*(08), 1507–1519. doi:10.1017/S0007114513003875 PMID:24299712

Sanfilippo, L., Li, C. K., Seth, R., Balwin, T. J., Menozzi, M. G., & Mahida, Y. R. (2000). *Bacteroidesfragilis*enterotoxin induces the expression of IL-8 and transforming growth factor-beta (TFG-_) by human colonic epithelial cells. *Clinical and Experimental Immunology, 119*(3), 456–463. doi:10.1046/j.1365-2249.2000.01155.x PMID:10691917

Schiffrin, E. J., & Blum, S. (2002). Interactions between the microbiota and the intestinal mucosa. *European Journal of Clinical Nutrition, 56*(S3), S60–S64. doi:10.1038j.ejcn.1601489 PMID:12142966

Schultz, M., Timmer, A., Herfarth, H. H., Sartor, R. B., Vanderhoof, J. A., & Rath, H. C. (2004). *Lactobacillus GG* in inducing and maintaining remission of Crohn's disease. *BMC Gastroenterology, 4*(1), 5. doi:10.1186/1471-230X-4-5 PMID:15113451

Schwiertz, A., Taras, D., Schäfer, K., Beijer, S., Bos, N. A., Donus, C., & Hardt, P. D. (2010). Microbiota and SCFA in lean and overweight healthy subjects. *Obesity (Silver Spring, Md.), 18*(1), 190–195. doi:10.1038/oby.2009.167 PMID:19498350

Sekirov, I., Russell, S. L., Antunes, L. C., & Finlay, B. B. (2010). Gut microbiota in health and disease. *Physiological Reviews*, *90*(3), 859–904. doi:10.1152/physrev.00045.2009 PMID:20664075

Sgouras, M., Maragkoudakis, P., Petraki, K., Martinez-Gonzalez, B., Eriotou, E., Michopoulos, S., ... Mentis, A. (2004). *In vitro* and *in vivo* inhibition of *Helicobacter pylori* by Lactobacillus casei strain Shirota. *Applied and Environmental Microbiology*, *70*(1), 518–526. doi:10.1128/AEM.70.1.518-526.2004 PMID:14711683

Shornikova, A. V., Casas, I. A., Isolauri, E., Mykkanen, H., & Vesikari, T. (1997). *Lactobacillus reuteri* as a therapeutic agent in acute diarrhea in young children. *Journal of Pediatric Gastroenterology and Nutrition*, *24*(4), 399–404. doi:10.1097/00005176-199704000-00008 PMID:9144122

Simpson, A., Tan, V. Y. F., Winn, J., Svensén, M., Bishop, C. M., Heckerman, D. E., ... Custovic, A. (2010). Beyond atopy: Multiple patterns of sensitization in relation to asthma in a birth cohort study. *American Journal of Respiratory and Critical Care Medicine*, *181*(11), 1200–1206. doi:10.1164/rccm.200907-1101OC PMID:20167852

Sivieri, K., Spinardi-Barbusan, A. L. T., Barbisan, L. F., Bedani, R., Pauly, N. D., Carlos, I. Z., ... Rossi, E. A. (2008). Probiotic Enterococcus faecium CRL 183 inhibit chemically induced colon cancer in male Wistar rats. *European Food Research and Technology*, *228*(2), 231–237. doi:10.100700217-008-0927-6

Strachan, P. (2000). Family size, infection and atopy: the first 416 decade of the "hygiene hypothesis". *Thorax, 417*(55-1), S2–S10.

Surawicz, C. M., McFarland, L. V., Greenberg, R. N., Rubin, M., Fekety, R., Mulligan, M. E., ... Elmer, G. W. (2003). The search for a better treatment for recurrent Clostridium difficile disease: Use of high-dose vancomycin combined with *Saccharomyces boulardii. Clinical Infectious Diseases*, *31*(4), 1012–1017. doi:10.1086/318130 PMID:11049785

Sýkora, J., Valecková, K., Amlerová, J., & ... . (2005). Effects of a specially designed fermented milk product containing probiotic *Lactobacillus casei* dn-114 001 and the eradication of *H. pylori* in children: A prospective randomized double-blind study. *Journal of Clinical Gastroenterology*, *39*, 692–698. doi:10.1097/01.mcg.0000173855.77191.44 PMID:16082279

Szajewska, H., Kotowska, M., Mrukowicz, J. Z., Armańska, M., & Mikołajczyk, W. (2001). Efficacy of *Lactobacillus* GG in prevention of nosocomial diarrhea in infants. *The Journal of Pediatrics*, *138*, 361–365. doi:10.1067/mpd.2001.111321 PMID:11241043

Szyman'ski, H., Pejcz, J., Jawien´, M., Chmielarczyk, A., Strus, M., & Heczko, P. B. (2006). Treatment of acute infectious diarrhoea in infants and children with a mixture of three *Lactobacillus rhamnosus*strains—a randomized, double-blind, placebo-controlled trial. *Alimentary Pharmacology & Therapeutics*, *23*(2), 247–253. doi:10.1111/j.1365-2036.2006.02740.x PMID:16393304

Taylor, A. L., Hale, J., Wiltschut, J., Lehmann, H., Dunstan, J. A., & Prescott, S. L. (2006). Effects of probiotic supplementation for the first 6 months of life on allergen- and vaccine-specific immune responses. *Clinical and Experimental Allergy*, *36*(10), 1227–1235. doi:10.1111/j.1365-2222.2006.02553.x PMID:17014429

Tung, J. M., Dolovich, L. R., & Lee, C. H. (2009). Prevention of *Clostridium difficile*infection with *Saccharomyces boulardii*: A systematicreview. *Canadian Journal of Gastroenterology*, *23*(12), 817–821. doi:10.1155/2009/915847 PMID:20011734

Turnbaugh, P. J., & Gordon, J. I. (2009). The core gut microbiome, energy balance and obesity. *The Journal of Physiology*, *587*(17), 4153–4158. doi:10.1113/jphysiol.2009.174136 PMID:19491241

Turnbaugh, P. J., Hamady, M., Yatsunenko, T., Cantarel, B. L., Duncan, A., Ley, R. E., ... Gordon, J. I. (2009). A core gutmicrobiome in obese and lean twins. *Nature*, *457*(7228), 480–484. doi:10.1038/nature07540 PMID:19043404

Tursi, A., Brandimarte, G., Giorgetti, G. M., Forti, G., Modeo, M. E., & Gigliobianco, A. (2004). Low-dose balsalazide plus a high-potency probiotic preparation is more effective than balsalazide alone or mesalazine in the treatment of acute mild-to-moderate ulcerative colitis. *Medical Science Monitor*, *10*, PI126–PI131. PMID:15507864

Vandenplas, Y., Brunser, O., & Szajewska, H. (2009). *Saccharomyces boulardii*in childhood. *European Journal of Pediatrics*, *168*(3), 253–265. doi:10.100700431-008-0879-7 PMID:19096876

Vandenplas, Y., Huys, G., & Daube, G. (2015). Probiotics: An update. *Jornal de Pediatria*, *91*(1), 6–21. doi:10.1016/j.jped.2014.08.005 PMID:25458874

Viljanen, M., Savilahti, E., Haahtela, T., Juntunen-Backman, K., Korpela, R., Poussa, T., ... Kuitunen, M. (2005). Probiotics in the treatment of atopic eczema/dermatitis syndrome in infants: A double-blind placebo-controlled trial. *Allergy*, *60*(4), 494–500. doi:10.1111/j.1398-9995.2004.00514.x PMID:15727582

Vizoso Pinto, M. G., Rodríguez Gómez, M., Seifert, S., Waltz, B., Holzapfel, W. H., & Franz, C. M. (2009). Lactobacilli stimultates the innate immune response and modulate TLR expression of HT29 intestinal epithelial cells in vitro. *International Journal of Food Microbiology*, *133*(1-2), 86–93. doi:10.1016/j.ijfoodmicro.2009.05.013 PMID:19523707

Wang, J. Z., Du, W. T., Xu, Y. L., Cheng, S. Z., & Liu, Z. J. (2017). Gut microbiome-based medical methodologies for early-stage disease prevention. *Microbial Pathogenesis*, *105*, 122–130. doi:10.1016/j.micpath.2017.02.024 PMID:28219830

Wullt, M., Hagslätt, M. L., & Odenholt, I. (2003). Lactobacillus plantarum 299v forthe treatment of recurrent Clostridium difficile-associated diarrhoea: A doubleblind,placebo-controlled trial. *Scandinavian Journal of Infectious Diseases*, *35*(6-7), 365–367. doi:10.1080/00365540310010985 PMID:12953945

Yarandi, S. S., Peterson, D. A., Treisman, G. J., Moran, T. H., & Pasricha, P. J. (2016). Modulatory effects of gut microbiota on the central nervous system: How gut could play a role in neuropsychiatric health and diseases. *Journal ofNeurogastroenterology and Motility*, *22*(2), 201–212. doi:10.5056/jnm15146 PMID:27032544

Chapter 2
Impact of Probiotics in Human Health and Disease Treatment

Jagan Mohan Rao Tingirikari
Chungbuk National University, South Korea

Muthu Vijaya Sarathy
Bharathiar University, India

Ashok Kumar Karthigarani
Bharathiar University, India

ABSTRACT

Probiotics have become the major breakthrough in therapeutic applications due to their various health promoting effects in humans by maintaining the homeostasis of the intestine and prevent microbial imbalance (dysbiosis) without any side effects. Dysbiosis in the microbial population is the major cause for several diseases in humans. Treatment of diseases using antibiotics is not recommended due to high cost, side effects, and the loss of intestinal friendly bacteria. Probiotics work in symbiotic association with the intestine and produce several metabolites which not only regulate the growth of pathogenic bacteria but also provide vital nutrients which contribute to human health. The present chapter highlights about the role of probiotics in treatment and prevention of different human diseases.

INTRODUCTION

Probiotics are generally defined as *live microorganisms when administered in adequate amounts confer a health benefit on the host* (UNFAO/WHO, 2001). The concept of probiotics was evident from earlier reports dating back in 1907, when Ellie Metchnikoff reported a relationship between ingestion of yogurt containing

DOI: 10.4018/978-1-5225-3267-5.ch002

lactic acid bacteria and enhanced longevity in Bulgarian peasants (Bron, Baarlen, & Kleerebezem, 2012). Probiotics exist naturally in several fermented foods such as beverages, yogurt, cheese and pickles (Amara & Shibl, 2015). The common microbes which are used as probiotics belong to bacteria, yeast or molds (Bron, Baarlen, & Kleerebezem, 2012). Among the copious number of strains identified with probiotic features *Lactobacillus*, *Bifidobacterium*, and *Saccharomyces* species were most frequently, used with major health benefits and good market value (Turroni, Ventura, Buttó, Duranti, O'Toole, Motherway, & Van Sindere, 2014).

Consumption of probiotics as functional foods has become more popular among the consumers in recent years. They are available in variety of sources such as dietary supplements, food products, ointments, and nasal sprays (Tripathi & Giri, 2014). Modulation of gut bacteria during the diseases condition can be accelerated by consumption of probiotics. Pioneering studies on probiotics have shown their therapeutic applications on human health by maintaining the microbial balance and homeostasis in the intestine (Kechagia, Basoulis, Konstantopoulou, Dimitriadi, Gyftopoulou, Skarmoutsou, & Fakiri, 2012). The primary criteria for standard probiotics include: stable shelf life; survival during intestinal transit, and production of beneficial products such as bacterocin, short chain fatty acids, and other inhibitory metabolites which can regulate the growth of pathogenic bacteria in the intestine (Vandenplas, Huy, & Daube, 2015).

The key mechanism of probiotics in controlling the disease is mediated by enhanced epithelial barrier function, increased adhesion to intestinal mucosa, and competitive exclusion of pathogenic microorganisms, production of antimicrobial, immune-modulatory substances (Kechagia, Basoulis, Konstantopoulou, Dimitriadi, Gyftopoulou, Skarmoutsou, & Fakiri, 2012). The present chapter is focused on the properties, mechanism of action, global prospects, and different dairy and non-dairy based probiotics available in the market will be addressed. Role of probiotics in treatment and prevention of different diseases associated due to the microbial dysbiosis will be discussed. In addition, safety issues related to probiotics will also be highlighted along with future prospects and development.

BACKGROUND

Human health and diseases are mainly driven by the microbial balance of the body, homeostasis of microbial population is considered as beneficial, while the dysbiosis causes many health problems (Gareau, Sherman, & Walker, 2010). The distinction between research aimed at health and disease treatment has unique regulatory implications, the former can be applied with foods and supplements, whereas the latter is confined to therapeutics (Sanders, Guarner, Guerrant, Holt, Quigley, Sartor, & Mayer, 2013). Despite number of factors contribute to human health and diseases patterns, but recent research has shown the predominant role of gut microbiota in several diseases (Li, Wang, Wang, Hu, & Chen, 2016). There are number of standing evidences revealing the health benefits of probiotics on gastrointestinal infections, antimicrobial activity, improvement in lactose metabolism, reduction in serum cholesterol, immune system stimulation, anti-mutagenic, anti-carcinogenic, anti-diarrheal, improvement in inflammatory bowel disease and suppression of *Helicobacter pylori* infection by addition of selected strains to food products (Faujdar, Mehrishi, Bishnoi, & Sharma, 2016). A recent report has shown the wide application of probiotics in treatment of many diseases as a result the market value of probiotics is increasing tremendously. The current market value of probiotic is 28.8 billion US$ which is expected to rise by 100 billion $USD by 2020 (Queen, Surette, & Moayyedi, 2017). Increasing market value of probiotics clearly states the significance and the role of probiotics in disease treatment and prevention.

DIFFERENT REGIONS OF HUMAN BODY COLONISED BY MICROBES

Different regions of human body is colonized by different microbes (skin, mouth, pharynx, intestinal tract, and urogenital tract) and the distribution of microbes is influenced by several factors such as antibiotics, diet, immunosuppressive agents, and external environmental conditions (Li, Wang, Wang, Hu, & Chen, 2016). Among all the regions maximum colonisation of microbes are found in human intestine with large and diverse community members such as bacteria, archaea, eukarya, viruses and parasites with total number of microbial cells constituting around 10^{13} - 10^{14} whereas very low population was found in stomach typically harbouring upto 10^{3} colony forming units (CFU) per gram of contents, comprising of *Lactobacilli*, *Streptococci*, and yeasts because of its very low pH (Li, Wang, Wang, Hu, & Chen, 2016). Different regions of human body are inhabited by specific phyla of microbiota: skin by *Actinobacteria, Firmicutes* and *Proteobacteria*; oral cavity by *Bacteroidetes*, *Firmicutes*, *Fusobacteria*, and *Proteobacteria*; while lungs by *Bacteroidetes*, *Firmicutes*, and *Proteobacteria*; gastrointestinal tract by *Bacteroidetes* and *Firmicutes*; and urogenital tract by *Firmicutes* (Wang & Kasper, 2014). Distribution of different microbial population in the human body has been mentioned in Figure 1.

Figure 1. Different regions of human body colonised by normal microbial flora and probiotics

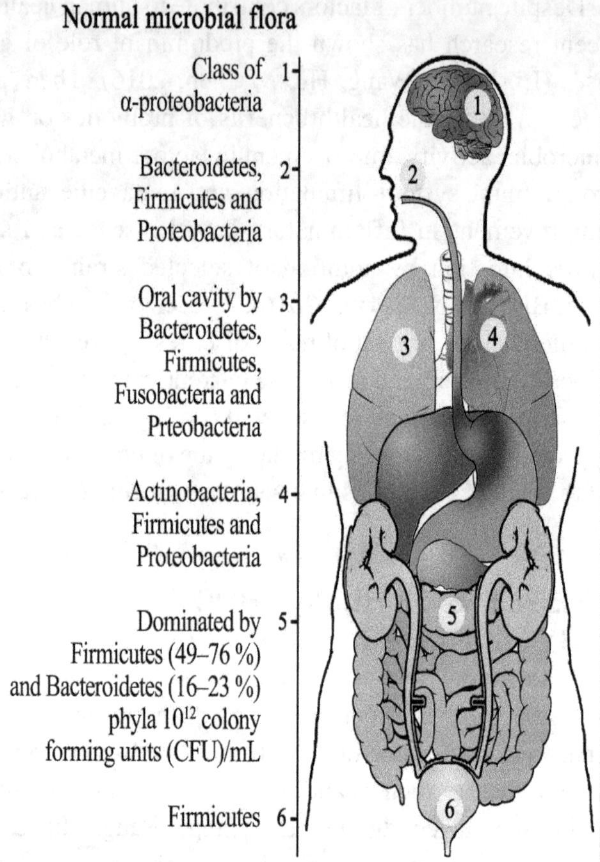

CHARACTERISTIC FEATURES AND PROPERTIES OF PROBIOTICS

In order to provide beneficial effects probiotic bacteria must be stable to physiological conditions such as acidic pH in stomach, intestinal bile secretions, and digestive enzymes in active form and parellely they must provide health benefit to the host. Some of the ideal properties of probiotics are as follows:

- At first, it should be non-pathogenic, nontoxic and sensitive to antibiotics and generally recognised as safe (GRAS).
- In order to confer desired health benefit on host the concentration of probiotics should be at least 10^6 CFU/mL of at the expiry date. While the recommended dosage required per day is 10^8–10^9 cells

- Should be able to taken through regular diet with adequate number of viable cells, capable of fermenting the food to confer the health benefit.
- Should arrest the virulent compounds which are harmful to the host system and able to bind the walls of intestine (anchoring and adhering) by means of exo-polysaccharide production.

The best approach to develop probiotics is by evaluating specific studies with target population and physiologic function (Franz, Huch, Abriouel, Holzapfel, & Gálvez, 2011).

MECHANISM OF ACTION OF PROBIOTICS

The functional activity of probiotics depends on the type of microbial strain employed and the site of action. The mechanism of action of probiotics are summarised in Figure 2.

PRODUCTION OF ENZYMES

Humans consume variety of carbohydrates (digestible and non-digestible) from plant and animal origin. Humans lack the enzymes required for the hydrolysis of non-digestible carbohydrates (Turroni, Ventura, Buttó, Duranti, O'Toole, Motherway, & Van Sinderen, 2014). However, several probiotic bacterial species has been reported to contain enzymes necessary for the hydrolysis of dietary fibres and non-digestible carbohydrates. The hydrolysed sugars and other metabolites may act as nutrients for colonocytes and other gut epithelial cells. Probiotics such as *Lb. bulgaricus* and *St. thermophiles* are reported to produce lactase (β-galactosidase) enzyme and help in fermentation of lactose to glucose and galactose, when administration to peoples suffering with lactose intolerance (Pandey, Naik, & Vakil, 2015) Protease produced by yeast (*Sa. boulardii*) capable of cleaving *Clostridium difficile* toxins and blocks the toxin intestinal receptors (Pandey, Naik, & Vakil, 2015). Turroni et al., (2014) reported that *Bifidobacterium longum* ssp. *infantis*, *Bi. bifidum*, and *Bi. Breve* will help in breakdown of human milk oligosaccharides using enzyme (fucosidases, sialidases, a type of β-hexosaminidase, and β-galactosidases).

Production of Antimicrobial Substance and Other Metabolites

The major antimicrobial substances produced by many probiotic bacteria were found to be short chain fatty acids (SCFA) and bacteriocins. SCFAs are generally

Figure 2. . Mechanism of action of probiotics. (1) Delivery of enzymes for digesting non-degradable carbohydrates; (2) Antimicrobial activity and production of SCFA; (3) Competition for nutrients and growth factors; (4) Improved barrier integrity function; (5) Regulation of immune system by direct communication with immune cells, (6) Production of beneficial products such as SCFA, vitamins, (7) Stimulation of mucous secretion.

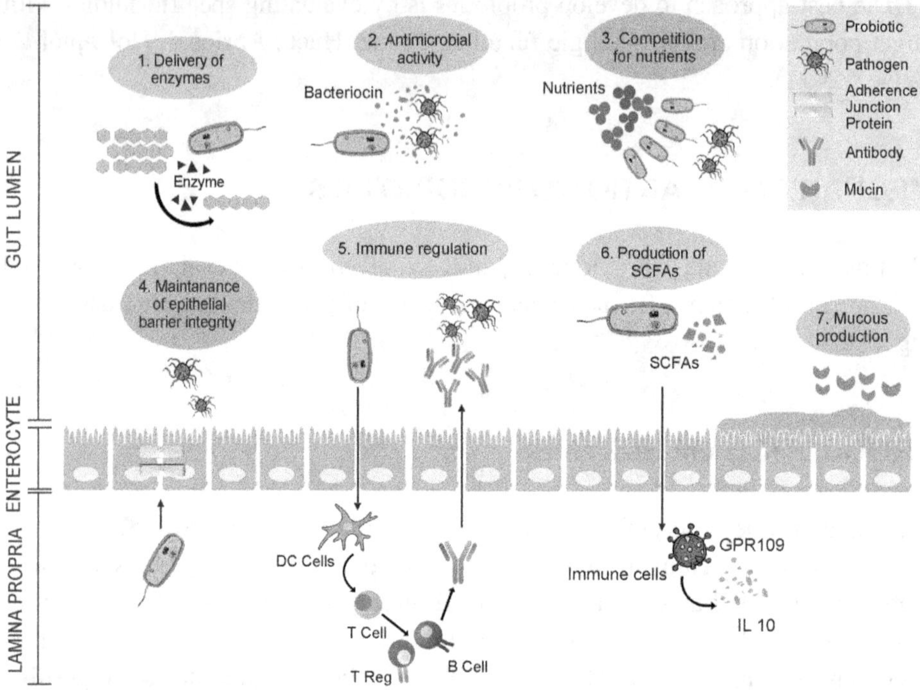

low molecular weight compounds such as lactate, acetate, propionate, and butyrate (Covian, Madiedo, Margolles, Gueimonde, Gavilan, & Salazar, 2016). SCFAs are highly permeable as a result they enter easily in to cytoplasm of the bacterial and decreases the pH which ultimately leads to death of the pathogen (Brito, Diaz, Quezada, Llorente, & Gil, 2012). Bacteriocins are short chain peptides produced by probiotic bacteria and shows lethal effect by destructing the target cells by pore formation or by inhibition of cell wall synthesis (Hemaiswarya, Raja, Ravikumar, & Isabel, 2013). Upon several investigations, bacteriocin-producing probiotic strains inhibit the growth of major pathogens including *E. coli*, *Salmonella*, *Campylobacter*, *Shigella*, *Vibrio*, *Clostridium*, *Candida albicans*, human immunodeficiency virus, and other viruses proved in several laboratory test (Brito, Diaz, Quezada, Llorente, & Gil, 2012). Some of the common bacterocins include lactacin B, acidolin, nisin, and plantaricin.

Probiotics also plays a crucial role in production of B-group vitamins especially in fermented milk products. For instance, *Lb. lactis* in yogurt has ability to synthesize folate (Vitamin B11), *Lb. reuteri* strains can synthesize Cobalamin (Vitamin B12), whereas Riboflavin (Vitamin B2) synthesis were observed strains harbouring rib operon such as *Lb. plantarum* strain NCDO 1752, *Lb. plantarum* strain JDMI isolated from cereals-derived products (Capozzi, Russo, Duenas, Lopez, & Spano, 2012).

Mucin Production and Competitive Exclusion

Mucous secretion is a kind of defence mechanism against pathogenic microbes. The primary component of mucous is mucin, a complex glycoprotein mixture secreted from intestinal epithelial cells (IECs). Several *in-vivo* experiments proved that many probiotic bacteria such as *lactobacillus species* increase mucin (MUC) expression in IECs either by adhesion dependent or independent mechanism. *Lb acidophilus* A4 cell extract is sufficient to increase MUC2 expression in human colon adenocarcinoma (HT29) cells independent of attachment (Brito, Diaz, Quezada, Llorente, & Gil, 2012). *Lb. plantarum* induces the expression of MUC2 and MUC3, which enhances the mucous layers and glycocalyx overlying the intestinal epithelium and provides protection against pathogen. *Lb. reuteri* has been reported to contain mucus-binding proteins and *Lb. fermentum* has mucous adhesion-promoting proteins which help in binding to IECs thereby preventing the adherence and invasion of entero-pathogenic *E. coli* (Brito, Diaz, Quezada, Llorente, & Gil, 2012).

Probiotic bacteria exert competitive exclusion of pathogens either by elimination of available bacterial receptor sites or competitive depletion of essential nutrients (Mohammadi, Mohammadi, Bagheri, & Roozbahani, 2013). Mainly probiotic bacteria express adhesiveness properties due to the interaction between its surface proteins and mucin secreted on epithelial cells. *Lactobacilli* and *Bifidobacteria* have specific receptors to bind to the host cells and prevent the binding of pathogens. The best example for this is *Lb. plantarum* a probiotic strain which has been reported to inhibit the internalization of pathogenic enterohemorrhagic *E. coli* in the human intestinal cell line by competitive exclusion mechanism (Brito, Diaz, Quezada, Llorente, & Gil, 2012).

Stabilization of Intestinal Epithelial Barrier

Intestinal epithelial barrier integrity is a major defence mechanism in human body which protects the intestine from the surrounding environment. The integrity of intestinal epithelial cells can be disturbed mainly by pathogenic bacteria, toxins, inflammation, or stress and causes activation of immune responses which can result in inflammatory and autoimmune disorders (Madsen, Cornish, Soper, McKaigney,

Jijon, Yachimec, Doyle, Jewell, & De Simone, 2001). Probiotic bacteria have been extensively studied for maintaining barrier integrity by expressing the genes responsible for tight junction signalling, promoting tissue repair, decreasing bacterial adhesion and secreting repair factors and nutrients (e.g., SCFA, polyamines, nitric acid, and stimulating production of secretary immunoglobulin A). Brito et al., (2012) reported that *Lactobacilli* can positively modulate epithelial barrier function when incubated with intestinal cells by inducing phosphorylation of adherence junction protein and protein kinase C (PKC)-δ. While, probiotic *E. coli Nissle* 1917 enhanced the expression and redistribution of tight junction proteins such as Zona occludens and PKC thereby repair damage by reconstruction of tight junction complex. Peptides (p 40, 75) isolated from *Lactobacillus rhamnosus* GG showed prevention of cytokine-induced cell apoptosis by activation of the anti-apoptotic protein kinase B in a phosphatidyl inositol-3-kinase-dependent pathway and by inhibiting the mitogen-activated protein kinase.

Immune Modulation

The host-microbial interaction plays a significant role in the proper functioning of the immune systems including development of immune cells, and production of effector molecules such as antibodies (Pandey, Naik, & Vakil, 2015). Probiotic bacteria have been reported to exert immune-modulatory effects by interactions with host cells such as epithelial (ECs) and dendritic cells (DCs) as well as monocytes or macrophages and lymphocytes (Brito, Diaz, Quezada, Llorente, & Gil, 2012). The primary response of host cells is triggered by pattern recognition receptors (PRRs) after binding to pathogen-associated molecular patterns (PAMPs), a common structure found in most of the pathogen. Probiotics interact with ECs and DCs through PRRs especially Toll like receptors (TLRs) family. In that TLR9 signalling is essential to mediate the anti-inflammatory effects of probiotic bacteria whereas TLR2 triggering by *Bifidobacterium breve* C50 induces maturation of DC cells thereby increase interleukin (IL)-10 production (Pandey, Naik, & Vakil, 2015).

GLOBAL PROSPECTS OF PROBIOTICS

Probiotics are highly prevalent in fermented foods, beverages and dietary supplements such as yogurt, sour milk or cheese. However, food industries are creating new medium for the delivery of probiotics which include whey, ice cream, breads, confectionary, soy products, meat and fermented vegetables (Franz, Huch, Abriouel, Holzapfel, &

Gálvez, 2011). According to the global market survey report, US, Europe and Japan are in leading state for marketing probiotic products for gut health. In 2013-14, Japan represented as single largest regional market for probiotics worldwide, with an estimated 34.2% of total global sales. In Western Europe, consumer market for probiotics is about 11.4 billion Euro (€), comprising biggest sector for sales of yogurt and desserts approximate €1 billion whereas probiotic milk products shares the major part and is forecast to grow annually at approximate 7-8% over the next five years (Sharma, Arora, & Baldi, 2013). In Asia-Pacific, China and Japan, dominate the market revenue for probiotics. In India, probiotic market was valued at $2 million as per 2010 estimates and revenues of India's dairy and probiotic market is expected to grow at the CAGR of around 5% during 2012-17. The market share of probiotics is expected to rise upto $522.8 million by 2018 (Sahib, Rakesh, Pal, Apoorva, & Nidhi, 2016). Currently milk and fermented milk products share 62% of the market value in probiotic products. Increase in health awareness among the people has contributed to a significant rise in the demand for probiotics. The global market presents a CAGR of 4.3%, to more than US$ 20 X 10^9 sales per year (Dash, 2014).

DAIRY AND NON-DAIRY BASED PROBIOTIC FOODS

Probiotics are consumed across the world in various commercialized formulation. Selection of suitable food matrix for the delivery of probiotics is the key for improving the stability of probiotics during processing and storage, and also in maintaining the interactions among microbes (Kumar, Vijayendra, & Reddy, 2015). Generally, probiotic can be classified into dairy and non-dairy based foods (Table 1). Dairy based are the most common fermented probiotic foods currently available in the market which include fermented milk, yoghurts, buttermilk, and kefir, while non-fermented products include sweet milk, and ice creams (Bansal, Mangal, Sharma, & Gupta, 2016). Numerous probiotic fermented milk products are available in all over the world. For instance, Yakult in Japan, Actimeal in Paris, Suntory Bikkle in Japan, Nestle LC1 in Switzerland, Vifit in Netherlands and Nesvita in Switzerland (Bansal, Mangal, Sharma, & Gupta, 2016). However, major drawbacks with dairy based products are lactose intolerance, allergy to milk proteins, high cholesterol content, and high amounts of saturated fatty acids which increases health concerns resulting in a shift towards non-dairy probiotic food products (Gupta & Abu-Ghannam, 2012). Also in recent years, the scientific studies have confirmed the probiotic potential of isolates in many of the traditional non-dairy based fermented foods luring the food scientist and researchers to concentrate more on the production of non-dairy

Table 1. Different types of Dairy and Non-dairy based probiotic foods

Probiotic Bacteria	Food Products	References
	Dairy Products	
Lb. acidophilus	Acidophilous milk	Ozden, (2008)
Bifidobacterium longum, Bi. bifidum	Bifidus Milk and Acidophilus-Bifidus milk	Kurnann et al., (1992)
Bi. breve, Bi.longum, and Lb. acidophilus	Mil-Mil	Kurnann et al., (1992)
Bi. bifidum	Kefir	Ozden, (2008)
Lb. delbrueckii ssp. bulgaricus, Lb. acidophilus, Lb.lactis	Acidophilin	Kurnann et al., (1992)
	Non-Dairy Products	
Lactobacillus sp	Sauerkraut	Bansal et al., (2016)
Lb. plantarum and *Lb. confusus*	Ogi and Baba	Johansson et al., (1995)
Lb. plantarum, Lb. sakei and Lb. kimchii	Kimchi	Bansal et al., (2016)
Lactobacillus and *Bacillus*	Stinky tofu or stinky soybean curd	Liu et al., (2011)
Lb. plantarum and *Lb. confusus*	fermented maize or sorghum porridge	Bansal et al., (2016)
Lb. lactis subsp. lactis, Bi. lactis, Lb. bulgaricus var delbruecki	Mahewu	Bansal et al., (2016)
Lb. plantarum and *Leuconostoc*	Boza	Moncheva et al., (2003)
Lb. plantarum, Lb. paracasei subsp. paracasei, Lb. brevis, Lb. fermentum, Lb. delbrueckii subsp. delbrueckii, St. thermophilus and *Enterococcus*	Bushera	Bansal et al., (2016)

based fermented foods (Gawkowski & Chikindas, 2013). Non-dairy fermented foods include foods derived from fruits, vegetable, cereals, and soy which are gaining importance in recent time (Kumar, Vijayendra, & Reddy, 2015). Due to increasing in health awareness among people the demand for probiotic based functional food is increasing rapidly (Tripathi & Giri, 2014).

ROLE OF PROBIOTICS IN REGULATION OF HUMAN DISEASES

Different diseases in human beings are governed by several metabolic and non-metabolic factors which can be addressed by the application of probiotics (Table 2). The pathophysiological conditions of different diseases are mentioned in Figure 3.

Table 2. Role of probiotics in treatment of human diseases

Diseases Type	Type of Probiotic Strains	Role of Probiotic or its Metabolites	Study in Human	References
Chronic Kidney Disease	*Bifidobacteria bifidum* A218, *Bi. catenulatum* A302, *Bi. longum* A101, and *Lb. plantarum* A87	Decreases serum TNF-α, IL-5, IL-6, and LPS Preservation of residual renal function	39 peritoneal dialysis patients, (21 patients treated with probiotics and 18 patients for placebo), for 6 months	Wang et al., (2015)
Cardio Vascular Disease	*Streptococcus thermophilus, Lactobacillis acidophilus, Lb. rhamnosus, Enterococcus faecium*	8.4% reduction in their LDL-cholesterol concentrations,	70 healthy, weight-stable, overweight and obese 20 males and 50 females, 18-55 years old	Kekkonen et al., (2008)
Diabetes Mellitus	*Lb. casei Shirota*	Glucose concentration increased by 10%, and whole body insulin sensitivity decreased by 27% in the control group, whereas normal insulin sensitivity was maintained in the probiotic group before and after overeating.	17 Healthy human subjects, 8 treated with Probiotic, and 9 were control	Hulston et al., (2015)
Antibiotic Associated Diarrhea	*Lb. plantarum* 299v	*Lb. plantarum* 299v shows preventive effects on some gastrointestinal symptoms during antibiotic treatment	163 patients, 80 were treated with *Lb. plantarum* 299v and 83 to placebo	Lonnermark, et al., (2010)
Helicobacter Pylori Infections	*Saccharomyces boulardii, Lb. reuteri*, and *Lb. rhamnosus* GG	Significant increase in eradication rate given along with triple therapy	90 children, the daily dose of *Saccharomyces boulardii* ranged from 500 mg to 1000 mg for 2-4 weeks	Szajewska et al., (2010)
Irritable Bowel Syndrome	VSL#3	reduces flatulence scores and retards colonic transit without altering bowel function in patients with IBS and bloating	48 patients, 24 treated with VSL#3 and 24 with placebo-controlled, for 8 weeks	Kim et al., (2005)
Food-Borne Diseases	*Lb. plantarum* LP 31	Inhibition of food pathogens by means of antimicrobial substances	*In vitro* studies	Muller et al., (2009)
Cancer	*Bi. longum*	Shows antitumor effects	tumor-bearing mice	Hu et al., (2009);
Autism Spectrum Disorder-(ASD)	*Lb. plantarum* WCFS1	Improves the disruptive antisocial behaviours, anxiety and communication problems	Randomized, double-blind, placebo controlled study in children with ASD, for 3 weeks	Parracho et al., (2010)
Oral Candidiasis	*Lb. rhamnosus* GG	Diminishing the *Candida albican* counts	294 patients, 145 treated with probiotics and 149 controls, for 16 weeks	Hatakka et al., (2007)
Cirrhosis with Ascites	VSL#3	Significantly reduced portal hypertension	12 patient's for 42–48 days.	Rincon et al., (2014)

Figure 3. Pathophysiological condition of different diseases in human beings. Adherent invasive E. coli (AIEC); Autism spectral disorder (ASD); Cardio-metabolic disease (CMD); Chronic kidney disease (CKD); Inflammatory bowel disorder (IBD); Irritable bowel syndrome (IBS); Major adverse cardiac event (MACE); Multiple sclerosis (MS); Short chain fatty acids (SCFA); Type 1 Diabetes (T1D)

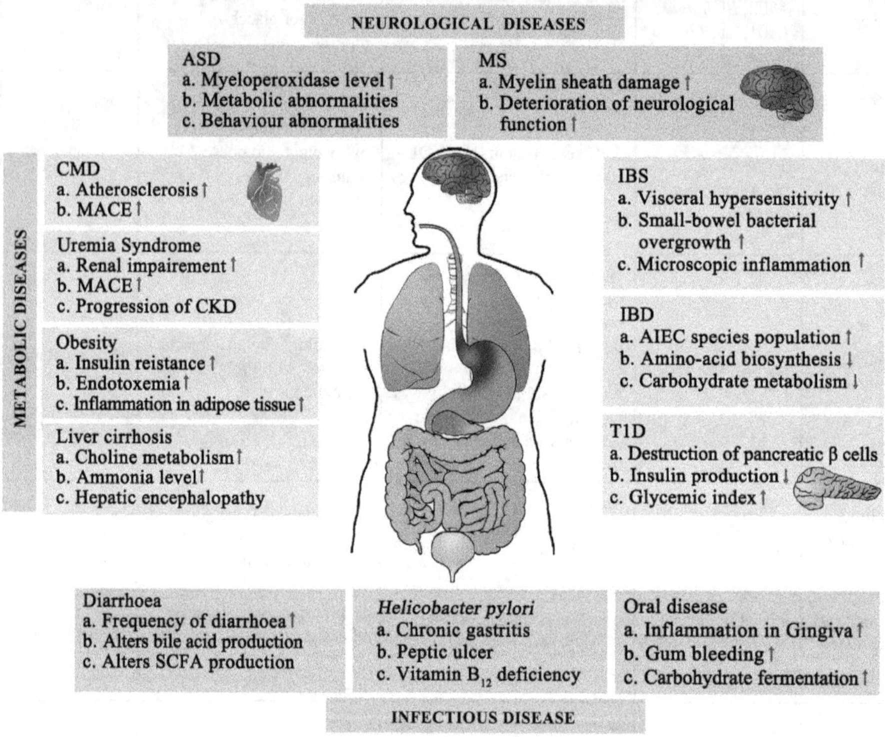

IMMUNIOLOGICAL DISEASES

Irritable Bowel Syndrome (IBS)

IBS is a multifactorial intestinal disorder with pathophysiological condition characterized by abdominal pain, bloating and altered bowel habits (constipation, and diarrhea) due to increased intestinal permeability, altered motility, visceral hypersensitivity, altered bacterial colonization, as well as other non-intestinal factors (Li, Wang, Wang, Hu, & Chen, 2016). IBS affects 15 - 20% of the population, with a highly increasing tendency in industrial nations (Guglielmetti, Mora, Gschwender, & Popp, 2011). *Pseudomonas aeruginosa* and *Staphylococcus aureus* are the two major bacteria responsible for the pathophysiology of IBS (Rinttilä, Lyra, Kurikka, & Palva, 2011). Patients suffering from IBS show a significant increase in the ratio of *Firmicutes* to *Bacteroidetes* (Jeffery, Toole, Human, Claesson, Deane, Quigley, & Simren, 2012). It was reported that there is a marked increase in population of pathogenic bacteria (*Dorea, Ruminococcus* and *Clostridium),* as well as lower numbers of commensals (*Faecalibacterium* and *Methanogens*), when compared with the healthy controls (Stojanovic, Biagi, Heilig, Kajander, Kekkonen, Tims, & De Vos, 2011). IBS patients on administration with probiotic bacteria like *Bi. infantis* strain 35624 exerts potent immunomodulatory effects like increased production of cytokine, interleukin (IL) 10 in peripheral blood mononuclear cells associated with reduced abdominal pain and bloating (Gareau, Sherman, & Walker, 2010). Also probiotic combinations such as VSL#3, [high concentration of probiotic preparation of eight live freezed bacterial species which include four strains of *Lactobacillus* (*Lactobacillus casei, Lb. plantarum, Lb. acidophilus, Lb. dulbrueckii* subsp. *bulgaricus),* three strains of *Bifidobacteria* (*Bi. longum, Bi. breve, Bi. infantis)* and *Streptococcus. salivarius* subsp. *Thermophilus*)], as well as SCM-III (combination of three probiotic bacteria which include *Lb. acidophilus, Lb. helveticus* and *Bifidobacterium* species) decreased the levels of flatulence and relieved abdominal bloating (Aragon et al., 2010). Consumption of *Bi. bifidum* MIMBb75 for 4 weeks effectively decreased the IBS and related symptoms (Guglielmetti, Mora, Gschwender, & Popp, 2011). Probiotic *E. coli Nissle* 1917 has been proved to be effective in IBS treatment, especially in patients with altered enteric microflora as a result of gastro-enterocolitis or administration of antibiotics (Kruis, Chrubasik, Boehm, Stange, & Schulze, 2012).

Inflammatory Bowel Diseases (IBD)

IBD involves chronic inflammation in mucosal surface of the gastro-intestinal tract and exhibits severe watery and bloody diarrhea with abdominal pain. IBD primarily includes Crohn's Disease (CD), Ulcerative colitis (UC), and pouchitis. CD is the most common form of IBD (Li, Wang, Wang, Hu, & Chen, 2016). CD patients have shown a marked increase in population of *Ruminococcus gnavus, Proteobacteria* as well as *Actinobacteria* and reduced level of anti-inflammatory commensal bacterium such as *Fb. prausnitzii,* a predominant butyrate producing bacteria (Matsuoka & Kanai, 2015). As a result a marked increase in levels of adherent invasive *E. coli* (AIEC) species was observed in patients suffering with Crohn's disease. Recent *in vitro* studies has shown that administration of *Lb. casei* DN-114 001 strains has significantly decreased the population of AIEC strains by preventing the interaction between the AIEC bacteria and epithelial cells (Gareau, Sherman, & Walker, 2010). In case of UC treatment, administration of either VSL# 3 or *E. coli Nissle* 1917 (DSM 6601*)* can be used in controlling and prevention of disease activity in mild to moderately severe UC (Veerappan, & Betteridge, & Young, 2012).

TYPE I DIABETES (T1D)

T1D is an autoimmune disease resulting in insulin deficiency by means of T-cell mediated destruction of pancreatic beta (β) cells. As a result the glycemic index of the body increases and requires insulin therapy (Li, Wang, Wang, Hu, & Chen, 2016). Intestinal permeability of antigens from dietary or pathogenic origin increases due to the action of Protein Kinase C-δ which triggers inflammation and immune responses to produce interferon's which damage the pancreatic β cells (Ebel, Lemetais, Beney, Cachon, Sokol, Langella, & Gervais, 2014). T1D suffering children displayed increase in virulence factors which significantly reduce the gut microbial diversity. Patients suffering from T1D show a marked increase in population of *Veillonella*, *Clostridium* and *Bacteroides* and decrease in number of *Lactobacillus*, *Prevotella* and *Bifidobacterium* as compared with healthy individuals (Li, Wang, Wang, Hu, & Chen, 2016). *Lactobacillus acidophilus, Lb. fermentum*, *Lb. gasseri*, and *Lb. rhamnosus* has been reported to modulate the expression of genes encoding junction and adhesion proteins in strengthening the complex E-cadherin / β-catenin, and reduce the expression of protein kinase C-δ (PKC-δ) (Gomes, Bueno, Souza, & Mota, 2014). Recently, VSL#3 administered non-obese diabetic (NOD) mice induced the over expression of inflammasome component such as indoleamine 2, 3-dioxygenase (IDO) and Interleukin (IL)-33 in the intestinal mucosa whereas IDO suppressed the activity of regulatory T-cells was by limiting the tryptophan concentration (Dolpady, Sorini, Pietro, Cosorich, Ferrarese, Saita, Clementi, Canducci, Falcone, 2016). *Bi. adolescentis* improves insulin sensitivity via increased production of glucagon-like peptide 1 (GLP-1). GLP-1 enhances glucose tolerance via complex mechanisms involving modulation of insulin secretion, pancreatic cell mass and food intake (Gomes, Bueno, Souza, & Mota, 2014).

METABOLIC DISEASES

Obesity

Changes in composition of gut microbiota, and imbalance in energy intake to energy expenditure are the major reasons for obesity (Stienstra, Tack, Kanneganti, Joosten, & Netea, 2012). Gut microbiota has been reported to influence the host metabolism in two possible pathways: by extracting energy and nutrients from food and another one is affecting the host gene expression levels involved in energy metabolism (Li, Wang, Wang, Hu, & Chen, 2016). For instance, the gut microbiota of obese mice has been reported to increase its energy capacity by digesting the indigestive dietary polysaccharides (starch) and other carbohydrates as compared to lean mice (Turnbaugh, Ley, Mahowald, Magrini, Mardis, & Gordon, 2006). Obesity is considered as the major risk for cardiovascular disease. *Lactobacillus* and *Bifidobacterial* strains are potent in controlling obesity by reducing the levels of low density lipoprotein and total cholesterol (Yadav, Lee, Lloyd, Walter, & Rane, 2013). Short chain fatty acids produced by the VSL#3 probiotic mixture, stimulate the release of glucagon like peptide (GLP-1) hormone which act as potent anti-hyperglycaemic hormone and induces the β-cells of pancreas to release insulin in response to rise in glucose levels, reduces food intake and improve glucose tolerance (Kimura, Inoue, Hirano, & Tsujimoto, 2014).

Uremia

It is a kind of metabolic syndrome caused due to retention of harmful bacterial metabolites such as phenols, indoles and amines affects the kidney functioning causing uremia (Koppe, Mafra, & Fouque, 2015). Generally, uremic illness was more prevalent in hemodialysis (HD) patient suffering with kidney failure or with chronic kidney disease (Evenepoel, Meijers, Bammens, & Verbeke, 2009). Recent investigation suggests that uremia is associated with abnormalities in the gastrointestinal mucosa and intestinal microbial imbalance (Koppe, Mafra, & Fouque, 2015). Factors which potentially modulate the intestinal homeostasis and metabolism in uremic patients include increase in colonic transit time, increase in blood ammonia concentrations, drug therapy and nutrient availability (Evenepoel, Meijers, Bammens, & Verbeke, 2009). HD patients show a marked decrease in population of saccharolytic species and parallel increases in proteolytic species, which results in formation of several toxic metabolites (Evenepoel, Meijers, Bammens, & Verbeke, 2009). Bacterial metabolites in HD patients were categorised into three different types: Small molecules (Urea, creatinine), Middle molecules (amines), and Protein bound molecules (Indole, p-cresol, p-cresyl sulphate (PCS) and indoxyl sulphate (IS)). Removal of protein bound molecules were the biggest challenge faced during dialysis (Fang, Lu, Chen, Wu, Chen, & Chen, 2014). Probiotics intervention is one of the most promising alternatives in reducing protein-bound uremic toxins by balancing the metabolism, inhibiting the growth of proteolytic bacteria or by metabolising the toxins (Koppe, Mafra, & Fouque, 2015). Pm1 (Consortium of *Lb. plantarum*, *Lb. paracasei*, *Streptocossus salivarius* subsp *thermophilus*) administration for 5 days significantly improved the renal functioning by binding/metabolising IS in cisplatin induced acute kidney injury (AKI) in rats (Fang, Lu, Chen, Wu, Chen, & Chen, 2014). Several single and multi-center randomised control trails in humans shows significant reduction in the generation PCs, IS, p-cresol, and urea (Koppe, Mafra, & Fouque, 2015).

Cardio Metabolic Diseases (CMD)

Cardio metabolic diseases are a class of medical disorders that include aneurysm, angina, atherosclerosis, cerebrovascular accident, cerebrovascular disease, congestive heart failure, coronary artery disease, myocardial infarction, and peripheral vascular disease (Ebel, Lemetais, Beney, Cachon, Sokol, Langella, & Gervais, 2014). It is estimated that about 20 million people died of CMD in 2015, providing CMD as the major contributor to mortality worldwide. Plasma levels of choline, as well as betaine, may be used as a prognostic value to determine the risk of developing a major adverse cardiac event, such as death, myocardial infarction, or stroke (Serino, Baque, Nicolas, & Burcelin, 2014). In another report, L-carnitine found in red meat induces trimethylamine (TMA) production and is associated with an increased risk of CMD (Wisnewsky & Clement, 2015). Several experimental evidence suggested that probiotic intervention could reverse the adverse metabolic phenotype in murine models (Hansen, Gobel, Hansen, & Pedersen, 2015). *Methanomassiliicoccus luminyensis* B10, a methanogenic bacterium decreases the levels of TMA by methanogenesis can be considered as probiotic for the treatment of CMD and other metabolic diseases (Serino, Baque, Nicolas, & Burcelin, 2014).

Liver Diseases

Liver receives 70% of blood from gut via portal vein along with gut-derived toxins such as lipopolysaccharide, flagellin, lipoteichoic acid, and other microbial products which may induce either intestinal inflammation or portal hypertension subsequently leading to the entry of large amount of pathogenic bacteria into the liver (Marchesi, Adams, Fava, Hermes, Hirschfield, Hold… Hart, 2016). Generally in liver, bacteria or their metabolites are mostly eliminated by kupffer cells. It was recently reported that damage to gut mucosal barrier leads to alteration in gut microbial composition which causes liver diseases such as nonalcoholic fatty liver disease (NAFLD), hepatic encephalopathy, alcohol-related liver disease, and hepatocellular carcinoma (Li, Wang, Wang, Hu, & Chen, 2016). Hepatic encephalopathy (HE) is often found in patients with advanced liver cirrhosis caused due to toxic substances produced by intestinal microbiota which affect the quality of life in the patients (Minemura et al., 2015). Although ammonia is thought to be the main factor responsible for HE, other factors such as mercaptans, phenols, short- and medium-chain fatty acids and benzodiazepine-like compounds which is derived from gut microbiota especially *Klebsiella* and *Proteus* species could contribute to the development of HE (Marchesi, Adams, Fava, Hermes, Hirschfield, Hold… Hart, 2016). Probiotics has been reported to show the promising results for treating ameliorating liver injury by reducing bacterial translocation and hepatic inflammation thereby reducing progression to chronic liver diseases (Minemura & Shimizu, 2015). Alteration of gut microbiota using probiotics such as *Lactobacillus, Bifidobacterium, E. coli Nissle* 1917, *Ct. butyricum, St. salivarius*, and *Sc. boulardii*, and VSL#3 could improve HE by means of decreasing the level of ammonia and improving the quality of life of those patients at secondary prophylaxis (Minemura & Shimizu, 2015).

INFECTIOUS DISEASES

Diarrhoea

Diarrhoeal is one among the major infectious disease manifested from gastrointestinal disorder especially due to microbial dysbiosis. Each year more than four billion incidence of diarrheal diseases was reported by WHO (Culligan, Hill, Sleator, 2009). Probiotics has shown potential application in treatment and prevention of diarrhoea caused due to dysbiosis (Kechagia, Basoulis, Konstantopoulou, Dimitriadi, Gyftopoulou, Skarmoutsou, & Fakiri, 2012). Two major types of diarrhoea which can be treated by probiotics are:

Acute Diarrhea (AD)

Acute diarrhoea is mainly associated with the clinical signs of acute enteritis and enterocolitis which occurs due to consumption of contaminated food and water (Gareau, Sherman, & Walker, 2010). There was a significantly increase the population of *Clostridium perfringens* and decrease in commensal population such as *Bacteroidetes*, *Faecalibacterium*, and *Ruminococcaceae*. The population of *Camphylobacter jejuni*, *Listeria monocytogenes*, and *Rota-virus* were more pronounced during the infection (Shen, Zhang, Li, Xie, Jiang, Wu, Ye, Yang, Mo, Situ, & Hu, 2016). Administration of *Lb. helveticus* r0052, inhibits the *Camphylobacter* species invasive by competitive exclusion and reduce diarrhoea (Wine, Gareau, Henry, & Sherman, 2009). Administration of *Lb. salivarius* uCC118, strain controls rapid colonization of *Li. monocytogenes* a food borne pathogens (Gareau, Sherman, & Walker, 2010). Probiotic species such as *Lb. rhamnosus* GG, *Lb. reuteri*, *Lb. casei shirota*, and *Bi. animalis* Bb12 can shorten the duration of acute rotavirus diarrhoea by following mechanism: competitive blockage of receptor site signals regulating secretory and motility defences, enhancement of the immune response, and production of substances that directly inactivate the viral particles (Kechagia, Basoulis, Konstantopoulou, Dimitriadi, Gyftopoulou, Skarmoutsou, & Fakiri, 2012).

Antibiotic Associated Diarrhoea (AAD)

Consumption of antibiotics in both short and long term, causes the dysbiosis of intestinal microbiota and subsequent alterations in the metabolism of carbohydrates, SCFA, and bile acids (Bartlett, 2002). Use of broad spectrum antibiotics are the major cause of AAD which suppresses the growth of normal microbiota, and promote the overgrowth of opportunistic or pathogenic strains such as *Clostridium difficile*. Usually, *Ct. difficile* is a cytotoxic strain which remain latent in most cases and increases the risk of diarrhea after antibiotic usage (Gareau, Sherman, & Walker, 2010). It was reported that approximately 15-60% of the patients are suffering with *Ct. difficile* mediated AAD. The efficacy of probiotic strains in the treatment of AAD were more pronounced for *Lb. rhamnosus* GG, *Saccharomyces cerevisiae* variant *boulardii*, and a mixture of *Bi. lactis*, and *St. thermophilus* which reduce the frequency of diarrhea in *Ct. difficile* infected patients (McFarland, 2008).

Helicobacter pylori Infection

Helicobacter pylori, is a Gram-negative pathogenic bacteria which majorly causes chronic gastritis, and peptic ulcer (Mohammadi, Mohammadi, Bagheri, & Roozbahani, 2013). It is highly adapted to gastric conditions in the stomach and induce increased inflammatory response particularly, Th17 inflammation (Homan, & Orel, 2015). Eradication of *He. pylori* infection by antibiotic treatment is 90% effective but it is very expensive and causes antibiotic resistance and some other side effects in diseased patients (Mohammadi, Mohammadi, Bagheri, & Roozbahani, 2013). Probiotics are capable of modifying immunologic response of the host with increased levels of pro-inflammatory cytokines, such as Interleukin IL-1β, IL-2, IL-6, IL-8 and tumor necrosis factor (TNF)- α in the gastric mucosa can regulate the *He. pylori* infection. Combination therapy (probiotics and antibiotic) reduced the side effects associated with *He. pylori* infection from 23% to 46% (Pantoflikova, Theulaz, & Blum, 2007). *Lb. bulgaricus* inhibited the activation of the Toll like receptor (TLR) 4 signalling pathway and IL-8 production induced by *He. pylori* lipopolysaccharide in SGC-7901 cells (Homan, & Orel, 2015).

ORAL HEALTH AND DISEASES

Dental Caries

Dental caries or tooth decay is mainly due to fermentation of carbohydrate by oral microorganisms characterized by acid production and causes demineralization in the tooth enamel (Faujdar, Mehrishi, Bishnoi, & Sharma, 2016). Continuous production of acid by *Streptococcus mutans* is the major reason for dental caries (Wade, 2013). The mounting evidence suggested that potential application of probiotics will balance the acid production from dietary sugars and help in maintaining homeostasis to prevent dental caries (Faujdar, Mehrishi, Bishnoi, & Sharma, 2016). *St. thermophilus* and *Lactobacillus* species were reported to integrate into a biofilm present on surface and interfere with development of the carcinogenic species such as *St. sobrinus*. *Lb. rhamnosus* GG, and *Lb. reuteri* has been reported to inhibit the tooth decay by preventing the colonization of carcinogenic *Streptococcal* species (Faujdar, Mehrishi, Bishnoi, & Sharma, 2016).

Periodontal Disease

Lack of oral hygiene leads to increase in population of Gram-negative, anaerobic bacteria which produce endotoxins and other enzymes which pass into the gingivae to induce structural changes and promote the activation of inflammatory mediators (Wade, 2013). *Porphyromonas gingivitis*, *Treponema denticola*, *Tannerella forsythia*, *Aggregatibacter*, and *Actinomycetem comitans*, are the main pathogens responsible for periodontitis (Faujdar, Mehrishi, Bishnoi, & Sharma, 2016). Variety of oral hygienic measures has been used throughout human history, but the application of probiotic bacteria in treatment of periodontal disease is increasing in the recent time (Wade, 2013). Probiotics like *Lb. reuteri* can decrease gum bleeding and reduce gingivitis in patients. Probiotic strains diminish the growth of most frequently isolated periodontal pathogens like *Bacteriodes* species, *Actinomyces* species, *Streptococcus intermedius*, and *Candida albicans*. Gingitivitis and periodontal diseases and pregnancy gingitivitis are locally treated with the culture supernatant of *Lb. acidophilus* (Faujdar, Mehrishi, Bishnoi, & Sharma, 2016).

Oral Candidiasis

Candida species are considered as commensals in oral flora in around 50% in healthy humans. It can cause clinically apparent lesions and infection in oral cavity in immuno compromised patients (Hatakka, Ahola, Yli-Knuuttila, Richardson, Poussa, Meurman, & Korpela, 2007). *Ca. albicans* produce organic acids (pyruvate and acetate) and are considered to have a significant impact on caries pathogenesis. Due to the high-level expression of putative virulence factors, *Ca. albicans* is considered more pathogenic than other *Candida* species. The pathogenicity of *Candida* species was mainly based on certain virulent factors such as adhesion to host surfaces, secretion of proteinase and hyphal formation apparently the most significant. *Candida* species can adhere to several host cell types such as epithelial, endothelial, and phagocytic cells. Consumption of probiotic cheese containing *Lb. rhamnosus* GG (10^7-10^9 CFU/mL) reduced the prevalence of *Cn. albicans* in the elderly patients (Hatakka, Ahola, Yli-Knuuttila, Richardson, Poussa, Meurman, & Korpela, 2007). All the *Lactobacilli* species except *Lb. acidophilus* La5, and *Lb. reuteri* PTA 5289 inhibited the *Candida* strains completely (Hasslof, Hedberg, Twetman, & Stecksén-Blicks, 2010).

NEUROLOGICAL DISEASES

Studies related to neuro-immune, and neuro-psychiatric disorders are correlated with variation of microbiome, microbiota-derived products, exogenous antibiotics and probiotics (Wang & Kasper, 2014). Several investigation states that microbe-mediated signals from the gut to the brain might be transduced directly via peripheral vagal afferent nerves (Cryan & Dinan, 2012). CNS disorders can be classified as immune mediated (exemplified by CNS autoimmune diseases such as multiple sclerosis) and non-immune-mediated (exemplified by neuro-psychiatric disorders such as autism, depression, anxiety and stress) according to main etiologies.

Multiple Sclerosis

Multiple sclerosis (MS) is an auto-immune disorder related to CNS which is mainly characterised by myelin sheath damage and progressive deterioration of neurological function (Li, Wang, Wang, Hu, & Chen, 2016). Epstein-Barr virus or human herpes virus has been suggested to trigger the human MS (Wang & Kasper, 2014). Several research reports revealed that intestinal microbiota might be an important regulator in the initiation of spontaneous demyelinating autoimmune disease (Berer, Mues, Koutrolos, Rasbi, Boziki, Johner, Wekerle, & Krishnamoorthy, 2011). Probiotics has been suggested to alleviate neuro-psychiatric disorders via hormonal and neuro-chemical mechanisms (Wang & Kasper, 2014). It was reported that administration of *Lb. rhamnosus* GG alleviated the anxiety-like behaviour in mice by modulating vagus nerve-dependent expression of GABA (γ-Aminobutyric acid) receptors in the brain. *Lactobacilli* (including *Lb. casei Shirota*), either administrated alone or in combination with other strains of *Bifidobacterium* genus, tend to alleviate murine EAE symptoms via reciprocal regulation of pro- and anti-inflammatory cytokine responses (Berer, Mues, Koutrolos, Rasbi, Boziki, Johner, Wekerle, & Krishnamoorthy, 2011). *Bifidobacterium animalis*, *Pediococcus acidilactici* R037, and *Bacteriodes fragilis* are the prominent probiotic strains which induced the expression of Foxp3 (Forkhead box protein) and Treg (Regulatory T cells) and significantly reduced susceptibility to EAE in mice model (Wang & Kasper, 2014).

Autism Spectrum Disorder (ASD)

ASD is a neurodevelopment disorder characterized by social and communication impairment and is often accompanied by behavioural symptoms, GI disturbance, and immune dysfunction (Ho & Ross, 2017). Disruption of gut microbiota might promote the over-colonization of neurotoxin-producing bacteria and thus contribute to autistic symptoms (Wang & Kasper, 2014). Presence of *Clostridium tetani* within the microbiome has been associated with impaired social behaviours in animals whereas in humans decreased stereotyped behaviours (Ho & Ross, 2017). Hsiao et al., (2013), reported that treatment with *Ba. fragilis* could correct behavioural abnormalities and metabolomic profile in ASD and ameliorate ASD-relevant GI barrier deficits in mice model. Consumption of *Lb. plantarum* has reduced disruptive behaviour, anxiety and communicative disturbance in children suffering with ASD (Navarro, Liu, & Rhoads, 2016).

COLORECTAL CANCER (CRC)

Colorectal cancer is the most common type of cancer across the world. Recent reports revealed that major factors for CRC are obesity and imbalanced diet (Sanders, Guarner, Guerrant, Holt, Quigley, Sartor, & Mayer, 2013). In addition, certain bacterial and viral infections are also strongly associated with some types of cancer (stomach cancers and cervical cancer). Catabolism of E-cadherin by entero-toxigenic *Ba. fragilis* generate intestinal inflammation thereby increasing the risk of CRC (Sanders, Guarner, Guerrant, Holt, Quigley, Sartor, & Mayer, 2013). Also β-glucosidase and urease convert pro-carcinogens into proximate carcinogens (Faujdar, Mehrishi, Bishnoi, & Sharma, 2016). Probiotics has been reported to reduce the risk associated with many cancers by altering the gut microbiota and its metabolites, changes in colonic pH, binding or inactivation of carcinogens, enhanced immune responses, reduced colonic inflammation, lowered epithelial proliferation and increased apoptosis (Sanders, Guarner, Guerrant, Holt, Quigley, Sartor, & Mayer, 2013). Supernatants of some probiotic bacteria strains such as *Bi. adolecenti* ATCC 15703, *Lb. plantarum* ATCC 8014 displayed inhibitory effects against mutagenic substance benzo[a]pyrene, and sodium azide (Mohammadi, Mohammadi, Bagheri, & Roozbahani, 2013). Probiotic bacteria (such as *Bifidobacterium*) shows anti-tumor activity by three proposed mechanisms includes: 1) Altering the immune functions associated with immune response; 2) Anti proliferative effects via regulation of apoptosis and cell differentiation, and; 3) Suppressing the production of enzymes like β-glucuronidase, urease, choloylglycine hydrolase, azedoreductase and nitro-reductase by pathogens especially entero-pathogens such as *E. coli* and *Ct. perfringens* (Pandey, Naik, & Vakil, 2015).

SAFETY CONSIDERATIONS OF PROBIOTICS

Increased consumption of probiotics raises the concerns for their safety. Safe use of probiotics depends on type of strains used, its preparation, its administration, dosage, and health status of the consumer. Following are some of the important risk factors to be considered while using probiotics for human consumption: (a) Bacteraemia and Endocarditis; (b) transfer of antimicrobial resistance; (c) Biogenic amines production; (d) D-Lactate acidosis, and; (e) Labelling of probiotics. Among the probiotics reported so far, lactic acid bacteria are generally recognised as safe. Also the infections in humans by these genera are extremely rare (Sanders, Akkermans, Haller, Hammerman, Heimbach… Mayer, 2010).

Bacteraemia and Endocarditis

A very negligible or less number of people suffering with bacteraemia and endocarditis upon administration of probiotics (*Lactobacillus*, and *Bifidobacteria*). Typically used foods, also contain a large population of *Streptococcus*, *Enterococcus*, and *Escherichia* which are pathogenic in nature. Probiotic supplements include broader range of intestine friendly or beneficial microbes (Sanders, Akkermans, Haller, Hammerman, Heimbach… Mayer, 2010). Hence in the safety assessment, accuracy of identification to the strain level is the critical step.

Transfer of Antibiotics Resistance

Certain probiotic strain shows inherent intrinsic resistance to some of the antibiotic because of their cell wall structure or other inherent physiological characteristics. Chances of transferring the antibiotic resistance genes from probiotic species to pathogenic microbial strains are very high (Sanders, Akkermans, Haller, Hammerman, Heimbach… Mayer, 2010). Although, antibiotic resistance is associated with transmissible genetic elements but use of such probiotic strains should be avoided for safety concerns (e.g., transmission of enterococcal resistance against the antibiotic, vancomycin).

Biogenic Amine's (BA's) Production

BA's are considered as undesirable metabolic products of some probiotic lactic acid bacteria such as *Lactobacillus*, *Bifidobacteria* and *Enterococcus* species with potential health risks to consumer. Histamine and Tyramine are the most studied BA's due to their toxic effects. Histamine causes histamine intoxication, while tyramine causes hypertension (Priyadarshani & Rakshit, 2011). Hence the probiotic bacteria must be screened for BA's before considering them for further studies.

D-Lactate Acidosis

It is a very rare clinical conditions manifest due to D-lactic acid producing probiotic bacteria. Ingestion of carbohydrate rich diet increases the saccharolytic activity in the intestine as a result a massive load of sugars increases which are metabolised by the intestinal bacteria to produce D-lactate. Humans metabolize D-lactate at a slower rate than the L-lactate isomer, increased absorption of D-lactate may lead to acidosis. This disease is characterised by decrease in absorption in the intestine and has been reported in patients suffering with intestinal bypass surgery or with short bowel syndrome (Sanders, Akkermans, Haller, Hammerman, Heimbach… Mayer, 2010). D-lactate-producing probiotics should be avoided by the subjects suffering with short bowel syndrome.

Labelling of Probiotics

Products labelled as probiotics should adhere to the guidelines established by a working group of the FAO (UNFAO/WHO, 2002). But, unfortunately the products currently labelled as probiotics neither are well defined nor substantiated with controlled human studies. Probiotic products currently available in the market fail to meet label claims with regard to numbers of viable microbes present in the product, thereby constituting illegally labelled products (Sanders, Akkermans, Haller, Hammerman, Heimbach… Mayer, 2010). Maintaining viability of microbes in commercial products through the end of shelf life can be a challenge. The critical part is that the microbes bear a consistent strain designation so that research can be tracked adequately for each strain even if the species name has been changed.

FUTURE RESEARCH DIRECTIONS

Treatment of diseases using antibiotics or drugs is costly and associated with several side effects. It also causes loss of intestine friendly bacteria. Several studies on probiotics have shown their therapeutic applications on human health without any side effects. Although there are several probiotic products currently available in the market, both as functional food and nutraceuticals; there is still uncertainty surrounding the regulation of these products. Since the area is still emerging and establishing in the global food industry, there is a need to change the existing regulatory process to serve the needs and safety of consumers globally. Further research is required to answer the key questions such as mode of action; optimal dosage and duration of probiotic therapy; origin and source of probiotic strain; strain specificity and stability of health claims; detection of antibiotic resistance and biogenic amines genes. Moreover functional properties, stability, taste, appeal and price are the crucial factors for successful commercialization of probiotics. Dairy based probiotics require cold chain storage which significantly affects the viability, shelf-life and cost of the product. Based on the available resources research must be focused on development of region specific probiotic foods. In future, food scientist must focus on the development of personalized probiotics or probiotics which can be used in prevention and treatment of different diseases.

CONCLUSION

Microbial dysbiosis in the intestine is the major reason for the development of several metabolic and non-metabolic diseases in human beings. In this regard probiotics have shown several functional benefits on host health and wellbeing by maintaining the homeostasis and parellely enhancing the population of beneficial bacteria in the intestine. As a result the global market for probiotics is increasing rapidly. There are several dairy and non-dairy based probiotics available in the market. Persons allergic to dairy based (lactose) probiotics can opt for non-dairy based products to boost their intestinal health. In view of the increasing use of probiotics as health supplements and therapeutic agents; all the risk factors, clinical studies, and safety measures must be addressed.

REFERENCES

Amara, A. A., & Shibl, A. (2015). Role of Probiotics in health improvement, infection control and disease treatment and management. *Saudi Pharmaceutical Journal*, *23*(2), 107–114. doi:10.1016/j.jsps.2013.07.001 PMID:25972729

Aragon, G., Graham, D. B., Borum, M., & Doman, D. B. (2010). Probiotic therapy for irritable bowel syndrome. *Gastroenterology & Hepatology*, *6*(1), 39–44. PMID:20567539

Bansal, S., Mangal, M., Sharma, S. K., & Gupta, R. K. (2016). Non-Dairy based probiotics: A healthy treat for intestine. *Critical Reviews in Food Science and Nutrition*, *56*(11), 1856–1867. doi:10.1080/10408398.2013.790780 PMID:25747894

Bartlett, J. G. (2002). Antibiotic-associated diarrhoea. *The New England Journal of Medicine*, *346*(5), 334–339. doi:10.1056/NEJMcp011603 PMID:11821511

Berer, K., Mues, M., Koutrolos, M., Rasbi, Z. A., Boziki, M., Johner, C., ... Krishnamoorthy, G. (2011). Commensal microbiota and myelin autoantigen cooperate to trigger autoimmune demyelination. *Nature*, *479*(7374), 538–541. doi:10.1038/nature10554 PMID:22031325

Brito, M. B., Diaz, J. P., Quezada, S. M., Llorente, C. G., & Gil, A. (2012). Probiotic mechanisms of action. *Annals of Nutrition & Metabolism*, *61*(2), 160–174. doi:10.1159/000342079 PMID:23037511

Bron, P. A., Baarlen, P. V., & Kleerebezem, M. (2012). Emerging molecular insights into the interaction between probiotics and the host intestinal mucosa. *Nature*, *10*(1), 66–78. PMID:22101918

Capozzi, V., Russo, P., Duenas, M. T., Lopez, P., & Spano, G. (2012). Lactic acid bacteria producing B-group vitamins: A great potential for functional cereals products. *Applied Microbiology and Biotechnology*, *96*(6), 1383–1394. doi:10.100700253-012-4440-2 PMID:23093174

Covian, D. R., Madiedo, P. R., Margolles, A., Gueimonde, M., Gavilan, C. G. D. L. R., & Salazar, N. (2016). Intestinal short chain fatty acids and their link with diet and human health. *Frontiers in Microbiology*, *7*(185), 1–9. PMID:26834723

Cryan, J. J., & Dinan, T. G. (2012). Mind-altering microorganisms: The impact of the gut microbiota on brain and behaviour. *Nature Reviews. Neuroscience*, *13*(10), 701–712. doi:10.1038/nrn3346 PMID:22968153

Culligan, E. P., Hill, C., Sleator, R. D., (2009). Probiotics and gastrointestinal disease: successes, problems and future prospects. *Gut Pathogens, 1*(19), 1-12.

Dash, S. K. (2014). Probiotics - an overview the value of chitosan healthful ingredients that address the major health concerns of aging consumers. *Nutraceuticals Now.* Retrieved from http://superbakrill.com/wp-content/uploads/2013/08/NN-pages-1.pdf

Dolpady, J., Sorini, C., Pietro, C. D., Cosorich, I., Ferrarese, R., Saita, D., Clementi, M., Canducci, F., Falcone, M. (2016). Oral probiotic *VSL#3* prevents autoimmune diabetes by modulating microbiota and promoting indoleamine 2,3-dioxygenase-enriched tolerogenic intestinal environment. *Journal of Diabetes Research*. .10.1155/2016/7569431

Ebel, B., Lemetais, G., Beney, L., Cachon, R., Sokol, H., Langella, P., & Gervais, P. (2014). Impact of probiotics on risk factors for cardiovascular diseases: A Review. *Critical Reviews in Food Science and Nutrition*, *54*(2), 175–189. doi:10.1080/10408398.2011.579361 PMID:24188267

Evenepoel, P., Meijers, B. K. I., Bammens, B. R. M., & Verbeke, K. (2009). Uremic toxins originating from colonic microbial metabolism. *Kidney International. Supplement*, *114*, S12–S19. doi:10.1038/ki.2009.402 PMID:19946322

Fang, C. Y., Lu, J. R., Chen, B. J., Wu, C., Chen, Y. P., & Chen, M. J. (2014). Selection of uremic toxin-reducing probiotics *in vitro* and *in vivo*. *Journal of Functional Foods*, *7*(1), 407–415. doi:10.1016/j.jff.2014.01.018

Faujdar, S. S., Mehrishi, P., Bishnoi, S., & Sharma, A. (2016). Role of Probiotics in human health and disease: An update. *International Journal of Current Microbiology and Applied Sciences*, *5*(3), 328–344. doi:10.20546/ijcmas.2016.503.040

Franz, C. M., Huch, M., Abriouel, H., Holzapfel, W. H., & Gálvez, A. (2011). *Enterococci* as probiotics and their implications in food safety. *International Journal of Food Microbiology*, *151*(2), 125–140. doi:10.1016/j.ijfoodmicro.2011.08.014 PMID:21962867

Gareau, M. G., Sherman, P. M., & Walker, W. A. (2010). Probiotics and the gut microbiota in intestinal health and disease. *Nature Reviews. Gastroenterology & Hepatology*, *7*(9), 503–514. doi:10.1038/nrgastro.2010.117 PMID:20664519

Gawkowski, D., & Chikindas, M. L. (2013). Non-dairy probiotic beverages: The next step into human health. *Beneficial Microbes*, *4*(2), 127–142. doi:10.3920/BM2012.0030 PMID:23271064

Gomes, A. C., Bueno, A. A., Souza, R. G. M. D., & Mota, J. F. (2014). Gut microbiota, probiotics and diabetes. *Nutrition Journal*, *13*(60), 1–13. PMID:24939063

Granato, D., Branco, G. F., Cruz, A. G., Faria, J. A. F., & Shah, N. P. (2010). Probiotic dairy products as functional foods. *Comprehensive Reviews in Food Science and Food Safety*, *9*(5), 455–470. doi:10.1111/j.1541-4337.2010.00120.x

Guglielmetti, S., Mora, D., Gschwender, M., & Popp, K. (2011). Randomised clinical trial: *Bifidobacterium bifidum* MIMBb75 significantly alleviates irritable bowel syndrome and improves quality of life a double-blind, placebo-controlled study. *Alimentary Pharmacology & Therapeutics*, *33*(10), 1123–1132. doi:10.1111/j.1365-2036.2011.04633.x PMID:21418261

Gupta, S., & Abu-Ghannam, N. (2012). Probiotic fermentation of plant based products: Possibilities and opportunities. *Critical Reviews in Food Science and Nutrition*, *52*(2), 183–199. doi:10.1080/10408398.2010.499779 PMID:22059963

Hansen, T. H., Gobel, R. J., Hansen, T., & Pedersen, O. (2015). The gut microbiome in cardio-metabolic health. *Genome Medicine*, *7*(1), 1–16. doi:10.118613073-015-0157-z PMID:25825594

Hasslof, P., Hedberg, M., Twetman, S., & Stecksén-Blicks, C. (2010). Growth inhibition of oral mutans *streptococci* and candida by commercial probiotic *lactobacilli* an *in vitro* study. *BMC Oral Health*, *10*(18), 1–6. PMID:20598145

Hatakka, K., Ahola, A. J., Yli-Knuuttila, H., Richardson, M., Poussa, T., Meurman, J. H., & Korpela, R. (2007). Probiotics reduce the prevalence of oral *Candida* in the elderly-A randomized controlled trial. *Journal of Dental Research*, *86*(2), 125–130. doi:10.1177/154405910708600204 PMID:17251510

Hemaiswarya, S., Raja, R., Ravikumar, R., & Isabel, S. C. (2013). Mechanism of action of probiotics. *Brazilian Archives of Biology and Technology*, *56*(1), 113–119. doi:10.1590/S1516-89132013000100015

Ho, P., & Ross, D. A. (2017). More than a gut feeling: The implications of the gut microbiota in psychiatry. *Biological Psychiatry*, *81*(5), e35–e37. doi:10.1016/j.biopsych.2016.12.018 PMID:28137375

Homan, M., & Orel, R. (2015). Are probiotics useful in *Helicobacter pylori* eradication? *World Journal of Gastroenterology*, *21*(37), 10644–10653. doi:10.3748/wjg.v21.i37.10644 PMID:26457024

Hsiao, E. Y., McBride, S. W., Hsien, S., Sharon, G., Hyde, E. R., McCue, T., ... Mazmanian, S. K. (2013). Microbiota modulate behavioral and physiological abnormalities associated with neurodevelopmental disorders. *Cell*, *155*(7), 1451–1463. doi:10.1016/j.cell.2013.11.024 PMID:24315484

Hu, B., Kou, L., Li, C., Zhu, L. P., Fan, Y. R., Wu, Z. W., ... Xu, G. X. (2009). *Bifidobacterium longum* as a delivery system of TRAIL and endostatin cooperates with chemotherapeutic drugs to inhibit hypoxic tumor growth. *Cancer Gene Therapy*, *16*(8), 655–663. doi:10.1038/cgt.2009.7 PMID:19229287

Hulston, C. J., Churnside, A. A., & Venables, M. C. (2015). Probiotic supplementation prevents high-fat, overfeeding-induced insulin resistance in human subjects. *British Journal of Nutrition*, *113*(4), 596–602. doi:10.1017/S0007114514004097 PMID:25630516

Jeffery, I. B., Toole, P. W. O., Human, L. O., Claesson, M. J., Deane, J., Quigley, E. M. M., & Simren, M. (2012). An irritable bowel syndrome subtype defined by species-specific alterations in faecal microbiota. *Gut*, *61*(7), 997–1006. doi:10.1136/gutjnl-2011-301501 PMID:22180058

Johansson, M. L., Sanni, A., Likner, C., & Molin, G. (1995). Phenotypically based taxonomy using API 50CH of lactobacilli from Nigerian ogi, and the occurrence of starch fermenting strains. *International Journal of Food Microbiology*, *25*(2), 159–168. doi:10.1016/0168-1605(94)00096-O PMID:7547147

Kechagia, M., Basoulis, D., Konstantopoulou, S., Dimitriadi, D., Gyftopoulou, K., Skarmoutsou, N., & Fakiri, E. M. (2012). *Health benefits of probiotics: A Review.* Hindawi Publishing Corporation ISRN Nutrition. .10.5402/2013/481651

Kekkonen, R. A., Sysi-Aho, M., Seppanen-Laakso, T., Julkunen, I., Vapaatalo, H., Oresic, M., & Korpela, R. (2008). Effect of probiotic *Lactobacillus rhamnosus* GG intervention on global serum lipidomic profiles in healthy adults. *World Journal of Gastroenterology*, *14*(20), 3188–3194. doi:10.3748/wjg.14.3188 PMID:18506924

Kim, H. J., Vazquez Roque, M. I., Camilleri, M., Stephens, D., Burton, D. D., Baxter, K., ... Zinsmeister, A. R. (2005). A randomized controlled trial of a probiotic combination *VSL#3* and placebo in irritable bowel syndrome with bloating. *Neurogastroenterology and Motility*, *17*(5), 687–696. doi:10.1111/j.1365-2982.2005.00695.x PMID:16185307

Kimura, I., Inoue, D., Hirano, K., & Tsujimoto, G. (2014). The SCFA receptor GPR43 and energy metabolism. *Frontiers in Endocrinology*, *5*(85), 7–14. PMID:24926285

Koppe, L., Mafra, D., & Fouque, D. (2015). Probiotics and chronic kidney disease. *Kidney International*, *88*(5), 958–966. doi:10.1038/ki.2015.255 PMID:26376131

Kruis, W., Chrubasik, S., Boehm, S., Stange, C., & Schulze, J. (2012). A double-blind placebo-controlled trial to study therapeutic effects of probiotic *Escherichia coli Nissle* 1917 in subgroups of patients with irritable bowel syndrome. *International Journal of Colorectal Disease*, *27*(4), 467–474. doi:10.100700384-011-1363-9 PMID:22130826

Kumar, B. V., Vijayendra, S. V. N., & Reddy, O. V. S. (2015). Trends in dairy and non-dairy probiotic products - a review. *Journal of Food Science and Technology*, *5*(10), 6112–6124. doi:10.100713197-015-1795-2 PMID:26396359

Kurmann, J. A., Rasic, J. L. J., & Kroger, M. (1992). *Encyclopedia offermentedfresh milk products: An International inventory of fermented milk, Cream, Buttermilk, Whey, and related products*. New York: Van Nostrand Reinhold, Springer.

Li, D., Wang, P., Wang, P., Hu, X., & Chen, F. (2016). The gut microbiota: A treasure for human health. *Biotechnology Advances*, *34*(7), 1210–1224. doi:10.1016/j.biotechadv.2016.08.003 PMID:27592384

Liu, S., Han, Y., & Zhou, Z. (2011). Lactic acid bacteria in traditional fermented Chinese foods. *Food Research International*, *44*(3), 643–651. doi:10.1016/j.foodres.2010.12.034

Lonnermark, E., Friman, V., Lappas, G., Sandberg, T., Berggren, A., & Adlerberth, I. (2010). Intake of *Lactobacillus plantarum* reduces certain gastrointestinal symptoms during treatment with antibiotics. *Journal of Clinical Gastroenterology*, *44*(2), 106–112. doi:10.1097/MCG.0b013e3181b2683f PMID:19727002

Madsen, K., Cornish, A., Soper, P., McKaigney, C., Jijon, H., Yachimec, C., ... De Simone, C. (2001). Probiotic bacteria enhance murine and human intestinal epithelial barrier function. *Gastroenterology*, *121*(3), 580–591. doi:10.1053/gast.2001.27224 PMID:11522742

Marchesi, J. R., Adams, D. H., Fava, F., Hermes, G. D., Hirschfield, G. M., Hold, G., ... Hart, A. (2016). The gut microbiota and host health: A new clinical frontier. *Gut*, *65*(2), 330–339. doi:10.1136/gutjnl-2015-309990 PMID:26338727

Matsuoka, K., & Kanai, T. (2015). The gut microbiota and inflammatory bowel disease. *Seminars in Immunopathology*, *37*(1), 47–55. doi:10.100700281-014-0454-4 PMID:25420450

McFarland, L. V. (2008). Antibiotic-associated diarrhoea: Epidemiology, trends and treatment. *Future Microbiology*, *3*(5), 563–578. doi:10.2217/17460913.3.5.563 PMID:18811240

Minemura, M., & Shimizu, Y. (2015). Gut microbiota and liver diseases. *World Journal of Gastroenterology*, *21*(6), 1691–1702. doi:10.3748/wjg.v21.i6.1691 PMID:25684933

Mohammadi, F., Mohammadi, M., Bagheri, A., & Roozbahani, H. (2013). Probiotics in human health. *European Journal of Experimental Biology*, *3*(2), 116–120.

Moncheva, P., Chipeva, V., Kujumzieva, A., Ivanova, I., Dousset, X., & Gocheva, B. (2003). The composition of the microflora of boza, an original Bulgarian beverage. *Biotechnology, Biotechnological Equipment*, *17*(1), 164–168. doi:10.1080/13102818.2003.10819214

Muller, D. M., Carrasco, M. S., Tonarelli, G. G., & Simonetta, A. C. (2009). Characterization and purification of a new bacteriocin with a broad inhibitory spectrum produced by *Lactobacillus plantarum* lp 31 strain isolated from dry-fermented sausage. *Journal of Applied Microbiology*, *106*(6), 2031–2040. doi:10.1111/j.1365-2672.2009.04173.x PMID:19302495

Navarro, F., Liu, Y., & Rhoads, J. M. (2016). Can probiotics benefit children with autism spectrum disorders? *World Journal of Gastroenterology*, *22*(46), 10093–10102. doi:10.3748/wjg.v22.i46.10093 PMID:28028357

Ozden, A. (2008). Other fermented dairy products: Bioyogurt-probioitc yogurt. *Guncel Gastroenteroloji*, *12*(3), 169–181.

Pandey, K. R., Naik, S. R., & Vakil, B. V. (2015). Probiotics, prebiotics and synbiotics- a review. *Journal of Food Science and Technology*, *52*(12), 7577–7587. doi:10.100713197-015-1921-1 PMID:26604335

Pantoflikova, D. L., Theulaz, I. C., & Blum, A. L. (2007). *Helicobacter pylori* and probiotics. *The Journal of Nutrition*, *137*(3), 812S–818S. doi:10.1093/jn/137.3.812S PMID:17311980

Parracho, H. M., Gibson, G. R., Knott, F., Bosscher, D., Kleerebezem, M., & McCartney, A. L. (2010). A double-blind, placebo-controlled, crossover-designed probiotic feeding study in children diagnosed with autistic spectrum disorders. *International Journal of Probiotics & Prebiotics*, *5*(2), 69–74.

Priyadarshani, W. M. D., & Rakshit, S. K. (2011). Screening selected strains of probiotic lactic acid bacteria for their ability to produce biogenic amines (histamine and tryamine). *International Journal of Food Science & Technology*, *46*(10), 2062–2069. doi:10.1111/j.1365-2621.2011.02717.x

Queen, G. M., Surette, M., & Moayyedi, P. (2017). The gut microbiota and psychiatric illness. *Journal of Psychiatry & Neuroscience*, *42*(2), 75–77. doi:10.1503/jpn.170028 PMID:28245172

Rincon, D., Vaquero, J., Hernando, A., Galindo, E., Ripoll, C., Puerto, M., ... Banares, R. (2014). Oral probiotic *VSL#3* attenuates the circulatory disturbances of patients with cirrhosis and ascites. *Liver International*, *34*(10), 1504–1512. doi:10.1111/liv.12539 PMID:24661740

Rinttilä, T., Lyra, A., Kurikka, L. K., & Palva, A. (2011). Real-time PCR analysis of enteric pathogens from faecal samples of irritable bowel syndrome subjects. *Gut Pathogens*, *3*(1), 1–9. doi:10.1186/1757-4749-3-6 PMID:21281494

Sahib, P., Rakesh, P. K., Pal, S. S., Apoorva, S., & Nidhi, G. (2016). Awareness and knowledge of people towards probiotics products in punjab region Kaur. *International Journal of Applied Biology and Pharmaceutical Technology*, *7*(1), 154–160.

Sanders, M. E., Akkermans, L. M., Haller, D., Hammerman, C., Heimbach, J., Hörmannsperger, G., ... Vaughan, E. (2010). Safety assessment of probiotics for human use. *Gut Microbes*, *1*(3), 164–185. doi:10.4161/gmic.1.3.12127 PMID:21327023

Sanders, M. E., Guarner, F., Guerrant, R., Holt, P. R., Quigley, E. M. M., Sartor, R. B. E. A., & Mayer, P. M. S. (2013). An update on the use and investigation of probiotics in health and disease. *Gut*, *62*(5), 787–796. doi:10.1136/gutjnl-2012-302504 PMID:23474420

Serino, M., Baque, V. B., Nicolas, S., & Burcelin, R. (2014). Far from the eyes, close to the heart: Dysbiosis of gut microbiota and cardiovascular consequences. *Current Cardiology Reports*, *16*(11), 1–7. doi:10.100711886-014-0540-1 PMID:25303894

Sharma, S., Arora, M., & Baldi, A. (2013). Probiotics in India: Current status and future prospects. *Pharm Aspire*, *4*(1), 1–11.

Shen, H., Zhang, J., Li Y., Xie, S., Jiang, Y., Wu, Y., Ye, Y., Yang, H., Mo, H., Situ, C., & Hu, Q. (2016). The 12 gastrointestinal pathogens spectrum of acute infectious diarrhea in a sentinel hospital, Shenzhen, China. *Frontiers in Microbiology, 7*(1926), 1-9.

Stienstra, R., Tack, C. J., Kanneganti, T. D., Joosten, L. A., & Netea, M. G. (2012). The inflammasome puts obesity in the danger zone. *Cell Metabolism*, *15*(1), 10–18. doi:10.1016/j.cmet.2011.10.011 PMID:22225872

Stojanovic, M. R., Biagi, E., Heilig, H. G., Kajander, K., Kekkonen, R. A., Tims, S., & De Vos, W. M. (2011). Signatures in fecal samples from patients with irritable bowel syndrome. *Gastroenterology*, *141*(5), 1792–1801. doi:10.1053/j.gastro.2011.07.043 PMID:21820992

Szajewska, H., Horvath, A., & Piwowarczyk, A. (2010). Meta-analysis: The effects of *Saccharomyces boulardii* supplementation on *Helicobacter pylori* eradication rates and side effects during treatment. *Alimentary Pharmacology & Therapeutics*, *32*(9), 1069–1079. doi:10.1111/j.1365-2036.2010.04457.x PMID:21039671

Tripathi, M. K., & Giri, K. (2014). Probiotic functional foods: Survival of probiotics during processing and storage. *Journal of Functional Foods*, *9*(1), 225–241. doi:10.1016/j.jff.2014.04.030

Turnbaugh, P. J., Ley, R. E., Mahowald, M. A., Magrini, V., Mardis, E. R., & Gordon, J. I. (2006). An obesity-associated gut microbiome with increased capacity for energy harvest. *Nature*, *444*(7122), 1027–1031. doi:10.1038/nature05414 PMID:17183312

Turroni, F., Ventura, M., Buttó, L. F., Duranti, S., O'Toole, P. W., Motherway, M. O., & Van Sinderen, D. (2014). Molecular dialogue between the human gut microbiota and the host: A *Lactobacillus* and *Bifidobacterium* perspective. *Cellular and Molecular Life Sciences*, *71*(2), 183–203. doi:10.100700018-013-1318-0 PMID:23516017

United Nations Food and Agriculture Organization of the United Nations/World Health Organization (UNFAO/WHO). (2002). *Guidelines for the Evaluation of Probiotics in Food.* Retrieved from http://ftp.fao.org/es/esn/food/wgreport2.pdf

United Nations Food and Agriculture Organization of the United Nations/World Health Organization (UNFAO/WHO). (2001). *Health and Nutritional Properties of Probiotics in Food including Powder Milk with Live Lactic Acid Bacteria*. Retrieved from http://ftp.fao.org/es/esn/food/probio_report_en.pdf

Vandenplas, Y., & Huy, G. (2015). Probiotics: An update. *Jornal de Pediatria*, *91*(1), 6–21. doi:10.1016/j.jped.2014.08.005 PMID:25458874

Veerappan, G. R., Betteridge, J., & Young, P. E. (2012). Probiotics for the treatment of inflammatory bowel disease. *Current Gastroenterology Reports*, *14*(4), 324–333. doi:10.100711894-012-0265-5 PMID:22581276

Wade, W. G. (2013). The oral microbiome in health and disease. *Pharmacological Research*, *69*(1), 137–143. doi:10.1016/j.phrs.2012.11.006 PMID:23201354

Wang, I. K., Wu, Y. Y., Yang, Y. F., Ting, I. W., Lin, C. C., Yen, T. H., ... Lin, H. C. (2015). The effect of probiotics on serum levels of cytokine and endotoxin in peritoneal dialysis patients: A randomised, double-blind, placebo-controlled trial. *Beneficial Microbes*, *6*(4), 423–430. doi:10.3920/BM2014.0088 PMID:25609654

Wang, Y., & Kasper, L. H. (2014). The role of microbiome in central nervous system disorders. *Brain, Behavior, and Immunity, 38*(5), 1–12. doi:10.1016/j.bbi.2013.12.015 PMID:24370461

Wine, E., Gareau, M. G., Henry, J. K., & Sherman, P. M. (2009). Strain-specific probiotic (*Lactobacillus helveticus*) inhibition of *Campylobacter jejuni* invasion of human intestinal epithelial cells. *FEMS Microbiology Letters, 300*(1), 146–152. doi:10.1111/j.1574-6968.2009.01781.x PMID:19765084

Wisnewsky, A. J., & Clément, K. (2016). The gut microbiome, diet, and links to cardiometabolic and chronic disorders. *Nature Reviews. Nephrology, 12*(3), 169–181. doi:10.1038/nrneph.2015.191 PMID:26616538

Yadav, H., Lee, J. H., Lloyd, J., Walter, P., & Rane, S. G. (2013). Beneficial metabolic effects of a probiotic via butyrate induced GLP-1 secretion. *The Journal of Biological Chemistry, 288*(35), 25088–25097. doi:10.1074/jbc.M113.452516 PMID:23836895

Section 2
Obesity

Chapter 3
Recent Trends in Functional Foods for Obesity Management

Amrita Poonia
Banaras Hindu University, India

ABSTRACT

Obesity is a medical condition caused by the accumulation of excess fat in the body. The main causes of obesity are lifestyle, less physical activity, and increased health problems. Overweight and obesity have increased over the past 20 years in many regions of the world, particularly the prevalence of obesity in childhood. It is not only a problem of developed countries but also becoming a growing burden for the developing countries. Functional foods might play important role in prevention or treatment of overweight. Functional foods for obesity influences the energy balance equation regulated by the control of energy intake or of energy dissipated as heat (thermogenesis).

INTRODUCTION

Obesity is a medical condition in which accumulation of excess body fat deposits in adipose tissues. As a condition, obesity is associated with reduced life expectancy and increased health problems (Haslam, & James, 2005). Obesity not only triggers diabetes but it is also associated with reduced life expectancy and many other health problems. Numerous studies indicate that higher levels of body fat are associated with an increased risk of many adverse health conditions. The problem of obesity arises from an energy imbalance whereby energy intake exceeds energy expenditure.

DOI: 10.4018/978-1-5225-3267-5.ch003

Dealing with obesity by either prevention or treatment requires modification of one or both components of energy balance. It is a multifactor disease where several factors cause its onset like heredity, metabolic, behavioural, environmental, cultural etc. All these factors may play together in different grades of contribution, which may differ between patients and may influence treatment objectives in each individual. Low BMR is a risk factor for later obesity (Griffiths, Payne, Stunkard, Ribers, & Cox, 1990; Ravussin, & Swinburn, 1993). Astrup et al. (1996) reported that formerly obese (post-obese) patients have a 5- fold higher risk of having a low BMR than the never obese.

Weight loss is increasingly recognized as bringing major health benefits to overweight people and is linked with increases in life expectancy of people having obesity-related complications (Rayalam, Della-Fera, & Baile, 2008). Overweight and obesity have increased over the past 20 years in many regions of the world, particularly the prevalence of obesity in childhood. Obesity is not only restricted to the developed world; it is also becoming a growing burden for the developing countries (Martorell, Kettel Khan, Hughes, & Grummer-Strawn, 2000). Data from the International Obesity Task Force (IOTF, 2005) indicates that worldwide, over 20 million children under the age of six are obese. Obesity is a multi-factorial problem and its development is due to multiple interactions between genes and environment.

Worldwide obesity has become a serious problem. Use of drugs in obesity management affects one of the fundamental processes of the weight regulation in human body and causes serious side effects which overcome over their beneficial effects. Now the clinical and non-clinical researchers are facing a challenge to search for non-pharmacological alternatives for the prevention and treatment of obesity. Diet modification, use of functional foods & nutraceuticals and changes in the life style are some options to prevent obesity. This chapter focuses on the importance and use of functional food ingredients for obesity management and various problems associated with it.

Since long time the fight against obesity and food manufactures has offered many food products like dietetic foods in which fat and sugars are substituted by artificial sweeteners and fat replacers, respectively. Recently many products are available in the market with low energy density, products with bioactive compounds, functional foods and nutraceuticals that are effective in obesity management. The main points in the evaluation of functional foods would be the safety and efficacy, thereby avoiding misleading advertisements to the consumer. The new European regulation regarding food labelling, may encourage the food industry to carry out more investment in research and in the determination of the effectiveness of the functional products launched to the market at biochemical, molecular, genomic and psychological levels.

CAUSES OF OBESITY

Increase Energy Intake

Obesity arises from an energy imbalance whereby energy intake exceeds energy expenditure. Prevention or treatment of obesity is associated with modifications of energy intake and energy expenditure. In weight management approaches, functional food approach can target multiple aspects of the energy balance systems like food intake, energy expenditure and energy storage. Pharmaceutical companies have adopted all of these approaches for developing foods for weight management. The relationship of physical activity and energy balance has shown in Figure 1.

Decrease in Energy Expenditure

Due to advancement in technologies, urbanization, transport and availability of a large range of domestic electrical appliances have resulted in substantial decline in the energy spent in these activities in most of the jobs. It is well documented

Figure 1. Energy balance for weight management

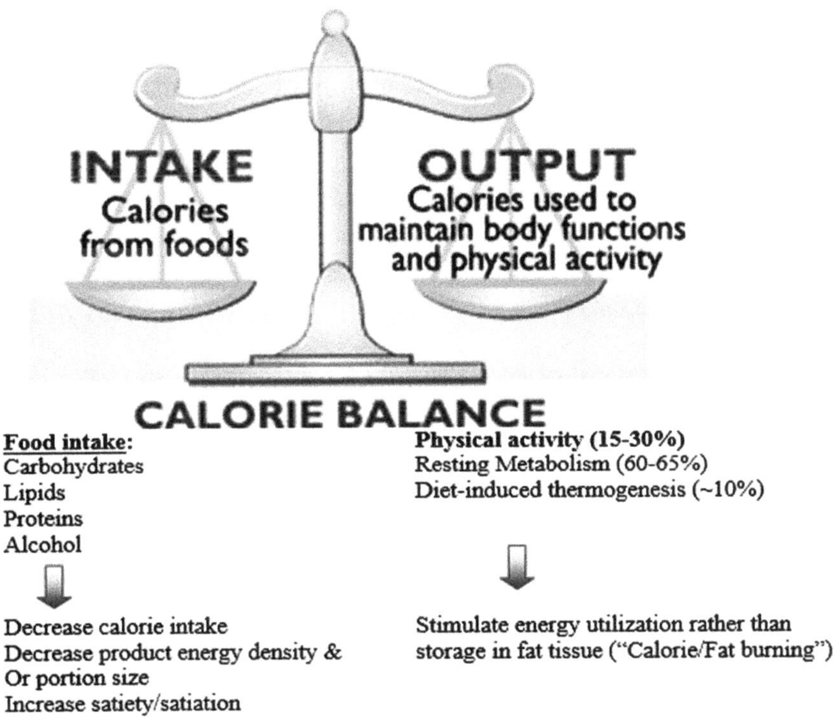

that regular physical activity is protective against unhealthy weight gain whereas sedentary lifestyles, particularly sedentary occupations and inactive recreation such as watching television, promote obesity (WHO, 1998).

Stress Full and Unhealthy Life Style

Stress has been identified as a barrier to the uptake of behaviour changes although some studies suggest it may need to reach a threshold level before impacting on behaviour. High levels of psychological distress are associated with psychopathology such as depression and anxiety.

Macronutrient Distribution and High Fat Diets

Excess body fat deposition is a result of an energy imbalance between calorie intake and energy expenditure. High energy density and high palatability of fat rich diets are considered to increase energy intake as compared to low fat diets. Commercial availability of high fat-based food items is another reason of increased energy intake.

Genetic Predisposition

BMI is a determinant act as a genetic factor affecting energy balance. More than 300 genes, markers, and chromosomal regions have been found to be associated with various human obesity phenotypes and it has been estimated that 30–70% of the variance in BMI in humans can be explained by genetic factors (Loos & Bouchard, 2003). The discovery of the leptin gene has dramatically changed our understanding of the role that adipose tissue plays in the regulation of energy balance and appetite. Leptin acts within the arcuate nucleus of the hypothalamus to decrease the expression of orexigenic signals and increase the levels of anorexigenic signals and thus reduce food intake.

Socio-Economic Status and Level of Education

Obesity is a common feature in migrants, where a population with a common genetic heritage live under new socio-economic and cultural conditions. Studies have found that BMI is significantly higher among low socioeconomic than middle and high socio-economic groups with lower socio-economic status (SES) being associated with accelerated weight gain during adulthood. Level of education is inversely associated with obesity especially in women, while husband's education is found to be correlated negatively with the prevalence of obesity in their wives.

Psychological Factors

Psychological status of human beings can influence eating habits, because most people eat more when they are in stress. Stress also shifts consumption toward high caloric foods that are normally avoided. It is thought that the effect of stress on food intake is mediated via increased adrenal glucocorticoid (GC) output. Chronically increased GC levels can give rise to increased intake of 'comfort foods' which in turn leads to abdominal obesity. Depression and some neurological problems can also promote overeating which will ultimately lead to increased fat accumulation in the body.

Other Factors

The causes of obesity are obviously multi-factorial. Sleep duration, smoking, pharmaceuticals, maternal age, increased life expectancy, endocrine disruptors, environmental temperature and reproductive fitness are some factors which are also responsible for obesity.

STRATEGIES FOR DEVELOPMENT OF FUNCTIONAL FOODS FOR OBESITY

Reduction of Energy Intake

The combination of energy reduced foods with functional ingredients that stimulate satiety peptides release may be an interesting and ambitious approach. It should be taken in consideration that the release of satiety peptides is normally proportional to the energy intake and energy density of food. In this sense, it seems difficult to design energy reduced food with the ability to stimulate satiety. Currently there are a variety of food ingredients that can be used with the purpose to replace fat and sugar in foods formulations. Dairy products, beverages, cakes, pastries, etc., target products for the replacement of simple sugars with non-nutritive sweeteners, contributed to 68% and 62% of the total intake of simple sugars, respectively. Its replacement with non-nutritive sweeteners could result in a reduction in energy intake. Some strategies to reduce energy intake are decreasing the energy density of foods by adding water or fiber, using appropriate palatability enhancers in nutritionally valuable foods (e.g. foods with low energy density or low glycemic index), serving reasonable food portions and avoiding excessive portions of high energy density foods. Replacement of food components with ingredients of lower energy content or reduced absorption rate are some other possibilities in reduction of energy intake. Different methods of satiety induction are discussed in Figure 2.

Satiety Peptides

Recently it has been reported that short and long-term satiety and hunger feelings may be regulated by several neural circuits at the ventromedial, dorsomedial and paraventricular hypothalamic nuclei for satiety sensations and at the lateral hypothalamus for hunger sensations. Although the hypothalamus is an important centre in the energy balance regulation, there are other brain regions such as the medulla oblongata and cortical and striatal structures, essential for the eating behaviour modulation. For example, some neural circuits of the medulla oblongata seem to have an important role in autonomic eating regulation, limiting the quantity of ingested food through the satiety responses regulation.

Short-term regulation of food intake results from an integrated response from neural and humoral signals that originate mainly at the brain, gastrointestinal tract and adipose tissue. Ingested food evokes satiety in the gastrointestinal tract primarily

Figure 2. Showing induction of satiety

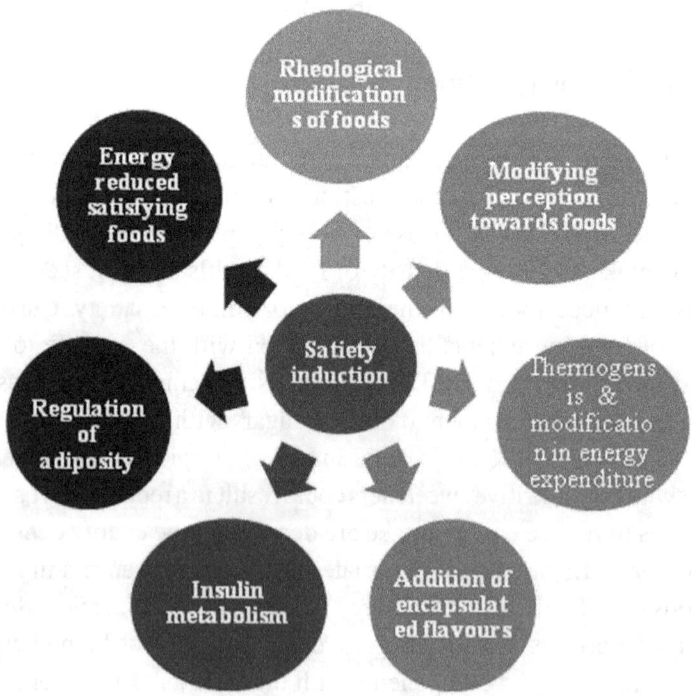
Rheological modifications of foods
Modifying perception towards foods
Thermogenesis & modification in energy expenditure
Addition of encapsulated flavours
Insulin metabolism
Regulation of adiposity
Energy reduced satisfying foods
Satiety induction

by two distinct ways, i.e. by mechanical stimulation and therefore stimulation of the nerve endings; and by the release of satiety peptides. These satiety peptides are discussed below:

Ghrelin

Ghrelin is a hormone secreted by the stomach. It is a fast-acting hormone and playing an important role in meal initiation. Human prepro-ghrelin consists of 117 amino acids. Mature ghrelin peptide is constituted of 28 amino acids with a fatty acid chain modification (octanoyl group) on the third amino acid. It attenuates leptin-induced reduction in food intake and body weight by modulating the expression of various hypothalamic peptides. It works as an appetite stimulating signal. Besides playing a role in short-term regulation of food intake, ghrelin might also play a role in long-term regulation of energy balance.

Cholecystokinin (CCK)

The inhibitory effect of CCK on food intake has been confirmed in numerous species, including humans. It is however short-lived, lasting less than 30 min. Therefore, CCK may inhibit food intake within the meal by reducing meal size and duration but does not affect the onset of a next meal. Thus it may have an important role in the causal chain leading to satiation or meal termination. Gastric distension augments the anoretic effects of CCK in humans. However, other mechanisms including activation of duodenal chemosensitive fibres and activation of CCK receptor 1 in the pyloric sphincter that may slow down gastric may be implicated.

Glucose-Dependent Insulinotropic Polypeptide (GIP)

GIP is released in response to the presence of nutrients in the intestinal lumen. The major stimuli for GIP release are dietary fat and carbohydrates.

Glucagon-Like Peptide 1 (GLP-1)

GLP-1 is an incretin hormone released in response to food intake. GLP-1 is typically very low in the fasting state, but rise quickly after food intake, especially after carbohydrate intake. The rise of GLP-1 has been correlated with increased satiety and less hunger. GLP-1 is thought to play an important role in the "ileal break", a mechanism that regulates the flow of nutrients from the stomach into the small intestine.

Peptide Tyrosine-Tyrosine (PYY)

PYY is a member of the pancreatic polypeptide fold family including neuropeptide Y (NPY) and pancreatic polypeptide (PP). PYY mediates ileal and colonic breaks, mechanisms that ultimately slow gastric emptying and promote digestive activities to increase nutrient absorption. Plasma concentration of PYY increases after meals consistent with a meal-related signal of energy homeostasis. Nutrients stimulate PYY release within 30 minutes of ingestion, reaching usually a maximum within 60 min. The release is directly proportional to caloric intake; however meal composition may affect postprandial PYY release. Batterham et al., (2002) reported that in humans infusion of PYY3-36 (active form) comparable to those after a meal result in decreased energy intake at subsequent meals compared with a control group.

Amylin

Amylin is co-secreted together with insulin from pancreatic β-cells. It is a 37 amino acid peptide with anorexigenic effects that have shown to reduce meal size as well as the number of meals. The inhibitory effect of amylin on food intake is thought to be due to the inhibition of gastric emptying.

Pancreatic Polypeptide (PP)

PP is secreted by F-cells on the endocrine pancreas comprising approximately less than 5% of its volume. The main function of PP is thought to be the inhibition of exocrine pancreas. Its secretion is controlled by the parasympathetic nervous system and shows a biphasic manner in proportion to food intake.

Leptin

It is a hormone produced mainly by adipose tissue. It also plays helpful in regulating energy balance, suppressing food intake and thus induce weight loss. Leptin acts through the leptin receptor (*LEPR* or *OBR*). The *OBR* gene is located on chromosome 1 (1p31), is constituted of 18 exons and 17 introns, and encodes a protein consisting of 1162 amino acids. Leptin is released into the circulatory system by the adipose tissue as a function of the energy stores. Serum and plasma leptin levels are higher in subjects with a higher BMI and a higher per cent total body fat (Schwartz, Peskind, Raskind, Boyko, & Porte, 1996).

Plasma leptin can pass through the blood-brain barrier (BBB). On release of leptin by the adipose tissue into the bloodstream, it crosses the BBB and binds with the hypothalamic leptin receptors, which then initiates signals for the brain to exchange information about the status of the body energy stores. In rodents and in humans, this result in a decrease in food intake and an increase in energy expenditure to balance the quantum of body fat stored in these subjects.

Hypothalamus is the main organ of our body which regulates the food intake and hence the body weight is regulated. Levels of cerebral spinal fluid (CSF) leptin are also correlated with BMI.

Insulin

Insulin helps in signalling in the regulation of food intake and neuronal growth and differentiation. Moreover, insulin has been shown to regulate neurotransmitter release and synaptic plasticity. Insulin concentrations are increased at positive energy balance and decreased at the times of negative energy balance. Additionally, plasma insulin are largely determined by peripheral insulin sensitivity which is related to the amount and distribution of body fat in insulin-resistant patients. Insulin thus provides information to the central nervous system about the size and distribution of the adipose mass to regulate metabolic homeostasis.

RHEOLOGICAL MODIFICATIONS OF FOODS

The main purpose of rheological modification is to induce satiety by modifying the perception of consumers toward food. This can be done by the development of products with a high volume and low density in both weight and energy. Satiety can also be introduced through the stimulation of retro-nasal aroma by food. Microencapsulation of the flavours is another way to introduce satiety. Rheological modifications for satiety peptide release are mainly based in the induction of a higher gastric distension and a reduction in gastric emptying which may promote the release of CCK and the decrease of ghrelin levels. Viscous fibres are the main nutrient associated with the ability to slow gastric emptying.

Digestive Enzyme Inhibition and Gut Energy Absorption Inhibition

By controlling the action of digestive enzyme and interacting with them to physically interrupt its absorption in the intestinal tract. Use of high fibre diet which modulates the intestinal transit time resulting in increased satiety, reduced physical accessibility of nutrients for being absorbed and a reduced calorie intake of the formulation. Bioactive compounds (tannins) have the ability to inhibit the activity of digestive enzymes, which have the ability to precipitate proteins (including enzymes), reducing its action. Polyphones (for example from tea) have the ability to inhibit *in vitro* the translocation of glucose transporter, GLUT2, in the intestinal epithelial cells, thus inhibiting the absorption of glucose (Kwon, Eck, Chen, Corpe, Lee, Kruhlak, & Levine, 2007).

Thermogenesis and Possible Modifications in Energy Expenditure

Carbohydrates induced an increased adrenaline concentration, resulting in increased muscle thermogenesis (Astrup, Bulow, Christensen, Madsen, & Quaade, 1986). Green tea extracts have been also described to stimulate thermogenesis in brown adipose tissue, mainly due to the interaction between its high content of catechins and caffeine that may stimulate the noradrenaline released by the sympathetic nervous system. Overall, the action of caffeine and catechins may prolong the stimulatory effects of noradrenaline on energy metabolism and lipid. Functional foods against insulin resistance may also help to reduce obesity by increasing insulin sensibility thus optimizing the use of energy (Ruijschop & Burgering, 2007).

It is widely accepted fact that not all types of foods produce the same quality (flavour) or quantity (intensity) of sensory stimulation. The physical structure of these food products largely seems to be responsible for stimulating the aroma. For example, solids food products tend to produce a greater sense of satiety than liquid foods, which is attributed probably to the increased contact time of food in the oral cavity and therefore the greater sensory stimulation.

Insulin Metabolism and the Regulation of Adiposity

Increased plasma glucose levels increase the secretion of insulin from pancreatic β-cells. Other substrates such as free fatty acids, ketone bodies, and certain amino acids can also directly stimulate insulin's release or augment glucose's ability to trigger insulin release. It has been suggested that a low-glycemic diet can help control obesity because of the ability to reduce the rate of glucose uptake in the small intestine and therefore the insulin secretion, as well as to increase satiety value of food and appetite regulation (Brand-Miller, Holt, Pawlak, & McMillan, 2002; Roberts, 2003). For example, replacing simple sugars like sucrose with fructose, as a sweetener with low glycemic index, has been associated with increased body adiposity. After the ingestion of fructose, insulin is not increased, leptin is reduced, and ghrelin is not inhibited. Because these hormones play important roles in regulating food intake, the combined effects of excessive fructose intake could result in a lower induction of satiety and increase in total intake. Moreover, these foods should be low in saturated fatty acids, especially *trans* fatty acids, which are associated with a higher induction in adiposity. Addition of conjugated linoleic acid appears to have an effect based on the inhibition of the activity of lipoprotein lipase, which may reduce the uptake of lipids by the adipocyte.

FUNCTIONAL FOOD INGREDIENTS FOR MANAGEMENT OF OBESITY

Dietary Polyphenols(DPs)

DPs are classified as phenolic acids, flavonoids (include flavonols, flavones, isoflavones, flavanones, anthocyanidins, flavanols), lignans and stilbenes. DPs undergo biotransformation by gut microbial enzymes, which change their bioavailability and beneficial effects. Vegetables, fruits, whole grains, legumes, and other plant sources have thousands of polyphenols. There are various health benefits of dietary polyphenols. They act as antioxidants, inhibiting free radicals & reactive oxygen species, anti-inflammatory, antibacterial, anti-viral and anti-proliferative activity and DNA scission inhibitory activity beneficial against osteoporosis, neurodegenerative disease, cardiovascular disease, diabetes mellitus, obesity and other metabolic disorders. Fernandez et al., (2011) studied anti-obesity action of polyphenolic extracts and polyphenolic compounds using animal cell cultures (3T3-L1) of adipogenesis and HFD induced obese animals. They reported that DPs may inhibit pre-adipocyte to adipocyte differentiation, cause adipocyte apoptosis, decrease fat absorption from gut, uptake of glucose by skeletal muscles, suppress lipid biosynthesis and promote catabolism in adipose, liver and other tissues. They also reported that DPs may promote anti-inflammatory molecules in adipose tissue.

McCarty (2005) reported that polyphenols also induce a higher rate of secretion of satiety peptides like GLP-1 possibly because of its effects in the inhibition of glucose uptake by enterocytes. So the addition of antioxidant dietary fibre (fibres with associated antioxidant compounds) to food formulation may help to increase satiety feeling of foods. Glucose and fat are the main inductors of satiety peptides. However, it is widely accepted that the increase in glucose and fat uptake are strongly related with obesity.

Dietary Fibres and Prebiotics

DFs are non-digestible and non-starch polysaccharides and are widely distributed in plants and certain microbes. Some examples of dietary fibres are pectin, β-glucan, xylan, inulin, resistant starch and guar gum. Fruits, vegetables and whole grain cereals are rich in DFs and their intake significantly lowers the risk of coronary heart disease, stroke, hypertension, diabetes, obesity, gastrointestinal diseases and boosts the immune system and stimulates the growth of beneficial microbes in the colon. Viscous fibres have been related to satiety because of its effects in gastric distension and emptying rates which may increase CCK and reduce ghrelin secretion. Viscous fibre may regulate bolus transit time in small intestine, which may affect the total glycemic load, regulating glucose and insulin levels, hence inducing direct satiety stimulation in central nervous system satiety centre. In case of fibre colonic fermentation by-products like short-chain fatty acids are recognized to induce L-cells proliferation in the colon, which are the main cells where GLP-1 and PYY is produced. Thus, chronic fibre intake may chronically increase the amount of these satiety peptides in plasma. Several researchers suggest that the amount of fibre that may exert satiety feeling in humans should be higher than 8 g/day, which difficult its incorporation in technologically modified foods. They may produce acute satiety feeling (intrameal and intermeal satiety); whereas fermentable fibres may produce chronic satiety feeling after consumption for more than 9 months. Mechanism of action of dietary fibres has been shown in Box 1.

Prebiotics are oligosaccharide derivatives produced by enzymatic hydrolysis of polysaccharides or by transglycosylations. The most widely studied and European Union approved prebiotics are fructo-oligosaccharides; galacto oligosaccharides and lactulose. DFs and prebiotics are resistant to human digestion and are fermented to acetate; propionate and butyrate, short chain fatty acids, due to synergistic action of colonic microflora(Flint, 2012). Propionate stimulates expression of leptin andreduces the pro-inflammatory factor resist in human adiposetissues (Al-Lahham, Roelofsen, Priebe, Weening, Dijkstra, Hoek, Rezaee, Venema, & Vonk, 2010). Arora et al., (2011) reported that propionate suppresses appetite and combats the obesity. Butyrate may epigenetically regulate genes in cholesterolbiosynthesis by inhibiting histone deacetylase. DFs and prebiotics not only lower fat and body weight, that are pre-requisite for obesity management but also, brought about prebiotic changes ingut microflora. Dietary fibres and prebiotics significantly improve immune functions (more anti-inflammatory markers and less pro-inflammatory markers), gut barrier function, regulation of gut hormones (increases satiety) and alteration of gene expression in liver and adipose tissues. Modified or partiallybroken carbohydrates may signal at specific receptors to alter whole-body energy and glucose metabolism. DFs and prebiotics also regulate release of gut hormones that signals brain of satiety. So, for prevention or management of obesity, a careful dietary manipulation of gut associated microflora should be a top priority.

Mechanism of Action of Dietary Fibres

DFs and prebiotics are resistant to human digestion and are fermented to acetate; propionate and butyrate, short chain fatty acids, due to synergistic action of colonic microflora. Propionate stimulates expression of leptin and reduces the pro-inflammatory factor resist in human adipose tissues. Propionate suppresses appetite and combats the obesity. Butyrate may epigenetically regulate genes in cholesterol biosynthesis by inhibiting histone deacetylase. SCFAs may reduce risk of metabolic disorders via binding to G-protein-coupled receptors, GPR41 and GPR43 and alter their expression SCFA are recognized as potential mediators of intestinal inflammatory response. Therefore a good SCFA profile in colon is crucial for colonic health. This could be achieved by incorporating 15–20 g of DF/prebiotic or their combinations.

Omega 3 Fatty Acids

The type and amount of fats consumed affect obesity insulin resistance and atherosclerosis in animal models. Although both conjugated linoleic acid and conjugated linolenic acid reduced non- HDL-cholesterol, conjugated linolenic acid impaired the insulin function. Bovine milk contains conjugated linoleic acid, short and medium-chain fatty acids that may have anti-inflammatory, immune enhancing, antibacterial, anti-ulcerative colitis, anti-cancer, anti-atherosclerosis and anti-hypertension effects. By adopting the various strategies i.e.: (a)increasing physical activity; (b) consuming non-starch polysaccharides/fiber and micronutrient-rich plant products; (c) breast feeding; and (d) reducing energy-dense, micronutrient-poor diets, obesity can be managed. Clifton (2012) reported that high protein diets produce greater satiety and weight loss, lower plasma triglyceride, blood pressure and spare lean mass than high carbohydrate diets; with no harmful effects on bone density or renal function.

FUNCTIONAL FOOD GROUPS

Functional Foods can be regarded so if they prove to cause beneficial effect on one or more target functions in the body, beyond adequate nutritional effects, in such a way relevant to improved health and well-being, reduction of risk of diseases, or both. Functional foods might have a particularly high impact for prevention or treatment of obesity and diabetes for which, more than in many other fields, the link between nutrition, biological responses and diseases is well established. Functional foods for obesity reduction should be surely able to manage the energy balance equation regulated by the control of energy intake and of energy dissipated as heat (thermogenesis).

Increased satiety is one of the promising avenues to reduce energy intake using functional foods. The main aim is to develop and provide foods that enhance the sense of fullness and encourage the individual to stop eating sooner, thereby reducing the total energy intake. By modifying the energy density of the diet; macronutrient composition of the diet and the glycaemic index of the diet, satiety may be increased. The various functional food groups which play important role in obesity management are discussed below.

Fruits and Vegetables

Consumption of high amount of fruits and vegetables are helpful in maintenance of health as well as provide protection against various health diseases. The presence of bioactive compounds in fruits and vegetables offered various health benefits. High consumption of fruits and vegetables has been associated with maintenance of health as they offer protection against various chronic diseases. Varied bioactive components at different levels may be responsible for the offered health protection. Crujeiras et al, (2006) conducted an intervention study of 8-weeks in obese men and women who received enriched fruits with an energy-restricted regimen resulted in low oxidized LDL and improved antioxidant capacity. Prior et al., (2010) reported that black raspberries contain high anthocyanin levels and their consumption reduced body weight gain, fasting serum glucose, leptin, insulin levels and homeostasis assessment of insulin resistance (HOMA-IR) in mice fed high fat diet. Aprikian et al, (2010) studied that apples are associated with reduced body weight gain, fat deposits and glucose. The anti-obesity properties are due to modulation of genes responsible for lipolysis, adipogenesis and fat oxidation (Boque, Iglesia, Garza, Milagro, Olivares, Bañuelos, Soria, Rodríguez-Sánchez, Martínez, & Campión, 2013).

Apples, with relative high fibre content, lowered plasma lipid content and triacylglycerides in liver, as well as improved oxidative status by producing larger intestinal pool and greater faecal excretion of bile acids in obese rats. Matsunaga et al.,(2014) reported that onion peel tea (OPT), high in polyphenols, exhibited anti-obesity properties in high fat diet induced obese (BALB/c) mice, when they were feed with onion peel tea for 28 days after induction of obesity by feeding a high fat diet for 3 weeks. Pomegranates are rich in phytochemicals such as ellagitannins, anthocyanins, phenolic acids, and a variety of volatile compounds. Pomegranates exhibited anti-obesity properties in *in-vivo* and *in-vitro* studies exhibiting hypoglycaemic activity, increase insulin sensitivity, inhibit α-glucosidase enzyme activity, reduce total cholesterol, improve blood lipid profiles, and retard inflammation by modulating PPAR pathways (Medjakovic & Jungbauer, 2013).

Beverages

Green tea is unfermented and rich in polyphenolic compounds. Oolong tea is partially oxidized and possesses considerable amounts of polyphenols. Black tea is fermented and contains mostly the flavins and polyphenols. Black tea polyphenols are reported to inhibit pancreatic lipase and thereby affect lipid metabolism. Matsuyama et al., (2008) conducted studies with green tea (576 - 592.2 mg catechins) and they reported an increase in fat oxidation, reduction in body fat ratio and waist circumference. Green tea helps in increasing energy expenditure by inhibiting catechol O-methytransferase (COMT) enzyme which degrades norepinephrine, inhibiting enzyme phosphodiesterase which degrades intracellular cAMP, antagonizes the inhibitory effects of adenosine on lipolysis, increased expression of uncoupling proteins, and activation of PPARs (Westerterp-Plantenga, 2010). Lin et al., (2013) studied the effect on obese mice which were tested for their effect in offering protection against obesity in high fat fed mice. They were fed with Blueberry Juice (BBJ) and Mulberry Juice (MBJ). They reported that these juices reduced body weight (7% - 10%), epididymal fat and size of fat cells. Serum glucose and cholesterol level were lowered by BBJ, but not by MBJ. Juices altered lipid metabolism by suppressing fatty acid synthesis related genes (PPARγ and FAS) and inducing the expression of β-oxidation-related gene (CPT 1)

Grains and Legumes

Whole grains contain antioxidants, dietary fiber (inulin, beta-glucan, resistant starch), phenolics, phytate, phyto-estrogens, phytostanols, phytosterols, vitamins (carotenoids, tocotrienols, tocopherols) and minerals. Fibre-rich cereals consumption help reduce cholesterol, hypertension, constipation and obesity. Nuts (tree nuts and peanuts) are nutrient dense (rich in unsaturated fats, protein, fiber, minerals, tocopherols, phytosterols, phenolics and other bioactive compounds) but epidemiologic and intervention studies showed they do not contribute to weight gain. Sesame contains sesamol, the powerful antioxidant that alleviates diet-induced inflammation and cardiometabolic syndrome in mammals by up-regulating PPARγ, PPAR a and e-NOS. The polyphenol-rich black soybean seed coat extract containing cyanidin 3-glucoside, catechins, and procyanidins amongst others, suppressed abdominal fat accumulation, plasma glucose level, major inflammatory cytokines, tumor necrosis factor-a and monocyte chemoattractant protein-1 (Dai, Hsu, Huang, & Wu, 2013). Pigeon pea (*Cajanus cajanL.*) has linoleic acid and phytosterol (B-sitosterol, campesterol, stigmasterol) that synergistically produce antioxidant and anti-dyslipidemic effects by promoting cholesterol conversion to bile acid and increasing hepatic carnitine palmitoyltransferase-1 (CPT-1), LDL receptor, and cholesterol 7 a-hydroxylase (or cytochrome P450 7A1, CYP7A1) expression in high fat diet-fed hamsters.

Herbs and Spices

Many herbs and spices have good positive effects on blood sugar, insulin sensitivity, dyslipidaemia, weight gain and the cardiovascular system. They activate PPARa and PPARg, inhibit NF-KB activation, and enhance anti-inflammatory cytokines expression. Catharanthus roseus, Thymus vulgaris, Hypericum perforatum, and Artemisia annua are also potently antioxidative. Cinnamon extract helped safeguard against tissue changes by minimizing protein aggregation, preventing glycation and oxidative stress in fructose-fed rodents. Cumin, cinnamon, and black pepper, inhibited in vitro advanced glycation end-products (AGE) formation at 1.0 mg/ml. Clove aqueous extracts have insulin-like biological activity and can gradually lower fasting blood glucose levels. *Momordica charantia, Morinda citrifolia* fruit, and *Centella asiatica* extract have anti-pancreatic lipase and antioxidant activities that help to prevent obesity (Gooda, Abdul-Hamid, Saari, Abas, Pak Dek, & Rahim, 2012). Cinnamon water extract or polyphenols with doubly linked procyanidin type-a polymers display insulin-like activity to improve blood glucose and lipid profiles of diabetes patients.

Probiotics and Synbiotics

FAO/WHO defined probiotics as, *live microorganisms which when administered in amount confer health benefits to the host.* They get colonized in the gut of humans and certain animals, promote gastrointestinal health. They also have health promoting effects such as modulation of the host immune system, improving bioavailability of nutrients, decreasing lactose intolerance, helps in regulating the host metabolic processes, weight gain and obesity. *Lactobacillus* and *Bifidobacteria* are generally regarded as safe (GRAS) probiotic strains. The numbers of these beneficial microbes can be enhanced by using various dietary fibres and prebiotics. Indigenous gut microbes also secrete low molecular weight bioactive metabolites such as short chain fatty acids, peptides, endotoxins, vitamins, enzymes and co-enzymes that may influence epigenetic reprogramming and post translational modifications. Thus gut microbes may regulate host metabolism (Shenderov, 2012). Probiotic-mediated modulation of gut flora as a potential approach for obesity and other metabolic diseases management. Their combination with a non-digestible carbohydrate source (dietary fibre or prebiotic) may be a better choice. The synbiotics can provide double benefits of both the ingredients that may take a lead in the future management of this major health problem.

Table 1. Examples of foods or food ingredients that may potentially be considered as 'functional' in the field of body weight regulation

Food/Ingredient Functions	Target Functions	Measurements
Fiber-Rich Foods Low Glycemic Index Starchy Foods Medium-Chain Triglycerides Polyunsaturated Fat	Energy intake	Satiety, hunger (Visual analogue scale) Dietary records, nutrient intake
Fat Replacers Food Intake Non-Caloric Sweeteners	-	Dietary records, BMI, NMR of visceral fat
Caffeine, Capsaicin, Green Tea	Energy expenditure	Indirect calorimetry
Conjugated Linoleic Acid Medium-Chain Triacylglycerides Diacylglycerols Low Fat Dairy Products Nuts	Body fat	BMI, NMR of visceral fat

BMI -body mass index; NMR-nuclear magnetic resonance
Source: (Riccardi, Capaldo, & Vaccaro, 2005)

CURRENT STATUS OF NUTRACEUTICALS IN OBESITY MANAGEMENT

Obesity is very serious problem globally; hence the role of nutrition and exercise plays a key role in its prevention and treatment. Kasbia (2005), reported that nutraceuticals like conjugated linoleic acid (CLA), capsaicin, *Momordica Charantia* (MC), and Psyllium fibre possess potential anti-obese properties. A blend of glucomannan, chitosan, fenugreek, *G sylvestre*, and vitamin C in the dietary supplement significantly reduced body weight and promoted fat loss in obese individuals.

METABOLICALLY ACTIVE FUNCTIONAL FOOD INGREDIENTS FOR WEIGHT CONTROL

Metabolically active agents may also act to inhibit fat storage through decreased lipid uptake or formation, stimulate fat mobilization through increased lipolysis, or enhance rates of fat oxidation. However, to benefit weight control, these must ultimately alter energy balance through increased expenditure or feedback into appetite control, or perhaps influence the balance of protein and lipid metabolism in a way that affects body composition.

Table 2. Functional foods and nutraceutical agents associated with obesity

Functional Foods Which Increase Energy Intake	Mechanism of Action
Caffeine and ephedrine	A combination of caffeine and ephedrine effective in long term weight management due to different mechanisms that may operate synergistically, e.g., respectively inhibiting the phosphodiesterase-induced degradation of cAMP and enhancing the sympathetic release of catecholamines.
Capsaicin	Weight loss and fight fat buildup by triggering certain beneficial protein changes in the body
Green tea	Catechins and caffeine, may act through the inhibition of catechol O-methyl-transferase, and the inhibition of phosphodiesterase
Oolong tea	Flavonoids and polyphenolic content increases energy expenditure the catechins, has been shown to inhibit catechol O-methyltransferase (COMT), an enzyme that degrades norepinephrine
Calcium	Ca intake is associated with a lower BMI
Functional Foods Which Reduce Energy Intake	
Fibre rich foods	High fiber diets may trigger maximal sensory stimulation in the mouth due to the increased need for chewing. They also lead to slower gastric emptying and a slower rate of nutrient absorption. High fiber content reduces the energy density of the overall diet
Nutraceutical Agents	
Curcumin	Curcumin suppression of angiogenesisin adipocytes together with its effect on lipid metabolism in adipocytes may contribute to lower body fat and body weight gain
Polyunsaturated fatty acids () PUFA	Dietary n-3 polyunsaturated fatty acids modulate each of the components of the triad of adiposity, inflammation, and fattyacid metabolism, with particular attention to the role of the postprandial period as a contributor to the pathophysiology of metabolic syndrome
Psyllium fiber	Psyllium reduces adiposity and improves glucose homeostasis in pediatric and adolescent patients suffering from obesity
Momordica Charantia (MC)	MC has been implicated in the reduction of adiposity in mice, lowering lipoproteinlevels, and as well lowering blood glucosein streptozotocin (STZ) induced rats and human participants as well
Resveratrol	Resveratrol helps in reduction in mean systolic blood pressure, leptin levels, systemic markers ofinflammation, plasma glucose, and insulinincreased energy expenditure
Flavonoids	Citrus flavonoids decreases plasma lipid levels, improve plasma lipid levels, improve glucose tolerance, and attenuate obesity. They reduce hepatic levels of the mRNA for stearoyl CoA desaturase-1 (SCD- 1), leading to repression of hyperlipidemia.
Caralluma fimbriata (edible cactus)	Caralluma fimbriata induced significant and dose dependent inhibition of food intake, with dose-related prevention of gains in body weight, liver weight and fat pad mass. It also conferred protection against atherogenesis
Other Compounds	
Brain serotonin	Brain serotonin has an inhibitory effect on eating behaviour. Serotonin appears to influence both energy balance and the circadian patterns of eating (i.e., three times a day) by activating satiety neurons in the medial hypothalamus. Serotonin seems to interact antagonistically with norepinephrine to decrease appetite and carbohydrate consumption
Dietary chromium	It improves insulin utilization and aids in metabolism which may also lead to reductions in body fat.

Table 3. Examples of metabolically active functional food ingredients with their mechanism of action

Functional Food Ingredients	Mechanism of Action
Conjugated Linoleic Acid (CLA)	Conjugated linoleic acid has been suggested to reduce body fat. CLA has low oxidative stability. The *cis, cis* -CLA isomers are most susceptible to oxidative degradation and the *trans, trans* -CLA isomers are the most stable. Cyclodextrins has been shown to improve the oxidative stability of CLA.
Diglycerides (DG)	Dietary TG is hydrolysed by 1,3-specific lipase to form 1,2-DG, which is further hydrolysed to 2-monoglyceride (MG).The 2-MG and their hydrolysed fatty acids are absorbed and rapidly re-esterified to TG in the small intestine epithelial cell, and appear as chylomicrons in postprandialplasma.
Medium-Chain Triglycerides	Medium-chain triglycerides are readily hydrolysed by lingual and gastric lipases. They differ from long-chain triglycerides (LCT, having fatty acids of >12 carbons) in that the fatty acids of MCT are absorbed directly into the portal circulation and transported to the liver for rapid oxidation.
Green and Oolong Tea	Caffeine is understood to act primarily through inhibition of phosphodiesterase, an enzyme that degrades intracellular cyclic AMP, and by antagonizing the negative modulatory effect of adenosine on increased noradrenalin release. Tea catechins have been shown to inhibit catechol *O*methyl- transferase, the enzyme that degrades noradrenalin.
Ephedrine and Caffeine	The thermogenic, lipolytic and anorectic effects of ephedrineare mainly attributed to sympathetic activation ofthe central nervous system. Ephedrine hasbeen shown to delay gastric emptying. Caffeine actsthrough inhibition of phosphodiesterase and through adenosine antagonism, which would result in increased cyclic AMP concentration in the cell and prolonged noradrenalinrelease.
Capsaicin and Other Pungent Principles	Capsaicin has been reported to act by stimulating catecholamines secretion from the adrenal medulla, mainly through sympathetic activation of the central nervous system.
Dietary Calcium	Two plausible mechanisms have been proposed by which dietary calcium may reduce adiposity. According to *in vitro* studies, dietary calcium may reduce the stimulus for Ca^{2+}influx into the adipocyte by suppressing 1, 25-dihydroxyvitamin D production. This would inhibit lipogenesis and stimulate lipolysis, resulting in reduced adipocyte triglyceride stores. It also stimulation of increased faecal fat and energy losses attributable or due to formation of non-absorbed complexes of calcium and fat.

FUTURE RESEARCH DIRECTIONS

There is a need to research and understand about the interactions of functional food ingredients with brain; gut; gut microbiota; genes and pathways involved in adipose tissue development and function. This interrelation of host's brain-gut axis on energy metabolism can be explained by a combined approach of nutrigenomics, metagenomics and metabolomics.

This will allow for identification of novel molecular targets that could be relevant for future development of innovative therapies, preventive measures, customized dietary plan and functional food/nutraceutical supplements with reference to obesity and associated co-metabolic disorders.

CONCLUSION

Obesity is a result of the effect of various complex pathways. Use of drugs for managing obesity is a serious problem and causes side effects. Now the use of functional foods with some life style modifications is a good option. Increased intake of energy with decrease in energy expenditure, coupled with stressful lifestyle are some of the major contributors of obesity. Various strategies like reduction in energy intake, satiety peptides, and rheological modifications of foods play important role in development of foods. Dietary polyphenols, dietary fibres, probiotics and prebiotics are the functional ingredients which help in obesity management. Metabolically active functional food ingredients like CLA, DG, medium chain tri-glycerides act to inhibit fat storage through decreased lipid intake or formation. Some proposed ingredients e.g. calcium, green tea, oolong tea, capsaicin could be particularly attractive because they have a long history of safe consumption, and also may bring other added health benefits beyond weight control. Nutraceuticals has proven their health benefits and disease prevention capability, which should be taken according to their acceptable recommended intake.

REFERENCES

Al-Lahham, S. H., Roelofsen, H., Priebe, M., Weening, D., Dijkstra, M., Hoek, A., ... Vonk, R. J. (2010). Regulation of adipokine production in human adipose tissueby propionic acid. *European Journal of Clinical Investigation*, *40*(5), 401–407. doi:10.1111/j.1365-2362.2010.02278.x PMID:20353437

Aprikian, O., Duclos, V., Guyot, S., Besson, C., Manach, C., Bernalier, A., ... Demigne, C. (2003). Apple Pectin and a Polyphenol-Rich Apple Concentrate Are More Effective Together than Separately on Cecal Fermentations and Plasma Lipids in Rats. *The Journal of Nutrition*, *133*(6), 1860–1865. doi:10.1093/jn/133.6.1860 PMID:12771330

Arora, T., Sharma, R., & Frost, G. (2011). Propionate. Anti-obesity and satiety enhancing factor. *Appetite*, *56*(2), 511–515. doi:10.1016/j.appet.2011.01.016 PMID:21255628

Astrup, A., Bulow, J., Christensen, N. J., Madsen, J., & Quaade, F. (1986). Facultative thermogenesis induced by carbohydrate: A skeletal muscle component mediated by epinephrine. *The American Journal of Physiology, 250*, E226–E229. PMID:3513610

Batterham, R. L., Cowley, M. A., Small, C. J., Herzog, H., Cohen, M. A., & Deakin, C. L. (2002). Gut hormone PYY(3-36) physiologically inhibits food intake. *Nature, 418*(6898), 415–421. doi:10.1038/nature00887 PMID:12167864

Boque, N., Iglesia, R., Garza, A. L., Milagro, F. I., Olivares, M., Bañuelos, O., ... Campión, J. (2013). Prevention of Diet-Induced Obesity by Apple Polyphenols in Wistar Rats through Regulation of Adipocyte Gene Expression and DNA Methylation Patterns. *Molecular Nutrition & Food Research, 57*(8), 1473–1478. doi:10.1002/mnfr.201200686 PMID:23529981

Brand-Miller, J. C., Holt, S. H., Pawlak, D. B., & McMillan, J. (2002). Glycemic index and obesity. *The American Journal of Clinical Nutrition, 76*(1), 281S–285S. doi:10.1093/ajcn/76.1.281S PMID:12081852

Choumenkovitch, S. F., McKeown, N. M., Tovar, A., Hyatt, R. R., Kraak, V. I., Hastings, A. V., et al. (2013). Whole grain consumption is inversely associated with BMI Z-score in rural school-aged children. *Public Health and Nutrition, 16*(2), 212-218.

Clifton, P. (2012). Effects of a high protein diet on body weight and comorbidities associated with obesity. *British Journal of Nutrition, 108*(2), S122-S129.

Crujeiras, A. B., Parra, M. D., Rodríguez, M. C., Martínez de Morentin, B. E., & Martínez, J. A. (2006). A Role for Fruit Content in Energy-Restricted Diets in Improving Antioxidant Status in Obese Women during Weight Loss. *Nutrition (Burbank, Los Angeles County, Calif.), 22*(6), 593–599. doi:10.1016/j.nut.2006.03.008 PMID:16704952

Dai, F. J., Hsu, W. H., Huang, J. J., & Wu, S. C. (2013). Effect of pigeon pea (Cajanus cajan L.) on high-fat diet-induced hypercholesterolemia in hamsters. *Food Chemistry and Toxicology, 53*, 384-391.

Ferna'ndez-Sa'nchez, A., Madrigal-Santillán, E., Bautista, M., Esquivel-Soto, J., Morales-González, Á., Esquivel-Chirino, C., ... Morales-González, J. A. (2011). Inflammation, oxidative stress, and obesity. *International Journal of Molecular Sciences, 12*(5), 3117–3132. doi:10.3390/ijms12053117 PMID:21686173

Flint, H. J. (2012). The impact of nutrition on the human microbiome. *Nutrition Reviews, 70*(Suppl. 1), S10–S13. doi:10.1111/j.1753-4887.2012.00499.x PMID:22861801

Gooda, S. N., Abdul-Hamid, A., Saari, N., Abas, F., Pak Dek, M. S., & Rahim, M. (2012). Anti-pancreatic lipase and antioxidant activity of selected tropical herbs. *International Journal of Food Properties*, *15*(3), 569-578.

Griffiths, M., Payne, P. R. A. J., Rivers, J. P. W., Cox, M., & Stunkard, A. J. (1990). Metabolic rate and physical development in children at risk of obesity. *Lancet*, *336*(8707), 76–78. doi:10.1016/0140-6736(90)91592-X PMID:1975323

Haslam, D. W., & James, W. P. (2005). Obesity. *Lancet*, *366*(9492), 1197–1209. doi:10.1016/S0140-6736(05)67483-1 PMID:16198769

Hil, J. O., & Peters, J. C. (2002). Biomarkers and functional foods for obesity and diabetes. *British Journal of Nutrition*, *88*(S2), 213–218. doi:10.1079/BJN2002685 PMID:12495462

International Obesity Task Force (IOTF). (2005). *Obesity in Europe*. EU Platform Briefing Paper. Retrieved from http://www.iaso.org/

Jungbauer, A., & Medjakovic, S. (2012). Anti-inflammatory properties of culinary herbs and spices that ameliorate the effects of metabolic syndrome. *Maturitas*, *71*(3), 227-239.

Kasbia, G. S. (2005). Functional foods and nutraceuticals in the management of obesity. *Nutrition & Food Science*, *35*(5), 344–351. doi:10.1108/00346650510625557

Kwon, O., Eck, P., Chen, S., Corpe, C. P., Lee, J. H., Kruhlak, M., & Levine, M. (2007). Inhibition of the intestinal glucose transporter GLUT 2 by flavonoids. *The FASEB Journal*, *21*(2), 366–377. doi:10.1096/fj.06-6620com PMID:17172639

Lin, Y. L., Chang, Y. Y., Yang, D. J., Tzang, B. S., & Chen, Y. C. (2013). Beneficial Effects of Noni (*Morinda citrifolia* L.) Juice on Livers of High-Fat Dietary Hamsters. *Food Chemistry*, *140*(1-2), 31–38. doi:10.1016/j.foodchem.2013.02.035 PMID:23578611

Loos, R. J. F., & Bouchard, C. (2003). Obesity – is it a genetic disorder? *Journal of Internal Medicine*, *254*(5), 401–425. doi:10.1046/j.1365-2796.2003.01242.x PMID:14535962

Martorell, R., Kettel Khan, L., Hughes, M. L., & Grummer-Strawn, L. M. (2000). Overweight and obesity in preschool children from developing countries. *International Journal of Obesity and Related Metabolic Disorders*, *24*(8), 959–967. doi:10.1038j.ijo.0801264 PMID:10951533

Matsunaga, S., Azuma, K., Watanabe, M., Tsuka, T., Imagawa, T., Osaki, T., & Okamoto, Y. (2014). Onion Peel Tea Ameliorates Obesity and Affects Blood Parameters in a Mouse Model of High-Fat-Diet-Induced Obesity. *Experimental and Therapeutic Medicine*, *7*(2), 379–382. doi:10.3892/etm.2013.1433 PMID:24396409

Matsuyama, T., Tanaka, Y., Kamimaki, I., Nagao, T., & Tokimitsu, I. (2008). Catechin Safely Improved Higher Levelsof Fatness, Blood Pressure, and Cholesterol in Children. *Obesity (Silver Spring, Md.)*, *16*(6), 1338–1348. doi:10.1038/oby.2008.60 PMID:18356827

Matsuyama, T., Tanaka, Y., Kamimaki, I., Nagao, T., & Tokimitsu, I. (2008). Catechin Safely Improved Higher Levelsof Fatness, Blood Pressure, and Cholesterol in Children. *Obesity (Silver Spring, Md.)*, *16*(6), 1338–1348. doi:10.1038/oby.2008.60 PMID:18356827

McCarty, M. F. (2005). A chlorogenic acid-induced increase in GLP-1 production may mediate the impact of heavy coffee consumption on diabetes risk. *Medical Hypotheses*, *64*(4), 848–853. doi:10.1016/j.mehy.2004.03.037 PMID:15694706

Medjakovic, S., & Jungbauer, A. (2013). Pomegranate: a fruit that ameliorates metabolic syndrome. *Food Functions*, *4*(1), 19-39.

Medjakovic, S., & Jungbauer, A. (2013). Pomegranate: A Fruit That Ameliorates Metabolic Syndrome. *Food & Function*, *4*(1), 19–39. doi:10.1039/C2FO30034F PMID:23060097

Prior, R. L., Wilkes, S. E., Rogers, T. R., Khanal, R. C., Wu, X., & Howard, L. R. (2010). Purified Blueberry Anthocyanins and Blueberry Juice Alter Development of Obesity in Mice Fed an Obesogenic High-Fat Diet. *Journal of Agricultural and Food Chemistry*, *58*, 3970–3976. doi:10.1021/jf902852d PMID:20148514

Ravussin, E., & Swinburn, B. A. (1993). metabolic predictors of obesity cross-sectional versus longitudinal dataInt. *Journal of Obesity*, *17*, S28–S31. PMID:8124397

Rayalam, S., Della-Fera, M. A., & Baile, C. A. (2008). Phytochemicals and regulation of the adipocyte life cycle. *The Journal of Nutritional Biochemistry*, *19*(11), 717–726. doi:10.1016/j.jnutbio.2007.12.007 PMID:18495457

Riccardi, G., Capaldo, B., & Vaccaro, O. (2005). Functional foods in the management of obesity and type 2 diabetes. *Current Opinion in Clinical Nutrition and Metabolic Care*, *8*(6), 630–635. doi:10.1097/01.mco.0000171126.98783.0c PMID:16205464

Roberts, S. B. (2003). Glycemic index and satiety. *Nutrition in Clinical Care*, *6*, 20–26. PMID:12841427

Ruijschop, R. M., & Burgering, M. J. M. (2007). Aroma induced satiation possibilities to manage weight through aroma in food products. *Agro Food Industry Hi-Tech*, *18*, 37–39.

Schwartz, M. W., Peskind, E., Raskind, M., Boyko, E. J., & Porte, D. Jr. (1996). Cerebrospinal fluid leptin levels: Relationship to plasma levels and to adiposity in humans. *Nature Medicine*, *2*(5), 589–593. doi:10.1038/nm0596-589 PMID:8616722

Shenderov, B. A. (2012). Gut indigenous microbiota and epigenetics. *Microbial Ecology in Health and Disease*, *23*(0), 17195. doi:10.3402/mehd.v23i0.17195 PMID:23990811

Westerterp-Plantenga, M. S. (2010). Green Tea Catechins, Caffeine and Body-Weight Regulation. *Physiology & Behavior*, *100*(1), 42–46. doi:10.1016/j.physbeh.2010.02.005 PMID:20156466

Woodgate, D. E., & Conquer, J. A. (2003). Prevalence of self-treatment with complementary products and therapies for weight loss: A randomized, cross-sectional Study in Overweight and Obese Patients in Colombia. *Curr Thera Res*, *64*, 248–262. doi:10.1016/S0011-393X(03)00058-4

World Health Organization Fact Sheet: Obesity and Overweight. (n.d.). Retrieved from http://www.who.int/mediacentre/factsheets/fs311/en/

Chapter 4
Functional Foods for Treatment and Prevention of Obesity and Its Associated Disorders

Jagan Mohan Rao Tingirikari
Chungbuk National University, South Korea

ABSTRACT

Obesity has now become an epidemic affecting wide variety of population across the world. It is associated with a cluster of cardiovascular diseases and other related metabolic disorders such as diabetes, hypertension, and cancer which is mainly caused due to the dysbiosis in the energy intake and expenditure. Researchers have found a wide variety of functional foods from different sources which help in combating and prevention of obesity and its related diseases. Recent advancement in nutritional science has led to the development of several functional foods with low glycemic index. The present chapter highlights about the problems related to obesity and the importance of various functional foods which have great potential to be incorporated in our daily diet to curb the menace of obesity.

INTRODUCTION

Obesity is considered as the lack of energy balance in the body which results in increase of weight. It is considered as the fifth leading factor for the mortality rate across the world. Around 2.8 millions of people die every year due to obesity related complications. The diseases associated with obesity are diabetes (44%), heart disease

DOI: 10.4018/978-1-5225-3267-5.ch004

(23%), and different types of cancer (41%) (Cencic & Chingwaru, 2010). Obesity has been associated with chronic inflammation mediated by increase in production of cytokines such as tumor necrosis factor (TNF)-α, interleukin (IL)-6, and monocyte chemo attractant protein (MCP)-1 derived from adipose tissue (Hotamisligil, Shargill, & Spiegelman, 1993). Among the developing countries the number of overweight individuals have tripled in the last 30 years due to improper diet (over and under nutrition), and requires proper attention (Keats & Wiggins, 2014). The major risk factors which contribute to obesity are: 1) change in life style; 2) diet; 3) lack of physical activity, and; 4.) increase in sedentary life style. The cost for treatment of obesity in US was estimated to be around $147 billon (Finkelstein, Trogdon, Cohen, & Dietz, 2009). Very few drugs are available in the market for the treatment of obesity especially for treating advanced stage of obesity (Miller, 2013). Prolonged or long-term usage of these drugs is associated with the potential health hazards as a result there is a great need to search for alternative foods or anti-obesity agents which can serve the purpose of combating the obesity and its menace (Berthoud, Lenard, & Shin, 2011). The efficiency of dietary and naturally available bioactive compounds in modulating the pathophysiology of obesity is under consideration. Several functional foods or nutraceuticals are being developed by food industry which holds great potential to meet the health-conscious consumers. Functional foods are defined as the food components which can provide health benefits to the host (Sunkara & Verghese, 2014). These foods not only provide vital nutrients but also enhance the biological active components of the body to impart health benefits.

Obesity leads to increase in number and size of adipocytes differentiated in to pre-adipocytes. Functional foods regulate adipocyte differentiation by inducing cell cycle arrest and increase apoptosis (Rayalam, Della-Fera, & Baile, 2008). Obesity management must target both energy intake and expenditure and should have the ability to induce satiety, reduce appetite increase lipid metabolism and induce thermogenesis. Increasing the satiety levels will help in decreasing the energy intake and absorption in the gut mediated by the complex interaction of neural and hormonal interactions (Wynne, Stanley, McGowan, & Bloom, 2005). Fibers enhance the satiety levels by increasing gastric load and emptying time by increasing the levels of cholecystokinin and reduce glurelin (Serrano, Cassanyé, & Portero-Otin, 2012). The lipase inhibitors in the intestine prevent fat digestion and absorption and thus help in weight management. It was reported that polyphenols, anthocyanins, tannins present in tea and di-caffeoyl quinic acids (di-CQA), caffeine from coffee displayed inhibitory effect on several digestive enzymes (maltase, sucrase and lipase) thus help in post-prandial hyperglycemic and hyper-insulinemia (Murase, Yokoi, Misawa, Ominami, Suzuki, Shibuya, & Hase, 2012). Body weight can be regulated by increasing the energy expenditure. Brown adipocytes regulate heat production by uncoupled proteins at mitochondria, while capaisin induce thermogenesis by increasing lipid metabolism and can be used as anti-obesity agent (Rayalam, Della-Fera, & Baile, 2008). Food components which can target the inflammatory regulators such as C-Jun amino-terminal kinase (JNK), and nuclear factor (NF)-kB plays a vital role in controlling obesity related pathologies (Hirai, Takahashi, Goto, Lin, Uemura, Yu, & Kawada, 2010).

The present chapter highlights about various pathophysiology factors, metabolic diseases associated with obesity, and their treatment by the application of functional foods. The role and mechanism of action of different functional foods in regulating obesity, cholesterol and triacylglycerol levels will be highlighted. Apart from the above the future prospects of various functional foods in combating obesity will be discussed.

BACKGROUND

Obesity is considered as one of the major global burden for several chronic diseases and disorders. It was estimated that around 1 billion adults are suffering with overweight problem and among them 300 million people are clinically obese (WHO, 2010). Obesity is a serious socioeconomic problem affecting all age groups. Individuals suffering with obesity has nearly doubled in past 30 years (WHO, 2010; Hil & Peter, 2002). The major diseases associated with obesity are listed in Table 1. Efficient systematic strategies for the prevention and treatment of obesity is key aspects. Functional foods are similar to conventional foods but the major difference is they provide additional physiological benefits to reduce the risk associated with chronic diseases and maintaining gut health (FAO, 2010). Apart from the above they also provide the body with essential nutrients required for proper functioning and healthy survival. Some of the most common functional foods include green tea, psyllium fiber, capsaicin, polyunsaturated fatty acids, flavonoids, probiotics, prebiotics, calcium, and chromium rich food (FAO, 2010).

PATHOPHYSIOLOGY OF OBESITY

Obesity is accompanied by adipose tissue hyperplasia. Adipose tissue serves as an important initiator for chronic inflammatory response characterized by infiltration of macrophages, and other immune cells. It causes the release of pro-inflammatory

Table 1. Major metabolic diseases associated with obesity

Diseases	Disorder	References
Chronic Inflammation	Increase in proinflammatory cytokine MCP-1 causes macrophage activation in adipocytes, NF-kB signaling pathway	Suganami et al., (2005)
Colorectal Cancer	Activation of IGF-1 mediated PI3K/Akt pathway; Increase in proinflammatory cytokine TNF-α, and IL-6	Clayton et al., (2011); Szlosarek et al., (2006)
Hepatocellular Carcinoma	Activation of IGF-1; Increase in proinflammatory cytokine TNF-α, and IL-6, leptin	Powell et al., (2005); Siegel et al., (2009)
Hyper-Cholesteriemia	Increase in TNF-α, IL-6, activation of NF-kB signaling pathway	Kim et al., (2008)
Hyperglycemia	Increase in IGR-1, IGR-2, TNF-α, and IL-6 levels	Rains et al., (2011); Qin et al., (2010)
Hypertension/High Blood Pressure	Cyclooxygenase activation, Increase in platelet aggregation, and sodium levels	Bose et al., (2008)
Type 2 Diabetes	MCP-1 mediated activation of macrophages produce TNF-α interfere with insulin signaling pathway	Suganami et al., (2007)

Abbreviations: Tumor necrosis factor-TNF; Interleukin-IL; Insulin like growth factor-IGF; Phosphatidylinositol 3-kinase-PI3K; Monocyte chemo attractant protein-MCP; Nuclear factors (NF)-kB; Toll-like receptor (TLR).

cytokines such as interleukin (IL)-1, tumor necrotic factor (TNF)-α, IL-6, plasmogen activator inhibitor (PAI)-1, leptin, monocyte chemo attractant protein (MCP)-1, serum amyloid A, retinol binding protein (RBP)-4, macrophage inflammatory protein (Hotamisligil, Shargill, & Spiegelman, 1993). The activation of above factors leads to increase in insulin resistance, energy imbalance and vascular homeostasis (Schenk, Saberi, & Olefsky, 2008). Plasma levels of vitamins and antioxidants are low in obese individuals (Aasheim, Hofso, Hjelmesaeth, Birkeland, & Bohmer, 2008). An inverse relationship has been reported between serum antioxidants levels and waist size (Chrysohoou, Panagiotakos, Pitsavos, Skoumas, Papademetriou, Economou, & Stefanadis, 2007). Treatment of obesity using drugs and surgical procedure is expensive and is associated with several side effects. Modification of diet or nutrition has been considered as one of the effective method in maintaining the right energy balance and combating the menace of obesity. In this aspect functional foods plays a physiological role in decreasing the chronic disease by lowering the levels of saturated fat and regular exercise will hold a key to the treatment of the metabolic syndrome which has crippled much of the world today (Dao, Frelut, Oberlin, Peres, Bourgeois, & Navarro, 2004).

MAJOR DISEASES ASSOCIATED WITH OBESITY

Obesity has been reported to affect the human health and causes several metabolic diseases such as chronic inflammation, hepatic and colorectal carcinoma, type 2 diabetes, hyper tension and cardiovascular diseases. The diseases associated with obesity are provided in Figure 1.

Obesity Induced Chronic Inflammation and Type 2 Diabetes

Adipose tissue plays a vital role in inducing chronic inflammatory response in obese people. The adipose tissue comprises of adipocytes and stromal vascular cells which in turn contains several cell types such as pre-adipocytes, endothelial cells, fibroblasts, and various immune cells especially macrophage infiltration which is common in obesity. The distribution of macrophages in adipose tissue depends on the body mass index, total amount of body fat and size of adipose tissue (Xu, Barnes, Yang, Tan, Yang, Chou…Chen, 2003). It was reported that type 2 diabetes is associated with obesity. A comparative study performed using a lean and, obese

Figure 1. Obesity induced metabolic disorders. (Tumor necrosis factor-TNFα; Interleukin-IL6; Insulin like growth factor-IGF)

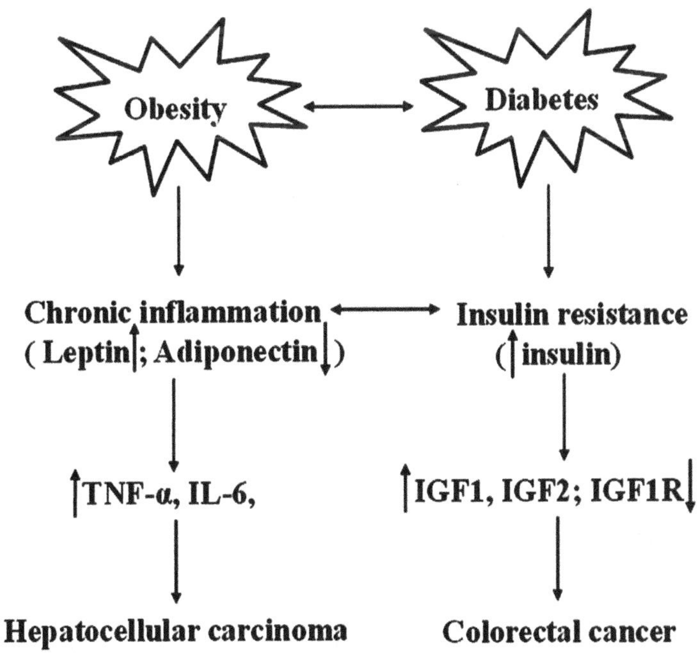

mouse showed a marked increase in production of pro-inflammatory cytokine MCP-1, which is the key for the macrophage activation and infiltration in the adipose tissue (Suganami, Nishida, & Ogawa, 2005). The activated macrophages produce inflammatory mediators like TNF-α which interfere with insulin signaling pathway and promotes fatty acid lipolysis in adipocytes. As a result the concentration of saturated fatty acid levels increases in the adipose tissue during obesity and induce inflammatory response by toll-like receptor (TLR)-4 (Tanimoto-Koyama, Nishida, Itoh, Yuan, Mizuarai, Kotani...Ogawa, 2007). Adipocytes and macrophages interact in paracrine manner and activate the cycle of chronic inflammation accompanied by insulin resistance to cause type 2 diabetes (Suganami, Nishida, & Ogawa, 2005).

Obesity Induced Colorectal Cancer (CRC)

Obesity is considered as the major risk factor for insulin resistance or hyper-insulinemia (Chang & Ulrich, 2003). Insulin and its signal transduction network play an important role in oncogenesis by stimulating the growth of CRC cells to promote CRC tumor growth (Tran, Medline, & Bruce, 1996). Insulin resistance increases the biological activity of insulin-like growth factor (IGF)-1 which is an important endocrine and paracrine regulator involved in tissue growth and metabolism. Binding of insulin and IGF-1 to the cell surface receptors of precancerous cells or tumor cells activates the phosphatidylinositol 3-kinase (PI3K/Akt) pathway responsible for cell growth, proliferation and survival (Clayton, Banerjee, Murray, & Renehan, 2011). The levels of IGF-1 depend on body mass index and waist circumference (Kajantie, Fall, Seppälä, Koistinen, Dunkel, Ylihärsilä... Eriksson, 2003). Increase in insulin resistance and adipose mass creates the oxidative stress in the tissue and increases the expression of pro-inflammatory cytokines such as TNF- α, and IL-6 which stimulate the tumor growth and progression (Hotamisligil, Peraldi, Budavari, Ellis, White, & Spiegelman, 1996). The excess production of saturated fatty acid causes adipocytokine imbalance leading to increase in the levels of leptin and decrease in production of adiponectin which is related to obesity induced carcinogenesis (Barb, Williams, Neuwirth, & Mantzoros, 2007). TNF-α, and IL-6 increases the level of leptin which in turn stimulates the cell growth in CRC and triggers the release of TNF-α, and IL-6. The above studies indicated that abnormalities caused due to obesity increases the risk of cancers and CRC.

Obesity Related Liver Carcinogenesis

Obesity has been considered as one of the major risk factor for the development of steatosis and hepatocellular carcinoma (HCC). Obesity induced insulin resistance causes the increased expression of TNF-α, IL-6, and serum leptin which is associated with the development of steatosis and inflammation in liver (Powell, Jonsson, & Clouston, 2005). Activation of IGF-1 promotes the liver carcinogenesis, while high levels of serum leptin concentration increases the risk of HCC. Non-alcoholic fatty liver disease is the most common form of chronic liver disease which covers non-alcholic steatohepatitis which progress to cirrhosis and finally to HCC (Siegel & Zhu, 2009). Insulin resistance and increase in free saturated fatty acid levels in liver are considered as the major risk factor for the liver carcinogenesis (Feldstein, Werneburg, Canbay, Guicciardi, Bronk, Rydzewski, Burgart, & Gores, 2004).

Obesity Induced Cardiovascular Diseases (CVD)

CVD is the name given to group of disorders related to heart and blood vessel and includes hypertension, coronary heart disease, cerebrovascular disease, heart failure and peripheral vascular disease. The major risk factors associated with CVD are obesity, high blood pressure, lack of physical activity, smoking, alcohol intake, and dyslipidemia (high levels of LDL) (Saetan, Grove, & Lambert, 2011).

ROLE OF FUNCTIONAL FOODS IN STRIKING ENERGY BALANCE

Functional foods play a vital role in obesity control and management either by reducing the energy intake or by increasing the energy expenditure.

Functional Foods to Reduce Energy Intake

One of the promising avenues to reduce obesity is by decreasing the energy intake and increasing the satiety levels. The main goal of functional foods is to increase the sense of satiety levels and promote the individual to stop eating which can be achieved by, modifying the food, macronutrient composition, and decrease the glycemic index of the diet. Foods with either high water or fiber content have a low energy density (Bruun, Lihn, Pedersen, & Richelsen, 2005). High fiber diet enhances maximum sensory stimulation in the mouth, slow rate of nutrient absorption, and gastric emptying (Yu, Kim, Kwon, & Kawada, 2006). Diets rich in polyunsaturated fatty acid stimulate the total fat oxidation than diet with saturated fatty acids (Ricote, Li, Willson, Kelly, & Glass, 1998). Polyphenols, tannins, and anthocyanins present in green tea, berries, and peas act as lipase inhibitors and prevent fat digestion and absorption in the intestine (Murase, Yokoi, Misawa, Ominami, Suzuki, Shibuya, & Hase, 2012). The polyphenols, di-caffeoyl quinic acids from coffee inhibit the action of digestive enzymes (maltase, sucrase, and lipase) and plays a role in postprandial hyperglycemia and hyper-insulinemia (Murase, Yokoi, Misawa, Ominami, Suzuki, Shibuya, & Hase, 2012). It was reported that food intake is directly related to the glycemic index. Foods with low glycemic index are preferred in weight management (Suganami, Nishida, & Ogawa, 2005).

Functional Foods to Increase Energy Expenditure

The other possible way to burn the extra calories is by increasing the energy expenditure. Some of the functional foods which have shown positive effect on calorie burning by inducing thermogenesis are caffeine, green tea, capsaicin. Obesity is mainly characterized by increase in adipocyte population which is mediated by chronic inflammatory cytokines. Hence, food components which can target the regulators involved in inflammation (NF-kB, and C-Jun amino-terminal kinase) will be the best strategy to control obesity related metabolic disorders (Rayalam, Della-Fera, & Baile, 2008).

FUNCTIONAL FOODS FOR REGULATING OBESITY

Obesity can be controlled & regulated by the use of wide variety of nutraceuticals & functional foods obtained different plant and animal sources. A brief outline on the role of different functional foods derived from different sources along with their mechanism of action is provided in Table 2. Some of the most common functional foods involved in regulating obesity are as follows:

Curcumin

It is an active component of turmeric with multiple pharmacological benefits. It is used in treatment of chronic inflammation associated with obesity, diabetes, and atherosclerosis (Aggarwal, 2010). Adipose tissue is the site for the secretion of leptin, adiponectin, and other inflammatory cytokines such as TNF-α, IL-1, IL-6 which play vital role obesity induced insulin resistance and chronic inflammation (Iyer, Panchal, Poudyal, & Brown, 2009). Curcumin interacts directly with cyclooxygenease-2, DNA polymerase, lipoxygenase, glycogen synthase, kinase 3b, TNF-α and indirectly with PPAR-γ (Aggarwal, 2010). Several clinical studies performed on humans have shown the safety aspects of curcumin. But the major obstacle in development of curcumin capsules is its poor absorption, rapid excretion, and low bioavailability which limit its therapeutic potential (Shehzad, Khan, & Sup-Lee, 2012).

Table 2. Mechanism of functional foods in combating obesity and its associated disorders

Source	Active Compound	Functional Affect	Mechanism of Action	Reference
Blue Berry, Apple, Grapes	Anthocyanin	Lipase inhibitor	Prevent fat digestion and absorption in the intestine	Tsuda, (2008)
Red Chilli Pepper	Capsiacin	Anti-oxidant, antibesity, anti- inflammatory, and anticancer activity	Inhibit the expression of MCP-1, IL-6, TNF-α; inactivation of NF-kB and C-Jun amino-terminal kinase pathway by activation of PPAR-γ.	Kang et al., (2007); Rayalam et al., (2008)
Ginger	6-Shogaol	Anti-inflammatory	Inhibits the expression of TNF-α in adipocytes	Isa et al., (2008)
Grandfir, Lodgepole Pine	Abetic acid, and Dehydroabetic acid	Anti-inflammatory, anti-diabetic, anti- hyper cholesteremic, and antitumoral activities	Suppress the expression of MCP-1, TNF- α and activation of PPAR-γ	Tsuchida et al., (2005)
Green Tea	Catechin, and Epigallocatechin-3-gallate	Antioxidant, anti-inflammatory, anti-obesity, anti-diabetic, reduced risk of hypertension and cardiovascular diseases, decrease in atherosclerosis, prevention of colorectal and liver cancer.	down regulate the signaling pathways related to Ras and P13 kinase; inhibiting the activity of IGF-1, IGF-2, TNF-α, IL-6, IL-1β, IL-18.	Yasuda et al., (2009); Qin et al., (2010); Shimizu et al., (2011)
Turmeric	Curcumin	Treatment of chronic inflammation associated with obesity, diabetes, and atherosclerosis	Prevent the activation of inflammatory cytokines such as TNF-α, IL-1, IL-6; inhibit the activity of cyclooxygenase, and lipoxygenase	Aggarwal, (2010); Shehzad et al., (2012)
Nuts, Oils, and Flax Seeds	Conjugated linoleic acid	Anti-obesity and prevention of cardiovascular diseases	Decrease the concentration of LDL by inhibiting the activity of C-AMP	Dauchy et al., (2003)
Fish Oil (ω-3 PUFA)	DHA and EPA	Anti-inflammatory	Activation of G-protein receptor 120 on macrophages helps in inactivation of TNF-α, IL-6, MCP-1, and lipopolysaccharides receptors present on macrophages	Oh et al., (2010)
Psyllium Seeds	Psyllium fiber	Increase satiety levels, decrease glycemic index	Prevents the secretion of digestive enzymes by altering gut hormones, decreased absorption of glucose	Slavin, (2005)
Grape Skin	Resveratrol, Vitisin-A	Anti-inflammatory, anti-adipogenic, anti- cholesterolemic antioxidant and anticancer effect	Inhibit the activity of TNF-α, NF-kB by preventing the expression of TLR 2/4, HMG-CoA and cyclooxygenase	Kim et al., (2011); Kumar and Sharma, (2010); Koom et al., (2008)
Milk, Yoghurt, and Cheese	Dietary calcium	Regulate body weight by decreasing body fat	Calcium forms fatty acid soaps in the intestine which reduces fat absorption; enhance lipolysis in adipocytes	Zemel and Miller, (2004)

continued on following page

Table 2. Continued

Source	Active Compound	Functional Affect	Mechanism of Action	Reference
Exoskeleton of Crustace, Cell Wall of Fungi	Chitosan	Reducing fat and cholesterol absorption	Positively charged chitosan binds to negatively bile acid and prevents fat digestion	Ikeda et al., (1993)
Cheese, Milk, Asparagus, Fish and Chicken	Carnitine	Remove excess fat and fatty acids	Promote β-oxidation of fatty acids to form acetyl CoA	Cha, (2008)
Vigna Mungo	Non-digestible fibers, proteins, and amino acids	Increase satiety levels, decrease glycemic index, prevents insulin resistance associated with type 2 diabetes	-	Duranti, (2006)
Emblica Officinalis	Vitamin C, minerals, and amino acids	Anti-inflammatory, diuretic, antioxidant, antihyper cholesterolemic, prevention of atherosclerosis and cardiovascular diseases	Increase in PPAR-α, reduce the levels of total cholesterol, LDL, triglycerides	Bhandari and Kamdod, (2010)
Lagenaria Siceraria	Vitamins, minerals, fibers and other essential nutrients	Anti-inflammatory, anti-hyperlipidemic, antioxidant, and anti-hyperglycemic activity; reduces total cholesterol, triglycerides, LDL levels	-	Katare et al., (2011)
Trigonella Foenum Graecum	Steroidal sapogenins; galactomannans, and isoleucine	Anti-hypercholesterolemia, decreases the glycemic index by decrease in glucose absorption, decrease levels of LDL, triglycerides	Sapogenins increase the levels of cholesterol excreting enzymes and increase insulin receptors	Basch et al.,(2003)
Probiotics	Lactobacillus, Bifidobacteria species	Anti-hyperglycemic, anti-inflammatory, anti-allergic, decrease glycemic index, promote satiety levels, increase SCFA, produce bacteriocins.	Stimulate GLP-1 which induce β- cells of pancreas to release insulin and promote glucose tolerance	Rijkers et al., (2010)
Prebiotics	Oligosaccharides (Malto,gluco,galacto, arabino, xylo, fructo, human milk) and inulin	Promote the growth of probiotic bacteria, increase satiety levels, enhance production of SCFA, maintain gut homeostasis	SCFA mediated activation of G-protein receptor 41, 43, and 109a which helps in secretion of gut satiety hormone PYY and GLP-1; activation of β-cells of pancreas	Kimura et al., (2014)

Abbreviations: Tumor necrosis factor-TNF; Interleukin-IL; Insulin like growth factor-IGF; Phosphatidylinositol 3-kinase-PI3K; monocyte chemo attractant protein-MCP; nuclear factors (NF)-kB; Toll-like receptor-TLR; Short chain fatty acid-SCFA; Low density lipoproteins-LDL; Adenosine triphosphate-ATP; Docosahexanoic acid-DHA; Eicosapentaenoic acid-EPA; Glucagon like peptide-GLP; Peptide YY-PYY; Peroxisome proliferator-activated receptor-PPAR; Hydroxymethylglutaryl-Coenzyme A-HMG Co. A.

Conjugated Linoleic Acid (CLA)

CLA is rich in nuts, oils, flax seeds and poultry eggs. It is sensitive to temperature as a result it should be consumed directly in the form of salad dressing. Consumption of CLA decreases the concentration of LDL in comparison to HDL by lowering the plasma triacylglycerol via decrease in very low density lipoprotein or apo-lipoprotein B. Fatty acid uptake was inhibited in rodents when fed with CLA, melatonin and eicosapentanoic acid (EPA) (Dauchy, Blask, Sauer, Davidson, Krause, Smith, & Dauchy, 2003). The activity of cyclic-AMP (adenosine monophosphate) was inhibited by CLA and melatonin which promoted the uptake of fat as major source of energy. Administration of CLA to high fat diet rodents prevented the onset of obesity induced insulin resistance (Dyck, 2000). Further studies on humans need to be performed to evaluate the exact mechanism by which CLA helps in weight management.

Poly Unsaturated Fatty Acid (PUFA)

Fatty acids play a vital role in regulating inflammatory response. Saturated fatty acids promote inflammation by activating toll-like receptor (TLR)-4 and macrophages. While, unsaturated fatty acids display pro-inflammatory response (Shi, Kokoeva, Inouye, Tzameli, Yin, & Flier, 2006). Omega-3 PUFA produced from fish oil has docosahexanoic acid (DHA) and eicosapentaenoic acid (EPA) which show anti-inflammatory response (Batetta, Griinari, Carta, Murru, Ligresti, Cordeddu… Banni, 2009). DHA and EPA activates G-protein receptor (GPR) 120 present on macrophages and fat cells of adipose tissue to inactivate TNF-α, IL-6, MCP-1, and lipopolysaccharides present on macrophages (Oh, Talukdar, Bae, Imamura, Morinaga, Fan…Olefsky, 2010). Activated GPR 120 induces insulin sensitization by repressing macrophage induced inflammation. Omega-3 PUFA mediated activation of PPAR-γ prevented the chronic inflammation of adipose tissue caused by obesity or high fat diet (Todoric, Löffler, Huber, Bilban, Reimers, Kadl…Stulnig, 2006).

Psyllium Fiber

The fiber is extracted from the husk of the psyllium seeds. Psyllium helps delay gastric emptying. The fiber promotes satiety by expanding in the intestine and decrease glucose absorption. The fiber has low glycemic index which help in decreasing the postprandial insulin and glycemic response. The fiber alters the secretion of gut hormones and inhibits the action of digestive enzymes. It also decreases the levels of total cholesterol and LDL levels in humans by decreasing the adipocytes (FAO, 2010; Slavin, 2005).

Momordica Charantia (MC)

It helps in reduction of adipocytes, and inflammatory mediators released by adipocytes (TNF-α, IL-6). It promotes the breakdown of lipids by hepatic enzymes such as glutathione S-transferase and increases the levels of cytochrome P-450 helps in decreasing the levels of triglycerides (Irizar, Barnett, Flatt, & Ioannides, 1995). Consumption of MC along with regular exercise will help in increasing insulin sensitivity (Miura, Itoh, Iwamoto, Kato, & Ishida, 2004).

Vigna Mungo

It is commonly known as black gram. Generally grain legumes are considered as important source of proteins as they are rich in non-digestible fibers, proteins, and amino acids. Frequent intake of black gram helps in regulating the lipid metabolism and significantly reduces the risk and development of cardiovascular disease. The legume has low glycemic index and comprises of some minor components like phytosterols, saponins, and oligosaccharides which further enhances its nutritional value and helps in preventing insulin resistance associated with type 2 diabetes. They also increase the satiety levels, thus help in controlling the overall bodyweight (Duranti, 2006).

Emblica Officinalis

It belongs to *Euphorbiaceae* family popularly known as Amla. It is a rich source of vitamin C, minerals, and amino acids. Amla has been reported to exhibit anti-inflammatory, diuretic, antioxidant, anti-hypercholesterolemic effects. It is also used in the treatment of peptic ulcer. Consumption of amla has significantly reduced the cholesterol, and triacylglyceride levels in serum and liver. Apart from the above it also increases the levels of PPAR-α in the liver. It has also shown to reduce the levels of total cholesterol, LDL, and triglycerides. Thus helps in protecting against atherosclerosis and coronary heart disease (Bhandari & Kamdod, 2010).

Langenaria Siceraria

It is popularly known as bottle gourd which belongs to Cucurbitaceae family. It is a rich source of vitamins, minerals, fibers and other essential nutrients which show anti-inflammatory, anti-hyperlipidemic, antioxidant, and anti-hyperglycemic activity. It also reduces total cholesterol, triglycerides, low density lipoproteins and increases the level of high density lipoproteins (Katare, Agrawal, Jain, Rani, Saxena, Prakash, & Godavarthi, 2011).

Trigonella Foenum Graecum (TFG)

TFG is commonly known as fenugreek which is quite popular in India and North African countries. It comprises of: 1) steroidal sapogenins; 2) galactomannans, and; 3) isoleucine. Steroidal sapogenin is effectively used in treatment of hypercholesterolemia related to diabetes. Galactomannans are highly viscous solution which decreases the absorption of glucose in the intestine as a result it helps in controlling calorie intake and type 2 diabetes associated with obesity. Human studies have shown the reduction in serum glucose levels, increase in insulin receptors, and decrease in serum triglycerides, LDL and total cholesterol caused due to cholesterol excreting enzymes produced by sapogenins (Basch, Ulbricht, Kuo, Szapary, & Smith, 2003).

Resveratrol

It is a polyphenolic compound commonly found in the grape skin. It has been reported to prevent cardiovascular disease, cancer, inflammation, and oxidative stress. It has anti-inflammatory and anti-adipogenic effect on TNF-α induced MCP-1 expression by inhibiting NF-kB activity in adipocytes (Kim, Jin, Choi, & Park, 2011). In animal models it inhibited the NF-kB signaling pathway and prevented the expression of TLR2/4 in adipose tissue (Kumar & Sharma, 2010). In rats the vascular levels of nitric oxide was maintained by decreasing the expression of TNF-α. It plays a major role in prevention of cardiovascular diseases by inhibiting the inflammatory markers, the cyclooxygenase (COX)-1 enzyme (Szewczuk, Forti, Stivala, & Penning, 2004). Vitisin A (tetramer of resveratrol) extracted from the skin of grape trees significantly reduced the expression of lipopolysaccharide stimulated macrophages and decreased adipocytes differentiation by inhibiting PPAR-γ activation. Vitisin A has anti-inflammatory, anti-adipogenic, and anti-cholestrolemic activities (Kim, Park, Lee, Cho, Kim, Hwang… Kwon, 2008). The tetramer also inhibited the cellular levels of 3-hydroxy methyl glutaryl co enzyme A (HMG CoA) reductase which prevented the cholesterol biosynthesis. Thus, leading to decrease in serum cholesterol levels and other pro-inflammatory cytokines produced by NF-kB expression (Koo, Kim, Lee, Yoo, Ryu, Kwon, & Kim, 2008).

Calcium Rich Foods

Dietary calcium has been reported to play a major role in regulating body weight (Zemel & Miller, 2004). A wide variety of calcium rich foods are available in the market which include margarines and dairy products (milk, yoghurt, and cheese). Calcium binds with fat present in the intestine to form calcium fatty acid soaps which reduce fat absorption (Welberg, Monkelbaan, de Vries, Muskiet, Cats, Oremus…

Kleibeuker, 1994). Increase in dietary calcium reduces the concentration of 1, 2, 5-dihydroxy vitamin D which causes the down regulation of calcium transfer into adipose and pancreatic tissues. Decrease in intracellular calcium levels in adipocytes causes decrease in fatty acid synthase which results in lowering of lipogenesis and increased lipolysis. While, decrease in intracellular calcium levels in pancreas decreases insulin output and reduces lipogenesis and enhance lipolysis in adipocytes (Zemel & Miller, 2004).

FUNCTIONAL FOODS FOR OBESITY INDUCED METABOLIC DISORDERS

Chronic Inflammation and Type 2 Diabetes

It was reported that peroxisome proliferation activated receptor (PPAR)-γ, helps in attenuation of inflammation in activated macrophages by interfering NF-kB signaling pathway. Thiazolidinediones (TZDs) is a synthetic ligand for PPAR- γ, which help in suppressing pro-inflammatory cytokines such as TNF- α in stimulated macrophages. TZDs is widely used as anti-diabetic drug and helps in activation of PPAR-γ which in turn help in differentiation of adipocytes. TZDs enhance the uptake of glucose by adipocytes and induce the production of adiponectin (insulin sensitive promoting factor) which suppress the TNF-α production (Maeda, Shimomura, Kishida, Nishizawa, Matsuda, Nagaretani…Matsuzawaet, 2002). Functional foods which can act as ligand for the PPAR-γ will act as both anti-diabetic and anti-inflammatory agents. Based on the mechanism involved we can broadly divide functional foods in to PPAR-γ dependent and independent.

PPAR- γ Dependent Functional Foods

Spices derived from plant source have been reported for their antioxidant, anticancer, anti-obesity, and anti-inflammatory activities. The anti-inflammatory compounds produced by the spices helps in regulating the inflammation in adipose tissue and thus improve obesity related pathology and insulin resistance (Kang, Kim, Han, Kawada, & Yu, 2007).

a. Capsaicin

It is produced by red chili pepper which induces oxidation of fat and thermogenesis. It was reported that capsaicin (8-25 mM per day), inhibits the expression and secretion of IL-6, TNF-α, and MCP-1 in adipose tissue and adipocytes of obese mice. Thereby inducing thermogenesis and fat oxidation. It enhances the production of adiponectin and inactivation of NF-kB pathway mediated by activation of PPAR-γ (Kang, Kim, Han, Kawada, & Yu, 2007). Capsaicin prevents the migration of macrophages in to adipocytes but also produce proinflammatory cytokines which help in prevention of insulin resistance.

b. Ginger

It is a rhizome plant (*Zingiber officinale Roscoe*), which belongs to Zingiberaceae family and it produces 6-Shogaol compound which has anti-inflammatory activity. As it is a potent agonist for PPAR-γ which enhances the expression of adiponectin and inhibits the expression of TNF-α in adipocytes (Isa, Miyakawa, Yanagisawa, Goto, Kang, Kawada, Morimitsu, Kubota, & Tsuda, 2008). Isoprenoids (terpenoid) such as abietic acid (AA), and dehydroabetic acid (DAA) produced mainly by herbal plants grandfir (*Abies grandis*) and lodgepole pine (*Pinus contorta*) display anti-inflammatory, anti-diabetic, anti-hypercholesteremic, and antitumoral activities (Aranda & Villalain 1997). It was reported that AA show anti-inflammatory effect on macrophage mediated by activation of PPAR-γ. While, DAA has been reported to suppress the expression of MCP-1, TNF-α and prevents the infiltration of macrophages into adipocytes by increased production of adiponectin. DAA strongly activate PPAR-γ which is involved in lipid metabolism (Tsuchida, Yamauchi, Takekawa, Hada, Ito, Maki, & Kadowaki, 2005). Auraptene (monoterpene derived from citrus fruit) is a dual agonist of PPAR α/γ and regulate the expression of PPAR-γ genes and induces the secretion of adiponectin which inhibit the MCP-1 (Kuroyanagi, Kang, Goto, Hirai, Ohyama, Kusudo…Kawada, 2008). It also prevents the infiltration of macrophages into the adipocytes while the co-application of PPAR α/γ treatment causes efficient glucose uptake in adipocyte and decrease the blood glucose levels without increase in bodyweight (Tsuchida, Yamauchi, Takekawa, Hada, Ito, Maki, & Kadowaki, 2005).

PPAR-γ Independent Functional Foods

Flavanoids are the plant metabolites comprising of C6-C3-and C6 structure. Most of the flavonoids are metabolized to flavone, dihydroflavonol, flavanol, leucoanthocyanidin, catechin, and anthocyanin by oxidation and reduction reactions. These flavonoids have anti-inflammatory, antitumor, and antioxidant activities. Recently, luteolin a flavone inhibited the chronic inflammation of adipocytes and macrophages. It inhibits the phosphorylation of c-Jun N-terminal kinase (JNK) in the macrophages derived from adipocytes (Ando, Takahashi, Hirai, Nishimura, Lin, Uemura…Kawada, 2009). Luteolin may affect directly or indirectly via a PPAR-γ independent mechanism.

Similar effect was reported in naringenin flavaonol which is abundant in tomato and citrus fruits. Anthocyanin flavonoids found in grapes, blueberries, apple, and beans are rich in anti-oxidants and anti-inflammatory activity in obese adipose tissue. Cyanidin 3-glucoside induces improvement in insulin sensitivity may also inhibit inflammatory mediators (Tsuda, 2008). The 6-Gingerol is a derivative of ginger and it has been reported to inhibit TNF-α mediated suppression of adiponectin in adipocytes by affecting JNK pathway in TNF-α induced adipocytes (Isa, Miyakawa, Yanagisawa, Goto, Kang, Kawada, Morimitsu, Kubota, & Tsuda, 2008). Unlike saturated fatty acids which promote inflammatory response in macrophages, the long chain ω-3 polyunsaturated fatty acids (PUFA) such as docosahexaenoic acid (DHA) and eicosapentaenoic acid (EPA) has been reported for their anti-obesity and anti-inflammatory property (Stulnig, 2003). Fish oil has been reported to be rich in DHA and EPA. As PUFA requires many cofactors such as folic acid, vitamins, minerals and other essential components for their activity (Das, 2003).

Obesity Induced Colorectal Cancer (CRC)

Tea can be generally grouped in to three main types black, oolong, and green tea. Among them the green tea (*Camelia sinensis*) is one of the most popular beverage consumed worldwide and its medical properties have been studied extensively. Green tea is rich in polyphenol compounds such as catechin, and epigallocatechin-3-gallate (EGCG) which play a vital role in combating and prevention of several chronic diseases including heart, neurodegenerative and cancer. Studies conducted on rodent model suffering with obesity and diabetes showed a significant decrease in bodyweight and improved hyper insulinemia, hyperglycemia, hyperleptimia, hepatic steratosis, and liver dysfunction (Bose, Lambert, Ju, Reuhl, Shapses, & Yang, 2008). Plasma levels of insulin, TNF-α, and IL-6 were decreased in mouse model (Qin, Polansky, Harry, & Anderson, 2010). Several studies have shown the antioxidant, anti-inflammatory, anti-cancer effects of green tea catechins (GTCs) and EGCG (Figure 2). It was reported that EGCG inhibit the proliferation and development of cancer cells by modulating the activity of different receptor tyrosine kinase (RTK) and down regulating the signaling pathways related to Ras and P13 kinase. EGCG also suppress the growth of CRC and HCC cells by inhibiting the activity of IGR-1R. It also decreases the expression of IGF1/2 and prevents the expression of hepatic fibrosis induced by carbon tetrachloride mediated by inhibition of IGF-1R expression (Yasuda, Shimizu, Sakai, Iwasa, Kubota, Adachi, Osawa, Tsurumi, Hara, & Moriwaki, 2009).

Figure 2. Role of green tea (catechine, and epigallocatechin-3-gallate (EGCG)) in prevention of (a) colorectal cancer and; (b) hepatocellular carcinoma (Tumor necrosis factor-TNF; Interleukin-IL; Insulin like growth factor-IGF; Glycogen synthase kinase-GSK)

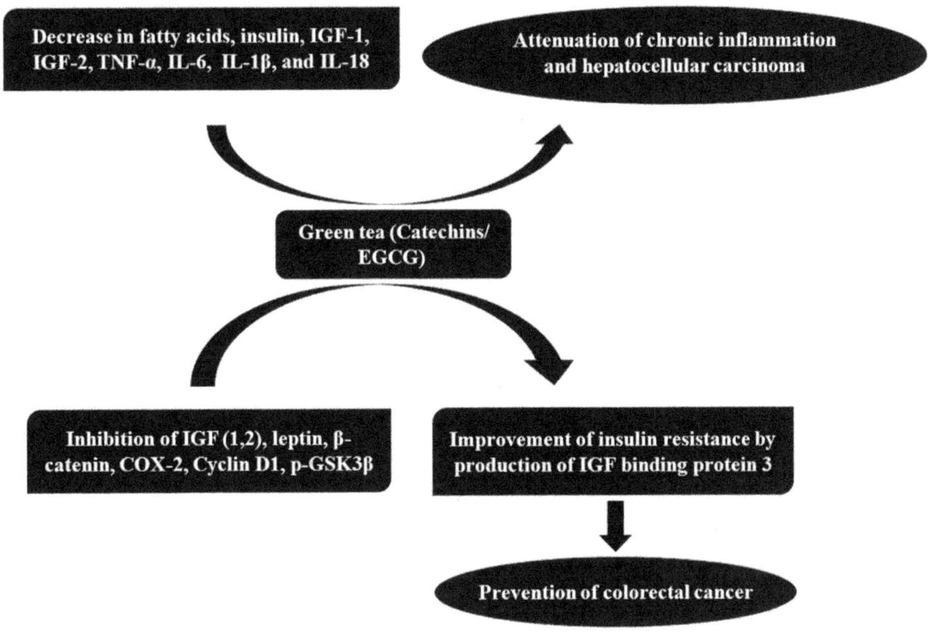

Hepatocellular Carcinogenesis (HCC)

EGCG is the major component of green tea which plays a vital role in inhibiting hepatic adenoma, and hepatic steatosis (Figure 2). Consumption of green tea rich in EGCG decreased the serum levels of free fatty acids, insulin, IGF-1, IGF-2, TNF-α, IL-6, IL-1β, IL-18, and causes the phosphorylation of IGF-1R in the liver and prevented the obesity related liver tumorigenesis (Shimizu, Sakai, Shirakami, Yasuda, Kubota, Terakura…Moriwak, 2011).

Cardiovascular Disorders (CVD)

Green tea (*Camellia sinensis*) is one of the most popular beverages consumed worldwide. It comprises of xanthine bases (Caffeine, and theophylline), essential oils, and polyphenols or flavonoids (Catechins, and EGCG). The medicinal and pharmacological properties of green tea have been studied extensively. Consumption of green tea (120 ml/day) by older women in China has significantly reduced the risk of developing hypertension. It was reported that administration of green tea is inversely related to the development of atherosclerosis (Bose, Lambert, Ju, Reuhl, Shapses, & Yang, 2008).

Diet rich in antioxidants, PUFA, polyphenols, flavonoids, and dietary fibers along with regular physical activity (exercise) helps in reducing the risk associated with CVD (Hu & Willett, 2002). Flavonoids were found to be highly effective in treatment of CVD by blocking the angiotensin converting enzymes which raise the blood pressure by blocking the suicide enzyme cyclooxygenase that hydrolyze prostaglandins, and helps in prevention of platelet aggregation (Hollman, Hertog, & Katan, 1996). Flavanoids also protect the vascular system and strengthen the capillaries which carry oxygen and other essential nutrients to all the cells (Cook & Sammam, 1996). Green tea rich in flavonoids (EGCG, and catechins) has been reported to reduce the risk associated with CVD. Epigallocatechin-3-gallate (EGCG) present in green tea inhibits the oxidation of LDL-cholesterol. While green tea rich in catechins significantly reduced body weight and fat among individuals suffering with obesity as compared to normal individuals by improvement of systolic blood pressure and decrease in LDL cholesterol levels (Saetan, Grove, & Lambert, 2011). Consumption of green tea (>6 cups per day) rich in EGCG has significantly decreased the plasma glucose and fructosamine levels in patients suffering with type 2 diabetes. Green tea catechins and EGCG has been proven for their anti-obesity, anti-inflammatory, antioxidant, anti-diabetic in both animals and humans (Rains, Agarwal, & Maki, 2011).

OTHER FUNCTIONAL FOODS

Chitosan

It is the exoskeleton of crustacean and is present in cell wall of fungi. It is a soluble dietary fiber produced by de-acetylation of chitin. It helps in delayed gastric emptying and inhibit uptake of lipids by increase in thickness of lumen of the intestine. Chitosan is positively charged due to the presence of less acetyl groups therefore it binds to negatively charged bile acids. Thus, inhibit the circulation of bile acid as a result fat is not digested thereby reducing fat and cholesterol absorption (Ikeda, Sugano, Yoshida, Sasaki, Iwamoto, & Hatano, 1993).

Carnitine

It is a quaternary ammonium compound synthesized from the amino acids lysine and methionine. It is present several foods such as cheese, milk, asparagus, fish and chicken. Carnitine helps in β-oxidation of fatty acids in the mitochondrial matrix to form acetyl Coenzyme A, to obtain energy from citric acid cycle. It also helps in removing excess fat and fatty acids, increase muscle mass and reduce fatigue. Thus all the above factors contribute in weight loss (Cha, 2008).

Niacin Bound Chromium (NBC)

NBC helps in regulating appetite and energy production. A human study performed using 400 and 600 mg of NBC for two months along with regular exercise has significantly reduced the body fat sparing the muscle. This study also demonstrated an improved insulin response to oral administered glucose (Perricone, Bagchi, Echard, & Preuss, 2010).

Probiotics

Human gut is populated with a wide variety of bacterial species which play a vital role in metabolic and immune function. Dysbiosis in the population of *Firmicutes* to *Bacteroides* causes obesity and type-1 diabetes. Increase in population of proteobacteria in the intestine causes type 2 diabetes (Figure 3). Gut microbiota influence the host metabolism in two possible pathways: 1) Extracting energy and nutrients from the food, and; 2) Effecting the gene expression level of host which are involved in energy metabolism. Probiotics are defined as live microbial supplements

Figure 3. Dysbiosis of intestinal bacteria causing obesity and diabetes

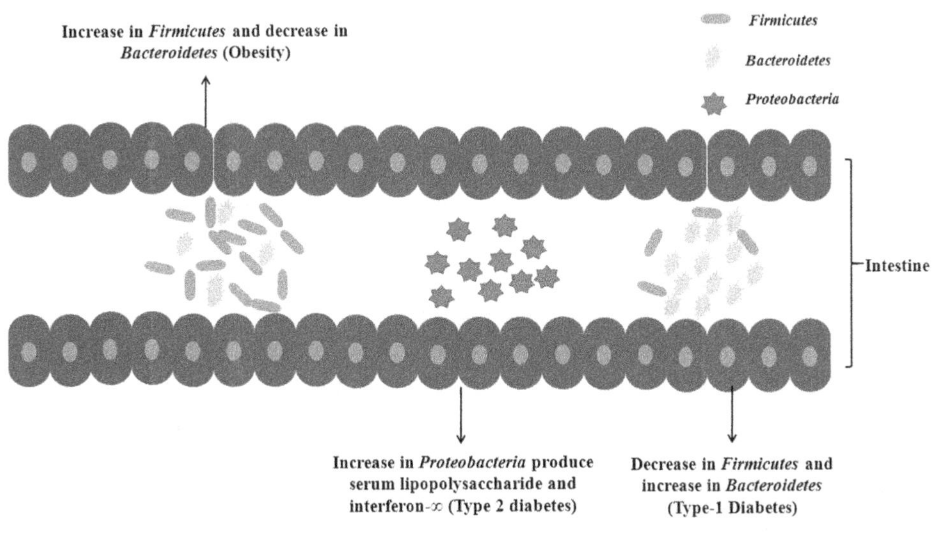

which upon ingestion provide health benefit beyond inherent basic nutrition (De verse & Schrezenmeir, 2008). Numerous probiotic microorganisms belonging to *Lactobacillus* and *Bifidobacterial* species are potent in regulating obesity by reducing the levels of LDL and cholesterol (Kobyliak, Conte, Cammarota, Haley, Styriak, Gaspar, Fusek, Rodrigo, & Kruzliak, 2016). VSL#3, is a probiotic mixture comprising of eight live bacterial species which include four strains of *Lactobacillus* (*Lactobacillus casei, Lb. plantarum, Lb. acidophilus, Lb. dulbrueckii subsp. Bulgaricus),* three strains of *Bifidobacteria (Bifidobacterium longum, Bi. Breve, Bi. Infantis*), and *Streptococcus salivarius subsp. Thermophilus* which is helpful in regulating obesity by producing SCFA. The SCFA produced by the probiotic bacteria stimulate the release of glucagon like peptide (GLP-1) a potent anti-hyperglycemic hormone and induce the β cells of pancreas to release insulin in response to glucose levels, promote satiety and improve glucose tolerance (Yadav, Lee, Lloyd, Walter, & Rane, 2013; Kimura, Inoue, Hirano, & Tsujimoto, 2014). Probiotics influence the human health by altering the intestinal microbiota. The concentration of probiotics required to show clinical effect in small intestine is $\geq 10^6$ colony forming unit (cfu) per milliliter and in colon is $\geq 10^8$ cfu/gram. Probiotics plays a vital role in treatment of several metabolic, chronic intestinal inflammation, infections, and allergy (Rijkers, Bengmark, Enck, Haller, Herz, Kalliomaki…Antoine, 2010).

Prebiotics

These are non-digestible yet fermentable carbohydrates which allow specific changes, both in the composition and/or activity in the gastrointestinal microflora to confer benefits upon host wellbeing and health (Gibson, Probert, van Loo, Rastall, & Roberfroid, 2004). To be considered as prebiotic, the compound must show resistance to human digestive enzymes such as salivary, pancreatic amylases, and gastric juice to reach the colon without degradation or alteration (Vitali, Ndagijimana, Maccaferri, Biagi, Guerzoni, & Brigidi, 2012). Prebiotic components are fermented by specific enzymes produced bacteria present in the intestine and promote the growth of probiotic bacteria which inhibit the growth of pathogenic bacteria by producing bacteriocins and short chain fatty acids (Broekaert, Courtin, Verbeke, Vandewiele, Verstraete, & Delcour, 2011). Currently available prebiotic ingredients in the market are inulin, and wide variety of malto, fructo, galacto, arabino, arabinoxylan and human milk oligosaccharides respectively (Younis, Ahmad, & Jahan, 2015). The consumption of prebiotics has been associated with reduced risks diarrhea caused due to intestinal infections; prevention of osteoporosis by promoting the uptake of calcium; lowered threats of obesity and Type 2 diabetes; neutralization of toxic products and decreased frequency of colon cancer; stimulation of immunity and protection of the urogenital system (Yasmin, Butt, Afzaal, van Baak, Nadeem, &

Shahid, 2015). With increase in awareness and growing demand the market value of prebiotic ingredients is expected to reach U.S $ 5.5 million by 2020 (Market and Standard Market, 2015). The increase in SCFA levels by the probiotic bacteria mediated by fermentation of prebiotic ingredients in the colon are sensed by G-protein coupled receptor present on the surface of colonocytes, liver and skeletal muscle and activates G-protein receptors (GPR 41, 43 and 109a). GPR 43 promotes the L cells of gastrointestinal tract to secrete the gut satiety hormones peptide YY (PYY) and glucagon like peptide-1 (GLP-1). The levels of PYY increases during food ingestion, while GLP-1 act as potent anti-hyperglycemic hormone and induces the β-cells of pancreas to release insulin in response to rise in glucose levels (Kimura, Inoue, Hirano, & Tsujimoto, 2014).

Synbiotics

These are the synergistic combination of both pro and prebiotics (De verse & Schrezenmeir, 2008). Regular consumption of probiotics or prebiotics either individually or in combination helps in maintaining the gut health and wellbeing of humans. Prebiotics provides the nutrients required for the growth of probiotic bacteria, while probiotic bacteria modulate the host immune system by affecting other microorganisms directly or indirectly by producing SCFA, bacteroicins, and by competitive inhibition strategy (Oelschlaeger, 2010).

FUTURE RESEARCH DIRECTIONS

Obesity occurs due to defect in various complex pathways. As a result there is a great need to target different markers involved in obesity. The current research available so far highlights the potential application of functional foods in treatment of metabolic disorders associated with obesity. But the real challenge for the food industry is to develop products that are effective and sensitive enough to target multiple mechanisms. Lack of potential biomarkers to test the efficacy of the compounds is the biggest challenge in developing the functional foods for obesity and its associated metabolic disorders. Current studies involved in development of function food ingredients should focus on determining the optimum level of intake, efficacy and safety of products for long-term consumption. Although many of these functional foods have been found to have high therapeutic potential, future studies must include well-designed clinical trials assessing different combinations of these nutrients to enhance the possible additive and/or synergistic effects on human health and wellbeing.

CONCLUSION

Obesity has become epidemic across the world affecting adults and children in equal proportion. With change in lifestyle, and food habits individuals are becoming more prone to cardiovascular and obesity associated disorders which are known to be silent killers. Researchers have understood the importance of functional foods in prevention, restriction and cure of various diseases is undeniable. The success rate of functional foods greatly depends on their purity, safety and efficacy. The information available currently on the application of established and emerging functional foods pose a challenge for nutritionists, physicians, food technologists, plant physiologists and public health personnel. The role of functional foods in clinical practice is still emerging. Long term clinical research is required to scientifically validate their role in different diseases. With a little bit of careful handling, the future of both plant and animal origin functional foods holds exciting opportunities in the medical field.

REFERENCES

Aasheim, E. T., Hofso, D., Hjelmesaeth, J., Birkeland, K. I., & Bohmer, T. (2008). Vitamin status in morbidly obese patients: A cross-sectional study. *The American Journal of Clinical Nutrition, 87*(2), 362–369. doi:10.1093/ajcn/87.2.362 PMID:18258626

Aggarwal, B. B. (2010). Targeting inflammation-induced obesity and metabolic diseases by curcumin and other nutraceuticals. *Annual Review of Nutrition, 21*(30), 173–199. doi:10.1146/annurev.nutr.012809.104755 PMID:20420526

Ando, C., Takahashi, N., Hirai, S., Nishimura, K., Lin, S., Uemura, T., ... Kawada, T. (2009). Luteolin, a food derived flavonoid, suppresses adipocyte-dependent activation of macrophages by inhibiting JNK activation. *FEBS Letters, 583*(22), 3649–3654. doi:10.1016/j.febslet.2009.10.045 PMID:19854181

Aranda, F. J., & Villala, J. (1997). The interaction of abietic acid with phospholipid membranes. *Biochimica et Biophysica Acta, 1327*(2), 171–180. doi:10.1016/S0005-2736(97)00054-0 PMID:9271259

Barb, D., Williams, C. J., Neuwirth, A. K., & Mantzoros, C. S. (2007). Adiponectin in relation to malignancies: A review of existing basic research and clinical evidence. *The American Journal of Clinical Nutrition, 86*(3), s858–s866. doi:10.1093/ajcn/86.3.858S PMID:18265479

Basch, E., Ulbricht, C., Kuo, G., Szapary, P., & Smith, M. (2003). Therapeutic applications of fenugreek. *Alternative Medicine Review*, *8*(1), 20–27. PMID:12611558

Batetta, B., Griinari, M., Carta, G., Murru, E., Ligresti, A., Cordeddu, L., ... Banni, S. (2009). Endo-cannabinoids may mediate the ability of (n-3) fatty acids to reduce ectopic fat and inflammatory mediators in obese Zucker rats. *The Journal of Nutrition*, *139*(8), 1495–1501. doi:10.3945/jn.109.104844 PMID:19549757

Berthoud, H. R., Lenard, N. R., & Shin, A. C. (2011). Food reward, hyperphagia, and obesity. *American Journal of Physiology. Regulatory, Integrative and Comparative Physiology*, *300*(6), R1266–R1277. doi:10.1152/ajpregu.00028.2011 PMID:21411768

Bhandari, P. R., & Kamdod, M. A. (2012). *Emblica officicalis* (Amla): A review on potential therapeutic applications. *International Journal of Green Pharmacy*, *6*(4), 257–269. doi:10.4103/0973-8258.108204

Bose, M., Lambert, J. D., Ju, J., Reuhl, K. R., Shapses, S. A., & Yang, C. S. (2008). The major green tea polyphenol, (-)-epigallocatechin-3-gallate, inhibits obesity, metabolic syndrome, and fatty liver disease in high-fat-fed mice. *The Journal of Nutrition*, *138*(9), 1677–1683. doi:10.1093/jn/138.9.1677 PMID:18716169

Broekaert, W. F., Courtin, C. M., Verbeke, K., Vandewiele, T., Verstraete, W., & Delcour, J. A. (2011). Prebiotic and other health-related effects of cereal-derived arabinoxylans, arabinoxylan-oligosaccharides, and xylooligosaccharides. *Critical Reviews in Food Science and Nutrition*, *51*(2), 178–194. doi:10.1080/10408390903044768 PMID:21328111

Bruun, J. M., Lihn, A. S., Pedersen, S. B., & Richelsen, B. (2005). Monocyte chemoattractant protein-1 release is higher in visceral than subcutaneous human adipose tissue (AT): Implication of macrophages resident in the AT. *The Journal of Clinical Endocrinology and Metabolism*, *90*(4), 2282–2289. doi:10.1210/jc.2004-1696 PMID:15671098

Cencic, A., & Chingwaru, W. (2010). The role of functional foods, nutraceuticals, and food supplements in intestinal health. *Nutrients*, *2*(6), 611–625. doi:10.3390/nu2060611 PMID:22254045

Cha, Y. S. (2008). Effects of l-carnitine on obesity, diabetes, and as an ergogenic aid. *Asia Pacific Journal of Clinical Nutrition*, *17*(1), 306–308. PMID:18296364

Chang, C. K., & Ulrich, C. M. (2003). Hyperinsulinaemia and hyperglycaemia: Possible risk factors of colorectal cancer among diabetic patients. *Diabetologia*, *46*(5), 595–607. doi:10.100700125-003-1109-5 PMID:12764580

Chrysohoou, C., Panagiotakos, D. B., Pitsavos, C., Skoumas, I., Papademetriou, L., Economou, M., & Stefanadis, C. (2007). The implication of obesity on total antioxidant capacity in apparently healthy men and women: The ATTICA study. *Nutrition, Metabolism, and Cardiovascular Diseases*, *17*(8), 590–597. doi:10.1016/j.numecd.2006.05.007 PMID:16901682

Clayton, P. E., Banerjee, I., Murray, P. G., & Renehan, A. G. (2011). Growth hormone, the insulin-like growth factor axis, insulin and cancer risk. *Nature Reviews. Endocrinology*, *7*(1), 11–24. doi:10.1038/nrendo.2010.171 PMID:20956999

Cook, N. C., & Samman, S. (1996). Flavonoids - Chemistry, metabolism, cardioprotective effects, and dietary sources. *The Journal of Nutritional Biochemistry*, *7*(2), 66–76. doi:10.1016/0955-2863(95)00168-9

Dao, H. H., Frelut, M. L., Oberlin, F., Peres, G., Bourgeois, P., & Navarro, J. (2004). Effects of a multidisciplinary weight loss intervention on body composition in obese adolescents. *International Journal of Obesity and Related Metabolic Disorders*, *28*(2), 290–299. doi:10.1038j.ijo.0802542 PMID:14970838

Das, U. N. (2003). Folic acid says NO to vascular diseases. *Nutrition (Burbank, Los Angeles County, Calif.)*, *19*(7-8), 686–692. doi:10.1016/S0899-9007(02)01044-4 PMID:12831960

Dauchy, R. T., Blask, D. E., Sauer, L. A., Davidson, L. K., Krause, J. A., Smith, L. C., & Dauchy, E. M. (2003). Physiologic melatonin concentration, omega-3-fatty acids, and conjugated linoleic acid inhibit fatty acid transport in rodent hind limb skeletal muscle in vivo. *Comparative Medicine*, *53*(2), 186–190. PMID:12784853

De vrese, M., & Schrezenmeir, J. (2008). Probiotics, prebiotics, and synbiotics. In *Advances in Biochemical Engineering and Biotechnology: Food Biotechnology* (pp. 1-66). Springer Publishing.

Duranti, M. (2006). Grain legume proteins and nutraceutical properties. *Fitoterapia*, *77*(2), 67–82. doi:10.1016/j.fitote.2005.11.008 PMID:16406359

Dyck, D. J. (2000). Dietary fat intake, supplements, and weight loss. *Canadian Journal of Applied Physiology*, *25*(6), 495–523. doi:10.1139/h00-033 PMID:11187927

Feldstein, A. E., Werneburg, N. W., Canbay, A., Guicciardi, M. E., Bronk, S. F., Rydzewski, R., ... Gores, G. J. (2004). Free fatty acids promote hepatic lipotoxicity by stimulating TNF-alpha expression via a lysosomal pathway. *Hepatology (Baltimore, Md.)*, *40*(1), 185–194. doi:10.1002/hep.20283 PMID:15239102

Finkelstein, E. A., Trogdon, J. G., Cohen, J. W., & Dietz, W. (2009). Annual medical spending attributable to obesity: Payer and service-specific estimates. *Health Affairs (Project Hope)*, *28*(5), 822–831. doi:10.1377/hlthaff.28.5.w822 PMID:19635784

Food and Agriculture Organization of the United Nations. (2007). *Report on functional foods, food quality and standards service (AGNS)*. Retrieved November 25, 2007, from http://www.fao.org/ag/agn/agns/files/Functional_Foods_Report_Nov 2007.pdf

Gibson, G. R., Probert, H. M., van Loo, J. A. E., Rastall, R. A., & Roberfroid, M. B. (2004). Dietary modulation of the human colonic microbiota: Updating the concept of prebiotics. *Nutrition Research Reviews*, *17*(2), 259–275. doi:10.1079/NRR200479 PMID:19079930

Hil, J. O., & Peters, J. C. (2002). Biomarkers and functional foods for obesity and diabetes. *British Journal of Nutrition*, *88*(2), 213–218. doi:10.1079/BJN2002685 PMID:12495462

Hirai, S., Takahashi, N., Goto, T., Lin, S., Uemura, T., Yu, R., & Kawada, T. (2010). Functional food targeting the regulation of obesity-induced inflammatory responses and pathologies. *Mediators of Inflammation. Article ID, 367838*. doi:10.1155/2010/367838

Hollman, P. C. H., Hertog, M. G. L., & Katan, M. B. (1996). Analysis and health effects of flavonoids. *Food Chemistry*, *57*(1), 43–46. doi:10.1016/0308-8146(96)00065-9

Hotamisligil, G. S., Peraldi, P., Budavari, A., Ellis, R., White, M. F., & Spiegelman, B. M. (1996). IRS-1-mediated inhibition of insulin receptor tyrosine kinase activity in TNF-alpha- and obesity-induced insulin resistance. *Science*, *271*(5249), 665–668. doi:10.1126cience.271.5249.665 PMID:8571133

Hotamisligil, G. S., Shargill, N. S., & Spiegelman, B. M. (1993). Adipose expression of tumor necrosis factor-α: Direct role I obesity-linked insulin resistance. *Science*, *259*(5091), 87–91. doi:10.1126cience.7678183 PMID:7678183

Ikeda, I., Sugano, M., Yoshida, K., Sasaki, E., Iwamoto, Y., & Hatano, K. (1993). Effects of chitosan hydrolyzates on lipid absorption and on serum and liver lipid concentration in rats. *Journal of Agricultural and Food Chemistry*, *41*(3), 431–435. doi:10.1021/jf00027a016

Irizar, A., Barnett, C. R., Flatt, P. R., & Ioannides, C. (1995). Defective expression of cytochrome P450 proteins in the liver of the genetically obese Zucker rat. *European Journal of Pharmacology*, *293*(4), 385–393. doi:10.1016/0926-6917(95)90059-4 PMID:8748692

Isa, Y., Miyakawa, Y., Yanagisawa, M., Goto, T., Kang, M. S., Kawada, T., ... Tsuda, T. (2008). 6-Shogaol and 6-gingerol, the pungent of ginger, inhibit TNF-α mediated down regulation of adiponectin expression via different mechanisms in 3T3-L1 adipocytes. *Biochemical and Biophysical Research Communications*, *373*(3), 429–434. doi:10.1016/j.bbrc.2008.06.046 PMID:18577375

Iyer, A., Panchal, S., Poudyal, H., & Brown, L. (2009). Potential health benefits of Indian spices in the symptoms of the metabolic syndrome: A review. *Indian Journal of Biochemistry & Biophysics*, *46*(6), 467–481. PMID:20361710

Kajantie, E., Fall, C. H., Seppälä, M., Koistinen, R., Dunkel, L., Ylihärsilä, H., ... Eriksson, J. (2003). Serum insulin-like growth factor (IGF)-I and composition, size at birth, and childhood growth. *The Journal of Clinical Endocrinology and Metabolism*, *88*(3), 1059–1065. doi:10.1210/jc.2002-021380 PMID:12629086

Kajantie, E., Fall, C. H., Seppala, M., Koistinen, R., Dunkel, L., Yliharsila, H., ... Yu, R. (2007). Capsaicin, a spicy component of hot peppers, modulates adipokine gene expression and protein release from obese mouse adipose tissues and isolated adipocytes, and suppresses the inflammatory responses of adipose tissue macrophages. *FEBS Letters*, *581*(23), 4389–4396. doi:10.1016/j.febslet.2007.07.082 PMID:17719033

Katare, C., Agrawal, S., Jain, M., Rani, S., Saxena, S., Prakash, S. B., & Godavarthi, B. K. S. P. (2011). Lagenaria siceraria: A potential source of anti-hyperlipidemic and other pharmacological agents. *Current Nutrition and Food Science*, *7*(4), 1–7. doi:10.2174/157340111804586501

Keats, S., & Wiggins, S. (2014). *The overseas development institute (ODI). Future diets: Implications for agriculture and food prices*. Retrieved January 20, 2014, from http://www.odi.org.uk/sites/odi.org.uk/files/odi-assets/publications-opinion-files/8776.pdf

Kim, S., Jin, Y., Choi, Y., & Park, T. (2011). Resveratrol exerts anti-obesity effects via mechanisms involving down-regulation of adipogenic and inflammatory processes in mice. *Biochemical Pharmacology*, *81*(11), 1343–1351. doi:10.1016/j.bcp.2011.03.012 PMID:21439945

Kim, S. H., Park, H. S., Lee, M. S., Cho, Y. J., Kim, Y. S., Hwang, J. T., ... Kwon, D. Y. (2008). Vitisin A inhibits adipocyte differentiation through cell cycle arrest in 3T3-L1 cells. *Biochemical and Biophysical Research Communications*, *372*(1), 108–113. doi:10.1016/j.bbrc.2008.04.188 PMID:18482581

Kimura, I., Inoue, D., Hirano, K., & Tsujimoto, G. (2014). The SCFA receptor GPR43 and energy metabolism. *Frontiers in Endocrinology*, *5*, 85. doi:10.3389/fendo.2014.00085 PMID:24926285

Kobyliak, N., Conte, C., Cammarota, G., Haley, A. P., Styriak, I., Gaspar, L., ... Kruzliak, P. (2016). Probiotics in prevention and treatment of obesity: A critical view. *Nutrition and Metabolism*, *13*(1), 14. doi:10.118612986-016-0067-0 PMID:26900391

Koo, M., Kim, S. H., Lee, N., Yoo, M. Y., Ryu, S. Y., Kwon, D. Y., & Kim, Y. S. (2008). 3-Hydroxy-3-methylglutaryl-CoA (HMG-CoA) reductase inhibitory effect of Vitis vinifera. *Fitoterapia*, *79*(3), 204–206. doi:10.1016/j.fitote.2007.11.005 PMID:18191910

Kumar, A., & Sharma, S. S. (2010). NF-kB inhibitory action of resveratrol: A probable mechanism of neuro protection in experimental diabetic neuropathy. *Biochemical and Biophysical Research Communications*, *394*(2), 360–365. doi:10.1016/j.bbrc.2010.03.014 PMID:20211601

Kuroyanagi, K., Kang, M. S., Goto, T., Hirai, S., Ohyama, K., Kusudo, T., ... Kawada, T. (2008). Citrus auraptene acts as an agonist for PPARs and enhances adiponectin production and MCP-1 reduction in 3T3-L1 adipocytes. *Biochemical and Biophysical Research Communications*, *366*(1), 219–225. doi:10.1016/j.bbrc.2007.11.119 PMID:18060855

Maeda, N., Shimomura, I., Kishida, K., Nishizawa, H., Matsuda, M., Nagaretani, H., ... Matsuzawa, Y. (2002). Diet-induced insulin resistance in mice lacking adiponectin/ACRP30. *Nature Medicine*, *8*(7), 731–737. doi:10.1038/nm724 PMID:12068289

Market and Standard Market. (2015). Retrieved September 25, 2015, from http://www.marketsandmarkets.com/Market-Reports/ prebiotics-ingredients-market-219677001.html

Miller, L. E. (2013). Lorcaserin for Weight Loss: Insights into US Food and drug administration approval. *Journal of the Academy of Nutrition and Dietetics*, *113*(1), 25–30. doi:10.1016/j.jand.2012.08.028 PMID:23260720

Miura, T., Itoh, Y., Iwamoto, N., Kato, M., & Ishida, T. (2004). Suppressive activity of the fruit of Momordica charantia with exercise on blood glucose in type 2 diabetic mice. *Biological & Pharmaceutical Bulletin*, *27*(2), 248–250. doi:10.1248/bpb.27.248 PMID:14758046

Murase, T., Yokoi, Y., Misawa, K., Ominami, H., Suzuki, Y., Shibuya, Y., & Hase, T. (2012). Coffee polyphenols modulate whole-body substrate oxidation and suppress postprandial hyperglycaemia, hyperinsulinaemia and hyperlipidaemia. *British Journal of Nutrition*, *107*(12), 1757–1765. doi:10.1017/S0007114511005083 PMID:22017960

Oelschlaeger, T. A. (2010). Mechanisms of probiotic actions - A review. *International Journal of Medical Microbiology*, *300*(1), 57–62. doi:10.1016/j.ijmm.2009.08.005 PMID:19783474

Oh, D. Y., Talukdar, S., Bae, E. J., Imamura, T., Morinaga, H., Fan, W., ... Olefsky, J. M. (2010). GPR120 is an ω-3 fatty acid receptor mediating potent anti-inflammatory and insulin-sensitizing effects. *Cell*, *142*(5), 687–698. doi:10.1016/j.cell.2010.07.041 PMID:20813258

Perricone, N. V., Bagchi, D., Echard, B., & Preuss, H. G. (2010). Long-term metabolic effects of different doses of niacin-bound chromium on Sprague-Dawley rats. *Molecular and Cellular Biochemistry*, *338*(1-2), 91–103. doi:10.100711010-009-0342-8 PMID:20012467

Powell, E. E., Jonsson, J. R., & Clouston, A. D. (2005). Steatosis: Co-factor in other liver diseases. *Hepatology (Baltimore, Md.)*, *42*(1), 5–13. doi:10.1002/hep.20750 PMID:15962320

Qin, B., Polansky, M. M., Harry, D., & Anderson, R. A. (2010). Green tea polyphenols improve cardiac muscle mRNA and protein levels of signal pathways related to insulin and lipid metabolism and inflammation in insulin-resistant rats. *Molecular Nutrition & Food Research*, *54*(1), S14–S23. doi:10.1002/mnfr.200900306 PMID:20112301

Rains, T. M., Agarwal, S., & Maki, K. C. (2011). Antiobesity effects of green tea catechins: A mechanistic review. *The Journal of Nutritional Biochemistry*, *22*(1), 1–7. doi:10.1016/j.jnutbio.2010.06.006 PMID:21115335

Rayalam, S., Della-Fera, M. A., & Baile, C. A. (2008). Phytochemicals and regulation of the adipocyte life cycle. *The Journal of Nutritional Biochemistry*, *19*(11), 717–726. doi:10.1016/j.jnutbio.2007.12.007 PMID:18495457

Ricote, M., Li, A. C., Willson, T. M., Kelly, C. J., & Glass, C. K. (2009). The peroxisome proliferator-activated receptor-γ is a negative regulator of macrophage activation. *Nature*, *391*(6662), 79–82. doi:10.1038/34178 PMID:9422508

Rijkers, G. T., Bengmark, S., Enck, P., Haller, D., Herz, U., Kalliomaki, M., ... Antoine, J. M. (2010). Guidance for substantiating the evidence for beneficial effects of probiotics: Current status and recommendations for future research. *The Journal of Nutrition*, *140*(3), 671S–676S. doi:10.3945/jn.109.113779 PMID:20130080

Saetan, S., Grove, K. A., & Lambert, J. D. (2011). Weight control and prevention of metabolic syndrome by green tea. *Pharmacological Research*, *64*(2), 146–154. doi:10.1016/j.phrs.2010.12.013 PMID:21193040

Schenk, S., Saberi, M., & Olefsky, J. M. (2008). Insulin sensitivity: Modulation by nutrients and inflammation. *The Journal of Clinical Investigation*, *118*(9), 2992–3002. doi:10.1172/JCI34260 PMID:18769626

Serrano, J. C., Cassanyé, A., & Portero-Otin, M. (2012). Trends in functional food against obesity. In B. Valdez (Ed.), *Scientific, Health and Social Aspects of the Food Industry* (pp. 279–294). Intech Publishing.

Shehzad, A., Khan, S., & Sup-Lee, Y. (2012). Curcumin molecular targets in obesity and obesity-related cancers. *Future Oncology (London, England)*, *8*(4), 179–190. doi:10.2217/fon.11.145 PMID:22335582

Shi, H., Kokoeva, M. V., Inouye, K., Tzameli, I., Yin, H., & Flier, J. S. (2006). TLR4 links innate immunity and fatty acid-induced insulin resistance. *The Journal of Clinical Investigation*, *116*(11), 3015–3025. doi:10.1172/JCI28898 PMID:17053832

Shimizu, M., Sakai, H., Shirakami, Y., Yasuda, Y., Kubota, M., Terakura, D., ... Moriwaki, H. (2011). Preventive Effects of (-)-Epigallocatechin gallate on diethylnitrosamine-induced liver tumorigenesis in obese and diabetic C57BL/KsJ-*db/db* mice. *Cancer Prevention Research (Philadelphia, Pa.)*, *4*(3), 396–403. doi:10.1158/1940-6207.CAPR-10-0331 PMID:21372039

Siegel, A. B., & Zhu, A. X. (2009). Metabolic syndrome and hepatocellular carcinoma: Two growing epidemics with a potential link. *Cancer*, *115*(24), 5651–5661. doi:10.1002/cncr.24687 PMID:19834957

Slavin, J. L. (2005). Dietary fiber and body weight. *Nutrition (Burbank, Los Angeles County, Calif.)*, *21*(3), 411–418. doi:10.1016/j.nut.2004.08.018 PMID:15797686

Stulnig, T. M. (2003). Immunomodulation by polyunsaturated fatty acids: Mechanisms and effects. *International Archives of Allergy and Immunology*, *132*(4), 310–321. doi:10.1159/000074898 PMID:14707462

Suganami, T., Nishida, J., & Ogawa, Y. (2005). A paracrine loop between adipocytes and macrophages aggravates inflammatory changes: Role of free fatty acids and tumor necrosis factor α. *Arteriosclerosis, Thrombosis, and Vascular Biology*, *25*(10), 2062–2068. doi:10.1161/01.ATV.0000183883.72263.13 PMID:16123319

Suganami, T., Tanimoto-Koyama, K., Nishida, J., Itoh, M., Yuan, X., Mizuarai, S., ... Ogawa, Y. (2007). Role of the toll-like receptor 4/NF-κB pathway in saturated fatty acid induced inflammatory changes in the interaction between adipocytes and macrophages. *Arteriosclerosis, Thrombosis, and Vascular Biology*, *27*(1), 84–91. doi:10.1161/01.ATV.0000251608.09329.9a PMID:17082484

Sunkara, R., & Verghese, M. (2014). Functional foods for obesity management. *Food and Nutrition Sciences*, *5*(14), 1359–1369. doi:10.4236/fns.2014.514148

Szewczuk, L. M., Forti, L., Stivala, L. A., & Penning, T. M. (2004). Resveratrol is a peroxidase mediated inactivator of COX-1 but not COX-2: A mechanistic approach to the design of COX-1 selective agents. *The Journal of Biological Chemistry*, *279*(21), 22727–22737. doi:10.1074/jbc.M314302200 PMID:15020596

Todoric, J., Löffler, M., Huber, J., Bilban, M., Reimers, M., Kadl, A., ... Stulnig, T. M. (2006). Adipose tissue inflammation induced by high-fat diet in obese diabetic mice is prevented by n-3 polyunsaturated fatty acids. *Diabetologia*, *49*(9), 2109–2119. doi:10.100700125-006-0300-x PMID:16783472

Tran, T. T., Medline, A., & Bruce, W. R. (1996). Insulin promotion of colon tumors in rats. *Cancer Epidemiology, Biomarkers & Prevention*, *5*(12), 1013–1015. PMID:8959325

Tsuchida, A., Yamauchi, T., Takekawa, S., Hada, Y., Ito, Y., Maki, T., & Kadowaki, T. (2005). Peroxisome proliferator-activated receptor (PPAR) α activation increases adiponectin receptors and reduces obesity-related inflammation in adipose tissue: Comparison of activation of PPARα, PPARγ, and their combination. *Diabetes*, *54*(12), 3358–3370. doi:10.2337/diabetes.54.12.3358 PMID:16306350

Tsuda, T. (2008). Regulation of adipocyte function by anthocyanins; possibility of preventing the metabolic syndrome. *Journal of Agricultural and Food Chemistry*, *56*(3), 642–646. doi:10.1021/jf073113b PMID:18211021

Vitali, B., Ndagijimana, M., Maccaferri, S., Biagi, E., Guerzoni, M. E., & Brigidi, P. (2012). An *in vitro* evaluation of the effect of probiotics and prebiotics on the metabolic profile of human microbiota. *Anaerobe*, *18*(4), 386–391. doi:10.1016/j.anaerobe.2012.04.014 PMID:22579985

Welberg, J. W., Monkelbaan, J. F., de Vries, E. G., Muskiet, F. A., Cats, A., Oremus, E. T., ... Kleibeuker, J. H. (1994). Effects of supplemental dietary calcium on quantitative and qualitative fecal fat excretion in man. *Annals of Nutrition & Metabolism*, *38*(4), 185–191. doi:10.1159/000177810 PMID:7832578

World Health Organization. (2010). *Global strategy on diet, physical activity and health*. Retrieved from http://www.who.int/dietphysicalactivity/publications/facts/obesity/en/

Wynne, K., Stanley, S., McGowan, B., & Bloom, S. (2005). Appetite control. *The Journal of Endocrinology*, *184*(2), 291–318. doi:10.1677/joe.1.05866 PMID:15684339

Xu, H., Barnes, G. T., Yang, Q., Tan, G., Yang, D., Chou, C. J., ... Chen, H. (2003). Chronic inflammation in fat plays a crucial role in the development of obesity-related insulin resistance. *The Journal of Clinical Investigation*, *112*(12), 1821–1830. doi:10.1172/JCI200319451 PMID:14679177

Yadav, H., Lee, J. H., Lloyd, J., Walter, P., & Rane, S. G. (2013). Beneficial metabolic effects of a probiotic via butyrate induced GLP-1 secretion. *The Journal of Biological Chemistry*, *288*(35), 25088–25097. doi:10.1074/jbc.M113.452516 PMID:23836895

Yasmin, A., Butt, M. S., Afzaal, M., van Baak, M., Nadeem, M. T., & Shahid, M. Z. (2015). Prebiotics, gut microbiota and metabolic risks: Unveiling the relationship. *Journal of Functional Foods*, *17*, 189–201. doi:10.1016/j.jff.2015.05.004

Yasuda, Y., Shimizu, M., Sakai, H., Iwasa, J., Kubota, M., Adachi, S., ... Moriwaki, H. (2009). (-)-Epigallocatechin gallate prevents carbon tetrachloride-induced rat hepatic fibrosis by inhibiting the expression of the PDGFR beta and IGF-1R. *Chemico-Biological Interactions*, *182*(2-3), 159–164. doi:10.1016/j.cbi.2009.07.015 PMID:19646978

Younis, K., Ahmad, S., & Jahan, K. (2015). Health benefits and application of prebiotics in foods. *Journal of Food Processing & Technology*, *6*, 433. doi:10.4172/2157-7110.1000433

Yu, R., Kim, C. S., Kwon, B. S., & Kawada, T. (2006). Mesenteric adipose tissue-derived monocyte chemo-attractant protein-1 plays a crucial role in adipose tissue macrophage migration and activation in obese mice. *Obesity (Silver Spring, Md.)*, *14*(8), 1353–1362. doi:10.1038/oby.2006.153 PMID:16988077

Zemel, M. B., & Miller, S. L. (2004). Dietary calcium and dairy modulation of adiposity and obesity risk. *Nutrition Reviews*, *62*(4), 125–131. doi:10.1111/j.1753-4887.2004.tb00034.x PMID:15141427

Section 3
Cardiovascular

Chapter 5
Roles of Nutraceuticals and Functional Food in Prevention of Cardiovascular Disease:
Sustaining Health

Shahrul Bariyah Hamid
Universiti Sains Malaysia, Malaysia

Auni Fatin Abd Hamid
Universiti Sains Malaysia, Malaysia

ABSTRACT

The chapter provides an overview of cardiovascular disease, a major cause of mortality worldwide. It relates economic and social impacts to the disease, especially in developing countries. One of the approaches to addressing this challenge is increasing awareness within society, through implementation of education programs. It is important for society to understand the types and roles of the risk factors leading to cardiovascular disease. Emphasis is on the role of functional food and nutraceuticals as dietary sources that could prevent development of cardiovascular disease. The chapter highlights roles of nutraceuticals and functional food sources from medical plants, seeds, berries, and tropical fruits in lowering risk factors. Key findings from trials conducted in Asia, China, Europe, and America provide supporting evidence for the importance of functional food to health, and its potential for modifying the level of risk factors related to cardiovascular diseases.

DOI: 10.4018/978-1-5225-3267-5.ch005

INTRODUCTION

Noncommunicable disease is on the public health agenda of the World Health Organization (WHO). The healthcare burden has been rising due to various diseases primarily related to lifestyle and dietary habits. According to the World Health Organization, cardiovascular disease is the major cause of disability and premature throughout the world (WHO, 2007). Addressing behavioral risk factors, such as tobacco use, unhealthy diet and obesity, physical inactivity, and harmful use of alcohol, can prevent most cardiovascular diseases, using population-wide strategies (Mendis, Puska, & Norrving, 2011). The percentage of premature death from cardiovascular diseases (CVDs) range from 4% in high income countries and 42% in low-income countries, indicating differences between countries and populations. Halting premature deaths from CVDs and other noncommunicable diseases will require global solidarity and broad alliances that go beyond national, cultural and ethnic boundaries (Mendis, Shanthi, Puska, Pekka, & Norrving, 2011). As a preventive measure against contracting the disease later in life, individuals must understand the root causes of cardiovascular disease. Increased knowledge sharing and dissemination programs on the importance of nutraceuticals in treating and preventing disease should be in place in schools and communities. In the long term, this would assist in reducing the economic burden due to increasing healthcare costs of noncommunicable diseases. Over the last 35 years, a trend toward use of natural products has increased worldwide (Newman & Cragg, 2007). Discovery of the various health benefits of natural compounds has led to their use in clinical applications, supported by emerging reports on the medicinal benefits of plant-derived products (Alves-Silva, Monica, Carla, Ligia, & Henrique, 2016; Guo, Gan, Haist, Rajapurohitam, Zeidan, Faruq, & Karmazyn, 2011; Hu, Koon, Chan, Lau, & Fung, 2012). They indicate the need for greater emphasis on exploring the healing qualities of nutraceutical and functional food products deemed safe for consumption, and with minimal adverse effects (Alam, Subhan, Rahman, Uddin, Reza, & Sarker, 2014; Alam, Kauter, & Brown, 2013; Ashraful, Kathleen & Lindsay, 2013; Kristen, Lehrke, Buss, Mereles, Steen, Ehlermann, . . . Katus, 2012; Sobenin, Pryanishnikov, Kunnova, Rabinovich, Martirosyan, & Orekhov, 2010). Increase in society's awareness could prevent diseases due to modifiable risk factors. Priority must be given to fostering healthy dietary practices in younger generations. Prevention occurs by inculcating knowledge and developing daily practices that focus on healthy food selection. This could lead to modification of lifestyle, long-term outcomes of which lead to achieving the goal of sustainable health.

In addition, this chapter gives an overview of cardiovascular disease prevalence, discussing multiple risk factors to provide a better understanding of how they cause cardiovascular diseases. The risks include lifestyle, dietary habits, genetics, and environmental factors reportedly related to coronary artery disease. The chapter introduces metabolic diseases (hypertension, obesity, diabetes mellitus) related to lipid abnormalities (i.e., dyslipidaemia, hypercholesterolemia). Similar to dyslipidaemic nondiabetic subjects, Type 2 diabetes mellitus (DM) patients show marked increased risk of CAD complications. The American Heart Association has designated DM as a "CHD risk equivalent." Furthermore, the International Diabetic Foundation (IDF) predicts that by the year 2025, the Southeast Asia Region will have the highest prevalence of diabetes.

We emphasize lipids, one of the potential risk factors for developing cardiovascular diseases according to data available from meta-analysis and clinical research findings. The chapter also includes the pathophysiology of atherosclerosis and its relation to the development of coronary artery diseases. This leads to a description of the role of lipids as a dietary source, their structure and functions, abnormalities in blood lipid levels, causes of dyslipidaemia, monitoring technologies, and highlighting the importance of self-monitoring. The National Education Program (NCEP ATP III) and other related guidelines are cited as references for the healthy population, diabetic patients, and cardiovascular disease patients.

The literature on disease prevention through the molecular mechanisms of functional food and nutraceuticals is described. Findings from cytotoxicity, antilipidemic, and other studies from the literature with regard to nutraceuticals and functional food are cited, as they relate to existing knowledge on the roles of nutraceuticals in the prevention of atherosclerosis.

Existing research approaches in genomics and proteomics provide methods of analysis at the cellular level. This involves application of both *in vivo* and *in vitro* techniques in studying these mechanisms. These techniques provide a platform to explore the potential of new natural compounds derived from nutraceutical and functional foods, which may play a cardio-protective role.

Generally, readers will know the differences in structure and function of the lipids, lipoprotein, and cardiac markers in human physiology. To enable better understanding, findings gathered from previous research provide information on roles that trans-fatty acids, triglycerides, oxidized low-density lipoprotein, high-density lipoprotein, chylomicrons, and intermediate-density lipoprotein play in health. This would enable readers from various walks of life to gauge basic knowledge, such as lipid sources, calories, and intake, on daily basis. It is important to address the limits of cholesterol intake as a preventive measure within the society. Individuals could control this modifiable risk factor, and it is practical for each individual to achieve recommended levels. The chapter also presents current technology for monitoring lipid level, or gadgets available for self-monitoring as a prevention measure. Individuals will be able to monitor their own cholesterol level and refer to recognized guidelines. Intake of nutraceuticals and functional food would ultimately contribute to improving their health status.

BACKGROUND

Cardiovascular disease incidence has been increasing. It occurs even among the younger generation, with an increased incidence of sudden cardiac death (SCD). Several risk factors have been related to the onset of cardiovascular diseases, including smoking, sedentary lifestyle, and eating habits. This indicates the need for modification of lifestyle and dietary habits, which play crucial roles in sustaining health. In order to achieve such goals, the society, and especially the younger generation, must acquire knowledge of healthy dietary practices and increased physical activity. Cardiovascular disease (CVD) is reported worldwide as the major cause of death, and is becoming a health burden to developing countries. Countries have taken various steps to control the increasing number of cases through health education, counseling on nutritional aspects, and promoting healthy lifestyle. Nonetheless, CVD is expected to increase. Deaths related to noncommunicable diseases are estimated to rise to 52 million by 2030. The major noncommunicable diseases (cardiovascular diseases, cancer, chronic respiratory diseases, and diabetes) account for 82% of total deaths (Mendis, 2014). According to the Global Status Report on noncommunicable diseases in 2014, low- and middle-income countries should target a 25% reduction in mortality (Mendis, 2014). The World Health Organization (WHO) has provided guidelines to policymakers and healthcare workers on how to target individuals at high risk of developing CVD, at all levels of the health system and in different resource settings, using evidence-based and cost-effective approaches to preventive measures, and for development of health policies. Its activities target common risk factors shared by CVD, cancer, diabetes, and chronic respiratory disease, and their implementation is critical to controlling the growing burden of noncommunicable diseases (WHO, 2007) . Socioeconomic, geographic, ethnic, and gender disparities in CVD risk, morbidity, and mortality persist, and influence individual behaviors (Harper, Lynch, & Smith, 2011). Thus, health disparities research is moving toward implementing culturally appropriate community-focused efforts to improve opportunities, resources, healthcare practices, and the built environment, to foster heart-healthy lifestyles (Glik, Deborah, Sharif, Mienah Zulfacar, Tucker, Katherine, Tejada, Shirley, Prelip, Michael, Ammerman, Alice . . . Stephanie, 2016).

The development of CVD is related to atherosclerosis, a process that occurs due to accumulation of lipids in the intima of capillary vessels (Nakashima, Fujii, Sumiyoshi,

Wight, & Sueishi, 2007). This implies that high levels of lipids in blood circulation or dyslipidaemia promote the initiation of atherosclerosis. Multiple factors have been linked to development of CVD, including high fat or carbohydrate-rich food intake, obesity, tobacco smoking, diabetes mellitus, and hypertension. Reportedly, public-health approaches effectively slow down the development of atherosclerosis, and reduce the incidence of some cancers and chronic respiratory diseases in young people, thus reducing the likelihood of future epidemics of CVD (WHO, 2007).

MAIN FOCUS OF THE CHAPTER

The chapter's focal point is to introduce cardiovascular disease prevalence and its socioeconomic impact on patients, their livelihood, and healthcare cost to their countries. Numerous studies on prevention *in vivo* and *in vitro* are highlighted to elucidate the underlying mechanisms by which nutraceuticals and functional food exhibit cardio-protective effects. Focusing on specific tropical fruits, citrus, berries, honey, seed, and oil highlights their importance as preventive agents against cardiovascular disease, and further describes the role of lipids as one of the risk factors of cardiovascular disease. The reader should have general knowledge of the link between cardiovascular diseases and lipids, as well as type 2 DM. Roles of specific nutraceuticals and functional food, not only in reducing the risks but also as preventive agents, enable the reader to understand their benefits to health. To achieve this goal, health-education initiatives play a vital role in creating awareness within all levels of society. NCEP ATP III and Dietary Guidelines provide knowledge on recommended target levels for lipid profile and dietary source. The latest gadgets for lipid detection are described briefly to address self-monitoring. Education among children on the importance of health aspects would instill knowledge at an early age. New generations would have a better understanding of curative and preventive effects of functional food and nutraceuticals. In the long run, each individual should be able to implement healthy dietary plans and inculcate healthy eating habits within their families. Hence, continuous and concerted efforts by the respective authorities would hinder further rises in the prevalence of cardiovascular disease.

Issues, Controversies, Problems

Cardiovascular disease is one of the costliest diseases, and a major economic burden to healthcare systems (Tarride, Jean-Eric, Lim, Morgan, DesMeules, Marie, Luo, Wei, Burke, Natasha, O'Reilly, Daria, . . . Ron, 2009). In addressing the burden of CVD, low- and middle-income countries must face the challenges of limited healthcare budgets and infrastructure, as well as constrained professional health workforce capacity (Lee, Edward, Vedanthan, Rajesh, Jeemon, Panniyammakal, Kamano, Jemima, Kudesia, Preeti, Rajan, Vikram, . . . Moran, Andrew, 2016). The Prospective Urban Rural Epidemiology (PURE) study reported that only 25% of patients with established cardiovascular disease were taking aspirin, 17% β blockers, 20% ACE inhibitors or ARBs, and 15% statins. In high-income countries, 11% of eligible patients were not taking any of these medicines, compared with 80% in low-income countries (Yusuf, Salim, Islam, Shofiqul, Chow, Clara K, Rangarajan, Sumathy, Dagenais, Gilles, Diaz, Rafael, . . . Avezum, Alvaro, 2011).

Of patients with known cardiovascular disease across 18 countries studied in PURE, only 686 (10%) used three of the recommended medicines, and 205 (3%) used all four medicines. In low-income and middle-income countries, there is a strong association between scarce availability and low affordability of these medicines and their use. This finding suggests that improvements in the availability and affordability of these medicines are prerequisites for increasing their use. However, use of the recommended medicines was low in low-income and middle-income countries even when the medicines were potentially available and affordable, and only reached about 18% use in high-income countries where these medicines are widely available and affordable. Thus, although the availability and affordability of medicines are prerequisites for their use, correcting these factors alone might not be sufficient to increase to optimum coverage the proportion of patients receiving all medicines. Other factors affecting medicine use could include patients' attitudes and knowledge related to taking medicines for prevention, and healthcare providers' attitudes and prescribing patterns (Khatib, McKee, Shannon, Chow, Rangarajan, Teo, . . . Yusuf, 2016).

A study in Europe showed that the largest contributors to total costs are hospital stay and revascularization procedures. Pharmaceuticals are estimated at 14–25% of total cost of acute coronary syndrome (ACS). The survey showed that the countries with higher expenditures for ACS patients tended to have lower case-fatality rates, and countries with the lowest incidence of ACS also had the lowest cost per capita (Taylor, Scuffham, McCollam, & Newby, 2007). Furthermore, CVD has significant socioeconomic effects on the livelihood of patients and their families.

According to the National Cholesterol Education Program (NCEP) ATP III guideline, individuals with type 2 DM have a CHD risk equivalent (Williams, 2002). Currently, out of 382 million diabetics, almost 175 million (46%) are undiagnosed cases (Linnenkamp, Guariguata, Beagley, Whiting, & Cho, 2014). These groups may be at potential risk of developing cardiovascular diseases. The majority of patients with diabetes are between 40 and 59 years old, and live in low- and middle-income countries (Linnenkamp, Guariguata, Beagley, Whiting, & Cho, 2014). In addition, evaluation of selected nutrients and food-group intakes among 2,757 overweight

U.S. adults diagnosed with type 2 DM, an established risk factor of CVD, showed that less than 50% of subjects consumed the minimum recommended servings of fruits and vegetables (Vitolins, Mara, Anderson, Andrea, Delahanty, Linda, Raynor, Hollie, Miller, Gary, Mobley, Connie, . . . Look, 2009).

Potentials of Nutraceutical and Functional Food in Prevention of Coronary Artery Diseases

Nutraceuticals and Functional Food

It is well known that a greater intake of fruit and vegetables can help prevent heart disease and mortality. Several components found in fruit, berries, and vegetables are probably involved in their protective effects against CVD. Potentially beneficial substances include antioxidant vitamins, folate, fibre, and potassium. Antioxidant compounds found in fruit and vegetables, such as vitamin C, carotenoids, and flavonoids, may influence the risk of CVD by preventing the oxidation of cholesterol in arteries (Voutilainen, Nurmi, Mursu, & Rissanen, 2006).

Honey

Honey, a natural sweetener, can be considered a natural therapy for atherosclerosis and CVDs. The probable mechanisms by which honey exhibits protective and curative actions against myocardial damage are improved antioxidative status and lowered plasma-cholesterol level. Major contributing agents of cardio-protective and antiatherosclerotic effects of honey may be flavonoid constituents commonly present in natural honey (Afroz, Tanvir, & Little, 2016)

Olive Oil

Olive oil consumption continues to be a major source of monounsaturated fatty acid (MUFA) in Mediterranean countries. Previous study suggests that the traditional Mediterranean diet, as it is usually defined, confers substantial cardiovascular protection among initially healthy middle-aged adults (Martínez-González, García-López, Bes-Rastrollo, Toledo, Martínez-Lapiscina, Delgado-Rodriguez, . . . Beunza, 2011). Trans-fatty acids (TFA) are unsaturated fatty acids that contain at least one nonconjugated double bond in the trans configuration, resulting in a straighter shape. TFA present in our diet can be either industrially produced or ruminant/natural. The major process contributing to formation of industrial TFA is hydrogenation of vegetable oils. Thermal processes such as edible oil refining and frying also lead to the formation of TFA, while ruminant/natural TFA forms in the rumen of ruminant animals through biohydrogenation. Industrial TFA poses severe threats to our health, such as cardiovascular problems, insulin resistance, infertility in women, compromised fetal development, and cognitive decline (Bhardwaj, Passi, & Misra, 2011).

Compared to other seed oils, olive oil has low levels of saturated (~16%) and high levels of monounsaturated (~70%) fatty acids. Cold-press extra-virgin olive oil is mechanically extracted from the olive (*Olea europaea sativa H.*) fruit without any thermal or chemical exposure (Yang & Irudayaraj, 2001). A Latin square–designed study among Italian subjects divided into three groups gave each one a different kind of oil (extra virgin olive oil, EVOO; olive oil, OO; or corn oil, CO, together with 150g of potatoes), with two-week washout periods between treatments. Blood samples were drawn at baseline and after one, two, and six hours after the meal. A significant decrease in inflammatory markers was noted for thromboxane B_2 (TXB_2) and leukotriene B_4 (LTB_4), after two and six hours after EVOO (but not OO or CO) consumption, and a concomitant increase of serum antioxidant capacity was recorded. These data reinforce the notion that the Mediterranean diet reduces the incidence of coronary heart disease, partially due to the protective role of its phenolic components, including those of extra virgin olive oil (Bogani, Galli, Villa, & Visioli, 2007).

Nigella Sativa

Nigella sativa is one of the most extensively studied plants in both *in vivo* and *in vitro* models. In 2014, application of this compound was noted in a clinical trial in the United States, initiated to determine its effect as an antihypertensive agent. Likewise, there are several ongoing clinical trials to elucidate its therapeutic function in dyslipidaemia, asthma, hypertension, and various diseases (NIH, 2012).

Nigella sativa (NIH, 2012) is a plant that belongs to the family *Ranunculaceae*, commonly grown in the Middle East and certain parts of Asia and Europe. Commonly known as black cumin, it has been used for centuries as a spice, preservative, and curative remedy in the Middle East, Asia, and parts of Europe (Awad & Binder, 2005). *N. sativa* seeds (called black seeds or black cumin) have been used for edible and medicinal purposes in many countries (Hosseinzadeh & Parvardeh, 2004). The medicinal properties attributed to black cumin seeds extract or oil include antihistaminic, antihypertensive, analgesic and anti-inflammatory, hypoglycemic, antibacterial, and antifungal (Ahmad, Aftab, Husain, Asif, Mujeeb, Mohd. . . Firoz, 2013; Hanafy & Hatem, 1991), as well as anthelmintic and antitumour effects.

Cardiovascular benefits of *Nigella sativa* have been reported previously. El-Bahai et al. reported evidence of physiological and beneficial cardiac hypertrophy in rats induced by long term *Nigella sativa* supplementation (El-Bahai, Al-Hariri, Yar, & Bamosa, 2009). The critical role of modified LDL in atherogenesis suggests the need to control its progression. Therefore, the modulatory effect of *Nigella sativa* oil on the progression of monocyte-derived macrophage growth was investigated. Previous study reported that treatment with a combination of *Nigella sativa* and oxidized LDL showed no visible intracellular lipid vesicle, and the monocyte surface was seen coated with oil red O. In addition, the morphological characteristics did not show significant development of monocyte into macrophage. The cells treated with oxidized LDL alone had intracellular stained lipid in several vesicles. Reduction of lipid stained deposits in combined treatment may be explained by the presence of *Nigella sativa* oil. It may functionally block the oxidized LDL from inducing differentiation of monocyte into macrophages, hence blocking the uptake by scavenger receptors. However, the actual mechanism on its action requires further study (Mat, Mohamed, & Hamid, 2011). The lipid deposits in the aorta had also been observed in studies to see the effect of *Nigella sativa*. Animal-model study indicated supplementation of either powder or oil form of *Nigella sativa* to hypercholesterolemic rabbits reduced lipid deposits on the intimal surface of the aorta, indicating inhibition of plaque formation (Al-Naqeep, Al-Zubairi, Ismail, Amom, & Esa, 2011).

Berries

In berries, the most abundant class of flavonoids is the anthocyanins. The most common anthocyanidin aglycones are pelargonidin, cyanidin, delphinidin, peonidin, petunidin, and malvidin. They form conjugates with sugars and organic acids to generate numerous anthocyanins. Berries have different types of anthocyanins; strawberries have only pelargonidin conjugates, but blueberries contain cyanidin, delphinidin, malvidin, petunidin, and peonidin conjugates (Crozier, Alan, Yokota, Takao, Jaganath, Indu, Marks, Serena, Saltmarsh, Michael, Clifford, & Michael, 2007).

Randomized controlled studies (RCTs) have shown improvements in several surrogate markers of cardiovascular risk, such as blood pressure, endothelial function, arterial stiffness, and blood lipids, after acute and short-term consumption of blueberries, strawberries, cranberries, or purified anthocyanin extracts in healthy or diseased individuals (Rodriguez-Mateos, Heiss, Borges, & Crozier, 2014). A double-blind, randomized, placebo-controlled trial was done using anthocyanin (also called Medox), which contains 80mg anthocyanin comprised of 17 different natural anthocyanins purified from the bilberry (*Vaccinium myrtillus*) and black currant (*Ribes nigrum*). A total of 122 hypercholesterolemic subjects aged 40–65 years were recruited into this clinical trial between November 2008 and December 2010. The study showed that serum HDL cholesterol concentration increased significantly more in the anthocyanin group than in the placebo group [11.39% (95% CI 9.64%, 13.13%) and −1.46% (95% CI −3.19%, 0.27%), respectively; $P < .018$] after the 24-week intervention. However, serum LDL cholesterol concentration significantly decreased by 9.72% (95% CI −13.80%, −5.63%) in the anthocyanin group and was reduced by 2.18% (95% CI −5.85%, 1.50%) in the placebo group by the end of the intervention. The change in both HDL cholesterol and LDL cholesterol were significantly different between the two groups (both $P < 0.05$) (Zhu, Yanna, Huang, Xiuwei, Zhang, Yuhua, Wang, Yun, Liu, Yan, Sun, Ruifang, & Xia, 2014).

The consumption of berry fruits and their contribution to improving cardiovascular condition is a subject of considerable interest. The commonly consumed berries in the United States include blackberry, black raspberry, blueberry, cranberry, red raspberry, and strawberry. Human intervention studies using chokeberries, cranberries, blueberries, and strawberries (fresh, as juice, or freeze-dried), or purified anthocyanin extracts have demonstrated significant improvements in LDL oxidation, lipid peroxidation, total plasma antioxidant capacity, dyslipidaemia, and glucose metabolism. Benefits were seen in healthy subjects and in those with existing metabolic risk factors. Underlying mechanisms for these beneficial effects are believed to include upregulation of endothelial nitric oxide synthase, decreased activities of carbohydrate digestive enzymes, decreased oxidative stress, and inhibition of inflammatory gene expression and foam cell formation (Arpita Basu, Rhone, & Lyons, 2010).

The Kuopio Ischemic Heart Disease Risk Factor Study (KIHD) showed a significantly lower risk of CVD-related deaths among 1,950 men in the highest quartile of berry intake (>408g/day) versus men with the lowest intake (<133g/day) during a mean follow-up of 12.8 years. These findings were based on a model adjusted for major CVD risk factors, which further showed an inverse correlation between intakes of fruits, berries, and vegetables and serum haptoglobin, a marker of inflammation (Rissanen, Voutilainen, Virtanen, Venho, Vanharanta, Mursu, & Salonen, 2003). A systemic review based on several studies, including prospective studies, recommended an increased intake of a mix of fruits and vegetables to reduce the risk of IHD. The maximum beneficial amount seems to be about 800g per day (Ovesen, 2005).

A 12-week randomized controlled trial with 60 subjects showed better effects of higher-dose freeze-dried strawberries (50g fresh reconstituted in two cups [474 mL] of water) compared to lower-dose freeze-dried strawberries (LD-FDS; 25g reconstituted in two cups [474 mL] of water). Higher-dose intake exhibited lowering of conventional serum total and LDL cholesterol, and NMR-derived small LDL particle concentrations, when compared with a lower dose in obese adults. They reported that strawberries exerted antioxidant effects by decreasing lipid peroxidation, although no effects were noted on adiposity, blood pressure, glycemic control, or inflammation (Basu, Betts, Nguyen, Newman, Fu, & Lyons, 2014).

Oxidative stress is thought to be responsible for the oxidative damage observed in various human diseases, including cardiovascular disease, atherosclerosis, and dyslipidaemia (Valko, Leibfritz, Moncol, Cronin, Mazur, & Telser, 2007). The results from epidemiology studies have demonstrated the protective role of antioxidants through diet rich in fruits and vegetables against the development and progression of metabolic syndromes (Santhakumar & Singh, 2016). Cranberries are reported to contain high antioxidant content and able to inhibit low-density lipoprotein (LDL) oxidation (Chu & Liu, 2005). There are two kinds of cranberry (CB) fruit. The small-fruited or European CB (*Vaccinium oxycoccos*) is found in marshy land in northern North America, northern Asia, and northern and central Europe. The study indicated that the 100% juices (with no added sugar) contained the most antioxidants. Cranberry juice inhibits the absorption of glucose and the *in vivo* formation of triglycerides from fructose, and thus decreases oxidative stress (Vinson, Bose, Proch, Al Kharrat, & Samman, 2008). Similarly, another study based on a 14-day intervention with intake of cranberry juice at 7 mL/kg body weight per day showed an increase in plasma antioxidant capacity, and a decrease in oxidized LDL (Ruel, Pomerleau, Couture, Lamarche, & Couillard, 2005).

Goji berry (wolfberry) is a member of the *Solanacea* family, and has recently been introduced in Western countries (Monzon Ballarin, Lopez-Matas, Saenz Abad, Perez-Cinto, & Carnes, 2011). A randomized, double-blind, placebo-controlled clinical trial was conducted in China, on general effects of the orally consumed goji berry, *Lycium barbarum*, as a standardized juice. The trial showed significant differences between day 1 and day 15 in the study group ($N = 16$), with an increase in ratings for energy level, athletic performance, quality of sleep, ease of awakening, ability to focus on activities, mental acuity, calmness, and feelings of health, contentment, and happiness. Goji juice also significantly reduced fatigue and stress, and improved regularity of gastrointestinal function. However, no significant changes in musculoskeletal or cardiovascular complaints were observed in either group (Amagase & Nance, 2008). Another randomized, double-blind, placebo-controlled study was done with 50 Chinese healthy adults aged 55 to 72 years. It found that 30 days of Goji berry consumption caused antioxidant markers to be significantly increased by 8.4% for superoxide dismutase (SOD), and 9.9% for glutathione peroxidase (GSH-Px) between the preintervention and postintervention measurements, whereas malondialdehyde (MDA) was significantly decreased by 8.7% (Amagase, Sun, & Borek, 2009). These preliminary results suggest that further research is required to confirm effects of *Lycium barbarum* after long-term intake.

Tropical Fruits

Tropical and subtropical countries have diverse genera and species of plants in the rainforest, which need further exploration. Fruit-bearing trees contain rich sources of nutrients, minerals, and vitamins vital for health (Moo-Huchin, Moo-Huchin,

Estrada-Leon, Cuevas-Glory, Estrada-Mota, Ortiz-Vazquez, . . . Sauri-Duch, 2015; Shofian, Hamid, Osman, Saari, Anwar, Dek, & Hairuddin, 2011). Besides fruits, most plant components—leaf, bark, root, and stem—have medicinal value. Hundreds of fruit-bearing trees are native to Southeast Asia, but many are indigenous or underutilized. They have potential for commercial development and medicinal uses (Khoo, Azlan, Kong, & Ismail, 2016). Seeds are among by-products of processing fruit-based products. Instead of discarding seeds as waste, seeds with high potential as antioxidants could be utilised for commercial purposes. A study done with tropical fruit seeds of guava (*Psidium guajava*), mango (*Mangifera indica L.*) and papaya (*Carica papaya L.*) found that the mango seed has the highest relative antioxidant level and primary antioxidant activity, followed by guava seeds and papaya seeds. (Norshazila, Zahir, Suleiman, Aisyah, & Rahim, 2010).

Guava

Guava is a tropical fruit that grows in Southeast Asia, Brazil, Costa Rica, India, and Africa. Guava leaf extract exhibits antioxidant activity through free-radical scavenging and reducing power. These effects are linked to the total phenolic compounds existing in the extracts (Chen & Yen, 2007; Flores, Gema, Dastmalchi, Keyvan, Wu, Shi-Biao. . . Edward, 2013; Nantitanon, Yotsawimonwat, & Okonogi, 2010). Lycopene is one of the antioxidant compounds found in guava (Kaliora, Dedoussis, & Schmidt, 2006). Antioxidants used nowadays are obtained through either chemical synthesis or natural living-source extraction. The use of synthetic antioxidants is tending to decrease, due to adverse effects, and other safer compounds must replace it (Nantitanon, Witayapan, Yotsawimonwat, Songwut, Okonogi, & Siriporn, 2010). Strawberry guavas were found to be superior to common guavas in antioxidant and antimicrobial activities, total phenolic, vitamin C, and high fibre content (McCook-Russell, Nair, Facey, & Bowen-Forbes, 2012).

A recent study provided 400g of ripe guava (with peel and without peel) fruit supplementation to healthy subjects in India. After six weeks, there was significant reduction in serum total cholesterol, triglycerides, and low-density lipoprotein cholesterol (LDLC) levels ($p<0.05$). The level of high-density lipoprotein cholesterol (HDLC) was increased, which suggests that guava pulp without peel may have a favourable effect on lipid levels (Kumari, Rakavi, & Mangaraj, 2016). Similarly, another randomized, single-blind, controlled trial was done with hypertensive subjects. Intake of 0.5-1kg daily of guava for four weeks caused reduction in blood pressure and blood lipids, but no decrease in HDLC, due to its higher potassium and soluble-fibre content (Singh, Rastogi, Singh, Ghosh, Gupta, & Niaz, 1993). Takahashi et al. (2015) tested effects of guava tea leaves in mice, and found that the administration of extracts from guava tea leaves to apoE-deficient mice significantly attenuated atherogenic lesions in the aorta and aortic sinus (Takahashi, Otsuki, Mori, Kawakami, & Ito, 2015).

Guava leaf extract was found to inhibit xanthine oxidase (XO) (Irondi, Emmanuel Anyachukwu, Agboola, Samson Olalekan, Oboh, Ganiyu… Francis, 2016). This enzyme catalyzes the terminal steps in the catabolism of purines, in which hypoxanthine is converted to xanthine and eventually to uric acid, during which molecular oxygen is reduced to superoxide, a reactive oxygen species (ROS) (Berry & Hare, 2004).

Papaya

Papaya is a delicious tropical fruit rich in flavor and nutrients. The decoction of *Carica papaya* Linn. leaf is used in folklore medicine in certain parts of Malaysia and Indonesia (Zunjar, Dash, Jivrajani, Trivedi, & Nivsarkar, 2016). One of the most significant and abundant carotenoids found in nature is lycopene, which has gained attention among nutritionists. Papaya is reportedly the best source of lycopene, obtained through simple-solvent based extraction (Jamal, Akbar, Yumi, & Irwandi, 2016). However, the fruit ethyl acetate fraction (FEAF) was found to contain the highest total amount of phenols (Khor & Wong, 2014). *C. papaya* leaves were extracted with methanol in a Soxhlet apparatus, and later with a liquid–liquid extraction (LLE), with the aim of identifying and quantifying secondary metabolites from this plant, using gas chromatography–mass spectrometry (GC–MS) in the selected ion-monitoring (SIM) mode. Results showed the presence of phenolic acids as the main compound, while chlorogenic acid was found in trace amounts in comparison to the flavonoids and coumarin compounds (Canini, Alesiani, D'Arcangelo, & Tagliatesta, 2007).

A study conducted in Hawaii showed that the vitamin C content of papaya was 51.2mg/100g, with no differences among cultivars. The provitamin A carotenoids averaged 232.3 microgram β-carotene and 594.3 microgram β-cryptoxanthin/100g; whereas the amount of vitamin A ranged from 18.7 to 74.0 microgram RAE/100g. Lycopene was not detected in the yellow-fleshed cultivars, Kapoho, Laie Gold, and Rainbow, but the red-fleshed Sunrise and SunUp fruit contained 1350–3674 microgram lycopene/100g (Wall, 2006). The Health Vegetarian Eating pattern guide suggests that the amount of fruit intake is between 1.5 and 2.5 cups daily for adults, in the form of all fresh, frozen, canned, or dried fruits, or fruit juices (Nelson, 2015).

A meta-analysis found that lycopene is effective in reducing LDL cholesterol and total serum cholesterol when taken in doses higher than 25mg daily, and is able to reduce systolic blood pressure in hypertensives. The LDL cholesterol-reducing effect of lycopene of about 10% is reportedly comparable to the effect of low-dose statins. Lycopene may be considered as an alternative to low-dose statins, without side effects in patients with slightly elevated cholesterol levels (Ried & Fakler, 2011). A study using human macrophages showed that lycopene was able to reduce the expression of HMG-CoA reductase in a dose-dependent manner (Palozza, Paola, Simone, Rossella, Catalano, Assunta... Franco, 2011). The enzyme 3-hydroxy-3-methylglutaryl coenzyme A (HMG-CoA) reductase catalyzes the conversion of HMG-CoA to mevalonate, a four-electron oxidoreduction that is the rate-limiting step in the synthesis of cholesterol (Friesen & Rodwell, 2004). Furthermore, the pulp and leaves of *Carica papaya* are sources of β-carotene and vitamin C. The level of these compounds varies in different varieties (Nwofia, Ojimelukwe, & Eji, 2012). Both lycopene and β-carotene have been demonstrated to also inhibit macrophage HMG-CoA reductase activity (Fuhrman, Elis, & Aviram, 1997). A preliminary study of the effect of vitamin C on endothelial function demonstrated improved acetylcholine-mediated vasodilation in hypercholesterolemic subjects (Perticone, Ceravolo, Maio, Cloro, Candigliota, Scozzafava, . . . Mattioli, 2000). In 2015, a meta-analysis was done on clinical trials focused on vitamin supplementations and endothelial functions. One of the findings showed that the supplementation of vitamin C provides moderate protective effect on endothelial function (Ashor, Ammar, Siervo, Mario, Lara, Jose, Oggioni, Clio, Afshar, Sorena, Mathers, & John, 2015).

Citrus

Citrus grow in many countries from the Northern Hemisphere to the Southern Hemisphere. Citrus and olive oil are the integral components in Mediterranean food (Harats, Dror, Chevion, Shlomit, Nahir, Menahem... Ellio, 1998). Types of citrus include Sweet Orange, Mandarin orange, Grapefruit, Pummelo, Lemon, Acid Lime, Sweet Lime, Citron, Calamadin, Natsudaidai, Hassaku, Kumquat, and Bael (Ladanyia & Ladaniya, 2010). Citrus fruits are a rich source of flavanones, available in both fruit and juice (Alam, Subhan, Rahman, Uddin, Reza, & Sarker, 2014; Mulvihill & Huff, 2012). Data suggests that these flavonoids can reach significant levels in plasma. Therefore, studies involving citrus flavonoids have begun to focus on identifying and delineating their specific pharmacological properties (Mulvihill & Huff, 2012). Recent studies suggest an important role for citrus flavonoids in the treatment of dyslipidaemia, insulin resistance, hepatic steatosis, obesity, and atherosclerosis (Assini, Mulvihill, & Huff, 2013). A study involving 10,623 participants (4,147 men, 6,476 women) was done among the Japanese population to understand the potential protective effects of fruit intake on the incidence of CVD and its subtypes. It reported that the frequent consumption of citrus fruit was significantly inversely associated with CVD incidence, with marked reductions in all stroke and cerebral infarction risk, except hemorrhagic stroke risk. The study also suggested that the frequency of citrus-fruit intake was not associated with incidence of myocardial infarction (Yamada, Tomoyo, Hayasaka, Shinya, Shibata, Yosuke… Kazunori, 2011).

Orange-juice consumption has become a worldwide dietary habit, and the consumption of frozen concentrated juice has increased steadily over the years. A study was conducted in Brazil among 31 normocholesterolemic (NC; 12 males and 19 females) and 14 hypercholesterolemic (HCH; 6 males and 8 females, with LDL cholesterol >130mg/dL) subjects. These subjects were evaluated on the first and last day of the 60-day period of orange-juice consumption (750mL/d). The HCH subjects showed a 12% decrease in LDL-cholesterol after the orange-juice intake period; whereas HDL cholesterol and triglycerides remained unchanged (Cesar, Aptekmann, Araujo, Vinagre, & Maranhão, 2010). The concentrated product has a greater flavonoid content of flavanone, mainly hesperitin (Seema Bhagwat & Holden, 2014).

Bergamot differs from other citrus fruits, particularly with regard to its high content of flavonoids (Dugo, Presti, Öhman, Fazio, Dugo, & Mondello, 2005). A prospective, open-label, parallel-group, placebo-controlled study on patients with elevated serum LDL-C and triglycerides was done to investigate the effect of bergamot-derived polyphenolic fraction (BPF) in patients with mixed hyperlipidemia. The group that received BPF (1000mg daily, given orally) plus rosuvastatin (10mg daily for 30 days; $n = 15$) had reduced levels of total cholesterol, LDL-C, the LDL-C/HDL-C ratio, and urinary mevalonate in hyperlipidemic patients, compared to the control group. In addition, this was accompanied by reductions of malondialdehyde, oxyLDL receptor LOX-1, and phosphoPKB, which are all biomarkers of oxidative vascular damage in peripheral polymorphonuclear cells (Gliozzi, Micaela, Walker, Ross, Muscoli, Saverio… Vincenzo, 2013).

A cohort study of 3,932 individuals was done based on data from the Finnish Mobile Clinic Health Examination Survey, conducted in 1968–1972. The participants were 40–74 years of age, and free of cardiovascular diseases at baseline. Data on plant-food consumption were derived from a one-year dietary history interview. During a 24-year follow-up, 625 cases of cerebrovascular diseases occurred, leading to either hospitalization or death. The study found that the consumption of cruciferous vegetables predicted a reduced risk of cerebrovascular diseases (RR 0·79; 95% CI 0·63, 0·99), ischaemic stroke (RR 0·67; 95% CI 0·49, 0·92), and intracerebral haemorrhage (RR 0·49; 95% CI 0·25, 0·98). The study showed that the consumption of fruits—especially citrus—and cruciferous vegetables may protect against cerebrovascular diseases (Mizrahi, Anna, Knekt, Paul, Montonen, Jukka… Ritva, 2009). Research has shown that lemon juice has higher total phenol content (64.5mg/l), while lime juice has higher total flavonoid content (29.5mg/l). It was reported that the administration of the juices to rats fed with a high-cholesterol diet caused a significant reduction in plasma total cholesterol, triglyceride, and LDL cholesterol levels, and an increase in plasma HDL cholesterol levels. This was due to the inhibition of angiotensin-1-converting enzyme activity, and thus exhibits the hypocholesterolemic effect of the juices (Oboh, Bello, Ademosun, Akinyemi, & Adewuni, 2015).

Cardiovascular Diseases

Predominant cardiovascular diseases are ischemic heart disease (IHD), stroke, and congestive heart failure (CHF). Other forms of CVD include Chagas disease, congenital abnormalities or genetically based cardiomyopathies, and rheumatic heart disease. The two leading manifestations of IHD are angina and acute myocardial infarction. Angina is the characteristic pain of IHD, caused by atherosclerosis leading to stenosis (partial occlusion) of one or more coronary arteries. Stroke is caused by a disruption in the flow of blood to part of the brain, either because of the occlusion of a blood vessel (ischemic stroke) or the rupture of a blood vessel (hemorrhagic stroke). CHF is characterized by abnormalities in myocardial function and neurohormonal regulation, resulting in fatigue, fluid retention, and reduced longevity (Gaziano, 2010).

Cardiovascular Disease Risk Factors

CVD major independent risk factors are advancing age, elevated blood pressure, elevated serum total and low-density lipoprotein cholesterol levels, low serum high-density lipoprotein cholesterol level, diabetes mellitus, and cigarette smoking (Grundy, Pasternak, Greenland, Smith, & Fuster, 1999; Wilson, 1994). Levels of low-density lipoprotein and high-density lipoprotein, habits of smoking and lack of physical activity, diabetes mellitus, and hypertension are all modifiable risk factors, and modification can prevent CAD.

Age, education, current smoking, diabetes, hypertension, and elevated serum cholesterol levels were significant risk factors for ischemic heart disease mortality among all race and sex groups in an assessment of 10,766 subjects studied, including black and white, men and women, for the period from 1971 to 1992 in the United States of America (Chang, Hahn, Teutsch, & L.C., 2001). Within the period, 1,401 (13.0%) subjects died from ischemic heart disease. In patients presenting with acute coronary syndrome (ACS), half had diabetes, hyperlipidemia, smoking, and hypertension, the recognized cardiovascular risk factors (Chin, Jeyaindran, Azhari, Wan Azman, Omar, Robaayah, & Sim, 2008).

Role of Lipids and Lipoproteins in Development of Coronary Artery Disease

Blood Lipids

The major lipids present in plasma are fatty acids, triglycerides, cholesterol, and phospholipids. Elevated plasma concentration cholesterol (hypercholesterolemia) is related to the pathogenesis of atherosclerosis, and is also one of the most studied risk factors for atherosclerosis (Taylor, Burke, O'Malley, Farb, Malcolm, Smialek, & Virmani, 2000).

Serum cholesterol is carried in the blood by several lipoprotein particles that perform the complex physiologic tasks of transporting dietary and endogenously produced lipids. Chylomicrons provide the primary means of transport of dietary lipids (principally triglycerides), while transport of endogenous lipids are very low-density lipoproteins (VLDL), low-density lipoproteins (LDL) and high-density lipoproteins (HDL).

High-Density Lipoproteins (HDL)

HDL is the smallest and densest of all the lipoprotein classes. It has the highest density because HDL particles contain the highest proportion of protein to lipids, and its most abundant apolipoproteins are apo A-I and apo A-II (Yetukuri, Laxman, Söderlund, Sanni, Koivuniemi, Artturi… Matej, 2010). This lipoprotein is synthesized in the liver as disc-shaped complexes of apolipoproteins and phospholipids. Lecithin-cholesterol acyltransferase (LCAT) converts the free cholesterol into cholesteryl ester, which is then sequestered in the core of the lipoprotein particle, resulting in spherical newly synthesized HDL. These increase in size as they circulate in the bloodstream and incorporate more cholesterol and phospholipid molecules from cells and other lipoproteins (Rader, 2006).

HDL transports cholesterol from other tissues back to the liver (known as reverse cholesterol transport) or to steroidogenic organs such as adrenals, ovaries, and testes, through direct and indirect pathways. The gatekeeper of this reverse cholesterol transport pathway is an ATP-binding cassette (ABC) transporter called ABCA1. Mutations in ABCA1 cause Tangier disease (TD), a severe HDL deficiency syndrome characterized by accumulation of cholesterol in tissue macrophages and prevalent atherosclerosis (Oram & Lawn, 2001). In fact, the association between HDL cholesterol (HDL-C) and cardiovascular disease risk is significant and strong (Chirovsky, Fedirko, Cui, Sazonov, & Barter, 2009). Various epidemiological and clinical studies prove that a low level of HDL-C is a powerful risk factor for cardiovascular disease.

Low-Density Lipoproteins (LDL)

The core of an LDL particle is hydrophobic and consists of esterified cholesterol and triacylglycerol, while its outer surface layer of phospholipids is surrounded by a single apo B-100 protein. LDL carries mostly cholesterol, some protein, and minimal triglycerides throughout the blood circulation. It is also important for the synthesis of steroid hormones (Goldstein & Brown, 2009). LDL contains 5-9% triacylglycerols, 43–50% cholesterol, and 19–21% phospholipids (Jain, Jain, Kesharwani, & Jain, 2013).

Uptake of cholesterol by a cell occurs through receptor-mediated endocytosis, whereby LDL will bind to an LDL receptor (LDLR) and form a complex that will be internalized into the cells. LDL dissociates from the receptor when the pH drops. The receptor is then recycled to the surface of the cell, while LDL is transferred into the lysosomes for degradation to monomers, and released into the cytoplasm (Harisa & Alanazi, 2014).

LDL is often linked to atherosclerosis, and the main target of therapy for the prevention of coronary heart disease (Carmena, Duriez, & Fruchart, 2004). It is susceptible to oxidative modification (Levitan, Volkov, & Subbaiah, 2010), and oxidation of LDL is assumed to occur in two main stages. During the initial stages of LDL oxidation *in vitro*, oxidative modifications of LDL result in little change in apolipoprotein B100, and such modified LDL is called minimally oxidized LDL (Yoshida & Kisugi, 2010). In the second stage, LDL is further oxidized along with modification in the protein portion of LDL, resulting in loss of recognition by the LDL receptor and a shift to recognition by the scavenger receptors. This can give rise to foam cells and cause ox-LDL to be more atherogenic than native LDL (Steinberg, 1997).

Very Low-Density Lipoproteins (VLDL)

Unlike LDL, VLDL mainly transports triglycerides (TAG) and contains less cholesterol than LDL. The core of VLDL consists of hydrophobic and triacylglycerol molecules and cholesterol ester, coated by a relatively hydrophilic monolayer consisting of phospholipids, free-cholesterol, and apolipoproteins. The TAG core of the VLDL particle is synthesised by liver cells, using fatty acids derived from hydrolysis of adipose tissue TAG stores (lipolysis), fatty acids derived from peripheral hydrolysis of plasma lipoprotein (VLDL and chylomicron) TAG cleared by the liver, or newly synthesised fatty acids via hepatic *de novo* lipogenesis (Niu & Evans, 2011). VLDL particles are important as a transport vehicle responsible for redistribution of endogenous triglycerides, phospholipids, cholesterol, and cholesteryl esters, from liver to peripheral tissues.

Apolipoprotein (apo) B100 is the major structural protein of VLDL, while ApoE regulates the binding of VLDL particles to heparin and lipoprotein receptors on hepatocytes, as well as other cells (Fielding, Ishikawa, & Fielding, 1989). Besides apoB-100 and apoE, VLDL also contains apoC-I, apoC-II and apoC-III. A loss of these apoCs, together with the action of lipoprotein lipase, leads to the conversion of VLDL to intermediate-density lipoprotein (IDL) (Sacks, 2015).

Chylomicrons

Chylomicrons are triglyceride-rich lipoproteins with a central lipid core and a layer of phospholipids (6–12%), free cholesterol (1–3%), and apolipoproteins (1–2%). Chylomicrons are large and have the lowest protein-to-lipid ratio, and thus the lowest density of all the lipoproteins. They are essential for the transport of triglycerides and fat-soluble vitamins (Hamilton, 2004). A key structural component of chylomicrons is apoprotein B48 (ApoB48), a large, hydrophobic, nonexchangeable protein of the rough endoplasmic reticular membrane (Goodman, 2010).

The synthesis of chylomicrons is dependent on microsomal triglyceride transport protein (MTP), which catalyzes the transfer of the water-insoluble triglyceride to the enlarging lipid droplet and combines with a high-density, protein-rich particle in the rough endoplasmic reticulum. Subsequently, the ApoB48 and dense particle complex combines with a large light particle with attached apoprotein AIV from the smooth endoplasmic reticulum, to form a prechylomicron (Mansbach & Gorelick, 2007). After the prechylomicrons are synthesized, these intracellular particles leave the endoplasmic reticulum (ER) and are carried through the secretory pathway for further modification (Abumrad & Davidson, 2012).

Chylomicron metabolism is very similar to VLDL metabolism. Although LDL is known as the major contributor to plaque cholesterol, abnormalities of chylomicron metabolism could also add to the risk of atherosclerosis. Chylomicron remnants are taken up into the subendothelial space and degraded by lipoprotein lipase on the artery wall. They are attached to the endothelium by high-density lipoprotein-binding protein 1 (GPIHBP1) and heparin sulphate proteoglycans (HPSG), which facilitate their uptake into the subendothelial space. Chylomicron remnants become trapped in the artery wall and disintegrate to contribute cholesterol to the atherosclerotic plaque (Tomkin & Owens, 2011).

Atherosclerosis

Atherosclerosis is closely related to development of coronary artery disease (Libby, 2005; Nordestgaard & Zacho, 2009), as a result of a combination of abnormalities in lipoprotein metabolism, oxidative stress, chronic inflammatory process, and tendency to thrombosis. Endothelial dysfunction is an initial step in atherosclerosis (Kampoli, Tousoulis, Antoniades, Siasos, & Stefanadis, 2009). Increased formation of reactive oxygen species (ROS) is reported to contribute to atherogenesis and CVD progression. The generation of large amounts of ROS can overwhelm the intracellular antioxidant defense, causing activation of neutrophils, lipid peroxidation, protein modification, and DNA breaks. Based on the oxidation theory of atherosclerosis, dietary antioxidants have attracted considerable attention as preventive and therapeutic agents (Kaliora, Dedoussis, & Schmidt, 2006) Atherosclerosis is characterized by a multifocal, smoldering disease of medium-sized and large arteries fueled by lipids, resulting in the formation of fatty and fibrous lesions in the arterial wall (Ross, 1999). The rate of progression of atherosclerosis is influenced by cardiovascular risk factors such as tobacco use, an unhealthy diet, and physical inactivity (which together result in obesity), elevated blood pressure (hypertension), abnormal blood lipids (dyslipidaemia), and elevated blood glucose (Type 2 DM) (WHO, 2007).

The concept that atherosclerosis is an inflammatory disease is widely accepted. The process includes accumulation of intra- and extracellular lipids, foam cell formation, proliferation of smooth muscle cells, and accumulation of connective tissue components. The earliest event in atherogenesis appears to be endothelial cell dysfunction that can be caused by various insults such as hypertension, diabetes, smoking, dyslipidaemia, and hyperhomocysteinemia (Libby, 2002). After endothelial cell dysfunction, mononuclear cells, initially loosely attached to the endothelium, adhere firmly afterwards and pass through diapedesis into the subendothelial space. During the atherosclerotic process, numbers of cytokines and growth-regulatory molecules are formed and released from the cells in the lesions, which consist of endothelial cells, smooth muscle cells, macrophages and T-lymphocytes (Ross, 1993).

The earliest visible lesion of atherosclerosis is the fatty streak, an aggregation of cholesterol-loaded macrophages or foam cells within the arterial wall (Nagy, Tontonoz, Alvarez, Chen, & Evans, 1998). Fatty-streak formation is widely accepted as a precursor of clinically significant and complicated atherosclerotic lesions later on (Steinberg & Witztum, 1990). With time, the fatty streak progresses into a fibrous plaque, the hallmark of established atherosclerosis. The lesion will ultimately evolve to contain large amounts of lipids and become unstable, which can lead to thrombotic occlusion of the overlying artery (Crowther, 2005). If the progression of the process is rapid, as in the case of plaque rupture accompanied by superimposed thrombosis, it may cause devastating acute coronary and cerebrovascular events such as unstable angina, myocardial infarction, stroke, or sudden death (Patel, Celermajer, & Bao, 2008).

NCEP ATP III Guidelines and Dietary Guideline

The importance of low-density lipoprotein (LDL) cholesterol measurement has been stated in the National Cholesterol Education Program Adult Treatment Panel III (NCEP ATP III) guidelines. NCEP ATP III is the latest report of the NCEP guidelines, and measurement of LDL cholesterol had been identified as its first step in risk assessment, followed by high-density lipoprotein (HDL) and serum triglyceride (TG) measurements. Lowering LDL cholesterol has been the target for management. An LDL cholesterol level of <100mg/dL is defined as optimal for the whole population (Pasternak, 2002).

NCEP ATP III was a detailed and evidence-based approach to both diagnosis and management of hypercholesterolemia, and the guidelines emphasized the patient's risk of developing coronary artery disease. The ATP III guideline also emphasized therapeutic lifestyle changes (TLC), such as benefits of healthy diet, weight control, and exercise, especially in patients with lifestyle risk factors such as obesity, sedentary lifestyle, and elevated plasma glucose, as its risk-lowering strategy (Stone, Bilek, & Rosenbaum, 2005). *The Dietary Guideline for Americans 2015–2020* recommends limiting intake of saturated fat to less than 10% of daily total calories (Nelson, 2015).

Diabetes Mellitus and Its Association to Coronary Artery Disease

Type 2 DM is a disease associated with coronary artery disease. The number of individuals with diabetes is set to rise beyond 592 million within 25 years (Linnenkamp, Guariguata, Beagley, Whiting, & Cho, 2014). Prevalence of diabetes increased from 5.1% in 2003 to 6.0% in 2007, and is estimated to increase to 7.3% by 2025 (Shaw, Sicree, & Zimmet, 2010). The International Diabetic Foundation (IDF) predicts the Western Pacific will have more than 200 million individuals living with diabetes by 2030 (Linnenkamp, Guariguata, Beagley, Whiting, & Cho, 2014). Southeast Asia will have the second highest prevalence, with 123 million individuals (Linnenkamp, Guariguata, Beagley, Whiting, & Cho, 2014).

Diabetes mellitus is a vascular disease related to macrovascular and microvascular diseases. Nearly 75% of diabetic patients die of an atherosclerotic event, and the incidence of coronary artery disease is two to four times greater in the diabetic than in nondiabetic subjects (Hsueh & Law, 1998). The clustering of type 2 DM, a well-documented risk factor for cardiovascular disease (CVD), with other established risk factors such as dyslipidaemia, smoking, hypertension, and abdominal obesity, is well recognized (Pelikanova, 2009).

The relationship between traditional risk factors and CVD in Asia differs from that in Western societies, and CVD in Asia has some unique features with respect to risk factors and metabolic abnormalities (Sasayama, 2008). For example, hypertension plays a more important role in the development of heart disease and stroke in Asia than in Western countries. The prevalence of obesity and overweight in Asia has been increasing as a consequence of economic development in the past two to three decades. The rate of increase for diabetes has been even more substantial. Mean cholesterol levels are lower for adults in most Asian countries than in Western countries, but an increasing upward trend has been observed (Hong, 2009).

Genetic Linkage With Lipid Metabolism Defects

Among the factors of cardiovascular risk is genetic polymorphism, a nonmodifiable risk factor. Apolipoprotein E (apoE) is the key protein in transportation of lipids, and its polymorphism is recognized as one of the most important genetic determinants for CAD (Mahley, 1988). On a population basis, it has the strongest impact on plasma lipid levels presently known for a single gene polymorphism. Genetic polymorphism is an important cause of aberrant lipoprotein metabolism and increases the CAD risk (Kalix, Meynet, Garin, & James, 2001; Kataoka, Robbins, Cowan, Go, Yeh, Devereux, . . . Howard, 1996). The gene for apo E is polymorphic. It has three common alleles, which consist of *epsilon (ε)* 2, ε3, and ε4, and each code for three major isoforms, resulting in six common genotypes. Figure 1 shows five different genotypes. These isoforms vary in their receptor-binding affinity, with apoE4 having the greatest receptor binding, and apoE2 having less than 2% binding affinity. Individuals with apoE2 are reported to have higher levels of triglycerides. In homozygotes an even great increase in concentrations of remnants was observed, resulting in type III dyslipidaemia (Zhao, Smelt, Van den Maagdenberg, Van Tol, Vroom. . . Van 't Hooft, 1994). Individuals with *epsilon* 4, conversely, tend to have a striking increase in LDL cholesterol (Kesaniemi, Ehnholm, & Miettinen, 1987). A case control study was done to determine the frequency distribution of APOE genotypes and alleles in patients with Type 2 DM, with and without CAD. Frequency of APOE genotypes in the overall study population showed that the most frequent APOE genotype was E3/E3 (59.1%). The next most common APOE genotype observed was E3/E4 (21.7%), followed by E2/E3 (11.3%), E2/E2 (4.3%), and both E2/E4 and E2/44 (1.7%). Generally, there was no significant difference in APOE frequency distribution between the Type 2 DM without CAD group and the Type 2 DM with CAD group. Percentages of those with the ε3 carrier (E2/E3, E3/E3 and E3/E4) were higher in the Type 2 DM without CAD group. However, there was

Figure 1. Electrophoresis separation of HhaI for APOE gene polymorphism

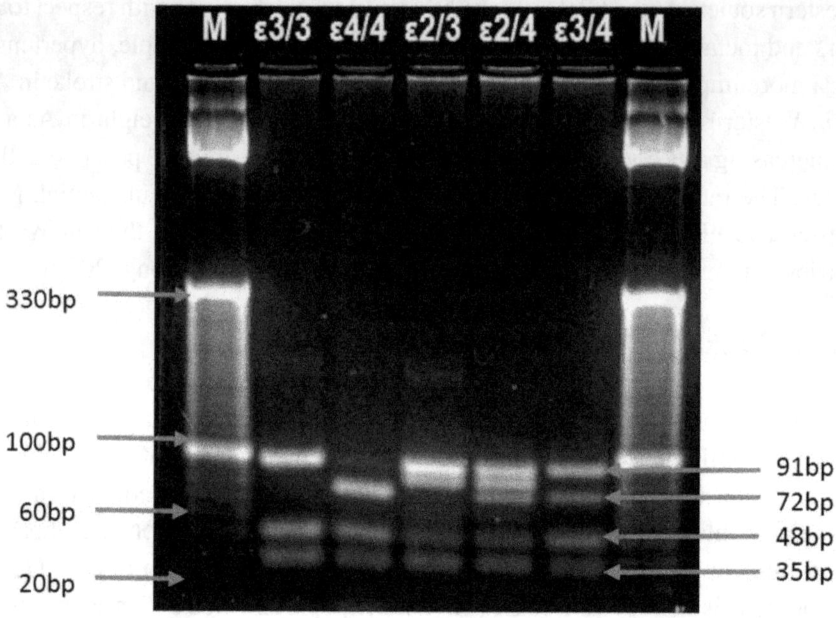

no significant difference in APOE genotypes distribution between the Type 2 DM without CAD group and the Type 2 DM with CAD group (Ashari, Omar, Hashim, & Hamid, 2016).

Monitoring of Blood Lipid Levels

Technology advancements have made health screening more accessible. Smartphone devices could be used as noninvasive methods to determine cholesterol. Easy to use and familiar to almost all age groups, their familiarity can dramatically reduce training requirements and potential user errors during testing. This lab-on-a-chip type of technology is reported to be potentially useful in both developed and developing countries (Erickson, David, O'Dell, Dakota, Jiang, Li . . . Saurabh, 2014). A trial was done using a smartphone accessory and software application for quantification of cholesterol levels in blood. The system accurately quantified total cholesterol levels in blood within 60 seconds by imaging standard test strips (Oncescu, Mancuso, & Erickson, 2014). On the other hand, an increasing number of products is now available on the market to monitor blood total cholesterol, HDL cholesterol, and triglycerides, such as the Cardiochek Starter Cholesterol Analyzer kit, Cardiochek Blood Testing Device kit, Cardiochek Triglycerides, and Cholestrak Total Cholesterol Home Testing kit.

SOLUTIONS AND RECOMMENDATIONS

Education plays a key role in prevention of disease. Healthcare agencies must increase the awareness within society of the importance of monitoring health status as a preventive measure. Regular screening activities should be organized in schools, both public and private, whether in rural or urban areas. Such effort would assist in identifying those potentially at risk of developing cardiovascular disease, diabetes mellitus type 2, or impaired glucose tolerance. Individuals identified as borderline must be monitored and provided with guidance on therapeutic lifestyle modification and nutrition counseling. The importance of nutraceuticals and functional food intake must be highlighted. It is important to inculcate healthy nutritional habits, beginning at a tender age.

Society must be encouraged to perform self-monitoring. Increase in advertisements and promotion activities to highlight current technologies for self-monitoring risk factors, and test methods that are cheap, reliable, and user friendly, would attract potential buyers.

WHO provides guidance on reducing disability and premature death from coronary heart disease, cerebrovascular disease, and peripheral vascular disease in people at high risk who have not yet experienced a cardiovascular event. It provides guidance to policymakers and healthcare workers on how to target individuals at high risk of developing CVD, at all levels of the health system and in different resource settings, using evidence-based and cost-effective preventive approaches.

FUTURE RESEARCH DIRECTIONS

Nutraceutical and functional food are great source of nutrients. They have potential to prevent cardiovascular diseases risk factors as reported in literature. Through policies and community-based activities, education on modification of risk factors will enable further assist in lowering the rate of cardiovascular incidence. The effects of functional food concoction could be further explored through clinical and pre-clinical studies as proof of concept. Evidences provided from such studies could support their role as preventive source of atherosclerosis initiation or progression. It is also reported that human studies focused on dose, bioavailability, efficacy, and safety are required to propel the use of these promising therapeutic agents into the clinical arena (Assini, Julia, Mulvihill, Erin, Huff, & Murray, 2013). In addition, community-level activities on improving food access and choices, including what restaurants, public schools, community events, and worksite wellness initiatives serve, should be listed and promoted in the community resource guide (Harper, Lynch, & Smith, 2011). The local social media and library could also play vital role in creating awareness of preventive measures and resources. Furthermore, there has to be consistent supply of fruits and vegetables to meet demands throughout the year. Policies should be in place for early screening of risk factors among younger generation. This could be a preventive measure and could reduce healthcare cost over time. With the current technology advancements, there is potential for investment into smart technology for development of simple and rapid non-invasive monitoring devices. User friendly gadgets would encourage self-monitoring. This would require designing software which could incorporate nutritional facts and guidelines on recommended levels of cardiovascular risk biomarkers.

CONCLUSION

Nutraceuticals and functional food are rich dietary sources with plenty of health benefits for prevention of CAD and SCD. Continuous health-education programs should be in place in schools, universities and community centers, to act as early preventive measures that could reduce the risk of cardiovascular disease. Evidence from numerous clinical and preclinical studies shows the significant roles of dietary sources in modulating these risk factors, particularly with regard to atherosclerosis. Consistent intake of healthy nutritional sources would have profound effects on lowering the risk of developing cardiovascular disease.

REFERENCES

Abumrad, N. A., & Davidson, N. O. (2012). Role of the gut in lipid homeostasis. *Physiological Reviews*, *92*(3), 1061–1085. doi:10.1152/physrev.00019.2011 PMID:22811425

Afroz, R., Tanvir, E., & Little, P. J. (2016). Honey-derived flavonoids: Natural products for the prevention of atherosclerosis and cardiovascular diseases. *Clinical & Experimental Pharmacology*, *6*(3).

Ahmad, A., Husain, A., Mujeeb, M., Khan, S. A., Najmi, A. K., Siddique, N. A., ... Anwar, F. (2013). A review on therapeutic potential of Nigella sativa: A miracle herb. *Asian Pacific Journal of Tropical Biomedicine*, *3*(5), 337–352. doi:10.1016/S2221-1691(13)60075-1 PMID:23646296

Al-Naqeep, Al-Zubairi, Ismail, Amom, & Esa. (2011). Antiatherogenic Potential of Nigella sativa Seeds and Oil in Diet-Induced Hypercholesterolemia in Rabbits. *Evidence-based Complementary and Alternative Medicine: eCAM, 2011*. doi: 10.1093/ecam/neq071

Alam, M. A., Kauter, K., & Brown, L. (2013). Naringin improves diet-induced cardiovascular dysfunction and obesity in high carbohydrate, high fat diet-fed rats. *Nutrients*, *5*(3), 637–650. doi:10.3390/nu5030637 PMID:23446977

Alam, S., Subhan, N., Rahman, M. M., Uddin, S. J., Reza, H. M., & Sarker, S. D. (2014). Effect of citrus flavonoids, naringin and naringenin, on metabolic syndrome and their mechanisms of action. *Advances in Nutrition*, *5*(4), 404–417. doi:10.3945/an.113.005603 PMID:25022990

Alves-Silva, J. M., Monica, Z., Carla, M., Ligia, S., & Henrique, G. (2016). Protective effects of terpenes on the cardiovascular system: Current advances and future perspectives. *Current Medicinal Chemistry*. PMID:27604093

Amagase, H., & Nance, D. M. (2008). A randomized, double-blind, placebo-controlled, clinical study of the general effects of a standardized Lycium barbarum (goji) juice, GoChi™. *Journal of Alternative and Complementary Medicine (New York, N.Y.)*, *14*(4), 403–412. doi:10.1089/acm.2008.0004 PMID:18447631

Amagase, H., Sun, B., & Borek, C. (2009). Lycium barbarum (goji) juice improves in vivo antioxidant biomarkers in serum of healthy adults. *Nutrition Research (New York, N.Y.)*, *29*(1), 19–25. doi:10.1016/j.nutres.2008.11.005 PMID:19185773

Ashari, A., Omar, J., Hashim, A., & Hamid, S. (2016). Apolipoprotein E Gene Polymorphism and Its Association with Cardiovascular Heart Disease Risk Factors in Type 2 Diabetes Mellitus. *World Academy of Science, Engineering and Technology, International Journal of Medical, Health, Biomedical. Bioengineering and Pharmaceutical Engineering*, *10*(9), 471–476.

Ashor, A. W., Siervo, M., Lara, J., Oggioni, C., Afshar, S., & Mathers, J. C. (2015). Effect of vitamin C and vitamin E supplementation on endothelial function: A systematic review and meta-analysis of randomised controlled trials. *British Journal of Nutrition*, *113*(08), 1182–1194. doi:10.1017/S0007114515000227 PMID:25919436

Assini, J. M., Mulvihill, E. E., & Huff, M. W. (2013). Citrus flavonoids and lipid metabolism. *Current Opinion in Lipidology*, *24*(1), 34–40. doi:10.1097/MOL.0b013e32835c07fd PMID:23254473

Awad, E. M., & Binder, B. R. (2005). In vitro induction of endothelial cell fibrinolytic alterations by Nigella sativa. *Phytomedicine*, *12*(3), 194–202. doi:10.1016/j.phymed.2003.09.008 PMID:15830841

Basu, A., Betts, N. M., Nguyen, A., Newman, E. D., Fu, D., & Lyons, T. J. (2014). Freeze-dried strawberries lower serum cholesterol and lipid peroxidation in adults with abdominal adiposity and elevated serum lipids. *The Journal of Nutrition*, *144*(6), 830–837. doi:10.3945/jn.113.188169 PMID:24670970

Basu, A., Rhone, M., & Lyons, T. J. (2010). Berries: Emerging impact on cardiovascular health. *Nutrition Reviews*, *68*(3), 168–177. doi:10.1111/j.1753-4887.2010.00273.x PMID:20384847

Berry, C. E., & Hare, J. M. (2004). Xanthine oxidoreductase and cardiovascular disease: Molecular mechanisms and pathophysiological implications. *The Journal of Physiology*, *555*(Pt 3), 589–606. doi:10.1113/jphysiol.2003.055913 PMID:14694147

Bhagwat, Haytowitz, & Holden. (2014). USDA Database for the Flavonoid Content of Selected Foods Release 3.1. U.S. Department of Agriculture Agricultural Research Service.

Bhardwaj, S., Passi, S. J., & Misra, A. (2011). Overview of trans fatty acids: Biochemistry and health effects. *Diabetes & Metabolic Syndrome*, *5*(3), 161–164. doi:10.1016/j.dsx.2012.03.002 PMID:22813572

Bogani, P., Galli, C., Villa, M., & Visioli, F. (2007). Postprandial anti-inflammatory and antioxidant effects of extra virgin olive oil. *Atherosclerosis*, *190*(1), 181–186. doi:10.1016/j.atherosclerosis.2006.01.011 PMID:16488419

Canini, A., Alesiani, D., D'Arcangelo, G., & Tagliatesta, P. (2007). Gas chromatography–mass spectrometry analysis of phenolic compounds from Carica papaya L. leaf. *Journal of Food Composition and Analysis*, *20*(7), 584–590. doi:10.1016/j.jfca.2007.03.009

Carmena, R., Duriez, P., & Fruchart, J.-C. (2004). Atherogenic Lipoprotein Particles in Atherosclerosis. *Circulation*, *109*(23suppl 1), III-2–III-7. doi:10.1161/01.cir.0000131511.50734.44 PMID:15198959

Cesar, T. B., Aptekmann, N. P., Araujo, M. P., Vinagre, C. C., & Maranhão, R. C. (2010). Orange juice decreases low-density lipoprotein cholesterol in hypercholesterolemic subjects and improves lipid transfer to high-density lipoprotein in normal and hypercholesterolemic subjects. *Nutrition Research (New York, N.Y.)*, *30*(10), 689–694. doi:10.1016/j.nutres.2010.09.006 PMID:21056284

Chang, M.-H., Hahn, R., Teutsch, S. M., & Hutwagner, L. C. (2001). Multiple risk factors and and population attributable risk for ischemic heart disease mortality in the United States, 1971-1992. *Journal of Clinical Epidemiology*, *54*(6), 634–644. doi:10.1016/S0895-4356(00)00343-7 PMID:11377125

Chen, H.-Y., & Yen, G.-C. (2007). Antioxidant activity and free radical-scavenging capacity of extracts from guava (Psidium guajava L.) leaves. *Food Chemistry*, *101*(2), 686–694. doi:10.1016/j.foodchem.2006.02.047

Chin, SP, Jeyaindran, S, Azhari, R, Wan Azman, WA, Omar, I, Robaayah, Z, & Sim, KH. (2008). Acute Coronary Syndrome (ACS) Registry - Leading the charge for National Cardiovascular Disease (NCVD) Database. *Med J Malaysia, 63 Supplemen C*, 29-36.

Chirovsky, D. R., Fedirko, V., Cui, Y., Sazonov, V., & Barter, P. (2009). Prospective studies on the relationship between high-density lipoprotein cholesterol and cardiovascular risk: A systematic review. *European Journal of Cardiovascular Prevention and Rehabilitation*, *16*(4), 404–423. doi:10.1097/HJR.0b013e32832c8891 PMID:19465856

Chu, Y.-F., & Liu, R. H. (2005). Cranberries inhibit LDL oxidation and induce LDL receptor expression in hepatocytes. *Life Sciences*, *77*(15), 1892–1901. doi:10.1016/j.lfs.2005.04.002 PMID:15982671

Crowther, M. A. (2005). Pathogenesis of Atherosclerosis. *Hematology*, *2005*(1), 436–441. doi:10.1182/asheducation-2005.1.436 PMID:16304416

Crozier, A., Yokota, T., Jaganath, I. B., Marks, S., Saltmarsh, M., & Clifford, M. N. (2007). *Secondary Metabolites in Fruits, Vegetables, Beverages and Other Plant-based Dietary Components. In Plant Secondary Metabolites* (pp. 208–302). Blackwell Publishing Ltd.

Dugo, P., Presti, M. L., Öhman, M., Fazio, A., Dugo, G., & Mondello, L. (2005). Determination of flavonoids in citrus juices by micro-HPLC-ESI/MS. *Journal of Separation Science*, *28*(11), 1149–1156. doi:10.1002/jssc.200500053 PMID:16116991

El-Bahai, M. N., Al-Hariri, M. T., Yar, T., & Bamosa, A. O. (2009, January 24). Cardiac inotropic and hypertrophic effects of Nigella sativa supplementation in rats. *International Journal of Cardiology*, *131*(3), e115–e117. doi:10.1016/j.ijcard.2007.07.075 PMID:17931720

Erickson, D., O'Dell, D., Jiang, L., Oncescu, V., Gumus, A., Lee, S., ... Mehta, S. (2014). Smartphone technology can be transformative to the deployment of lab-on-chip diagnostics. *Lab on a Chip*, *14*(17), 3159–3164. doi:10.1039/C4LC00142G PMID:24700127

Fielding, P. E., Ishikawa, Y., & Fielding, C. J. (1989). Apolipoprotein E mediates binding of normal very low density lipoprotein to heparin but is not required for high affinity receptor binding. *The Journal of Biological Chemistry*, *264*(21), 12462–12466. PMID:2745454

Flores, G., Dastmalchi, K., Wu, S.-B., Whalen, K., Dabo, A. J., Reynertson, K. A., ... Kennelly, E. J. (2013). Phenolic-rich extract from the Costa Rican guava (Psidium friedrichsthalianum) pulp with antioxidant and anti-inflammatory activity. Potential for COPD therapy. *Food Chemistry*, *141*(2), 889–895. doi:10.1016/j.foodchem.2013.03.025 PMID:23790863

Friesen, J. A., & Rodwell, V. W. (2004). The 3-hydroxy-3-methylglutaryl coenzyme-A (HMG-CoA) reductases. *Genome Biology*, *5*(11), 1. doi:10.1186/gb-2004-5-11-248 PMID:15535874

Fuhrman, B., Elis, A., & Aviram, M. (1997). Hypocholesterolemic effect of lycopene and β-carotene is related to suppression of cholesterol synthesis and augmentation of LDL receptor activity in macrophages. [Article]. *Biochemical and Biophysical Research Communications*, *233*(3), 658–662. doi:10.1006/bbrc.1997.6520 PMID:9168909

Gaziano, T., Reddy, K. S., Paccaud, F., Horton, S., & Chaturvedi, V. (2010). *Cardiovascular Disease Control Priorities in Developing Countries* (2nd ed.). Washington, DC: National Academies Press (US).

Glik, Sharif, Tucker, Tejada, Prelip, Ammerman, & ... Jilcott Pitts. (2016). Community-engagement to support cardiovascular disease prevention in disparities populations: Three case studies. *Journal of Health Disparities Research and Practice*, *9*(1), 6.

Gliozzi, M., Walker, R., Muscoli, S., Vitale, C., Gratteri, S., Carresi, C., ... Mollace, V. (2013). Bergamot polyphenolic fraction enhances rosuvastatin-induced effect on LDL-cholesterol, LOX-1 expression and protein kinase B phosphorylation in patients with hyperlipidemia. *International Journal of Cardiology*, *170*(2), 140–145. doi:10.1016/j.ijcard.2013.08.125 PMID:24239156

Goldstein, J. L., & Brown, M. S. (2009). The LDL Receptor. *Arteriosclerosis, Thrombosis, and Vascular Biology*, *29*(4), 431–438. doi:10.1161/ATVBAHA.108.179564 PMID:19299327

Goodman, B. E. (2010). Insights into digestion and absorption of major nutrients in humans. *Advances in Physiology Education*, *34*(2), 44–53. doi:10.1152/advan.00094.2009 PMID:20522896

Grundy, M., Pasternak, R., Greenland, P., Smith, S., & Fuster, V. (1999). Assessment of Cardiovascular Risk by Use of Multiple-Risk Factor Assessment Equations: A statement for Healthcare Professionals From The American Heart Association and The American College of Cardiology. *100*, 1481-1492.

Guo, J., Gan, X. T., Haist, J. V., Rajapurohitam, V., Zeidan, A., Faruq, N. S., & Karmazyn, M. (2011). Ginseng inhibits cardiomyocyte hypertrophy and heart failure via NHE-1 inhibition and attenuation of calcineurin activation. *Circulation: Heart Failure*, *4*(1), 79–88. doi:10.1161/CIRCHEARTFAILURE.110.957969 PMID:20971938

Hamilton, J. A. (2004). Fatty acid interactions with proteins: What X-ray crystal and NMR solution structures tell us. *Progress in Lipid Research*, *43*(3), 177–199. doi:10.1016/j.plipres.2003.09.002 PMID:15003394

Hanafy, M. S., & Hatem, M. E. (1991). Studies on the antimicrobial activity of Nigella sativa seed (black cumin). *Journal of Ethnopharmacology*, *34*(2-3), 275–278. doi:10.1016/0378-8741(91)90047-H PMID:1795532

Harats, D., Chevion, S., Nahir, M., Norman, Y., Sagee, O., & Berry, E. M. (1998). Citrus fruit supplementation reduces lipoprotein oxidation in young men ingesting a diet high in saturated fat: Presumptive evidence for an interaction between vitamins C and E in vivo. *The American Journal of Clinical Nutrition*, *67*(2), 240–245. doi:10.1093/ajcn/67.2.240 PMID:9459371

Harisa, G. I., & Alanazi, F. K. (2013). Low density lipoprotein bionanoparticles: From cholesterol transport to delivery of anti-cancer drugs. *Saudi Pharmaceutical Journal*. PMID:25561862

Harisa, G. I., & Alanazi, F. K. (2014). Low density lipoprotein bionanoparticles: From cholesterol transport to delivery of anti-cancer drugs. *Saudi Pharmaceutical Journal*, *22*(6), 504–515. doi:10.1016/j.jsps.2013.12.015 PMID:25561862

Harper, S., Lynch, J., & Smith, G. D. (2011). Social determinants and the decline of cardiovascular diseases: Understanding the links. *Annual Review of Public Health*, *32*(1), 39–69. doi:10.1146/annurev-publhealth-031210-101234 PMID:21219168

Hong, Y. (2009). Burden of Cardiovascular Disease in Asia: Big Challenges and Ample Opportunities for Action and Making a Difference. *Clinical Chemistry*, *55*(8), 1450–1452. doi:10.1373/clinchem.2009.125369 PMID:19498049

Hosseinzadeh, H., & Parvardeh, S. (2004). Anticonvulsant effects of thymoquinone, the major constituent of Nigella sativa seeds, in mice. *Phytomedicine*, *11*(1), 56–64. doi:10.1078/0944-7113-00376 PMID:14971722

Hsueh, W. A., & Law, R. E. (1998). Diabetes is a vascular disease. *Journal of Investigative Medicine*, *46*(8), 387–390. PMID:9805424

Hu, F., Koon, C. M., Chan, J. Y., Lau, K. M., & Fung, K. P. (2012). The cardioprotective effect of danshen and gegen decoction on rat hearts and cardiomyocytes with post-ischemia reperfusion injury. *BMC Complementary and Alternative Medicine*, *12*(1), 249. doi:10.1186/1472-6882-12-249 PMID:23228089

Irondi, E. A., Agboola, S. O., Oboh, G., Boligon, A. A., Athayde, M. L., & Shode, F. O. (2016). Guava leaves polyphenolics-rich extract inhibits vital enzymes implicated in gout and hypertension in vitro. *J Intercult Ethnopharmacol*, *5*(2), 122. doi:10.5455/jice.20160321115402 PMID:27104032

Jain, A., Jain, K., Kesharwani, P., & Jain, N. K. (2013). Low density lipoproteins mediated nanoplatforms for cancer targeting. *Journal of Nanoparticle Research*, *15*(9), 1–38. doi:10.100711051-013-1888-7

Jamal, P., & Akbar, I. (2016). Process Development for Maximum Lycopene Production from Selected Fruit Waste and its Antioxidant and Antiradical Activity. *Journal of Food Processing & Technology*, *07*(04). doi:10.4172/2157-7110.1000576

Kaliora, A. C., Dedoussis, G. V. Z., & Schmidt, H. (2006). Dietary antioxidants in preventing atherogenesis. *Atherosclerosis*, *187*(1), 1–17. doi:10.1016/j.atherosclerosis.2005.11.001 PMID:16313912

Kalix, B., Meynet, M. C., Garin, M. C., & James, R. W. (2001). The apolipoprotein epsilon2 allele and the severity of coronary artery disease in Type 2 diabetic patients. *Diabetic Medicine*, *18*(6), 445–450. doi:10.1046/j.1464-5491.2001.00497.x PMID:11472462

Kampoli, A.-M., Tousoulis, D., Antoniades, C., Siasos, G., & Stefanadis, C. (2009). Biomarkers of premature atherosclerosis. *Trends in Molecular Medicine*, *15*(7), 323–332. doi:10.1016/j.molmed.2009.06.001 PMID:19577961

Kataoka, S., Robbins, D. C., Cowan, L. D., Go, O., Yeh, J. L., Devereux, R. B., ... Howard, B. V. (1996). Apolipoprotein E polymorphism in American Indians and its relation to plasma lipoproteins and diabetes. The Strong Heart Study. *Arteriosclerosis, Thrombosis, and Vascular Biology*, *16*(8), 918–925. doi:10.1161/01.ATV.16.8.918 PMID:8696954

Kesaniemi, Y. A., Ehnholm, C., & Miettinen, T. A. (1987). Intestinal cholesterol absorption efficiency in man is related to apoprotein E phenotype. *The Journal of Clinical Investigation*, *80*(2), 578–581. doi:10.1172/JCI113107 PMID:3611358

Khatib, R., McKee, M., Shannon, H., Chow, C., Rangarajan, S., Teo, K., ... Yusuf, S. (2016). Availability and affordability of cardiovascular disease medicines and their effect on use in high-income, middle-income, and low-income countries: An analysis of the PURE study data. *Lancet*, *387*(10013), 61–69. doi:10.1016/S0140-6736(15)00469-9 PMID:26498706

Khoo, H. E., Azlan, A., Kong, K. W., & Ismail, A. (2016). Phytochemicals and Medicinal Properties of Indigenous Tropical Fruits with Potential for Commercial Development. *Evidence-Based Complementary and Alternative Medicine*, *7591951*. doi:10.1155/2016/7591951 PMID:27340420

Khor, E.-S., & Wong, N.-K. (2014). Potential antioxidant and cytotoxic properties of secondary metabolite extracts from Carica Papaya fruits and seeds. *International Journal of Pharmacy and Pharmaceutical Sciences*, *6*(7), 220–224.

Kristen, A. V., Lehrke, S., Buss, S., Mereles, D., Steen, H., Ehlermann, P., ... Katus, H. A. (2012). Green tea halts progression of cardiac transthyretin amyloidosis: An observational report. *Clinical Research in Cardiology; Official Journal of the German Cardiac Society*, *101*(10), 805–813. doi:10.100700392-012-0463-z PMID:22584381

Kumari, S., Rakavi, R., & Mangaraj, M. (2016). Effect of Guava in Blood Glucose and Lipid Profile in Healthy Human Subjects: A Randomized Controlled Study. *Journal of Clinical and Diagnostic Research: JCDR*, *10*(9), BC04–BC07. doi:10.7860/JCDR/2016/21291.8425 PMID:27790420

Ladanyia, M., & Ladaniya, M. (2010). *Citrus fruit: biology, technology and evaluation*. Academic press.

Lee, E. S., Vedanthan, R., Jeemon, P., Kamano, J. H., Kudesia, P., Rajan, V., ... Moran, A. E. (2016). Quality improvement for cardiovascular disease care in low- and middle-income countries: A systematic review. *PLoS One*, *11*(6), e0157036. doi:10.1371/journal.pone.0157036 PMID:27299563

Levitan, I., Volkov, S., & Subbaiah, P. V. (2010). Oxidized LDL: Diversity, Patterns of Recognition, and Pathophysiology. *Antioxidants & Redox Signalling*, *13*(1), 39–75. doi:10.1089/ars.2009.2733 PMID:19888833

Libby, P. (2002). Inflammation in atherosclerosis. *Nature*, *420*(6917), 868–874. doi:10.1038/nature01323 PMID:12490960

Libby, P. (2005). Act local, act global: Inflammation and the multiplicity of "vulnerable" coronary plaques. *Journal of the American College of Cardiology*, *45*, 1600–1602. doi:10.1016/j.jacc.2005.02.058 PMID:15893173

Linnenkamp, U., Guariguata, L., Beagley, J., Whiting, D. R., & Cho, N. H. (2014). The IDF Diabetes Atlas methodology for estimating global prevalence of hyperglycaemia in pregnancy. *Diabetes Research and Clinical Practice*, *103*(2), 186–196. doi:10.1016/j.diabres.2013.11.004 PMID:24300016

Mahley, R. W. (1988). Apolipoprotein E: Cholesterol transport protein with expanding role in cell biology. *Science*, *240*(4852), 622–630. doi:10.1126cience.3283935 PMID:3283935

Mansbach, C. M. II, & Gorelick, F. (2007). Development and Physiological Regulation of Intestinal Lipid Absorption. II. Dietary lipid absorption, complex lipid synthesis, and the intracellular packaging and secretion of chylomicrons. *American Journal of Physiology. Gastrointestinal and Liver Physiology*, *293*(4), G645–G650. doi:10.1152/ajpgi.00299.2007 PMID:17627968

Martínez-González, M. A., García-López, M., Bes-Rastrollo, M., Toledo, E., Martínez-Lapiscina, E. H., Delgado-Rodriguez, M., ... Beunza, J. J. (2011). Mediterranean diet and the incidence of cardiovascular disease: A Spanish cohort. *Nutrition, Metabolism, and Cardiovascular Diseases*, *21*(4), 237–244. doi:10.1016/j.numecd.2009.10.005 PMID:20096543

Mat, M. C., Mohamed, A. S., & Hamid, S. S. (2011). Primary human monocyte differentiation regulated by Nigella sativa pressed oil. *Lipids in Health and Disease*, *10*(1), 216–216. doi:10.1186/1476-511X-10-216 PMID:22104447

McCook-Russell, K. P., Nair, M. G., Facey, P. C., & Bowen-Forbes, C. S. (2012). Nutritional and nutraceutical comparison of Jamaican Psidium cattleianum (strawberry guava) and Psidium guajava (common guava) fruits. *Food Chemistry, 134*(2), 1069–1073. doi:10.1016/j.foodchem.2012.03.018 PMID:23107729

Mendis, S. (2014). *Global status report on non communicable diseases.* World Health Organization.

Mendis, S., Puska, P., & Norrving, B. (2011). *Global atlas on cardiovascular disease prevention and control.* World Health Organization.

Mizrahi, A., Knekt, P., Montonen, J., Laaksonen, M. A., Heliövaara, M., & Järvinen, R. (2009). Plant foods and the risk of cerebrovascular diseases: A potential protection of fruit consumption. *British Journal of Nutrition, 102*(7), 1075–1083. doi:10.1017/S0007114509359097 PMID:19646291

Monzon Ballarin, S., Lopez-Matas, M. A., Saenz Abad, D., Perez-Cinto, N., & Carnes, J. (2011). Anaphylaxis associated with the ingestion of Goji berries (Lycium barbarum). *Journal of Investigational Allergology & Clinical Immunology, 21*(7), 567–570. PMID:22312943

Moo-Huchin, V. M., Moo-Huchin, M. I., Estrada-Leon, R. J., Cuevas-Glory, L., Estrada-Mota, I. A., Ortiz-Vazquez, E., ... Sauri-Duch, E. (2015). Antioxidant compounds, antioxidant activity and phenolic content in peel from three tropical fruits from Yucatan, Mexico. *Food Chemistry, 166*, 17–22. doi:10.1016/j.foodchem.2014.05.127 PMID:25053022

Mulvihill, Erin E, & Huff, Murray W. (2012). Citrus flavonoids and the prevention of atherosclerosis. *Cardiovascular & Haematological Disorders-Drug Targets (Formerly Current Drug Targets-Cardiovascular & Hematological Disorders), 12*(2), 84-91.

Nagy, L., Tontonoz, P., Alvarez, J. G. A., Chen, H., & Evans, R. M. (1998). Oxidized LDL Regulates Macrophage Gene Expression through Ligand Activation of PPAR[3]. *Cell, 93*(2), 229–240. doi:10.1016/S0092-8674(00)81574-3 PMID:9568715

Nakashima, Y., Fujii, H., Sumiyoshi, S., Wight, T. N., & Sueishi, K. (2007). Early human atherosclerosis: Accumulation of lipid and proteoglycans in intimal thickenings followed by macrophage infiltration. *Arteriosclerosis, Thrombosis, and Vascular Biology, 27*(5), 1159–1165. doi:10.1161/ATVBAHA.106.134080 PMID:17303781

Nantitanon, W., Yotsawimonwat, S., & Okonogi, S. (2010). Factors influencing antioxidant activities and total phenolic content of guava leaf extract. *Lebensmittel-Wissenschaft + Technologie*, *43*(7), 1095–1103. doi:10.1016/j.lwt.2010.02.015

Nelson, B. M., Lichtenstein, A. H., Abrams, S., Adams-Campbell, L., & Anderson, C. J. (2015). 2015–2020 Dietary Guidelines for Americans (8th ed.). U.S. Department of Health and Human Services and the U.S. Department of Agriculture.

Newman, D. J., & Cragg, G. M. (2007). Natural Products as Sources of New Drugs over the Last 25 Years. *Journal of Natural Products*, *70*, 461–477.

NIH. (2012). *Clinical Trials*. NIH.

Niu, Y.-G., & Evans, R. D. (2011). Very-Low-Density Lipoprotein: Complex Particles in Cardiac Energy Metabolism. *Journal of Lipids*, *9*. doi:10.1155/2011/189876 PMID:21773049

Nordestgaard, B. G., & Zacho, J. (2009). Lipids, atherosclerosis and CVD risk: Is CRP an innocent bystander? *Nutrition, Metabolism, and Cardiovascular Diseases*, *19*(8), 521–524. doi:10.1016/j.numecd.2009.07.005 PMID:19695857

Norshazila, S. Jr, Syed Zahir, I., Mustapha Suleiman, K., Aisyah, M. R., & Kamarul Rahim, K. (2010). Antioxidant levels and activities of selected seeds of malaysian tropical fruits. *Malaysian Journal of Nutrition*, *16*(1), 149–159. PMID:22691862

Nwofia, G. E., Ojimelukwe, P., & Eji, C. (2012). Chemical composition of leaves, fruit pulp and seeds in some Carica papaya (L) morphotypes. *International Journal of Medicinal and Aromatic Plants*, *2*(1), 200–206.

Oboh, G., Bello, F. O., Ademosun, A. O., Akinyemi, A. J., & Adewuni, T. M. (2015). Antioxidant, hypolipidemic, and anti-angiotensin-1-converting enzyme properties of lemon (Citrus limon) and lime (Citrus aurantifolia) juices. *Comparative Clinical Pathology*, *24*(6), 1395–1406. doi:10.100700580-015-2088-x

Oncescu, V., Mancuso, M., & Erickson, D. (2014). Cholesterol testing on a smartphone. *Lab on a Chip*, *14*(4), 759–763. doi:10.1039/C3LC51194D PMID:24336861

Oram, J. F., & Lawn, R. M. (2001). ABCA1: The gatekeeper for eliminating excess tissue cholesterol. *Journal of Lipid Research*, *42*(8), 1173–1179. PMID:11483617

Ovesen, L. F. (2005). Increased consumption of fruits and vegetables reduces the risk of ischemic heart disease. *Ugeskr Laeger*, *167*(25-31), 2742-2747.

Palozza, P., Simone, R., Catalano, A., Parrone, N., Monego, G., & Ranelletti, F. O. (2011). Lycopene regulation of cholesterol synthesis and efflux in human macrophages. *The Journal of Nutritional Biochemistry*, *22*(10), 971–978. doi:10.1016/j.jnutbio.2010.08.010 PMID:21208793

Pasternak, R. (2002). Adult Treatment Panel II vs Adult Treatment Panel III: What has changed and why? *The American Journal of Cardiology*, *89*(5suppl), 3C–7C. doi:10.1016/S0002-9149(02)02221-X PMID:11900712

Patel, S., Celermajer, D. S., & Bao, S. (2008). Atherosclerosis-Underlying inflammatory mechanisms and clinical implications. *The International Journal of Biochemistry & Cell Biology*, *40*(4), 576–580. doi:10.1016/j.biocel.2007.11.017 PMID:18203647

Pelikanova, T. (2009). Treatment of diabetes in metabolic syndrome]. *Vnitrni Lekarstvi*, *55*(7-8), 637–645. PMID:19731868

Perticone, F., Ceravolo, R., Maio, R., Cloro, C., Candigliota, M., Scozzafava, A., ... Mattioli, P. L. (2000). Effects of atorvastatin and vitamin C on endothelial function of hypercholesterolemic patients. *Atherosclerosis*, *152*(2), 511–518. doi:10.1016/S0021-9150(00)00370-1 PMID:10998481

Rader, D. J. (2006). Molecular regulation of HDL metabolism and function: Implications for novel therapies. *The Journal of Clinical Investigation*, *116*(12), 3090–3100. doi:10.1172/JCI30163 PMID:17143322

Ried, K., & Fakler, P. (2011). Protective effect of lycopene on serum cholesterol and blood pressure: Meta-analyses of intervention trials. *Maturitas*, *68*(4), 299–310. doi:10.1016/j.maturitas.2010.11.018 PMID:21163596

Rissanen, T. H., Voutilainen, S., Virtanen, J. K., Venho, B., Vanharanta, M., Mursu, J., & Salonen, J. T. (2003). Low intake of fruits, berries and vegetables is associated with excess mortality in men: The Kuopio Ischaemic Heart Disease Risk Factor (KIHD) Study. *The Journal of Nutrition*, *133*(1), 199–204. doi:10.1093/jn/133.1.199 PMID:12514290

Rodriguez-Mateos, A., Heiss, C., Borges, G., & Crozier, A. (2014). Berry (Poly) phenols and Cardiovascular Health. *Journal of Agricultural and Food Chemistry*, *62*(18), 3842–3851. doi:10.1021/jf403757g PMID:24059851

Ross, R. (1993). The pathogenesis of atherosclerosis: A perspective for the 1990s. *Nature, 362*(6423), 801–809. doi:10.1038/362801a0 PMID:8479518

Ross, R. (1999). Atherosclerosis - An Inflammatory Disease. *The New England Journal of Medicine, 340*(2), 115–126. doi:10.1056/NEJM199901143400207 PMID:9887164

Ruel, G., Pomerleau, S., Couture, P., Lamarche, B., & Couillard, C. (2005). Changes in plasma antioxidant capacity and oxidized low-density lipoprotein levels in men after short-term cranberry juice consumption. *Metabolism: Clinical and Experimental, 54*(7), 856–861. doi:10.1016/j.metabol.2005.01.031 PMID:15988692

Sacks, F. M. (2015). The crucial roles of apolipoproteins E and C-III in apoB lipoprotein metabolism in normolipidemia and hypertriglyceridemia. *Current Opinion in Lipidology, 26*(1), 56–63. doi:10.1097/MOL.0000000000000146 PMID:25551803

Santhakumar, A. B., & Singh, I. (2016). Antioxidants as Functional Foods in Metabolic Syndrome. *Examining the Development, Regulation, and Consumption of Functional Foods*, 149.

Sasayama, S. (2008). Heart Disease in Asia. *Circulation, 118*(25), 2669–2671. doi:10.1161/CIRCULATIONAHA.108.837054 PMID:19106388

Shaw, J. E., Sicree, R. A., & Zimmet, P. Z. (2010). Global estimates of the prevalence of diabetes for 2010 and 2030. *Diabetes Research and Clinical Practice, 87*(1), 4–14. doi:10.1016/j.diabres.2009.10.007 PMID:19896746

Shofian, N. M., Hamid, A. A., Osman, A., Saari, N., Anwar, F., Dek, M. S., & Hairuddin, M. R. (2011). Effect of freeze-drying on the antioxidant compounds and antioxidant activity of selected tropical fruits. *International Journal of Molecular Sciences, 12*(7), 4678–4692. doi:10.3390/ijms12074678 PMID:21845104

Singh, R. B., Rastogi, S. S., Singh, N. K., Ghosh, S., Gupta, S., & Niaz, M. A. (1993). Can guava fruit intake decrease blood pressure and blood lipids? *Journal of Human Hypertension, 7*(1), 33–38. PMID:8383769

Sobenin, I. A., Pryanishnikov, V. V., Kunnova, L. M., Rabinovich, Y. A., Martirosyan, D. M., & Orekhov, A. N. (2010). The effects of time-released garlic powder tablets on multifunctional cardiovascular risk in patients with coronary artery disease. *Lipids in Health and Disease, 9*(1), 119. doi:10.1186/1476-511X-9-119 PMID:20958974

Steinberg, D. (1997). Low Density Lipoprotein Oxidation and Its Pathobiological Significance. *The Journal of Biological Chemistry*, *272*(34), 20963–20966. doi:10.1074/jbc.272.34.20963 PMID:9261091

Steinberg, D., & Witztum, J. L. (1990). Lipoproteins and Atherogenesis: Current Concepts. *Journal of the American Medical Association*, *264*(23), 3047–3052. doi:10.1001/jama.1990.03450230083034 PMID:2243434

Stone, N. J., Bilek, S., & Rosenbaum, S. (2005). Recent National Cholesterol Education Program Adult Treatment Panel III Update: Adjustments and Options. *The American Journal of Cardiology*, *96*(4suppl), 53E–59E. doi:10.1016/j.amjcard.2005.06.006 PMID:16098845

Takahashi, Y., Otsuki, A., Mori, Y., Kawakami, Y., & Ito, H. (2015). Inhibition of leukocyte-type 12-lipoxygenase by guava tea leaves prevents development of atherosclerosis. *Food Chemistry*, *186*, 2–5. doi:10.1016/j.foodchem.2015.03.105 PMID:25976783

Tarride, J.-E., Lim, M., DesMeules, M., Luo, W., Burke, N., O'Reilly, D., ... Goeree, R. (2009). A review of the cost of cardiovascular disease. *The Canadian Journal of Cardiology*, *25*(6), e195–e202. doi:10.1016/S0828-282X(09)70098-4 PMID:19536390

Taylor, A. J., Burke, A. P., O'Malley, P. G., Farb, A., Malcolm, G. T., Smialek, J., & Virmani, R. (2000). A Comparison of The Framingham Risk Index, Coronary Artery Calcification, and Culprit Plaque Morphology in Sudden Cardiac Death. *Circulation*, *101*(11), 1243–1248. doi:10.1161/01.CIR.101.11.1243 PMID:10725282

Taylor, S., Scuffham, P. A., McCollam, P. L., & Newby, D. E. (2007). Acute coronary syndromes in Europe: 1-year costs and outcomes. *Current Medical Research and Opinion*, *23*(3), 495–503. doi:10.1185/030079906X167462 PMID:17355731

Tomkin, G. H., & Owens, D. (2011). The chylomicron: Relationship to atherosclerosis. *International Journal of Vascular Medicine*. PMID:22007304

Valko, M., Leibfritz, D., Moncol, J., Cronin, M. T., Mazur, M., & Telser, J. (2007). Free radicals and antioxidants in normal physiological functions and human disease. *The International Journal of Biochemistry & Cell Biology*, *39*(1), 44–84. doi:10.1016/j.biocel.2006.07.001 PMID:16978905

Vinson, J. A., Bose, P., Proch, J., Al Kharrat, H., & Samman, N. (2008). Cranberries and Cranberry Products: Powerful in Vitro, ex Vivo, and in Vivo Sources of Antioxidants. *Journal of Agricultural and Food Chemistry*, *56*(14), 5884–5891. doi:10.1021/jf073309b PMID:18558697

Vitolins, M. Z., Anderson, A. M., Delahanty, L., Raynor, H., Miller, G. D., Mobley, C., ... Mayer-Davis, E. (2009). Action for Health in Diabetes (Look AHEAD) Trial: Baseline evaluation of selected nutrients and food group intake. *Journal of the American Dietetic Association*, *109*(8), 1367–1375. doi:10.1016/j.jada.2009.05.016 PMID:19631042

Voutilainen, S., Nurmi, T., Mursu, J., & Rissanen, T. H. (2006). Carotenoids and cardiovascular health. *The American Journal of Clinical Nutrition*, *83*(6), 1265–1271. doi:10.1093/ajcn/83.6.1265 PMID:16762935

Wall, M. M. (2006). Ascorbic acid, vitamin A, and mineral composition of banana (Musa sp.) and papaya (Carica papaya) cultivars grown in Hawaii. *Journal of Food Composition and Analysis*, *19*(5), 434–445. doi:10.1016/j.jfca.2006.01.002

WHO. (2007). *Prevention of cardiovascular disease*. World Health Organization.

Williams, L. (2002). Third report of the National Cholesterol Education Program (NCEP) expert panel on detection, evaluation, and treatment of high blood cholesterol in adults (Adult Treatment Panel III) final report. *Circulation*, *106*(25), 3143–3143. PMID:12485966

Wilson, W. (1994). Established Risk Factors And Coronary Artery Disease. *American Journal of Hypertension*, *7*(7_Pt_2), 7S–12S. doi:10.1093/ajh/7.7.7S PMID:7946184

Yamada, T., Hayasaka, S., Shibata, Y., Ojima, T., Saegusa, T., Gotoh, T., ... Kayaba, K. (2011). Frequency of Citrus Fruit Intake Is Associated With the Incidence of Cardiovascular Disease: The Jichi Medical School Cohort Study. *Journal of Epidemiology*, *21*(3), 169–175. doi:10.2188/jea.JE20100084 PMID:21389640

Yang, H., & Irudayaraj, J. (2001). Comparison of near-infrared, fourier transform-infrared, and fourier transform-raman methods for determining olive pomace oil adulteration in extra virgin olive oil. *Journal of the American Oil Chemists' Society*, *78*(9), 889. doi:10.100711746-001-0360-6

Yetukuri, L., Söderlund, S., Koivuniemi, A., Seppänen-Laakso, T., Niemelä, P. S., Hyvönen, M., ... Orešič, M. (2010). Composition and lipid spatial distribution of HDL particles in subjects with low and high HDL-cholesterol. *Journal of Lipid Research*, *51*(8), 2341–2351. doi:10.1194/jlr.M006494 PMID:20431113

Yoshida, H., & Kisugi, R. (2010). Mechanisms of LDL oxidation. *Clinica Chimica Acta*, *411*(23–24), 1875–1882. doi:10.1016/j.cca.2010.08.038 PMID:20816951

Yusuf, S., Islam, S., Chow, C. K., Rangarajan, S., Dagenais, G., Diaz, R., ... Avezum, A. (2011). Use of secondary prevention drugs for cardiovascular disease in the community in high-income, middle-income, and low-income countries (the PURE Study): A prospective epidemiological survey. *Lancet*, *378*(9798), 1231–1243. doi:10.1016/S0140-6736(11)61215-4 PMID:21872920

Zhao, S. P., Smelt, A. H., Van den Maagdenberg, A. M., Van Tol, A., Vroom, T. F., Gevers Leuven, J. A., ... Van 't Hooft, F. M. (1994). Plasma lipoprotein profiles of normocholesterolemic and hypercholesterolemic homozygotes for apolipoprotein E2(Arg158-->Cys) compared. *Clinical Chemistry*, *40*(8), 1559–1566. PMID:8044997

Zhu, Y., Huang, X., Zhang, Y., Wang, Y., Liu, Y., Sun, R., & Xia, M. (2014). Anthocyanin Supplementation Improves HDL-Associated Paraoxonase 1 Activity and Enhances Cholesterol Efflux Capacity in Subjects With Hypercholesterolemia. *The Journal of Clinical Endocrinology and Metabolism*, *99*(2), 561–569. doi:10.1210/jc.2013-2845 PMID:24285687

Zunjar, V., Dash, R. P., Jivrajani, M., Trivedi, B., & Nivsarkar, M. (2016). Antithrombocytopenic activity of carpaine and alkaloidal extract of Carica papaya Linn. leaves in busulfan induced thrombocytopenic Wistar rats. *Journal of Ethnopharmacology*, *181*, 20–25. doi:10.1016/j.jep.2016.01.035 PMID:26812680

Chapter 6
Nutraceutical Intervention of Phytosterols in Cardiovascular Aging

Charu Gupta
Amity University, India

Dhan Prakash
Amity University, India

Sneh Gupta
RGPG College, India

ABSTRACT

Phytosterols and phytostanols are a large group of compounds that are found exclusively in plants. They are structurally and functionally related to cholesterol but differ from cholesterol in the structure of the side chain. Phytosterols lower total and low-density lipoprotein (LDL) blood cholesterol by preventing cholesterol absorption from the intestine, so they have been known as blood cholesterol-lowering agents. Phytosterols are naturally found in fruits, vegetables, nuts, and mainly oils. Dietary phytosterol intakes normally range from 160-400 mg/day with variations depending on food culture and major food sources. Dairy foods remain a food of choice for use as delivery vehicle for many functional ingredients including phytosterols and there are many dairy products available in the global markets which are enriched with phytosterols. The use of phytosterols in commonly consumed dairy products may soon provide an effective tool against CVD and its introduction to our food products is worth anticipating in the near future as nutraceuticals for healthy ageing.

DOI: 10.4018/978-1-5225-3267-5.ch006

INTRODUCTION

Cardiovascular diseases were collectively the number one cause of death in the United States in 2007, accounting for one third of deaths (Xu, Kochanek, Murphy, & Tejada-Vera, 2010). Most of these deaths were attributable to ischemic heart diseases, in which a portion of the muscle in the heart does not receive adequate blood flow. A major cause of ischemia is atherosclerosis, which is characterized by inflammation and lipid accumulation in the lumen of arteries, which decreases blood flow by narrowing the artery and can eventually lead to thrombosis, thereby completely blocking the artery with a blood clot. The Framingham Heart Study is often credited with being the first to systematically investigate the links between blood cholesterol concentrations as a risk factor for cardiovascular diseases, and particularly the effects of low-density lipoprotein cholesterol (LDL-C), high-density lipoprotein cholesterol (HDL-C), and total cholesterol (Castelli, 1988). The Framingham Heart Study, a long-term observational study, is now observing the third generation of participants from residents in Framingham, MA. The data from this study have allowed a number of prediction models of cardiovascular disease risk associated with a variety of risk factors, and has worked to separate environmental, genetic, and other effects through epidemiological modeling. In one such model, cholesterol concentrations were determined to be such a significant risk factor for coronary heart disease that all other risk factors, such as diabetes, smoking, and blood pressure, were converted into either cholesterol or LDL-C risk points, which were then compared to categories on a risk chart (Wilson, D'Agostino, Levy, Belanger, Silbershatz, & Kannel, 1998). Clearly, LDL-C concentrations are an important risk factor for heart disease.

Cholesterol in the body mainly comes from two sources- endogenous synthesis and dietary consumption. Dietary cholesterol contributes a relatively minor proportion of the cholesterol in the system, with an average of only 276 mg of cholesterol consumed per day (Agricultural Research Service USDA, 2010). In addition, dietary cholesterol minimally affects blood cholesterol, with estimates of only a 0.022-0.027 mg/dL difference in blood cholesterol for every 1 mg of dietary cholesterol consumed (McNamara, 2000). To put this into perspective, an individual with high cholesterol (>240 mg/dL) would need to consume an additional 100 mg of cholesterol per 6 day to increase their blood cholesterol by about 1%. Although dietary cholesterol alone seems to have little effect on blood cholesterol, dietary cholesterol is not the only source of cholesterol in the intestinal lumen. The gall-bladder secretes approximately 1000 mg of cholesterol per day into the small intestine. Of the total cholesterol in the intestinal lumen, approximately 50% is absorbed, making inhibition of intestinal cholesterol absorption, not just decreasing dietary cholesterol, an important target for lowering blood cholesterol concentrations (McNamara, 2000).

Cardiovascular diseases (CVDs) inflict a huge burden in terms of mortality and morbidity, contributing to disability and decline of quality of life (Niccoli & Partridge, 2012; North & Sinclair, 2012). In addition, aging itself produces numerous changes in human heart, at structural, molecular, and functional levels. The most important age-related alterations are left ventricular (LV) hypertrophy, fibrosis, denervation, and maladaptive remodeling that frequently lead to diastolic dysfunction (Rengo, Pagano, Vitale, Formisano, Komici, & Petraglia, 2016). Vascular aging is characterized by impaired endothelial function, chronic vascular inflammation, and augmented arterial stiffness (Ungvari, Kaley, de Cabo, Sonntag, & Csiszar, 2010). Endothelial dysfunction is mainly related to increased production of reactive oxygen species (ROS) partially due to an increased activity of NAD(P)H oxidases (NOX) (Csiszar, Ungvari, Edwards, Kaminski, Wolin… & Koller, 2002). Moreover, increased age-related oxidative stress and decreased production of nitric oxide (NO) constitute critical factors for the alteration of cardiovascular (CV) homeostasis (Ungvari, Buffenstein, Austad, Podlutsky, Kaley, & Csiszar, 2008). microRNAs (miRNAs) are small non-coding RNAs approximately 18–25 nucleotides long, which regulate gene expression at different levels. Importantly, miRNAs are emerging as key factors in the development and progression of CVDs. Notably several basic and clinical studies identified peculiar miRNAs expression profile in pathological conditions. Consequently, miRNA have been proposed as diagnostic/prognostic biomarkers and therapeutic targets (de Lucia, Komici, Borghetti, Femminella, Bencivenga, Cannavo… & Rengo, 2017).

Phytosterols have been known for almost 60 years to lower blood cholesterol in humans, with initial hypothesis pointing to a disruption of cholesterol absorption. Since then, many studies have been done to quantify the effects of phytosterols on blood cholesterol, with one meta-analysis indicating that phytosterols can lower LDL-C (which is considered atherogenic) by approximately 10% (Demonty, Chan, Pelled, & Jones, 2009). Phytosterols are therefore a powerful nutraceutical for lowering an atherosclerotic risk factor. In the decades since the initial discovery, a number of mechanisms have been proposed and investigated to explain the cholesterol-lowering properties of phytosterols.

Phytosterols, phytostanols and their esters are a group of steroid alcohols and esters that occur naturally in plants as non-saponifiable fraction of plant oils (Figure 1). Phytosterols (including plant sterols and stanols) cannot be synthesized by humans, and all plant sterols and stanols in the human body therefore originate from the diet (De Jong, Plat, Bast, Godschalk, Basu, & Mensink, 2008). They are known to have several bioactive qualities with possible implications for human health. Their properties for reducing blood cholesterol levels, as well as their other beneficial health effects, have been known for many years. It was recognized in

Figure 1. Structure of Cholesterol, Phytosterol and its derivatives

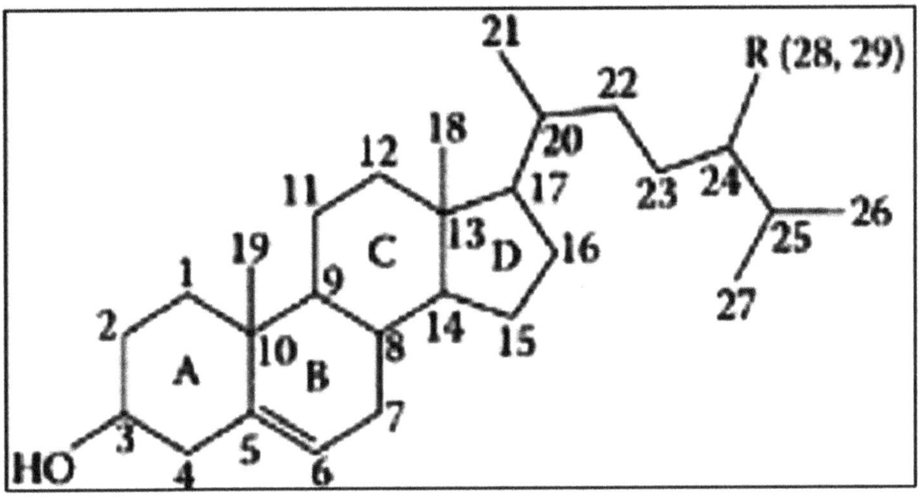

SCHEME 1. **Structure of cholesterol and phytosterols**
R=H: Cholesterol; R=CH3: Campesterol; R=C2H5: β-sitosterol; R=C2H5, Δ22

the 1950s that plant sterols lower serum concentrations of cholesterol. Plant sterols might also protect against certain types of cancer such as colon, breast and prostate (Awad & Fink, 2000).

People with high blood cholesterol levels are typically advised by health professionals to exercise and consume a diet high in fiber and low in saturated fats and cholesterol. Although these measures can reduce blood cholesterol but they are not self-sufficient. Other cholesterol-lowering interventions may be needed, including cholesterol lowering medicines or adding phytosterol esters to the diet. The primary phytosterols in the diet are sitosterol, stigmasterol and campesterol and typical consumption of plant sterols is approximately 160-400mg/day (Berger, Jones, & Abumweis, 2004). The enrichment of foods with phytosterols is one of the recent developments in functional foods to enhance the cholesterol lowering ability of traditional food products (Anon, 2005). Phytosterols compete with cholesterols to reduce their level and helps to restrict absorption in digestive system. They find applications in food additives in cold cuts, spicy sauces, milk sausages, yoghurts, spreads, bakery products and margarines. Government affirmation regarding phytosterols application as food additives to supplement the nutritional requirement in foods and beverages is expected to drive the global market growth over the next five years. Growing cardiovascular diseases ad heart attacks due to high cholesterol content is anticipated to shift consumers towards phytosterols content foods. This also expected to replace cholesterol market with phytosterol in the near future (Kuna, Raju, & Poshadri, 2011).

An estimated 50 to 55% of the milk produced is converted into a variety of traditional milk products, using processes such as coagulation (heat and/or acid), desiccation and fermentation. The major factors driving growth in dairy products consumption are increased demand due to population growth, growing household incomes, increased demand for value added milk products and the preference for liquid milk as a principle protein source, across all age groups. In 2009, the per capita availability of milk was 265g per day, close to the world's average. The preference for liquid milk is due to both its cultural significance as well as tradition of vegetarianism has left demand for dairy products relatively inelastic, despite increasing consumer prices over the past few years. The major milk producer countries are European Union, India, and US to name few. Keeping in view all these factors, dairy products have become the best vehicle for phytosterol enrichment.

CHEMICAL STRUCTURES OF PHYTOSTEROL

Sterols are an essential component of cell membranes, and both animals and plants produce them. They play an important role in cell membrane function. They are structurally related to cholesterol, but differ from cholesterol in the structure of the side chain (Law, 2000). Plant sterols include a wide variety of molecules that are structurally similar to cholesterol; the principal examples are 4-desmethyl sterols (Quilez, Garcia-Lorda, & Salas-Salvado, 2003). Plant sterols are C-28 or C-29 sterols, differing from cholesterol (C-27) by the presence of an extra methyl (campesterol) or ethyl (sitosterol) group on the cholesterol side chain. While over 40 plant sterols from seven different plant classes have been identified, campesterol (C-28), stigmasterol (C-29) and especially β-sitosterol (C-29) are the most abundant (Law, 2000). Saturated plant sterols, referred to as plant stanols have no double bond in the ring structure. Plant stanols are produced by the hydrogenation of sterols and are not abundant in nature (Law, 2000). Sitostanol and campastenol are saturated plant sterols which are found in nature in much smaller amounts than plant sterols (Jong et al., 2003).

STRUCTURE OF PHYTOSTEROLS

Phytosterols are sterols that are structurally similar to cholesterol but are synthesized in plants and phytoplankton. Usually, they are characterized by alkyl groups (methyl or ethyl group) at C-24, by side-chain double bonds at C-22 or C-24 or/and by nuclear double bonds at positions other than C-5 (Morreau, Whitaker, & Hicks, 2002). Among phytoplankton, the Dinophyceae are an exception because they can have a methyl group in the C-4 or C-23 position (Piretti, Giampiero, Boni, Pistocchi, Diamante, & Gazzotti, 1997). Some Chlorophyceae contain unusual Δ^7-sterols such as chondrillasterol (Thompson, 1996), whereas some Chlorophyceae in the order Chlamydomonadales have ergosterol (Brumfield, Moroney, Moore, Simms, & Donze, 2010), which is also found in Euglenophyceae (Patterson, 1991). There is a great diversity of sterols in Diatomophyceae, but none of them are found exclusively in diatoms (Rampen, Abbas, Schouten, & Sinninghe Damste, 2010). For example brassicasterol is also a major sterol in Cryptophyceae (Rampen, Abbas, Schouten, & Sinninghe Damste, 2010) and stigmasterol, and β-sitosterol is typical for Chrysophyceae and Raphidophyceae in addition to Diatomophyceae (Rampen, Abbas, Schouten, & Sinninghe Damste, 2010; Leblond, Dahmen, Lebret, & Rengefors, 2013; Taipale, Hiltunen, Vuorio, & Peltomaa, 2016).

In foods, cholesterol occurs as the free alcoholic sterol or as cholesteryl esters (Fenton, 1992), whereas plant sterols occurs as free plant sterols, esterified plant sterols, plant steryl glycosides and acylated plant steryl glycosides (Akihisa, Kokke, & Tamura, 1991). It is obvious that chemical, physical and nutritional properties of these phytosterol classes may be very different (Piironen, Toivo, & Lampi, 2000). The different fractions are assumed to exist in different parts of the plant cell. Free plant sterols are generally believed to be the storage products. They can be found in the cytosol of plant cells, in droplets or vesicles. The largest amount of plant steryl glycosides has been found in the microsomal fraction of the plant cell and acylated steryl glycosides are believed to exist in mitochondria (Anon, 1989).

DOSE EFFECTS OF DIETARY PHYTOSTEROLS ON CHOLESTEROL METABOLISM

Phytosterol supplementation of 2 g/d is recommended by the National Cholesterol Education Program to reduce LDL cholesterol (Racette, Lin, Lefevre, Spearie, Most, Ma, & Ostlund, 2010). However, the effects of different types of phytosterol intake on cholesterol metabolism are uncertain. In a study, the effects of 3 phytosterol intakes on whole-body cholesterol metabolism were evaluated. In this placebo-controlled, crossover feeding trial, 18 adults received a phytosterol-deficient diet (50 mg phytosterols/2000 kcal) plus beverages supplemented with 0, 400, or 2000 mg phytosterols/d for 4 weeks each, in random order. All meals were prepared in a metabolic kitchen; breakfast and dinner on weekdays were eaten on site. Primary outcomes were fecal cholesterol excretion and intestinal cholesterol absorption measured with stable-isotope tracers and serum lipoprotein concentrations. It was finally concluded that dietary phytosterols in moderate and high doses favorably alter whole-body cholesterol metabolism in a dose-dependent manner. A moderate phytosterol intake (459 mg/d) can be obtained in a healthy diet without supplementation. This trial was registered at clinicaltrials.gov as NCT00860054 (Racette, Lin, Lefevre, Spearie, Most, Ma, & Ostlund, 2010).

In yet another study, the objective was to test the hypothesis that intrinsic phytosterols present in unmodified foods alter whole-body cholesterol metabolism. Little was known about their effects on cholesterol metabolism when given in native, unpurified form and in amounts achievable in the diet. However, it was found that the extrinsic phytosterols supplemented to the diet reduce intestinal cholesterol absorption and plasma low-density lipoprotein (LDL)-cholesterol. In all, 20 out of 24 subjects completed a randomized, crossover feeding trial wherein all meals were provided by a metabolic kitchen. Each subject consumed two diets for 4 weeks each. The diets differed in phytosterol content (phytosterol-poor diet, 126 mg phytosterols/2000 kcal; phytosterol-abundant diet, 449 mg phytosterols/2000 kcal), but were otherwise matched for nutrient content. Cholesterol absorption and excretion were determined by gas chromatography/mass spectrometry after oral administration of stable isotopic tracers. It was concluded that intrinsic phytosterols at levels present in a healthy diet are biologically active and have large effects on whole-body cholesterol metabolism not reflected in circulating LDL. More work is still needed to assess the effects of phytosterol-mediated fecal cholesterol excretion on coronary heart disease risk in humans (Lin, Racette, Lefevre, Spearie, Most, Ma, & Ostlund, 2010).

In another study, preparation developed for human use containing different vitamins, minerals and trace elements enriched with phytosterol (VMTP) affecting the severity of experimental hyperlipidemia and myocardial ischemia/reperfusion injury was investigated and it was concluded that treatment of hyperlipidemic subjects with a VMTP preparation reduces serum cholesterol, the major risk factor for cardiovascular disease; however, it does not provide cardioprotection (Csont, Sárközy, Szűcs, Szűcs, Bárkányi, Bencsik… & Ferdinandy, 2013).

MECHANISM OF ACTION OF PHYTOSTEROLS

While phytosterols have been ascribed a number of biological functions in animals, including antioxidant capabilities (Loizou, Lekakis, Chrousos, & Moutsatsou, 2010), anti-carcinogenic properties (Woyengo, Ramprasath, & Jones, 2009) and immune regulation (Brüll, Mensink, van den Hurk, Duijvestijn, & Plat, 2010), the most common and prominent use of phytosterols is to lower blood cholesterol, with the end goal of lowering the risk of heart disease. The proposed mechanisms for the cholesterol-lowering properties of phytosterols have centered on pathways in which cholesterol is directly involved, including intestinal solubility, interaction with digestive enzymes, protein-mediated absorption, and gene regulation.

The exact mechanism by which phytosterols decrease serum cholesterol levels is not completely understood, but several theories have been proposed. One of them suggests that cholesterol in the intestine, already marginally soluble, is precipitated into a non-absorbable state in the presence of added phytosterols and stanols (Rozner & Garti, 2006). Another theory is based on the fact that phytosterols when consumed may reduce cholesterol absorption by competing with cholesterol for incorporation into the bile salts micelles or for up-taking of cholesterol by enterocytes through Niemann Pick C1 Like 1 (NPC1L1) transporter. In addition, phytosterols may enhance cholesterol excretion back into the intestinal lumen through the ATP binding cassette G5 (ABCG5) and G8 (ABCG8) transporters. Phytosterols could also prevent esterification of the free cholesterol into cholesterol esters and thus it's assembling into the chylomicrons. As a result of reducing cholesterol absorption by phytosterols, the cholesterol synthesis rate increase, but the net effect is a reduction in LDL-cholesterol levels (Jones & AbuMweis, 2009).

Cholesterol absorption is a very important physiological mechanism that regulates cholesterol metabolism. A recent trial showed that efficacy of phytosterols is not influenced by dietary cholesterol intake in hypercholesterolemic individuals (Kassis, Vanstone, AbuMweis, & Jones, 2008). Both dietary cholesterol and recirculating biliary cholesterol mixed in the intestine are partially absorbed. Failure to reabsorb intestinal cholesterol is the principle means of eliminating cholesterol from the body.

Some studies show that phytosterols compete with and displace cholesterol from bile salt/phospholipid micelles, the form from which cholesterol absorption occurs. During one trial, nine adults were fed a meal containing 500mg of cholesterol and 1g beta-sitosterol or 2g beta-sitosteryl oleate (Mattson, Grundy, & Crouse, 1982). The addition of beta-sitosterol resulted in a 42% decrease in cholesterol absorption, and the beta-sitosteryl oleate caused a 33% reduction compared to the control group, which resulted in a consequent decrease in plasma cholesterol. Sitosterol has increased affinity for biliary micelles compared with cholesterol, so sitosterol uptake by micelles is energetically favoured.

Unlike cholesterol, phytosterols and phytostanols are poorly absorbed and the small amount that is absorbed is actively re-excreted in bile. This results in low serum levels of these sterol molecules. The inhibition of cholesterol absorption is thought to produce a state of relative cholesterol deficiency that is followed by up-regulation of cholesterol biosynthesis and LDL receptor activity (Ling & Jones, 1995).

ABSORPTION OF PHYTOSTEROLS

Earlier studies showed that the phytosterols are not absorbed in rodents and rabbits including other mammals. However, initial studies by Salen *et al.* (1989) proved that 1.5-5% of phytosterol (sitosterol) is absorbed in human beings. Phytosterols reduce cholesterol absorption while being poorly absorbed them and the effects can be studied in human subjects in single-meal tests using stable isotopic tracers. Because phytosterols are insoluble and biologically inactive when purified, careful attention needs to be given to ensuring that commercial supplement products are rendered bioavailable by dissolution in fat or by emulsification. It has also been found that phytosterols in natural food matrices are also bioactive. The retention of phytosterols during food manufacturing and the use of foods with high phytosterol content may constitute an alternative to the use of supplements (Ostlund, 2007). Reported data also shows that some phytosterols get metabolized into acidic products (Kritchevsky & Chen, 2005).

DIETARY SOURCES AND INTAKES

Phytosterols can be found at widely varying concentrations in the fat-soluble fractions of seed, root stems, branches, leaves and blossoms. They are constituents of both edible and ornamental plants, including herbs, shrubs and trees (Clifton, 2002). As natural constituents of the human diet, phytosterols are naturally found in all food items of plant origin, principally oils and pulses and dried fruits (Piironen, Toivo, & Lampi, 2000). Their content is highest in edible oils, seeds and nuts. The total contents are variable and range from nearly 8g/kg in corn oil to 0.5g/kg in palm oil, with intermediate levels being found in commonly used oils (Phillips, Ruggio, Toivo, Swank, & Simpkins, 2002). Tall oil contains a higher proportion of plant stanols than do vegetable oils (Anon, 2005). The refining process in vegetable oils leads to a significant reduction in phytosterols content, and it would therefore be very interesting to develop industrial methods which minimize these losses (Quilez, Garcia-Lorda, & Salas-Salvado, 2003). Table 1 shows the total phytosterol contents of selected foods.

The dietary intake of phytosterols among and within different human population varies greatly, depending upon the type and amount of plant foods eaten. Although cooking oils, margarine and peanut butter are the main sources of phytosterols in the diet, phytosterols are also consumed from seeds, nuts, cereals and legumes (Tasan, Bilgin, Gecgel, & Demirci, 2006; Clifton, 2009).

Table 1. Total phytosterols contents of selected foods

Phytosterol Food Sources	Total Phytosterols Content (mg/100g)
Oils	
Rice bran	1055
Corn	952
Wheat germ	553
Flax seed	338
Cottonseed	327
Soybean	221
Peanut	206
Olive	176
Coconut	91
Palm	49
Vegetables	
Beet root	25
Brussels sprout	24
Cauliflower	18
Onion	15
Carrot	12
Cabbage	11
Yam	10
Fruits	
Orange	24
Banana	16
Apple	12
Cherry	12
Peach	10
Pear	8
Nuts	
Cashew	158
Almond	143
Pecan	108
Pistachio	108
Walnut	108
Legumes	
Pea	135
Kidney bean	127
Broad bean	124

(Source: Kuna, Raju, & Poshadri, 2011)

The daily doses, considered optimal for the purpose of lowering blood cholesterol levels are 2-3g of phytostanols and/or phytosterols, which translates to 3.4-5.2g in esterified form. This recommended daily dose is typically divided in 1-3 portions of food providing 1.7-5.2g ester, which equals 1-3g phytostanol and/or phytosterol equivalents.

The consumption of phytosterols can range between 170mg/day in populations eating a Western diet and 360mg/day in diets rich in vegetable products. The dietary intake of plant stanols is usually only about 50mg/day unless the diet is supplemented with tall oil, which is derived from conifers and is rich in sitostanol (Gilbert, Thompson, & Grundy, 2005). The normal dietary intake of plant stanols is much less than that of plant sterols.

Although people consume phytosterols every day in food, the amounts are often not great enough to have significant cholesterol lowering effect (Anon, 2003). Phytosterols can be incorporated into traditional food products. In order to achieve maximum cholesterol lowering benefit, doses of 2-3 g/day plant sterols or plant stanols need to be consumed (Isabelle, Rouyanne, Henk, Van der Knaap, Guus, Duchateau...& Trautwein, 2009; Kuna & Poshadri, 2012) which can be achieved by enriching the commonly consumed foods with phytosterols. Also, finding and cultivating varieties with higher phytosterol contents will increase consumption in the population. Genetic modification becomes a powerful tool for related purposes (Venkatramesh, Karunanandaa, Sun, Gunter, Boddupalli, & Kishore, 2003).

PHYTOSTEROLS AS NUTRACEUTICAL: ENRICHMENT OF DAIRY FOODS WITH PHYTOSTEROLS

The primary purpose of phytosterol supplementation is for improvement of plasma cholesterol levels. The use of foods containing phytosterols is a relatively recent development in human nutrition (Gilbert, Thompson, & Grundy, 2005). Phytosterols as functional ingredients in foods, appear to be a practical and safe option for decreasing cholesterol levels in the population suffering from coronary vascular diseases. These components are incorporated nowadays into a wide variety of dairy products such as yoghurt, yoghurt drinks, milk drinks, butter milk, acid milk, cream cheese and soy yoghurt drinks (Kuna, Raju, & Poshadri, 2011).

Dairy foods remain a choice delivery vehicle for functional ingredients such as antioxidants, fatty acids, fiber, probiotics and whey proteins for phytosterols because refrigerated and freezing temperatures assist with keeping many functional ingredients active. Commercially, phytosterols are currently contained in many dairy products all over the world (Cantrill & Kawamura, 2008). Phytosterols, phytostanols and their esters are incorporated into a variety of dairy based foods and beverages, produced by a growing number of food and beverage manufacturers. The main dairy product formats incorporated with phytosterol esters are yoghurts (1.25g per 125mL), yoghurt drinks (3.4g per 100mL), and milk (5g per litre) (Kuna, Raju, & Poshadri, 2011).

Commercially, phytosterols are isolated from vegetable oils, such as soybean oil, rapeseed (canola) oil, sunflower oil or corn oil, or from so-called "tall oil", a by-product of the manufacture of wood pulp. Phytosterols can be hydrogenated to obtain phytostanols. Phytosterols and phytostanols are high melting powders. Phytostanol and phytosterol esters are chemically stable materials, having comparable chemical and physical properties to edible fats and oils. The substances are insoluble in water, but soluble in non-polar solvents, such as hexane, iso-octane and 2-propanol. The esters are also soluble in vegetable fats and oils.

Phytosterols are also being sold with other functional ingredients such as: fiber (France), healthy oils (England), non-absorbable diacylglycerol (Israel), almonds, soy protein and viscous fibers and minerals (Berger, Jones, & Abumweis, 2004). In early studies of cholesterol-lowering efficacy of phytosterols, they were in the form of a crystalline powder (un-esterified form), and has to be used in relatively large quantities to achieve significant lowering of cholesterol. Un-esterified plant sterols are not water soluble and their solubility in fat is limited, their use in food applications is restricted (Salo & Wester, 2005). Plant sterol and stanol esters are far more lipid soluble than plant sterols and stanols. The commercial esterification of plant sterols and stanols with fatty acids from vegetable oil has made it possible to produce dairy products containing the desired esters and also well accepted sensory characters in all the designer dairy products (Salo & Wester, 2005).

Initially, esterified plant stanols and sterols were commercially used in fat-based foods such as margarines, shortenings and mayonnaise, but recent clinical studies have shown that the cholesterol-lowering efficacy of esterified plant sterols and stanols is independent of food matrix (Hyun, Kim, Kang, Lee, Jang, Liponkoski, & Salo, 2005). The use of a low fat vehicle for delivery of stanol esters was tested by Mensink *et al.*,(2002), who showed reductions in total and LDL cholesterol levels in individuals consuming stanol ester in low fat yoghurt were comparable to those observed with similar amounts of stanol ester taken in the form of margarine. Salo and Wester (2005) also showed that cholesterol-lowering efficacy of plant stanol esters was independent of the food type (meat based ready-made low fat meals, apsta, and low fat yoghurt drinks) in which it is incorporated. Gylling and Miettinen (1999) showed that plant stanols esterified with butter fatty acids (predominantly myristic acid) and extracted in butter was just as effective in lowering LDL cholesterol as was plant stanol esterified with rapeseed oil and dissolve in margarine. Low-fat yoghurt enriched with plant stanol ester was effective in reducing cholesterol level in a habitual diet without restriction of fat and cholesterol intake (Hyun, Kim, Kang,

Lee, Jang, Liponkoski, & Salo, 2005). With esterification of plant stanols, the food vehicle need not have a high fat content to be an effective means of delivery of plant stanol (Salo & Wester, 2005). Both phytosterol and phytostanol esters give an enhanced creamy texture to low fat dairy products (yoghurt/drinking yoghurt). They may also improve the taste of food products by masking bitterness and hence reduce the amount of sugar or other sweetener required to obtain a pleasant taste and mouth feel (e.g. in milk drinks, buttermilk, soy drinks etc.) (Salo & Wester, 2005).

MERITS OF PHYTOSTEROLS AS NUTRACEUTICALS IN FOODS

Phytosterols are Stable at High Temperature

The chief advantage of phytosterols and their fatty acid esters are that they are quite stable compounds and they undergo only limited degradation during oil processing. Only under harsh conditions, such as high temperatures (>100°C) in the presence of oxygen, oxidation of the phytosterol moiety may occur in the same way as cholesterol (Soupas, Huikko, Lampi, & Piironen, 2005; Soupas, 2006). Phytosterols are mono-unsaturated compounds (double bond in the B-ring), which are more stable than the mono-unsaturated fatty acids (e.g. oleic acid), because of steric hindrance by the ring structure. Therefore, even under severe conditions, such as during shallow frying, sterol oxidation products form only slowly (Thanh, Vergnes, Kaloustian, El-Moselhy, Amiot-Carlin, & Portugal, 2006). Under conditions of use for shallow frying by consumers, temperatures 160-200°C, 5-10 minutes of frying), the level of oxidation of sitosterol esters remains below 1.3% when the matrix consists of liquid oil or liquid margarine and if using free sterols these levels are somewhat higher at 2.5% and 5.1% respectively (Salta, Kalogeropoulos, Karavanou, & Andrikopoulos, 2008). Factors affecting phytosterol oxidation include not only temperature and heating time, but also the composition of the lipid matrix. Since dairy products such as dahi, misti dahi, paneer, butter milk, lassi etc. can be processed under 100°C, it is best option to use dairy products as vehicles for phytosterols fortification as compared to other vehicles which involves high temperature processing (Kuna, Raju, & Poshadri, 2011).

Stability of Phytosterols During Product Manufacturing and Storage

Phytosterols and phytostanols remain stable and ineffective as they are not affected by the fermentation process used to produce yoghurt as they are microbiologically inert (Monu, Blank, Holley, & Zawistowsk, 2008). Furthermore, the ester added to various food products shows excellent stability at different pH values during long term storage (up-to at least a year). Phytostanol and phytosterol esters are also stable in milk and fermented milk products with viable bacteria like yoghurts and yoghurt drinks (Cantrill & Kawamura, 2008; Kuna, Raju, & Poshadri, 2011).

Oxidative Stability of Phytosterols in Foods

Since phytosterols are chemically sterols, an unsaturated lipid compounds (steroid alcohols), and are thus susceptible to oxidation (Dutta, 2004). Their resistance to oxidation and thus to the formation of oxidation products, needs to be investigated.

Oxidized phytosterols are generally classified as cooked food mutagens, along with acrylamides, heterocyclic amines, nitrosoamines, and polyaromatic hydrocarbons (Jagerstad & Skog, 2005). Research on oxidation of phytosterols has not been as systematic and extensive as with cholesterol, but based on all information available, phytosterols seem to oxidize in a similar fashion to cholesterol. This can also be assumed from their structural similarities (Dutta, 2004). A foundation for understanding sterol oxidation mechanisms has been provided by studies conducted on fatty acid oxidation (Lercker & Rodriguez-Estrada, 2002). Sterol oxidation can proceed via non-enzymic or enzymic pathways (Dutta, 2004).

FACTORS AFFECTING EFFICACY OF PHYTOSTEROLS

The physical state of plant sterols may have an impact on their cholesterol-lowering effect. For example, in a double-blind randomized, placebo-controlled study, a crystallizing method was used to add plant sterols into dietary fats and oils homogeneously (Christiansen, Lahteenmaki, Mannelin, Seppänen-Laakso, Hiltunen, & Yliruusi, 2001). Hypercholesterolemic participants consuming 1.5 or 3.0 g/day of free un-esterified plant sterols in this 'microcrystalline' form experienced a 7.5–11.6% reduction in LDL-C levels.

However, conflicting data raise some doubts about the biologic activity of the microcrystalline phytosterols. During single-meal tests in humans, crystalline phytosterols (1000 mg) did not reduce absorption of labeled cholesterol consistently, whereas 300mg of phytosterols complexed with lecithin reduced cholesterol absorption by 34% (Ostlund, Spilburg, & Stenson, 1999). Despite the increased sterol purity, it has been suggested that the extremely stable state of the crystalline structure requires both energy and time to disrupt. Crystalline phytosterols took several days to reach an equilibrium state during solubilization in solutions of bile salts. There is almost no transfer of crystalline phytosterols from the solid state to the micelles of artificial bile solutions over periods of a few hours at physiologic temperature (Ostlund, Spilburg, & Stenson, 1999). These *in-vitro* findings suggest that it is unlikely that phytosterol crystals are biologically active.

PHYTOSTEROLS IN COMBINATION WITH OTHER AGENTS

A recent set of studies compared the cholesterol-lowering efficacy of different esters of plant sterols was reported (Chan, Demonty, Pelled, & Jones, 2006; Demonty, Chan, Pelled, & Jones, 2006). Participants were fed five different dietary sterols including olive oil, fish oil, and fatty acid plant sterol esters of sunflower oil, as well as olive oil, and fish oil at level of 1.7 g/day for 28 days, each separated by washout periods.

Diets were controlled precisely so that participants ate meals provided from a central metabolic kitchen to maintain weight balance. Plant sterol-fish oil ester reduced fasting and postprandial plasma triacylglycerol levels compared with plant sterol-sunflower oil ester by 39 and 40%, respectively. Compared with an olive oil diet, plant sterol-fish oil ester and plant sterol-sunflower oil ester lowered LDL-C levels by 3 and 6%, respectively.

HDL-cholesterol levels were not affected by any of the treatments. Fish oil and sunflower oil plant sterols resulted in lower total cholesterol: HDL-cholesterol ratio and lower apo-lipoprotein B levels than olive oil and fish oil. Phytosterols are also effective when combined with other dietary factors including psyllium (Shrestha, Volek, Udani, Wood, Greene, Aggarwal, Contois, Kavoussi, & Fernandez, 2006), fish oil (Micallef & Garg, 2008), beta-glucan (Theuwissen & Mensink, 2007), or statin drugs (De Jong, Plat, Bast, Godschalk, Basu, & Mensink, 2008) and could be useful in secondary prevention of heart disease when greater targeted reductions in LDL-C are needed.

PHYTOSTEROLS AND CANCER

Besides lowering the blood cholesterol level, phytosterols have also been shown to provide some protection against cancer (Awad & Fink, 2000). The proposed mode of action is inhibition of cell division, stimulating tumor cell death and modifying some hormones that are essential to tumor growth (Awad, Karen, Downie, & Fink, 2000). A long-term study shows an association between the amount of plant sterol consumed in the diet and developing cancer. It is estimated that about 9 million new cancer cases are diagnosed every year and over 4.5 million people die from cancer each year in the world (Reddy, 2012). However, the estimated number of new cancer patients in India per year is about 7 lakhs and over 3.5 lakhs people die of cancer each year. Phytosterols have been found useful in treating other conditions, including rheumatoid arthritis, but their widest application is in protecting the heart. However, reports also suggest that excessive intake of dietary phytosterols and stanols in plasma and tissues may contribute to the increased blood pressure (Chen, Gruber, Swist, Coville, Pakenham, Ratnayake, & Scoggan, 2010).

PHYTOSTEROLS: REGULATORY STATUS IN WORLD

Phytosterols, phytostanols and their esters have been evaluated globally by various authorities. Following through assessment, positive approval for phytosterols has been obtained in the European Union (EU), Australia, Switzerland, Norway, Iceland, Brazil, South Africa, Japan, Turkey and Israel. Furthermore in USA, a self-GRAS (Generally Recognized as Safe) procedure has been followed for both phytosterols and phytostanols, to which the US-FDA raised no objections. The first GRAS approval was obtained in 1999 for phytosterol esters for use as an ingredient in vegetable oil based spreads. In addition to receive approval by FDA, phytosterol esters have also been evaluated by major health organizations in the United States. In the European Union (comprising 27 countries), the use of phytosterols, phytostanols and their esters in foods is regulated under Regulation (EC) No. 258/97 of the European Parliament and of the Council of 27 January 1997 concerning novel foods and novel food ingredients (Cantrill & Kawamura, 2008). India and other Asian countries are yet to develop phytosterols enriched products and bring them onto market shelves with all regulatory approvals.

CONCLUSION

At the current growth rate of coronary vascular diseases throughout the world, it can be expected that the market demand for phytosterols enriched products will start in the near future. There is no doubt that phytosterols as functional food ingredients will be a new approach to reduce LDL cholesterol through dairy foods will hold great promise for long term health management. Over the past decade, the possibility of using phytosterols as a functional food ingredient has led to numerous research studies in relation to their ability to reduce blood cholesterol. Initially, phytosterol esters were commercially used in margarines, but recent clinical trials show that phytosterol esters effectively reduce blood cholesterol, even if used in food vehicles with a low fat content as well as dairy products. The use of phytosterols in commonly consumed dairy foods may soon provide an effective tool against many diseases and their introduction to Indian subcontinent is worth anticipating in the near future.

ACKNOWLEDGMENT

The authors are grateful to Dr. Ashok K. Chauhan, Founder President and Mr. Atul Chauhan, Chancellor, Amity University UP, Noida, India for the encouragement, research facilities and financial support. Further, we thankfully acknowledge Dr. Aparna Kuna, Department of Food & Nutrition, N.G. Ranga Agricultural University, Hyderabad and National Dairy Research Institute, Karnal (India) for the necessary research material and motivation.

REFERENCES

Agricultural Research Service USDA (2010). *What we eat in America.* NHANES 2007-2008.

Akihisa, T., Kokke, W., & Tamura, T. (1991). Naturally occurring sterols and related compounds from plants. In G. W. Peterson & W. D. Nes (Eds.), *Physiology and Biochemistry of Sterols* (pp. 172–178). Champaign, IL: AOCS.

Anon. (1989). Analysis of steryl glycosides. In W. D. Nes & E. J. Parish (Eds.), *Analysis of sterols and other biologically significant steroids*. San Diego, CA: Academic Press Inc.

Anon. (2003). *Functional foods fact sheet: Plant stenols and sterols*. Available: http://ific.org/

Anon. (2005). *Phytosterol esters (Plant sterols and stenols esters).* Available: http://www.ifst.org/hottop29.htm

Awad, A. B., & Fink, C. S. (2000). Phytosterols as anticancer dietary components: Evidence and mechanism of action. *The Journal of Nutrition*, *130*(9), 2127–2130. doi:10.1093/jn/130.9.2127 PMID:10958802

Awad, A. B., Karen, C. C., Downie, A. C., & Fink, C. S. (2000). Peanuts as a source of B-sitosterol, a Sterol with anticancer properties. *Nutrition and Cancer*, *36*(2), 238–241. doi:10.1207/S15327914NC3602_14 PMID:10890036

Berger, A., & Jones, P. J. H. (2004). Plant sterols: Factors affecting their efficacy and safety as functional food ingredients. *Lipids in Health and Disease*, *3*(1), 1–54. doi:10.1186/1476-511X-3-1 PMID:15070410

Brüll, F., Mensink, R. P., van den Hurk, K., Duijvestijn, A., & Plat, J. (2010). TLR2 activation is essential to induce a Th1 shift in human peripheral blood mononuclear cells by plant stanols and plant sterols. *The Journal of Biological Chemistry*, *285*(5), 2951–2958. doi:10.1074/jbc.M109.036343 PMID:19948716

Brumfield, K. M., Moroney, J. V., Moore, T. S., Simms, T. A., & Donze, D. (2010). Functional characterization of the *Chlamydomonas reinhardtii ERG3* Ortholog, a gene involved in the biosynthesis of ergosterol. *PLoS One*, *5*(1), e8659. doi:10.1371/journal.pone.0008659 PMID:20084111

Cantrill, R., & Kawamura, Y. (2008). Phytosterols, phytostanols and their esters Chemical and technical assessment. *Proceedings of 69th JECFA*, 1-13.

Castelli, W.P. (1988). Cholesterol and lipids in the risk of coronary artery disease--the Framingham Heart Study. *Canadian Journal of Cardiology, 4*(A), 5A-10A.

Chan, Y. M., Demonty, I., Pelled, D., & Jones, P. J. H. (2006). Olive oil containing olive oil fatty acid esters of plant sterols and dietary diacylglycerol reduces low-density lipoprotein cholesterol and decreases the tendency for peroxidation in hypercholesterolaemic subjects. *British Journal of Nutrition*, *98*(03), 563–570. doi:10.1017/S0007114507730775 PMID:17559697

Chen, Q., Gruber, H., Swist, E., Coville, K., Pakenham, C., Ratnayake, W. M. N., & Scoggan, K. A. (2010). Dietary phytosterols and phytostanols decrease cholesterol levels but increase blood pressure in WKY inbred rats in the absence of salt-loading. *Nutrition and Metabolism*, *7*(1), 11–20. doi:10.1186/1743-7075-7-11 PMID:20637058

Christiansen, L. I., Lahteenmaki, P. L. A., Mannelin, M. R., Seppänen-Laakso, T. E., Hiltunen, R. V., & Yliruusi, J. K. (2001). Cholesterol-lowering effect of spreads enriched with microcrystalline plant sterols in hypercholesterolemic subjects. *European Journal of Nutrition*, *40*(2), 66–73. doi:10.1007003940170017 PMID:11518201

Clifton, P. (2002). Plant sterol and stanols-comparison and contrasts. Sterol versus stanols in cholesterol lowering: Is there a difference? *Atherosclerosis*, *3*(3), 5–9. doi:10.1016/S1567-5688(02)00020-X PMID:12429167

Clifton, P. (2009). Lowering cholesterol: A review on the role of plant sterols. *Reprint from Australian Family Physician*, *38*(4), 218–221. PMID:19350071

Csiszar, A., Ungvari, Z., Edwards, J. G., Kaminski, P., Wolin, M. S., Koller, A., & .... (2002). Aging-induced phenotypic changes and oxidative stress impair coronary arteriolar function. *Circulation Research*, *90*(11), 1159–1166. doi:10.1161/01.RES.0000020401.61826.EA PMID:12065318

Csont, T., Sárközy, M., Szűcs, G., Szűcs, C., Bárkányi, J., Bencsik, P., ... Ferdinandy, P. (2013). Effect of a multivitamin preparation supplemented with phytosterol on serum lipids and infarct size in rats fed with normal and high cholesterol diet. *Lipids in Health and Disease*, *12*(1), 138. doi:10.1186/1476-511X-12-138 PMID:24063587

De Jong, A., Plat, J., Bast, A., Godschalk, R. W., Basu, S., & Mensink, R. P. (2008). Effects of plant sterol and stanol ester consumption on lipid metabolism, antioxidant status and markers of oxidative stress, endothelial function and low-grade inflammation in patients on current statin treatment. *European Journal of Clinical Nutrition*, *62*(2), 263–273. doi:10.1038j.ejcn.1602733 PMID:17487211

de Lucia, C., Komici, K., Borghetti, G., Femminella, G. D., Bencivenga, L., Cannavo, A., ... Rengo, G. (2017). microRNA in Cardiovascular Aging and Age-Related Cardiovascular Diseases. *Frontiers in Medicine*, *4*, 74. doi:10.3389/fmed.2017.00074 PMID:28660188

Demonty, I., Chan, Y. M., Pelled, D., & Jones, P. J. H. (2006). Fish-oil esters of plant sterols improve the lipid profile of dyslipidemic subjects more than do fish-oil or sunflower oil esters of plant sterols. *The American Journal of Clinical Nutrition*, *84*(6), 1534–1542. doi:10.1093/ajcn/84.6.1534 PMID:17158440

Demonty, I., Ras, R. T., van der Knaap, H. C. M., Duchateau, G. S. M. J. E., Meijer, L., Zock, P. L., ... Trautwein, E. A. (2009). Continuous dose-response relationship of the LDL-cholesterol-lowering effect of phytosterol intake. *The Journal of Nutrition*, *139*(2), 271–284. doi:10.3945/jn.108.095125 PMID:19091798

Dutta, P. C. (2004). Chemistry, analysis, and occurrence of phytosterol oxidation products in foods. In P. C. Dutta (Ed.), Phytosterols as Functional Food Components and Nutraceuticals (pp. 397–417). Academic Press.

Fenton, M. (1992). Chromatographic separation of cholesterol in foods. *Journal of Chromatography. A*, *624*(1-2), 369–388. doi:10.1016/0021-9673(92)85689-Q PMID:1494014

Gilbert, R., Thompson, M. D., & Grundy, S. M. (2005). History and development of plant sterol and stanol esters for cholesterol-lowering purposes. *The American Journal of Cardiology*, *96*(1suppl.), 3D–9D. doi:10.1016/j.amjcard.2005.03.013 PMID:15992509

Gylling, H., & Miettinen, T. A. (1999). Cholesterol reduction by different plant sterol and stanol esters for cholesterol lowering purposes. *The American Journal of Cardiology*, *96*(suppl.), 3D–9D.

Hyun, Y. J., Kim, O. Y., Kang, J. B., Lee, J. H., Jang, Y., Liponkoski, L., & Salo, P. (2005). Plant stanol esters in low-fat yoghurt reduce total and low density lipoprotein cholesterol and low-density lipoprotein oxidation in normocholesterolemic and mildly hypercholesterolemic subjects. *Nutrition Research (New York, N.Y.)*, *25*(8), 743–753. doi:10.1016/j.nutres.2005.08.004

Isabelle, D., Rouyanne, T. R., & Henk, C. M. (2009). Continuous dose-response relationship of the LDL-cholesterol-lowering effect of phytosterol intake. *The Journal of Nutrition*, *139*(2), 271–284. doi:10.3945/jn.108.095125 PMID:19091798

Jagerstad, M., & Skog, K. (2005). Genotoxicity of heat-processed foods. *Mutation Research*, *574*(1-2), 156–172. doi:10.1016/j.mrfmmm.2005.01.030 PMID:15914214

Jones, P. J. H. J., & AbuMweis, S. S. (2009). Phytosterols as functional food ingredients: Linkages to cardiovascular disease and cancer. *Current Opinion in Clinical Nutrition and Metabolic Care*, *12*(2), 147–151. doi:10.1097/MCO.0b013e328326770f PMID:19209468

Jong, A., Plat, J., & Mensink, R. P. (2003). Metabolic effects of plant sterols and stanols. *The Journal of Nutritional Biochemistry*, *14*(7), 362–369. doi:10.1016/S0955-2863(03)00002-0 PMID:12915216

Kassis, A. N., Vanstone, C. A., AbuMweis, S. S., & Jones, P. J. H. J. (2008). Efficacy of plant sterol is not influenced by dietary cholesterol intake in hypercholesterolemic individuals. *Metabolism: Clinical and Experimental*, *57*(3), 339–346. doi:10.1016/j.metabol.2007.10.008 PMID:18249205

Kritchevsky, D., & Chen, S. C. (2005). Phytosterols-health benefits and potential concerns: A review. *Nutrition Research (New York, N.Y.)*, *25*(5), 413–428. doi:10.1016/j.nutres.2005.02.003

Kuna, A., & Poshadri, A. (2012). Phytosterol- A functional ingredient for Indian food industry. *Indian Food Industry*, *30*(3), 21–28.

Kuna, A., Raju, P. N., & Poshadri, A. (2011). Phytosterols as functional ingredients for dairy foods. *Indian Journal of Dairy Science*, *64*(5), 359–367.

Law, M. (2000). Plant sterol and stanol margarines and health. *British Medical Journal, 320*(7238), 861–864. doi:10.1136/bmj.320.7238.861 PMID:10731187

Leblond, J. D., Dahmen, A. S., Lebret, K., & Rengefors, K. (2013). Sterols of the green-pigmented, freshwater raphidophyte, *Gonyostomum semen*, from Scandinavian lakes. *The Journal of Eukaryotic Microbiology, 60*(4), 399–405. doi:10.1111/jeu.12050 PMID:23731265

Lercker, G., & Rodriguez-Estrada, M. T. (2002). Cholesterol oxidation mechanisms. In F. Guardiola, P. C. Dutta, R. Codony, & G. P. Savage (Eds.), *Cholesterol and Phytosterol Oxidation Products* (pp. 1–25). Champaign, IL: AOCS Press.

Lin, X., Racette, S. B., Lefevre, M., Spearie, C. A., Most, M., Ma, L., & Ostlund, R. E. Jr. (2010). The effects of phytosterols present in natural food matrices on cholesterol metabolism and LDL-cholesterol: A controlled feeding trial. *European Journal of Clinical Nutrition, 64*(12), 1481–1487. doi:10.1038/ejcn.2010.180 PMID:20808333

Ling, W. H., & Jones, P. J. H. (1995). Dietary phytosterols; a review of metabolism, benefits and side effects. *Life Sciences, 57*(3), 195–206. doi:10.1016/0024-3205(95)00263-6 PMID:7596226

Loizou, S., Lekakis, I., Chrousos, G. P., & Moutsatsou, P. (2010). Beta-Sitosterol exhibits anti-inflammatory activity in human aortic endothelial cells. *Molecular Nutrition & Food Research, 54*(4), 551–558. doi:10.1002/mnfr.200900012 PMID:19937850

Mattson, F. H., Grundy, S. M., & Crouse, J. R. (1982). Optimizing the effect of plant sterols on cholesterol absorption in man. *The American Journal of Clinical Nutrition, 35*(4), 697–700. doi:10.1093/ajcn/35.4.697 PMID:7072622

McNamara, D. J. (2000). Dietary cholesterol and atherosclerosis. *Biochimica et Biophysica Acta, 1529*(1-3), 310–320. doi:10.1016/S1388-1981(00)00156-6 PMID:11111098

Mensink, R. P., Ebbing, S., Lindhout, M., Plat, J., & Heugten, M. M. (2002). Effects of plant-stanol esters supplied in low-fat yoghurt on serum lipids and lipoproteins, non-cholesterol sterols and fat soluble antioxidant concentrations. *Atherosclerosis, 160*(1), 205–213. doi:10.1016/S0021-9150(01)00562-7 PMID:11755939

Micallef, M. A., & Garg, M. L. (2008). The lipid-lowering effects of phytosterols and (n-3) polyunsaturated fatty acids are synergistic and complementary in hyperlipidemic men and women. *The Journal of Nutrition, 138*(6), 1086–1090. doi:10.1093/jn/138.6.1086 PMID:18492838

Monu, E., Blank, G., Holley, R., & Zawistowski, J. (2008). Phytosterol effects on milk and yoghurt microflora. *Journal of Food Science*, *00*, M1–M6. PMID:18387114

Morreau, R. A., Whitaker, B. D., & Hicks, K. B. (2002). Phytosterols, phytostanols, and their conjugates in foods: Structural diversity, quantitative analysis, and health-promoting uses. *Progress in Lipid Research*, *41*(6), 457–500. doi:10.1016/S0163-7827(02)00006-1 PMID:12169300

Niccoli, T., & Partridge, L. (2012). Ageing as a risk factor for disease. *Current Biology*, *22*(17), R741–R752. doi:10.1016/j.cub.2012.07.024 PMID:22975005

North, B. J., & Sinclair, D. A. (2012). The intersection between aging and cardiovascular disease. *Circulation Research*, *110*(8), 1097–1108. doi:10.1161/CIRCRESAHA.111.246876 PMID:22499900

Ostlund, R. E. Jr. (2007). Phytosterols, cholesterol absorption and healthy diets. *Lipids*, *42*(1), 41–45. doi:10.100711745-006-3001-9 PMID:17393209

Ostlund, R. E. Jr, Spilburg, C. A., & Stenson, W. F. (1999). Sitostanol administered in lecithin micelles potently reduces cholesterol absorption in humans. *The American Journal of Clinical Nutrition*, *70*(5), 826–831. doi:10.1093/ajcn/70.5.826 PMID:10539742

Patterson, G. W. (1991). Sterols of algae. In G. W. Patterson & D. W. Nes (Eds.), *Physiology and Biochemistry of Sterols* (pp. 118–156). Campaing, IL: American Oil's Chemists' Society.

Phillips, K. M., Ruggio, D. M., Toivo, J. I., Swank, M. A., & Simpkins, A. H. (2002). Free and esterified sterol composition of edible oils and fats. *Journal of Food Composition and Analysis*, *15*(2), 123–142. doi:10.1006/jfca.2001.1044

Piironen, V., Toivo, J., & Lampi, A. M. (2000). Natural sources of dietary plant sterols. *Journal of Food Composition and Analysis*, *13*(4), 619–624. doi:10.1006/jfca.2000.0898

Piretti, M. V., Giampiero, P., Boni, L., Pistocchi, R., Diamante, M., & Gazzotti, T. (1997). Investigation of 4-methyl sterols from cultured dinoflagellate algal strains. *Journal of Phycology*, *33*(1), 61–67. doi:10.1111/j.0022-3646.1997.00061.x

Quilez, J., Garcia-Lorda, P., & Salas-Salvado, J. (2003). Potential uses and benefits of phytosterols in diet: Present situation and future directions. *Clinical Nutrition (Edinburgh, Lothian)*, *22*(4), 343–351. doi:10.1016/S0261-5614(03)00060-8 PMID:12880600

Racette, S. B., Lin, X., Lefevre, M., Spearie, C. A., Most, M. M., Ma, L., & Ostlund, R. E. Jr. (2010). Dose effects of dietary phytosterols on cholesterol metabolism: A controlled feeding study. *The American Journal of Clinical Nutrition*, *91*(1), 32–38. doi:10.3945/ajcn.2009.28070 PMID:19889819

Rampen, S. W., Abbas, B. A., Schouten, S., & Sinninghe Damste, J. S. (2010). A comprehensive study of sterols in marine diatoms (Bacillariophyta): Implications for their use as tracers for diatom productivity. *Limnology and Oceanography*, *55*(1), 91–105. doi:10.4319/lo.2010.55.1.0091

Reddy, K. R. (2012). *Kidwai memorial institute of oncology*. Retrieved from http://kidwai.kar.nic.in/statistics.html

Rengo, G., Pagano, G., Vitale, D. F., Formisano, R., Komici, K., Petraglia, L., ... Ferrara, N. (2016). Impact of aging on cardiac sympathetic innervation measured by (123) I-mIBG imaging in patients with systolic heart failure. *European Journal of Nuclear Medicine and Molecular Imaging*, *43*(13), 2392–2400. doi:10.100700259-016-3432-3 PMID:27287990

Rozner, S., & Garti, N. (2006). The activity and absorption relationship of cholesterol and phytosterols. *Colloids and Surfaces. A, Physicochemical and Engineering Aspects*, *282*, 435–456. doi:10.1016/j.colsurfa.2005.12.032

Salen, G., Shore, V., Tint, G. S., Forte, T., Shefer, S., Horak, I., ... Kwiterovich, P. O. Jr. (1989). Increased sitosterol absorption, decreased removal, and expanded body pools compensate for reduced cholesterol synthesis in sitosterolemia with xanthomatosis. *Journal of Lipid Research*, *30*, 1319–1330. PMID:2600539

Salo, P. M. D., & Wester, I. M. S. (2005). Low fat formulations of plant stanols and sterols. *The American Journal of Cardiology*, *96*(1suppl.), 51D–54D. doi:10.1016/j.amjcard.2005.03.021 PMID:15992517

Salta, F. N., Kalogeropoulos, N., Karavanou, N., & Andrikopoulos, N. K. (2008). Distribution and retention of phytosterols in frying oils and fried potatoes during repeated deep and pan frying. *European Food Research and Technology*, *41*(2), 391–400. doi:10.100700217-007-0733-6

Shrestha, S., Volek, J. S., Udani, J., Wood, R. J., Greene, C. M., Aggarwal, D., ... Fernandez, M. L. (2006). A combination therapy including psyllium and plant sterols lowers LDL cholesterol by modifying lipoprotein metabolism in hypercholesterolemic individuals. *The Journal of Nutrition*, *136*(10), 2492–2497. doi:10.1093/jn/136.10.2492 PMID:16988115

Soupas, L. (2006). *Oxidative stability of phytosterols in food models and foods* (Academic dissertation). University of Helsinki, Helsinki, Finland.

Soupas, L., Huikko, L., Lampi, A. M., & Piironen, V. (2005). Esterification affects phytosterol oxidation. *European Journal of Lipid Science and Technology*, *107*(2), 107–118. doi:10.1002/ejlt.200401096

Taipale, S. J., Hiltunen, M., Vuorio, K., & Peltomaa, E. (2016). Suitability of Phytosterols alongside Fatty Acids as Chemotaxonomic Biomarkers for Phytoplankton. *Frontiers in Plant Science*, *7*, 212. doi:10.3389/fpls.2016.00212 PMID:26973664

Tasan, B.M., Bilgin, U., & Gecgel, A.S., & Demirci. (2006). Phytosterols as functional food ingredients. *Tekirdag Ziraat Fakültesi Dergisi*, *3*(2), 153–159.

Thanh, T. T., Vergnes, M. F., Kaloustian, J., El-Moselhy, T. F., Amiot-Carlin, M. J., & Portugal, H. (2006). Effect of storage and heating on phytosterol concentrations in vegetable oils determined by GC/MS. *Journal of the Science of Food and Agriculture*, *86*(2), 220–225. doi:10.1002/jsfa.2322

Theuwissen, E., & Mensink, R. P. (2007). Simultaneous intake of beta-glucan and plant stanol esters affects lipid metabolism in slightly hyper-cholesterolemic subjects. *The Journal of Nutrition*, *137*(3), 583–588. doi:10.1093/jn/137.3.583 PMID:17311944

Thompson, G. A. Jr. (1996). Lipids and membrane function in green algae. *Biochimica et Biophysica Acta*, *1302*(1), 17–45. doi:10.1016/0005-2760(96)00045-8 PMID:8695653

Ungvari, Z., Buffenstein, R., Austad, S. N., Podlutsky, A., Kaley, G., & Csiszar, A. (2008). Oxidative stress in vascular senescence: Lessons from successfully aging species. *Frontiers in Bioscience*, *13*(13), 5056–5070. doi:10.2741/3064 PMID:18508570

Ungvari, Z., Kaley, G., de Cabo, R., Sonntag, W. E., & Csiszar, A. (2010). A. Mechanisms of vascular aging: New perspectives. *The Journals of Gerontology. Series A, Biological Sciences and Medical Sciences*, *65*(10), 1028–1041. doi:10.1093/gerona/glq113 PMID:20576649

Venkatramesh, M., Karunanandaa, B., Sun, B., Gunter, C. A., Boddupalli, S., & Kishore, G. M. (2003). Expression of a streptomyces 3-hydroxysteroid oxidase geve in oilseeds for converting phytosterols to phytostanols. *Phytochemistry*, *62*(1), 39–46. doi:10.1016/S0031-9422(02)00431-4 PMID:12475617

Wilson, P. W., D'Agostino, R. B., Levy, D., Belanger, A. M., Silbershatz, H., & Kannel, W. B. (1998). Prediction of coronary heart disease using risk factor categories. *Circulation*, *97*(18), 1837–1847. doi:10.1161/01.CIR.97.18.1837 PMID:9603539

Woyengo, T. A., Ramprasath, V. R., & Jones, P. J. H. (2009). Anti-cancer effects of phytosterols. *European Journal of Clinical Nutrition*, *63*(7), 813–820. doi:10.1038/ejcn.2009.29 PMID:19491917

Xu, J., Kochanek, K., Murphy, S., & Tejada-Vera, B. (2010). Deaths: Final data for 2007. *National Vital Statistics Reports*, *58*, 1–136. PMID:25075874

Section 4

Hypertension and Hyperlipidemia

Chapter 7
Dietary Fibers and Nutraceuticals in Prevention of Hypertension

John Intru Disouza
Tatyasaheb Kore College of Pharmacy, India

Kiran Shivaji Patil
Tatyasaheb Kore College of Pharmacy, India

Pratik Shailendra Kakade
Institute of Chemical Technology, India

Vandana Bharat Patravale
Institute of Chemical Technology, India

ABSTRACT

Hypertension is the major cause of mortality amongst many cardiovascular risk factors causing 7.5 million deaths annually. Macronutrient and micronutrient deficiencies are very common in general population and have broad-ranging physiological effects in-vivo which lessen inflammatory cascades and vascular reactivity. A recent trend is to perform nutritional epidemiological studies linking overall diet pattern to the lifestyle, examining the link between food and nutrients of diet to risk of chronic diseases. This chapter would deal with pharmacological and pathological basis of hypertension, utilization of dietary fibers, functional foods, nutraceuticals for hypertensive populations as well as to those with increased cardiovascular risks.

DOI: 10.4018/978-1-5225-3267-5.ch007

INTRODUCTION

Cardiovascular diseases (CVD) are the leading cause of death globally accounting for more than 20 million deaths annually. 3.9 million Deaths in Europe and over 1.8 million deaths in the European Union (EU) occur due to (CVD) every year (*European Cardiovascular Disease Statistics*, 2017; EHN - European Heart Network, n.d.). Cardiovascular diseases are a group of disorders of the heart and blood vessels. People who are at high cardiovascular risk due to the presence of risk factors such as hypertension, diabetes, hyperlipidemia or already established disease, need early detection and management using counseling and medicines, as appropriate.

HYPERTENSION

Hypertension is a major risk factor for morbidity and mortality associated with stroke, heart failure and coronary artery disease and chronic kidney disease (CKD) (Mancia, Fagard, Narkiewicz, Redón, Zanchetti, & Böhm, 2013). Hypertension in adults of age 18 years and older is defined as systolic blood pressure (SBP) of 140 mmHg or greater and/or diastolic blood pressure (DBP) of 90 mmHg or greater or any level of blood pressure in patients taking antihypertensive medication (Chobanian, Bakris, Black, Cushman, Green, & Izzo, 2003).

CVD nevertheless remains the main cause of death, especially ischemic heart disease and cerebrovascular disease (CD)(Kearney et al., 2005; Zimmet, Alberti, & Shaw, 2001; Jackson, Lawes, Bennett, Milne, & Rodgers, 2005). Hypertension, was identified in a recent World Health Organization report as among the most important preventable causes of premature death. Atherosclerosis is the basic reason for high blood pressure, in which plaque builds inside the arteries. Several factors which lead to atherosclerosis are faulty food habits, lack of exercise, stress, sedentary lifestyle, etc. (McGill, 1979; He, Merchant, Rimm Rosner, Stampfer, Willett, & Ascherio,

Table 1. Types of hypertension

Category Pressure	Systolic Pressure mm Hg	Diastolic Pressure mm Hg
• Normal	90–119	60-79
• Pre-hypertension	120–139	80–89
• Stage 1	140–159	90–99
• Stage 2	≥160	≥100
• Isolated systolic Hypertension	≥140	<90

2003; Bernstein, Sun, Hu, Stampfer, Manson, & Willett, 2010). Smokers with obesity live 14 fewer years than nonsmokers with normal weight. Lifestyle-related conditions, such as obesity, hyperlipidemia, type II diabetes, and hypertension, are also widespread and becoming more prevalent globally(Alberti, Eckel, Grundy, Zimmet, Cleeman, & Donato, 2009). The origin of these CVD is multifactorial. The Cardiovascular risk factors (CVRF) are categorized in table 2 (Bertomeu & Castillo-Castillo, 2008; Olalla, Medrano, Sierra, & Almazán, 1999; Anderson, Wilson, Odell, & Kannel, 1991; Jeppesen, Hein, Suadicani, & Gyntelberg, 1998; Lehto, Rönnemaa, Pyörälä, & Laakso, 2000; Vartiainen, Laatikainen, Peltonen, Juolevi, Männistö, Sundvall, ... Puska, 2010).

EPIDEMIOLOGY

The global epidemic of cardiovascular disease is increasing as well as it is shifting from developed to developing nations. The disability-adjusted life year (DALY) is a measure of overall disease burden. It is expressed as the number of years lost due to ill-health, disability or early death. It indicates the total burden of a disease. 10% of DALYs are lost in low- and middle-income countries and 18% in high- income countries due to cardiovascular disease. Annually, 15 million people worldwide suffer a stroke. Of these, 5 million die and another 5 million are left permanently

Table 2. Underlying factors that associated with high blood pressure

Non-Modifiable Risk Factors	Metabolic Risk Factors	Lifestyle Risk Factors	Novel Risk Factors	Other Factors
• Advancing age • Male gender • Family history/ genotype • Susceptible ethnic origin • Dark skin colour • Low birth weight	• Hypertension • Hyperlipidemia • Diabetes mellitus • Metabolic syndrome • Obesity/ overweight • Excess salt intake • Low potassium intake • Fructose • Excess alcohol • VitaminD deficiency • Low folic acid intake • Hyperuricaemia	• Unhealthy diet, particular excess calories, fat and • Increased triglycerides • Smoking • Physical activity • Psychological stress • Sedentary occupation • Sleep deprivation • Long-term exposure to noise	• Elevated homocysteine level • Elevated lipoprotein (a) level • Small dense LDL-C • Elevated inflammatory markers levels • Elevated hemostatic factors levels • Elevated homocysteine level	• Obstructive sleep apnea • Increased arterial stiffness • Systemic pro inflammatory state • Prescription drugs • (eg, nonsteroidal anti-inflammatory drugs)

disabled. Hypertension epidemiology is mainly associated with diet and nutrient intake which plays an etiological role in vascular homeostasis. The shifting of paradigm from the "Paleolithic diet to our modern diet" has produced an epidemic of nutritionally-related diseases (Table 3).

It clearly signifies that hypertension, atherosclerosis, coronary heart disease (CHD), myocardial Infarction (MI), congestive heart failure (CHF), cerebrovascular accidents (CVA), renal disease, type 2 diabetes mellitus (T2DM), metabolic syndrome (MS) and obesity are an epidemic of nutritionally-related diseases (Eaton, Eaton, & Konner, 1997; *Review Paleolithic Nutrition Revisited*, 1997). Evolution from a pre-agricultural, hunter-gatherer milieu to an agricultural, refrigeration society has imposed an unnatural and unhealthful nutritional selection process. Morale of the story is our diet has changed more than our genetics can adapt.

The macronutrient and micronutrient variations, oxidative stress from radical oxygen species (ROS) and radical nitrogen species (RNS) and inflammatory mediators such as cell adhesion molecules (CAMs), cytokines, signaling molecules and autoimmune vascular dysfunction of T cells and B cells, contribute to the higher incidence of hypertension and other cardiovascular diseases through complex nutrient-gene interactions, epigenetic and nutrient-caveolae interactions and nutrient reactions with pattern recognition receptors (toll like receptors (TLR) and nod-like receptors) in the endothelium (Layne, Majkova, Smart, Toborek, & Hennig, 2011; Dandona, Ghanim, Chaudhuri, Dhindsa, & Kim, 2010; Houston, 2014; Berdanier, 1994; Zhao, Lee, & Hwang, 2011) (Figure 1).

Table 3. Diet of Paleolithic and contemporary humans

Nutrients and Dietary Characteristics	Paleolithic Intake	Modern Intake
• Sodium	< 50 mmol/d (1.2 g)	175 mmol/d (4 g)
• Potassium	> 10000 meq/d (256 g)	150 meq/d (6 g)
• Sodium/Potassium Ratio	< 0.13/d	> 0.67/d
• Calcium	1000-1500 mg/d	1000 mg/d
• Protein	37%	20%
• Carbohydrate	41%	40%-50%
• Fat	22%	30%-40%
• Polyunsaturated/Saturated Fat Ratio	1.4	0.4
• Fiber	> 100 g/d	9 g/d
• Omega 3 and 6 fat (g)	9.6 Roughly equal	Far more omega -6
• Cholesterol (Mg)	480 (Equal or more)	480

Source: Adapted from (Broadhurst, 1997; The Nutritional Characteristics of a Contemporary Diet Based Upon Paleolithic Food Groups Abstract 4 / Diet (Nutrition), n.d.; Melvin Konner).

Figure 1. Vascular inflammation, oxidative stress and immune dysfunction lead to endothelial dysfunction and vascular smooth muscle dysfunction
Source: Houston, 2014). The role of nutrition and nutraceutical supplements in the treatment of hypertension. World Journal of Cardiology, 6(2), 38–66.

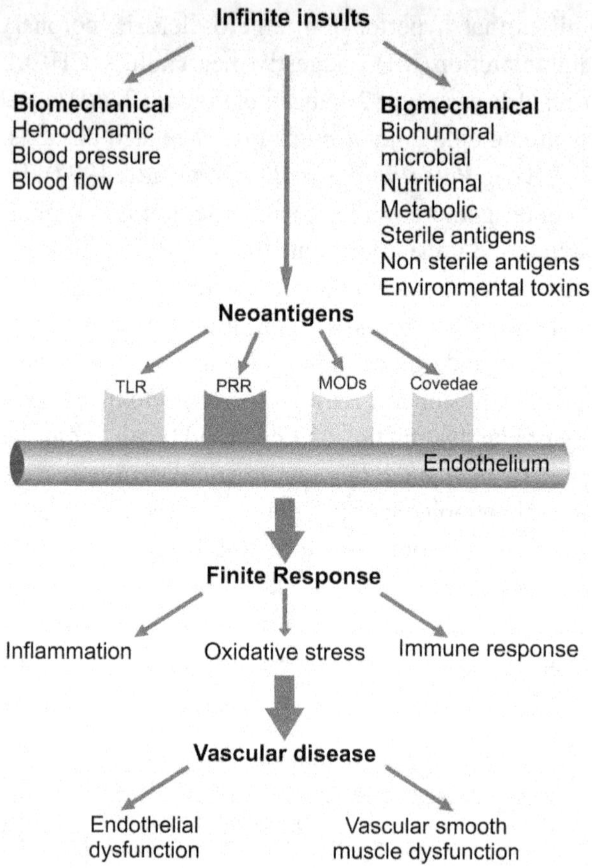

Reduction in nitric oxide bioavailability, increase in angiotensin II and endothelin coupled with endothelial activation initiate the vascular and cardiac dysfunction and hypertension. Poor nutrition, coupled with obesity and a sedentary lifestyle have resulted in an exponential increase in nutritionally-related diseases. In particular, the high Na+/K+ ratio of modern diets has contributed to hypertension, CVA, CHD, MI, CHF and renal disease (Houston & Harper, 2008; Buckland & Gonzalez, 2015) as have the relatively low intake of omega-3 PUFA, increase in omega-6 PUFA, saturated fat and trans fatty acids (Broadhurst, 1997).

PATHOPHYSIOLOGY

Vascular biology assumes a central role in the initiation and perpetuation of hypertension and cardiovascular disease. Oxidative stress (ROS and RNS), inflammation and autoimmune vascular dysfunction (T cells and B cells) are the main pathophysiological and functional mechanisms that induce vascular disease (Eftekhari, Mathiassen, Buus, Gotzsche, Mulvany, & Christensen, 2011; Houston, 2014; Touyz, 2012) (Figure 2). A Lethal combination of all three of these leads to, vascular smooth muscle, cardiac dysfunction, hypertension, vascular disease, atherosclerosis and CVD. This becomes a malfunctioning in the vascular system

Figure 2. process of Immune vascular dysfunction
Source: Houston, M. (2014). The role of nutrition and nutraceutical supplements in the treatment of hypertension. World Journal of Cardiology, 6(2), 38–66.

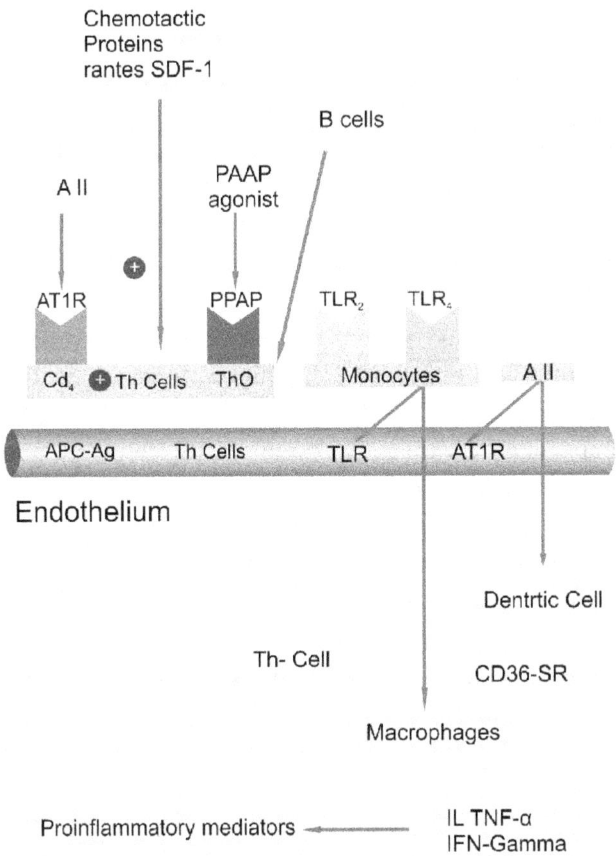

that was initially intended to provide a vascular defense to the endothelial insults (Houston, 2014; Touyz, 2012; Society, P. by: B. C., Society, B. H., Uk, D., Uk, H., Society, P. C. C., & Association, 2005).

In hypertensive patients, due to abnormal microvasculature small resistance in arteries is created leading to impaired vasodilatory capacity, increased vascular resistance, increased media to lumen ratio, decreased maximal organ perfusion and reduced flow reserve, especially in the heart with decreased coronary flow reserve (Eftekhari, Mathiassen, Buus, Gotzsche, Mulvany, & Christensen, 2011; Xing, Wang, Li, & Wang, 2012).

Oxidative Stress

Oxidative stress, with an imbalance between ROS and RNS and the anti-oxidant defense mechanisms, contributes to the etiology of hypertension (Eftekhari, Mathiassen, Buus, Gotzsche, Mulvany, & Christensen, 2011; Broadhurst, 1997). Radical oxygen species directly damage endothelial cells, degrade NO, influence eicosanoid metabolism, oxidize LDL, lipids, proteins, carbohydrates, DNA and organic molecules, increase catecholamines, damage the genetic machinery, influence gene expression and transcription factors (Kearney, Whelton, Reynolds, Muntner, Whelton, & He, 2005; Houston, 2014; Kizhakekuttu & Widlansky, 2010; Tse, Maxwell, Thomason, Blann, Thorpe, Waite, & Holder, 1994; Mansego, Solar, Alonso, Martínez, Sáez, Escudero, … Chaves, 2011). The increased oxidative stress, inflammation and autoimmune vascular dysfunction in human hypertension results from a combination of increased generation of ROS and RNS, an exacerbated response to ROS and RNS and a decreased antioxidant reserve(Rodríguez-Iturbe, Franco, Tapia, Quiroz, & Johnson, 2012; Quiroz, Johnson, & Rodríguez-Iturbe, 2012; Muller, Kvakan, & Luft, 2011; Marketou, Kontaraki, Zacharis, Kochiadakis, Giaouzaki, Chlouverakis, & Vardas, 2012; Luft, 2012; Herrada, Campino, Amador, Michea, Fardella, & Kalergis, 2011).

Activation of the AT1R in the RVLM increases NADPH oxidase and increases oxidative stress and superoxide anion, increases SNS outflow causing an imbalance of SNS/PNS activity with an elevation of BP, increased heart rate and alterations in heart rate variability and heart rate recovery time, which can be blocked by AT1R blockers(Nishihara, Hirooka, Matsukawa, Kishi, & Sunagawa, 2012; Konno, Hirooka, Araki, Koga, Kishi, & Sunagawa, 2008).

Inflammation

Increases in high sensitivity C-reactive protein (HS-CRP) as well as other inflammatory cytokines such as interleukin-1B, (IL-1B), IL-6, tumor necrosis alpha (TNF-α) and chronic leukocytosis occur in hypertension and hypertensive- related TOD, such as increased carotid IMT (Amer, Elawam, Khater, Omar, Mabrouk, & Taha, 2011). Elevated HS-CRP is both a risk marker and risk factor for hypertension and CVD. Nitric oxide and eNOS are inhibited by HS-CRP. The AT2R, which normally counterbalances AT1R, is downregulated by HS-CRP (Vongpatanasin, Thomas, Schwartz, Cassis, Osborne-Lawrence, Hahner, ... Shaul, 2007; Razzouk, Muntner, Bansilal, Kini, Aneja, Mozes, ... Farkouh, 2009). Angiotensin II (A-II) upregulates many of the cytokines, especially IL-6, CAMs and chemokines by activating nuclear factor Kappa B (NF- κb) leading to vasoconstriction. These events, along with the increases in oxidative stress and endothelin-1, elevate BP (Fa & A, 2007).

Autoimmune Dysfunction

Innate and adaptive immune responses are linked to hypertension and hypertension-induced CVD through at least three mechanisms: cytokine production, central nervous system stimulation and renal damage. This includes salt-sensitive hypertension with increased renal inflammation as a result of T cell imbalance, dysregulation of CD4+ and CD8+ lymphocytes and chronic leukocytosis with increased neutrophils and reduced lymphocytes(H, Fc, & Dn, 2009; Rodríguez-Iturbe, Franco, Tapia, Quiroz, & Johnson, 2012; Tian, Penman, Manning, Flessner, & Mawson, 2012) (Figure 2). Macrophages and various T-cell subtypes regulate BP, invade the arterial wall, activate TLRs and induce autoimmune vascular damage (Tian, Penman, Manning, Flessner, & Mawson, 2012; Muller, Kvakan, & Luft, 2011).

PHARMACOTHERAPY

In many people the BP remains high regardless of appropriate non-pharmacological measures, under these conditions pharmacological approaches must be taken into consideration. Higher the BP greater the risk of cardiovascular disease and, therefore, the JNC-7 defined BP of 120-139/80-89 mm Hg as pre-hypertension (Lewington, Clarke, Qizilbash, Peto, Collins, & Prospective Studies Collaboration, 2002; Chobanian, Bakris, Black, Cushman, Green, & Izzo, 2003). The newest category of pre-hypertension, was introduced to emphasize that patients whose BP was found to be greater than the 120/80 mm Hg mark were more likely to progress towards definite hypertension.

Table 4. Suggested targets for blood pressure control in various co-morbidity groups among adults with hypertension

Sub-Group	Target Systolic BP mm Hg	Target Diastolic BP mm Hg
• Usual care uncomplicated hypertension	<140	<90
• Diabetes	<130	<80
• Coronary heart disease	<130, preferably <120	<80
• Chronic renal disease	<130	<80
• Congestive heart failure	<120, preferably <110	<80 or <75
• Isolated systolic hypertension	<140	

Source: Adapted from Ref: (Lewington, Clarke, Qizilbash, Peto, Collins, & Prospective Studies Collaboration, 2002;European Society of Hypertension-European Society of Cardiology guidelines for the management of arterial hypertension., 2003; National Kidney Foundation, 2002;Expert Panel on Detection, Evaluation, and Treatment of High Blood Cholesterol in Adults, 2001) It was also hoped that health care providers will encourage persons with BP in pre-hypertension range to begin non-pharmacological lifestyle modifications. It has been recommended that pharmacological therapy should be initiated early if the targets are not achieved by lifestyle changes alone (Lewington, Clarke, Qizilbash, Peto, Collins, & Prospective Studies Collaboration, 2002).

PRIMARY MANAGEMENT OF HYPERTENSION

The overall goal of treatment in hypertensive patients is to lowering BP and reduces the risk of cardiovascular morbidity and mortality. In general, the goal is to lower BP to below 140/90 mm Hg. In patients with heart failure, diabetes, or renal disease, the goal is to lower BP to below 130/85 mm Hg (Table 4). In older patients with isolated systolic hypertension (ISH), the goal is to lower systolic BP to below 140 mm Hg. These goals can be achieved through lifestyle alteration or drug therapy. The initial drug management of hypertension is a contentious issue.

Examples of the main classes of antihypertensives that were recommended by JNC 8 include:

1. **Diuretics:** Chlorthalidone, Hydrochlorothiazide, Indapamide,Metolazone
2. **Thiazide (or thiazide-like):** Hydrochlorothiazide, chlortalidone, indapamide
3. **ACE inhibitors:** Lisinopril, enalapril, captopril
4. **Angiotensin-II Receptor Antagonists:** Candesartan, irbesartan, losartan, valsartan
5. **Calcium-channel blockers:** Amlodipine, diltiazem
6. **Beta-Blockers:** Metoprolol, atenolol

Some of these drugs are available in fixed-dose combination formulations. These single pill formulations simplify dosing regimens and improve adherence. Despite the considerable advances that have occurred over the past few decades in the management of hypertension yet it remains one of the major epidemics in the western as well as in developing world. Thus, efforts are ongoing to develop new strategies to combat this condition. (Pharmacotherapy: A Pathophysiologic Approach, 9e & Joseph, 2014; High Blood Pressure, 2014; James, Oparil, Carter, Cushman, Dennison-Himmelfarb, Handler…Ortiz, 2014.;Overview of Hypertension, 2015).

NUTRACEUTICALS AND FUNCTIONAL FOODS (NFFS) FOR HYPERTENSION

"Nutraceutical" is a term coined in 1979 by Stephen De Felice *(Nutraceuticals - Opportunities in an Emerging Market,* n.d.) It is defined *as a food or parts of food that provide medical or health benefits, including the prevention and treatment of disease* (Dillard & German, 2000).

Nutraceuticals are pharmaceutical grade dietary additives and supplements that are employed in maintaining well-being, enhancing health, modulating immunity and thereby preventing as well as treating specific diseases (Ramaa, Shirode, Mundada, & Kadam, 2006). Due to presumed safety and potential nutritional and therapeutic effects, nutraceuticals have received significant interest.

In recent years changing food consumption pattern has been scientifically proven to cause lifestyle-related diseases. As mentioned earlier, foods and nutrients play a vital role in normal functioning of the body and specifically heart.

A desirable therapeutic outcome with reduced side effects gains the popularity in Cardio protective bioactive foods and nutraceuticals. Cardiovascular nutraceuticals are helpful in maintaining the functioning of the heart and reducing the risk associated with cardiovascular diseases.

They are now part of nutrition supplements at nonprescription counters and self-prescription is also increased at large scale. Therefore, the discovery and production of nutraceuticals over pharmaceuticals is, well appreciated by the many pharmaceutical and biotechnology companies.

DIETARY FIBERS INTRODUCTION

Fibers are portions of plant or analogous carbohydrates that are impermeable to digestion and absorb or transport in to the human small intestine with comprehensive or partial fermentation in the large intestine. Fibers are parts or compounds of plants,

Table 5. Nutraceuticals lowering Blood cholesterol

Nutraceuticals Which Lower Blood Cholesterol	
Bioactive Compounds	**Nutraceuticals**
• Tocopherols, omega-3 fattyacids	Nuts (Sabate & Ang, 2009; Albert, Gaziano, Willett, & Manson, 2002)
• Fiber and polyphenols	Legumes (Erkkilä & Lichtenstein, 2006)
• Fiber (pectin)	Fruits and vegetables (He, Merchant, Rimm, Rosner, Stampfer, Willett, & Ascherio,2003)
• Phytosterols	Margarine (Darmadi-Blackberry, Wahlqvist, Kouris-Blazos, Steen, Lukito, Horie, & Horie, 2004)
• Omega-3 fatty acids	Fish oil (Moreau, Whitaker, & Hicks, 2002)
• Fiber and phytochemicals	Whole grains (Dyerberg, Eskesen, Andersen, Astrup, Buemann, Christensen, … Stender, 2004)
• Genistein and daidzein	Soy proteins (Lutsey, Jacobs, Kori, Mayer-Davis, Shea, Steffen… Tracy, 2007)
• Flavonoid	Dark chocolate (Masters, Liese, Haffner, Wagenknecht, & Hanley, 2010;Grassi, Lippi, Necozione, Desideri, & Ferri, 2005; Baba, Natsume, Yasuda, Nakamura, Tamura, Osakabe, … Kondo, 2007)
• B glucan	Oats (Chen, Wang, Zhang, & Yang, 2014)
• Bioactive Peptides from Hydrolysis of Fish Protein Sardine peptides	Fish skin- collagen (Cinq-Mars, Hu, Kitts, & Li-Chan, 2008)

Table 6. Nutraceuticals inhibiting oxidation of LDL-C

Inhibition of LDL-C oxidation	
Bioactive Compounds	**Nutraceuticals**
• Omega-3 fatty acids	Fish
• Carotenoids	Green leafy vegetables, fruits (Chopra, O'Neill, Keogh, Wortley, Southon, & Thurnham, 2000)
• Vitamin C	Citrus fruits and vegetables (Nayak, Karmen, Frishman, & Vakili, 2001)
• Lycopene	Tomato (Yussif, Abdul Aziz, & Abdel Rahman, 2016)
• Polyphenolics and oleic acid	Extravirgin olive oil (Engelhard, Gazer, & Paran, 2006)
• Tea polyphenolics	Green tea (Engelhard, Gazer, & Paran, 2006)
• Genistein, daidzein, andglycitein	Soy proteins (Wiseman, O'Reilly, Adlercreutz, Mallet, Bowey, Rowland, & Sanders, 2000)
• Flavonoid	Dark chocolate (Grassi, Lippi, Necozione, Desideri, & Ferri, 2005)
• Polyphenols	Pomegranate (Yussif, Abdul Aziz, & Abdel Rahman, 2016)

Table 7. Nutraceuticals lowering blood pressure

Decreasing Blood Pressure	
Bioactive Compounds	**Nutraceuticals**
• Omega-3 fatty acids	Fish, Walnuts, Flaxseed, Rapeseed, Soybeans, Oats (Konno, Hirooka, Araki, Koga, Kishi, & Sunagawa, 2008; Mozaffarian, 2008)
• Ascorbic acid	Citrus fruits (Block, Mangels, Norkus, Patterson, Levander, & Taylor, 2001)
• Ginsenosides	Ginseng (Mozaffarian, 2008)
• Quercetin	Onion and garlic (Grassi, Lippi, Necozione, Desideri, & Ferri, 2005)
• Tea polyphenolics	Green tea (Sumpio, Cordova, Berke-Schlessel, Qin, & Chen, 2006)
• Grape polyphenols	Grapes and red wine (Sumpio, Cordova, Berke-Schlessel, Qin, & Chen, 2006)
• Flavonoid	Dark chocolate (Pérez-Jiménez & Saura-Calixto, 2008)
• Chlorogenic Acid (CGA).	coffee beans, apples, pears, tomatoes,blueberry, potatoes, peanuts,Chinese parsley, and eggplants (Sumpio, Cordova, Berke-Schlessel, Qin, & Chen, 2006)
• (6)-shogaol and (6)-gingerol,	Ginger (Suekawa, Ishige, Yuasa, Sudo, Aburada, & Hosoya, 1984)
• Fiber	Legumes (He, Klag, Whelton, Chen, Qian, & Het, 1995)
• phytochemicals Fiber	Whole grains (Savica, Bellinghieri, & Kopple, 2010)

Table 9. Nutraceuticals with antioxidant action

Antioxidant Action	
Bioactive Compounds	**Nutraceuticals**
• Lycopene	Tomatoes (Engelhard, Gazer, & Paran, 2006)
• Carotenoids	Green leafy vegetables and fruits (Krinsky & Johnson, 2005)
• Tocopherol, tocotrienols	Vegetable oils (Nayak, Karmen, Frishman, & Vakili, 2001)
• Vitamin C	Citrus fruits and vegetables (Yussif, Abdul Aziz, & Abdel Rahman, 2016)
• Genistein and daidzein	Soy proteins (Lichtenstein, 1998)
• Tea polyphenols	Green and black teas (Sumpio, Cordova, Berke-Schlessel, Qin, & Chen, 2006)
• Anthocyanins, catechins,cyanidins, and flavonols,myricetin and quercetin	Grapes and red wines

which pass relatively unchanged through our abdominal track and intestines. The main role of fiber is to keep the digestive system healthy (Fibre in Food, 2017; Health Information, 2017) Dietary fibers include polysaccharides, oligosaccharides, lignin, and associated plant elements. Dietary fibers induce and promote beneficial

Table 10. Nutraceuticals with anti-inflammatory action

Anti-Inflammatory Action	
Bioactive Compounds	**Nutraceuticals**
• Vitamin E	Nuts, seeds, and oils(Singh, Devaraj, & Jialal, 2005; Kushi, Folsom, Prineas, Mink, Wu, & Bostick, 1996)
• Fish	Omega-3 fatty acids (Ueeda, Doumei, Takaya, Shinohata, Katayama, Ohnishi, … Kusachi, 2008)
• Polyphenols, Anthocyanins, catechins,	Legumes (Lutsey, Jacobs, Kori, Mayer-Davis, Shea, Steffen, … Tracy, 2007)
• cyanidins and flavonols, • myricetin and quercetin	Grapes and red wines (Yussif, Abdul Aziz, & Abdel Rahman, 2016)

Table 8. Nutraceuticals lowering blood homocysteine

Lowering Blood Homocysteine	
Bioactive Compounds	**Nutraceuticals**
• Folate Phytochemicals	Fruits and vegetables (Savica, Bellinghieri, & Kopple, 2010)
• Fiber and phytochemicals	Whole grains (Jenkins, Kendall, Marchie, Faulkner, Wong, de Souza, … Connelly, 2005)
• Vitamin C	Citrus fruits and vegetables (Broekmans, Klöpping-Ketelaars, Schuurman, Verhagen, van den Berg, Kok, & van Poppel, 2000)
• Vitamin E	Nuts, seeds and oils (Eidelman, Hollar, Hebert, Lamas, & Hennekens, 2004)

Table 11. Nutraceuticals improving endothelial function

Endothelial Function	
Bioactive Compounds	**Nutraceuticals**
• Polyphenols	Nuts (Ros, Núñez, Pérez-Heras, Serra, Gilabert, Casals, & Deulofeu, 2004)
• Fish	Omega-3 fatty acids (Ueeda, Doumei, Takaya, Shinohata, Katayama, Ohnishi, … Kusachi, 2008)
• Vitamin C	Citrus fruits and vegetables (Broekmans, Klöpping-Ketelaars, Schuurman, Verhagen, van den Berg, Kok, & van Poppel, 2000)
• cyanidins, flavonols, myricetin and quercetin	Grapes and red wines (Yussif, Abdul Aziz, & Abdel Rahman, 2016)
• Flavonoid	Dark chocolate (Grassi, Lippi, Necozione, Desideri, & Ferri, 2005)
• Hyperoside	Hawthorn (Koçyildiz, Birman, Olgaç, Akgün-Dar, Melikoğlu, & Meriçli, 2006)
• Anthocyanins, catechins, cyanidins, flavonols, myricetin and quercetin	Grapes and red wines(Sumpio, Cordova, Berke-Schlessel, Qin, & Chen, 2006)

physiological effects including laxation, attenuation of blood cholesterol levels, and/or reduction in blood glucose levels (Fibre in Food, 2017; Health Information, 2017; Hipsley, 1953).

Dietary fiber has been defined on the basis of the properties it reveals that have been characterized as part of the comprehensive worldwide research effort of the past 30 plus years (Dietary Reference Intakes, 2011). This research exertion has correlated the constructive health effects of dietary fiber with its augmented consumption. This definition makes reference to the plant constituents accepted as being contemporary in the defined dietary fiber that imparted the constructive health effects (Dietary Reference Intakes, 2011). Analogous fibers, in addition to the vital digestion and fermentation properties, must also reveal a positive budding health benefit that has been certified to dietary fiber. This inclusion undoubtedly acknowledges that certain food ingredients, whether they are plant extracts, distillates, reformed carbohydrates, or compounds produced by design, exist, and should be recognized as dietary fiber when considering their nutritional properties and labeling necessities when part of a food. The definition, as written, clearly delineates the meaning of dietary fiber and analogous fiber, and defines the chief and appropriate functional properties of all dietary fibers. Fibers are also known as 'bulk' and 'roughage'(Fiber in Food, 2017; Health Information, 2017). Current and future nondigestible carbohydrates in the food resources that are considered to be meaningful subdivisions of the potential substances. So, total fiber is nothing but Dietary Fiber (nondigestible carbohydrates and lignin that are intrinsic and intact in plants) and Added Fiber (isolated, nondigestible carbohydrates that have beneficial physiological effects in humans) (Dhingra, Michael, Rajput, & Patil, 2012; Hipsley, 1953; Fiber in Food, 2017).

MAIN TYPES OF FIBER

There are two types of fiber which categorized on the basis of its solubility:

- **Soluble Fiber**: Contains pectins, gums and mucilage, which are found mainly in plant cells. One of its key roles is to reduce LDL (bad) cholesterol levels. Noble sources of soluble fiber include fruits, vegetables, oat bran, barley, seed pods, flaxseed, psyllium, dehydrated beans, lentils, peas, soy milk and soy foodstuffs. Soluble fiber can also help to relieve constipation (Fibre in Food, 2017; Health Information, 2017; Dhingra, Michael, Rajput, & Patil, 2012).
- **Insoluble Fiber**: Contains cellulose, hemicelluloses, and lignin, which make up the structural parts of plant cell walls. A major role of insoluble fiber is

to add bulk to feces and to prevent constipation and related problems such as hemorrhoids. Good sources include bran (wheat, corn, rice), the skins of fruits and vegetables, nuts, seeds, dried beans and whole grain foods. (Fiber in Food, 2017; Health Information, 2017; Dhingra, Michael, Rajput, & Patil, 2012).

INTAKE OF DIETARY FIBER

The Heart Foundation recommends that adults should aim to ingest around 25–30 g daily. Youngsters aged between 4 and 8 years ought to consume 18 g of fiber day after day. Women aged 9 to 13, and 14 to 18 years, should consume 20 g and 22 g per day respectively. Boys aged 9 to 13, and 14 to 18 years, should consume 24 g and 28 g per day respectively. Women would like 25 grams of fiber per day, and men should consume 38 grams per day, according to the Institute of medicine (Fibre in Food, 2017; Health Information, 2017).

APPLICATION OF DIETARY FIBERS

Dietary fibers are categorized as high nutritional quality food, as they are able to cure many chronic as well as acute diseases and improve quality, physical characteristics, and shelf life of foods. Soluble Fibre is responsible for binding cholesterol and Insoluble Fibre increases faecal bulk and frequency. Fibre has also been implicated in a number of disease states, and increasing dietary fibre seeks to prevent some of these conditions: Diverticular Disease, Hypercholesterolemia, leading to heart disease and stroke, Cancer of the colon, Diabetes, Irritable Bowel Syndrome, Constipation, Haemorrhoids and Varicose Veins. (Fiber in Food, 2017; Health Information, 2017).

Target group i.e. fibers and its antihypertensive functionality plays important role in cardiovascular disease and/ or risk minimization. Several cross-sectional and prospective studies have investigated the relationship of fibre intake with hypertension. The outcomes of these studies are by and large consistent with a proposed blood pressure-lowering effect of dietary fibre (He, Streiffer, Muntner, Krousel-Wood, & Whelton, 2004). There has been significant variability in blood pressure response which changes as per changes in dietary fiber. Factors such age, sex, daily intake, source, purity of fiber and type of fibre as per its solubility parameter is an important consideration with respect to its physical and chemical or pathophysiological activities leads to disease attenuation or for treatment. (He, Streiffer, Muntner, Krousel-Wood, & Whelton, 2004; Whelton, Hyre, Pedersen, Yi, Whelton, & He, 2005 ;Dietary Fiber and Blood Pressure, 2004).

Its cholesterol lowering capacity plays active role in blood pressure management therapy as fibers are parts of the plant but they do not break down in the intestine by human digestive enzymes. Because it is not digested, fiber is not absorbed in the body i.e. bacteria in the intestines are able to ferment certain soluble fibers, changing their molecular structure to short-chain fatty acids that are absorbed. In general, however, the fiber itself is neither digested nor absorbed. This property has been exploited for disease control. Soluble fiber generally dissolves in the liquid environment of stomach and is found in foods like legumes, barley, oat bran and chia seeds. Insoluble fiber is found in foods like wheat, corn, oat bran, fruit peel, nuts and flaxseed. They do not dissolve in liquid environment of stomach and instead provides 'bulk' and can ease defecation.

Blood pressure-lowering effects of fibers have been attributed to a variety of factors with varying degrees of conclusiveness. These factors include increased nitric oxide release and improved endothelial function by inhibiting sodium absorption, so this mechanism works to control cardiovascular risk factors and minimize hypertension (Aljuraiban, Griep, Chan, Daviglus, Stamler, Horn,... Frost, 2015; Dietary Fiber and Blood Pressure, 2004). For a better health with the help of change in lifestyle i.e. yoga, change in habits, exercise, different dietary supplement and dedicated designed dietary patterns to control/treat acute/chronic diseases is a major working area in this era of health-conscious society. Especially, to control hypertension by using dietary fibers there are dietary pattern which works on the principle category of food, its intake frequency, actives of diet and its role in body system. On the basis of fiber actives, dietary patterns categories are Mediterranean Diet, Vegetarian Diet, Portfolio Diet and Okinawan Diet. As per body need, compliance and disease state diet control and food pattern applies to individual. Here, we are remarking details of dietary food and different dietary pattern for hypertension. (Beilin & Burke, 1995).

DIETARY PATTERNS AND REDUCED RISK OF HYPERTENSION

He J et. al., 2004 elaborates the results of a controlled trial designed to establish the efficacy of dietary fibres in hypertension. Nutritional as well as lifestyle factors are now responsible for major aspects of blood pressure. The dietary patterns and its practical approaches have a numbers of major strengths. Patterns generally gives overall idea of diet and its constituent foods, frequency of administration and nutrients in relationship to overcome health problem and to treat disease condition and/ or to control the health problems. (Adrienne Forman, 2015; Dietary Guidelines Advisory Committee, ODPHP USA gov., 2015) As per literature survey we found there are major four types of dietary patterns as follow,

Table 12. Applications of dietary fibers in hypertension

AREA	FIBERS ROLE	BENEFITES	REFERENCE
• Heart-Health Perks • Lowers cholesterol • Protects against strokes • Lowers blood pressure	-- • Helps in metabolism of cholesterol by inhibiting bile re-absorption • Antioxidant and vitamins which helps in oxidation of LDL and leads to help in prevention of stroke and death • DASH approach- especially Dietary protein and soluble fiber to control and presentation of blood pressure	-- • Reduces LDL, lower blood cholesterol • Reduces LDL level • Lowers BP & improves endothelial function	-- ("Foods That Lower Cholesterol," 2007) (Das, Bhaumik, Raychaudhuri, & Chakraborty, 2012) Foroughi et al., (2013) Al-Solaiman et al., (2010)
• Diabetes Management	• Glycemic cycle control and glucose level management	• Lower blood glucose level	Das et al., (2012)
• Kidney Disease	• Reduces oxidative stress in renal toxicity and treatment for renal failure • Reduced inflammation and related kidney problem	• Biological effects in the kidney are still not clear totally (scope for research)	("Foods That Lower Cholesterol," 2007) Aksoy et al., (2012)
• Obesity	• Reduce triglyceride, fatty acid levels and shows lipid lowering mechanism	• Cholesterol-lowering • Oxidation of body fat	(Badimon, Vilahur, & Padro, 2010)

MEDITERRANEAN DIET

Most of the burden of CVD is believed to be preventable through healthy lifestyles including a salutary dietary pattern· (Stampfer, Hu, Manson, Rimm, & Willett, 2000)· The current paradigm in nutritional epidemiology is used to analyze dietary patter instead of other traditional analytical approaches. A 2011 systematic review found that a Mediterranean diet appeared to be more effective than a low-fat diet in bringing about long-term changes to cardiovascular risk factors, such as lowering cholesterol level and blood pressure (Martínez-González, Corella, Salas-Salvadó, Ros, Covas, & Fiol, 2012). A meta-analysis in 2013 compared Mediterranean, vegan, vegetarian, low-glycemic index, low-carbohydrate, high-fiber, and high-protein diets with control diets. The research concluded that Mediterranean, low-carbohydrate, low-glycemic index, and high-protein diets are effective in improving markers of risk for cardiovascular disease and diabetes, while there was limited evidence for an effect of vegetarian diets on glycemic control and lipid levels unrelated to weight loss (Ajala, English, & Pinkney, 2013). The Mediterranean diet often is cited as beneficial for being low in saturated fat and high in monounsaturated fat and dietary fiber. One of the main explanations for health effects observed in the Mediterranean diet, is thought to be the inclusion of Olive oil. Olive oil contains monounsaturated fats, most notably oleic acid, which is under clinical research for its potential health benefits (Buckland & Gonzalez, 2015). The European Food Safety Authority Panel on Dietetic Products, Nutrition and Allergies approved health claims on olive oil, for protection by its polyphenols against oxidation of blood lipids (Buckland & Gonzalez, 2015) and for the contribution to the maintenance of normal blood LDL-cholesterol levels by replacing saturated fats in the diet with oleic acid (EFSA Panel on Dietetic Products, 2011). A study in 2014 concluded that increased consumption of olive oil is associated with reduced risk of many ailments including all-cause mortality, cardiovascular events and stroke, while monounsaturated fatty acids of mixed animal and plant origin showed no significant effects (EFSA Panel on Dietetic Products, Nutrition and Allergies (NDA), 2011). However, Consistent evidence suggests that the promotion of the Mediterranean dietary pattern can be an effective and feasible tool for the prevention of CVD.

VEGETARIAN DIET

There is enough evidence that demonstrates the health benefits of vegetarian and plant-based diets, which have been associated with a reduced risk of heart disease, obesity, diabetes and some types of cancer as well as increased longevity. Vegetarian diets are typically lower in fat, particularly saturated fat, and higher in dietary fibers. They are also likely to include more whole grains, legumes, nuts, and soy protein, and together with the absence of red meat, this type of eating plan may provide many benefits for the prevention and treatment of chronic health problems, including cardiovascular disease. The most consistent evidence for the health benefits of a vegetarian diet relates to a reduced risk of coronary heart disease (CHD) and coronary disease mortality. Several studies have demonstrated a lower incidence of CHD) (Appleby, Thorogood, Mann, & Key, 1999), and a combined analysis of 5 prospective studies reported a 24% lower risk of mortality from ischemic heart disease (IHD) in vegetarians compared with meat eaters, with lactoovo vegetarians having a 34% reduced risk and vegans a 26% reduced risk (Burr & Butland, 1988). The benefit was apparent in those who had followed their diet for at least 5 years and was greater in younger age groups. These findings are perhaps not surprising considering that vegetarians generally have a better cardiovascular risk profile than nonvegetarians, with lower total and low-density lipoprotein (LDL) cholesterol levels, a lower body weight (Chang-Claude, Hermann, Eilber, & Steindorf, 2005) and a lower incidence of diabetes and hypertension, all of which contribute to CVD risk. Some research has also suggested that a vegetarian diet may reduce the susceptibility of LDL to oxidation (Fraser, 1999). Nuts may protect against CHD through effects on lipids, lipid oxidation, inflammation, and vascular reactivity (De Biase, Fernandes, Gianini, & Duarte, 2007). Soy protein has been shown to reduce total and LDL cholesterol levels, and a recent meta-analysis of 30 studies demonstrated a small but significant reduction in both total and LDL cholesterol with the consumption of 25 g of soy protein per day (Chen, Lin, Lin, Lin, Chen, & Lin, 2008).

Since 1999, the US FDA has approved a health claim that foods high in soy protein may help lower heart disease risk (Rosell, Appleby, Spencer, & Key, 2006). Although individual components of a vegetarian diet may provide benefits for CVD risk, a combination of these foods is likely to provide the greatest effect. For example, a diet which includes items such as soluble fiber, soy protein, almonds, and plant sterols has been shown to reduce LDL cholesterol by a similar amount as 20 g of lovastatin does, over a 4-week administration period. Although some studies have linked red meat intake with CHD risk, a recent meta-analysis found that processed meat intake, rather than red meat intake, was associated with a higher risk of CHD (Spencer, Appleby, Davey, & Key, 2003). However, Improved health is one of the many reasons people choose to adopt a vegetarian diet, and there is now a wealth of evidence to support the health benefits of a vegetarian diet.

PORTFOLIO DIET

The portfolio diet is a new approach to lowering cholesterol that builds on a conventional cardio protective diet by including specific foods that are known to target abnormal lipids. Food for Thought and salt, and high in fibre and fruit and vegetables. The difference is that, once established on this cardio protective diet, the patient adds a combination of more specific foods including soya protein, almonds, stanols/sterols and plant fibers (*Lipid Modification*, n.d.). Clinical trials suggest that the portfolio diet can lower cholesterol by about 25%. There is also evidence that the diet can improve the entire lipid profile, reducing LDL-C by 28-35%, and improving both HDL-C and triglyceride levels. In a study comparing the diet with lovastatin 20 mg, the portfolio diet reduced LDL-C by 29.1% compared with 34.5% for the statin. Although LDLC was lower in patients taking the statin, this study confirms the effectiveness of the portfolio diet, and that it can achieve target treatment goals when used in primary prevention of uncomplicated patients with mild-moderate hypercholesterolemia. The different modes of action of the components of the portfolio diet are thought to contribute to the significant results seen in clinical trials. Almonds are rich in monounsaturated fatty acids that lower LDL-C, and also contain other nutrients involved in the regulation of cholesterol synthesis. Fibre reduces the concentration of bile acids, causing the liver to compensate by increasing the conversion of cholesterol to bile acids, which in turn reduces blood cholesterol (Jenkins, Kendall, Marchie, Faulkner, Wong, de Souza,... Connelly, 2005) (Resources From Heart - The Cholesterol Charity Expert Advice From Heart, UK). The portfolio diet may offer an alternative for these patients, and can also act in combination with a statin to reduce the amount of medication patients need to take. The idea that combinations of foods are more effective than a single dietary intervention reflects the current approach to medical treatment, which combines several drugs to reduce overall cardiovascular risk.

OKINAWAN DIET

Recently, the Okinawa diet plan, off late, has been the area of focus for discussion among nutrition scientists, and health-conscious individuals alike. These foods contain properties that are proving to be important to heart health such as the antioxidant vitamins A, C, and E, anthocyanin's and other polyphenols, carotenoids, flavonoids, and more. A recent analysis of the antioxidant activity of vegetables from Okinawa prefecture found high contents of phenolic compounds and strong radical scavenging activities in many traditional Okinawan vegetables (Maeda, Takara, Wada, Oki, Masuda, Ichiba,... Suda, 2006). Carotenoids are found mostly in the brightly colored yellow, orange, and green vegetables that are plentiful in Okinawa.

The beta-carotene in carrots and orange sweet potatoes and the lycopene in tomatoes, watermelon, and possibly Okinawan sweet potatoes are the best known of the more than 600 carotenoids. Flavonoids are antioxidant and hormone-like plant compounds that exist in more than 4000 varieties. They are found in soy foods, onions, broccoli, and red wine, and in green, black, and oolong teas, among other foods. Healthy omega-3 fat, found in fish and soy oil, is also an important part of the Okinawan diet, and like the other components mentioned, has been shown in well-conducted studies to play an important role in cardiovascular health. Results so far have been impressive and have revealed that increasing consumption of such types of vegetables, commonly consumed in the traditional dietary pattern, can increase potassium excretion (Walford, Mock, Verdery, & MacCallum, 2002) in normotensive healthy young women as well as raise levels of circulating endothelial progenitor cells (Tuekpe, Todoriki, Sasaki, Zheng, & Ariizumi, 2006). Changes in the endothelial progenitor cells level in these young women also inversely correlated with changes in both serum total cholesterol and LDL cholesterol level. Serum folic acid increases and plasma homocysteine decreases were also observed (Mano, Ishida, Ohya, Todoriki, & Takishita, 2009).

DELIVERY SYSTEM FOR CONVENTIONAL AS WELL AS MODIFIED NUTRACEUTICALS AND DIETARY FIBER

Need of Delivery Systems for Conventional Nutraceuticals and Dietary Fiber

Broad-scale research in last few years has revealed that most acute as well as chronic diseases, including cardiovascular diseases, pulmonary diseases, cancer, diabetes, are mediated through short/ long term tenderness (Nair, Sung, Yadav, Kannappan, Chaturvedi, & Aggarwal, 2010). For suppressing this acute/ chronic inflammation, prevention and its treatment to stop its recurrence; there is need of the novel delivery system which can significantly improve disease state in terms of patient compliance, safety and efficacy. General mechanism of novel drug delivery system is to give new life to existing drug molecule. Here, numbers of nutraceuticals and functional food obtained from pods, vegetables, vitamins, spices, legumes, traditional Chinese and Ayurveda have been shown to safely suppress proinflammatory pathways; however, their low bioavailability and in vivo limits their use in curing, preventing and treating acute or chronic diseases. The potential platform of nanotechnology to overcome all these limitations is a good modified novel approach and excellent delivery system. There as many nutraceuticals and foods which have been packaged as nanoparticles and confirmed to be useful in many disease states (Nair, Sung, Yadav, Kannappan, Chaturvedi, & Aggarwal, 2010).

Applications of Delivery Systems for Functional Foods and Dietary Fiber

Application of functional foods and dietary fiber provide health benefits, especially for the prevention and treatment of acute as well as chronic diseases like diabetes, obesity, cardiovascular disease, and cancer.

Enhancing bioavailability is a key step in ensuring bio- efficacy of bioactive food compounds. Therefore, several technologies and techniques have been investigated and developed to improve the bioavailability of xenobiotics including structural alterations, nanotechnology, and colloidal systems. These novel techniques have been successfully utilized for the treatment of hypertension and cardiac problems (Rein, Renouf, Cruz-Hernandez, Actis-Goretta, Thakkar, & da Silva Pinto, 2013). The dosage forms for the same could be tablets, capsules, sachets, pro and prebiotic powder formulations, lipidic systems, surfactant systems and biopolymer systems.

FUNCTIONAL FOOD AND DRUG INTERACTIONS

Food-drug interaction which generally affects the pharmacokinetic and dynamic effects of the drug because of food entities which alter the activity of drug by changing its metabolism. Food-drug interactions can result in two key clinical effects: either a decreased bioavailability of a drug, which predisposes to treatment failure, or an increased bioavailability, which increases the risk of adverse events and can precipitate toxicities. Food-drug interactions can result in a reduction in absorption of certain oral medicines and may lead to suboptimal drug concentrations at the site of action or infection. This influences the patient to treatment failure. Stimulation or inhibition of enzymes in the gut by nutrients may lead to a significant change in oral bioavailability of drugs or vice versa. For example, grapefruit juice which is a selective intestinal CYP3A4 inhibitor. Average exposure of some drugs can be increased by more than fivefold when taken with grapefruit juice and increase the risk of toxicity (Genser, 2008; Ling, Aziz, Wojnarowicz, Olkowski, & Alcorn, 2010). Pharmacokinetics refers to the quantitative description of drug disposition, which includes absorption, distribution, metabolism, and excretion. Pharmacodynamics refers to the physiologic or clinical effects of a drug (Chan, 2002).

TYPE-I AND TYPE-II FOOD AND DRUG INTERACTIONS

There are two types of functional food and drug interaction (Type I and Type II), Type I interactions because of its biochemical reaction like oxidation, reduction, precipitation and neutralization whereas, Type II is because of biotransformation mechanisms like complexation, binding, and/or other deactivating processes. Both this interaction cause either an increase or decrease of the oral bioavailability (Genser, 2008). Again considering the pre systemic metabolism and different pathways of body biochemistry/ physiology this types may affect the drug effects which leads to increase or decrease the drug bioavailability and its effect on target site. Example like grapefruit juice as above mentioned which causes drowsiness and prolonged sedation after taking the tranquillizers diazepam or midazolam in combination with grapefruit juice, Hypotension can result in people treated with calcium-channel blockers, cardiovascular symptoms in medication of erythromycin and consuming grapefruit together leads to cardiac dysrhythmias and they also altered metabolic function or macronutrient status (Genser, 2008; Chan, 2002; Chan, 2002). Another example of *Ginkgo biloba* Leaf extract, in rat model increased the bioavailability of Diltiazem via a mechanism-based inhibition for CYP3A Reason for all this is pre/post metabolic changes because of food-drug interactions (Ohnishi, Kusuhara, Yoshioka, Kuroda, Soga, Nishikawa, … Yokoyama, 2003).

CHARACTERIZATION OF NUTRACEUTICALS/ DIETARY FIBER

Analytical Methods: Characterization of Nutraceuticals/Dietary Fiber

Different innovative analytical techniques used to characterize nutraceuticals/ dietary fibers enriched in different families (carbohydrates, sterols, lipids, alkaloids, polyphenols, carotenoids etc.) From most of the research paper we noticed that most significant analytical techniques presently used for the characterization of nutraceuticals / dietary fibers, such as High-Performance Liquid Chromatography (HPLC), Gas Chromatography (GC) and Capillary Electrophoresis (CE), discussing the fundamentals of the separation, and the detectors coupled to these separation techniques for the analysis of bioactive composites (Genser, 2008).

Innovative high-performance anion-exchange chromatographic methods coupled with pulsed amperometric detection (HPAEC-PAD), which are specific for carbohydrate analysis or characterization of nutraceuticals/ dietary fibers and their metabolic profile which has been reported in recent trends of nutraceuticals/ dietary fibers characterization (Zierler-Brown, 2007; Corradini, Galanti, & Nicoletti, 2002).

Statistical Methods: for Characterization of the Dietary Pattern

There are so many papers where scientist have reported Index, *cluster* and *factor* are the three statistical tools for the characterization of the dietary pattern and effects of nutraceuticals/dietary fiber.

1. **Index Analysis:** Based on numerical scoring system defined on the basis of a priori knowledge. Indexes generate scores for different sets of dietary components based on the researcher's scoring approach and interpretation of dietary guidance.
2. **Cluster Analysis:** Methodology identifies aggregates of individuals in multidimensional space, where each food variable constitutes an axis (using the squared Euclidian distances between observations to determine cluster position). Each individual is positioned in space on the basis of consumption of numerous foods.
3. **Factor Analysis:** Also known as principal component analysis, examines the correlation matrix of food variables and searches for underlying factors that explain most of the variation in the information. Thus, a large number of food variables are reduced to a smaller set of variables that capture the major dietary factors in the population (Reedy, Wirfält, Flood, Mitrou, Krebs-Smith, Kipnis, … Subar, 2010).

Regulatory Aspects in Formulation of Nutraceuticals and Dietary Fibers

The Nutraceutical is an emerging business and having huge market capacity but still, there are no clear-cut regulations on nutraceuticals. Laws governing to Nutraceutical are country specefic. Even the names of nutraceuticals are different in some countries. Nutraceutical is known as a dietary supplement in the USA, Natural Health Product in Canada, Complementary medicines in Australia, Food Supplements in European, and in India it is known as Foods for Special dietary use. Globalization of nutraceutical industries presents significant challenges with respect to regulatory variance. Many of regulatory hurdles are yet to be overcome.

Dietary Supplement Health Education Act (DSHEA), 1994 act was introduced in the senate by senator Orrin. G. Hatch.

This law provides the information about the definition of the dietary supplement and the legal requirements necessary for the marketing of dietary supplement product in the US which is essential for marketing and sale of CVD nutraceuticals. 21 CFR 190 deals with Dietary supplements; For the registration of dietary supplement in U.S, the ingredients of dietary supplements is separated into two types, (i.e.) Active and Inactive ingredients. The active ingredient found in the product should meet the definition said by DSHEA, 1994.If it meets the definition, then it can be registered as a dietary ingredient.

FDA does not approve the dietary supplement as any other drug product; it is the responsibility of the manufacturer/Distributor to claim the safety of the product by submitting the relevance documents regarding the safety of the Dietary Supplement (Dietary Supplem, 2015; *Council for Responsible Nutrition,* 2003). Safety, efficacy issues world over in different populations need to be addressed. Food safety standard and standards act (FSSA): 2006 statutory body FSSA which regulates the manufacture, storage, distribution, sale and import, to ensure the availability of the food and food products within the country. (Ministry of Health and Family, New Delhi, India, 2006). The USFDA has released the GMP regulations for the Dietary supplements which are applied to all the foreign companies and domestic companies. This GMP regulation specifies the requirements for Manufacture, Package, label or hold of dietary supplements (*Dietary Supplement Regulation in the United States*, n.d.).

Regulatory framework governing nutraceuticals in major jurisdictions is evolving. Functional food interaction with commonly administered active pharmaceutical agents also needs to be studied. Quality standards have to be in built into products and Quality by design approaches utilizing design of experiments concept needs to be integrated.

FUTURE TRENDS AND CONCLUSION

In recent years' alternative medicine such as nutraceuticals, functional food, fibers and its manufacturing this large scale is a new and highly functional area of food as well as pharmaceutical industry. There are many alternative medicinal areas on which scientist are working because of its high commercial value. The market of nutraceuticals is growing very fast as per their high demand because of health-conscious people and change in lifestyle. Nutraceuticals and functional food in forms of tablets, capsules, sachets, powder formulation, lipidic systems (simple, multiple, multilayer, and solid lipid particle emulsions); surfactant systems (simple micelles, mixed micelles, vesicles, and microemulsions) and biopolymer systems (soluble complexes, coacervates, hydrogel droplets, and particles) are already available in market. In addition to these conventional dosage forms, scientists are developing novel varied other delivery system of nutraceuticals.

REFERENCES

Ajala, O., English, P., & Pinkney, J. (2013). Systematic review and meta-analysis of different dietary approaches to the management of type 2 diabetes. *The American Journal of Clinical Nutrition*, *97*(3), 505–516. doi:10.3945/ajcn.112.042457 PMID:23364002

Aksoy, N., Dogan, Y., Iriadam, M., Bitiren, M., Uzer, E., Ozgonul, A., & Aksoy, S. (2012). Protective and therapeutic effects of licorice in rats with acute tubular necrosis. *Journal of Renal Nutrition: The Official Journal of the Council on Renal Nutrition of the National Kidney Foundation*, *22*(3), 336–343. doi:10.1053/j.jrn.2011.07.002 PMID:22047711

Al-Solaiman, Y., Jesri, A., Mountford, W. K., Lackland, D. T., Zhao, Y., & Egan, B. M. (2010). DASH Lowers Blood Pressure in Obese Hypertensives Beyond Potassium, Magnesium and Fiber. *Journal of Human Hypertension*, *24*(4), 237–246. doi:10.1038/jhh.2009.58 PMID:19626043

Albert, C. M., Gaziano, J. M., Willett, W. C., & Manson, J. E. (2002). Nut Consumption and Decreased Risk of Sudden Cardiac Death in the Physicians' Health Study. *Archives of Internal Medicine*, *162*(12), 1382–1387. doi:10.1001/archinte.162.12.1382 PMID:12076237

Alberti, K. G. M. M., Eckel, R. H., Grundy, S. M., Zimmet, P. Z., Cleeman, J. I., & Donato, K. A. (2009). Harmonizing the metabolic syndrome: a joint interim statement of the International Diabetes Federation Task Force on Epidemiology and Prevention; National Heart, Lung, and Blood Institute; American Heart Association; World Heart Federation; International Atherosclerosis Society; and International Association for the Study of Obesity. *Circulation, 120*(16), 1640–1645. .19264410.1161/CIRCULATIONAHA.109

Aljuraiban, G. S., Griep, L. M. O., Chan, Q., Daviglus, M. L., Stamler, J., Horn, L. V., ... Frost, G. S. (2015). Total, insoluble and soluble dietary fibre intake in relation to blood pressure: The INTERMAP Study - CORRIGENDUM. *British Journal of Nutrition, 114*(9), 1534–1534. doi:10.1017/S0007114515003876 PMID:26388506

Amer, M. S., Elawam, A. E., Khater, M. S., Omar, O. H., Mabrouk, R. A., & Taha, H. M. (2011). Association of high-sensitivity C-reactive protein with carotid artery intima-media thickness in hypertensive older adults. *Journal of the American Society of Hypertension: JASH*, *5*(5), 395–400. doi:10.1016/j.jash.2011.03.004 PMID:21524639

Anderson, K. M., Wilson, P. W., Odell, P. M., & Kannel, W. B. (1991). An updated coronary risk profile. A statement for health professionals. *Circulation*, *83*(1), 356–362. doi:10.1161/01.CIR.83.1.356 PMID:1984895

Appleby, P. N., Thorogood, M., Mann, J. I., & Key, T. J. (1999). The Oxford Vegetarian Study: An overview. *The American Journal of Clinical Nutrition*, *70*(3Suppl), 525S–531S. doi:10.1093/ajcn/70.3.525s PMID:10479226

Baba, S., Natsume, M., Yasuda, A., Nakamura, Y., Tamura, T., Osakabe, N., ... Kondo, K. (2007). Plasma LDL and HDL cholesterol and oxidized LDL concentrations are altered in normo- and hypercholesterolemic humans after intake of different levels of cocoa powder. *The Journal of Nutrition*, *137*(6), 1436–1441. doi:10.1093/jn/137.6.1436 PMID:17513403

Badimon, L., Vilahur, G., & Padro, T. (2010). Nutraceuticals and atherosclerosis: Human trials. *Cardiovascular Therapeutics*, *28*(4), 202–215. doi:10.1111/j.1755-5922.2010.00189.x PMID:20633023

Beilin, L. J., & Burke, V. (1995). Vegetarian diet components, protein and blood pressure: Which nutrients are important? *Clinical and Experimental Pharmacology & Physiology*, *22*(3), 195–198. doi:10.1111/j.1440-1681.1995.tb01979.x PMID:7554413

Berdanier, C. D. (1994). Nutrient-gene interactions: Today and tomorrow. *The FASEB Journal*, *8*(1), 1. doi:10.1096/fasebj.8.1.8299881 PMID:8299881

Bernstein, A. M., Sun, Q., Hu, F. B., Stampfer, M. J., Manson, J. E., & Willett, W. C. (2010). Major dietary protein sources and risk of coronary heart disease in women. *Circulation*, *122*(9), 876–883. doi:10.1161/CIRCULATIONAHA.109.915165 PMID:20713902

Bertomeu, V., & Castillo-Castillo, J. (2008). Situación de la enfermedad cardiovascular en España. Del riesgo a la enfermedad. *Revista Espanola de Cardiologia*, *8*(Supl.E), 2–9.

Bhagwat, R. R. (2015). Novel drug delivery systems: an overview. *International Journal of Pharmaceutical Sciences and Research*. Retrieved April 12, 2017, from http://ijpsr.com/bft-article/novel-drug-delivery-systems-an-overview/?view=fulltext

Block, G., Mangels, A. R., Norkus, E. P., Patterson, B. H., Levander, O. A., & Taylor, P. R. (2001). Ascorbic acid status and subsequent diastolic and systolic blood pressure. *Hypertension (Dallas, Tex.: 1979)*, *37*(2), 261–267.

Broadhurst, C. L. (1997). Balanced intakes of natural triglycerides for optimum nutrition: An evolutionary and phytochemical perspective. *Medical Hypotheses*, *49*(3), 247–261. doi:10.1016/S0306-9877(97)90210-3 PMID:9293470

Broekmans, W. M., Klöpping-Ketelaars, I. A., Schuurman, C. R., Verhagen, H., van den Berg, H., Kok, F. J., & van Poppel, G. (2000). Fruits and vegetables increase plasma carotenoids and vitamins and decrease homocysteine in humans. *The Journal of Nutrition*, *130*(6), 1578–1583. doi:10.1093/jn/130.6.1578 PMID:10827213

Buckland, G., & Gonzalez, C. A. (2015). The role of olive oil in disease prevention: A focus on the recent epidemiological evidence from cohort studies and dietary intervention trials. *British Journal of Nutrition*, *113*(S2Suppl 2), S94–S101. doi:10.1017/S0007114514003936 PMID:26148926

Burr, M. L., & Butland, B. K. (1988). Heart disease in British vegetarians. *The American Journal of Clinical Nutrition*, *48*(3Suppl), 830–832. doi:10.1093/ajcn/48.3.830 PMID:3414590

Chan, L.-N. (2002). Drug-nutrient interaction in clinical nutrition. *Current Opinion in Clinical Nutrition and Metabolic Care*, *5*(3), 327–332. doi:10.1097/00075197-200205000-00014 PMID:11953660

Chang-Claude, J., Hermann, S., Eilber, U., & Steindorf, K. (2005). Lifestyle determinants and mortality in German vegetarians and health-conscious persons: Results of a 21-year follow-up. *Cancer Epidemiology, Biomarkers & Prevention, 14*(4), 963–968. doi:10.1158/1055-9965.EPI-04-0696 PMID:15824171

Chen, C.-W., Lin, Y.-L., Lin, T.-K., Lin, C.-T., Chen, B.-C., & Lin, C.-L. (2008). Total cardiovascular risk profile of Taiwanese vegetarians. *European Journal of Clinical Nutrition, 62*(1), 138–144. doi:10.1038j.ejcn.1602689 PMID:17356561

Chen, G., Wang, H., Zhang, X., & Yang, S.-T. (2014). Nutraceuticals and functional foods in the management of hyperlipidemia. *Critical Reviews in Food Science and Nutrition, 54*(9), 1180–1201. doi:10.1080/10408398.2011.629354 PMID:24499150

Chobanian, A. V., Bakris, G. L., Black, H. R., Cushman, W. C., Green, L. A., & Izzo, J. L. (2003). Seventh report of the Joint National Committee on Prevention, Detection, Evaluation, and Treatment of High Blood Pressure. *Hypertension (Dallas, Tex.: 1979), 42*(6), 1206–1252. 10.1161/01.HYP.0000107251.49515.c2

Chopra, M., O'Neill, M. E., Keogh, N., Wortley, G., Southon, S., & Thurnham, D. I. (2000). Influence of increased fruit and vegetable intake on plasma and lipoprotein carotenoids and LDL oxidation in smokers and nonsmokers. *Clinical Chemistry, 46*(11), 1818–1829. PMID:11067818

Cinq-Mars, C. D., Hu, C., Kitts, D. D., & Li-Chan, E. C. Y. (2008). Investigations into inhibitor type and mode, simulated gastrointestinal digestion, and cell transport of the angiotensin I-converting enzyme-inhibitory peptides in Pacific hake (Merluccius productus) fillet hydrolysate. *Journal of Agricultural and Food Chemistry, 56*(2), 410–419. doi:10.1021/jf072277p PMID:18163568

Corradini, C., Galanti, R., & Nicoletti, I. (2002). Characterization of nutraceuticals and functional foods by innovative HPLC methods. *Annali di Chimica, 92*(4), 387–396. PMID:12073884

Council for Responsible Nutrition. (2003). Retrieved April 15, 2017, from http://www.crnusa.org/

Dandona, P., Ghanim, H., Chaudhuri, A., Dhindsa, S., & Kim, S. S. (2010). Macronutrient intake induces oxidative and inflammatory stress: Potential relevance to atherosclerosis and insulin resistance. *Experimental & Molecular Medicine, 42*(4), 245–253. doi:10.3858/emm.2010.42.4.033 PMID:20200475

Darmadi-Blackberry, I., Wahlqvist, M. L., Kouris-Blazos, A., Steen, B., Lukito, W., Horie, Y., & Horie, K. (2004). Legumes: The most important dietary predictor of survival in older people of different ethnicities. *Asia Pacific Journal of Clinical Nutrition*, *13*(2), 217–220. PMID:15228991

Das, L., Bhaumik, E., Raychaudhuri, U., & Chakraborty, R. (2012). Role of nutraceuticals in human health. *Journal of Food Science and Technology*, *49*(2), 173–183. doi:10.100713197-011-0269-4 PMID:23572839

De Biase, S. G., Fernandes, S. F. C., Gianini, R. J., & Duarte, J. L. G. (2007). Vegetarian diet and cholesterol and triglycerides levels. *Arquivos Brasileiros de Cardiologia*, *88*(1), 35–39. doi:10.1590/S0066-782X2007000100006 PMID:17364116

Dhingra, D., Michael, M., Rajput, H., & Patil, R. T. (2012). Dietary fibre in foods: A review. *Journal of Food Science and Technology*, *49*(3), 255–266. doi:10.100713197-011-0365-5 PMID:23729846

Dietary fibre and blood pressure. (2004). Dietary fibre and blood pressure. *Journal of Hypertension*. Retrieved April 13, 2017, from http://journals.lww.com/jhypertension/Fulltext/2004/01000/Dietaryfibreandbloodpressure.5.aspx

Dietary Reference Intakes. (2011). *Dietary Reference Intakes: Proposed Definition of Dietary Fiber*. The National Academies Press. Retrieved April 13, 2017, from https://www.nap.edu/ catalog/10161/dietary-reference-intakes-proposed-definition-of-dietary-fiber

Dietary Supplem, C. for F. S. and A. (2015). U S Food and Drug Administration. Retrieved from https://www.fda.gov/Food/DietarySupplements/

Dietary Supplement Regulation in the United States. (n.d.). Retrieved from http://www.springer.com/in/book/9783319015019

Dillard, C. J., & German, J. B. (2000). Phytochemicals: Nutraceuticals and human health. *Journal of the Science of Food and Agriculture*, *80*(12), 1744–1756. doi:10.1002/1097-0010(20000915)80:12<1744::AID-JSFA7253.0.CO;2-W

Dyerberg, J., Eskesen, D. C., Andersen, P. W., Astrup, A., Buemann, B., Christensen, J. H., ... Stender, S. (2004). Effects of trans- and n-3 unsaturated fatty acids on cardiovascular risk markers in healthy males. An 8 weeks' dietary intervention study. *European Journal of Clinical Nutrition*, *58*(7), 1062–1070. doi:10.1038j.ejcn.1601934 PMID:15220949

Eaton, S. B., Eaton, S. B., & Konner, M. J. (1997). Paleolithic nutrition revisited: A twelve-year retrospective on its nature and implications. *European Journal of Clinical Nutrition*, *51*(4), 207–216. doi:10.1038j.ejcn.1600389 PMID:9104571

EFSA Panel on Dietetic Products, N. and A. (NDA). (2011). Scientific Opinion on the substantiation of health claims related to polyphenols in olive and protection of LDL particles from oxidative damage (ID 1333, 1638, 1639, 1696, 2865), maintenance of normal blood HDL cholesterol concentrations (ID 1639), maintenance of normal blood pressure (ID 3781), "anti-inflammatory properties" (ID 1882), "contributes to the upper respiratory tract health" (ID 3468), "can help to maintain a normal function of gastrointestinal tract" (3779), and "contributes to body defences against external agents" (ID 3467) pursuant to Article 13(1) of Regulation (EC) No 1924/2006. *EFSA Journal*, *9*(4). 10.2903/j.efsa.2011.2033

EFSA Panel on Dietetic Products. (2011). Scientific Opinion on the substantiation of health claims related to oleic acid intended to replace saturated fatty acids (SFAs) in foods or diets and maintenance of normal blood LDL-cholesterol concentrations (ID 673, 728, 729, 1302, 4334) and maintenanc: Health claims related to oleic acid intended to replace saturated fatty acids (SFAs) in foods or diets. *EFSA Journal*, *9*(4), 2043. doi:10.2903/j.efsa.2011.2043

Eftekhari, A., Mathiassen, O. N., Buus, N. H., Gotzsche, O., Mulvany, M. J., & Christensen, K. L. (2011). Disproportionally impaired microvascular structure in essential hypertension. *Journal of Hypertension*, *29*(5), 896–905. doi:10.1097/HJH.0b013e3283447a1c PMID:21330935

Eidelman, R. S., Hollar, D., Hebert, P. R., Lamas, G. A., & Hennekens, C. H. (2004). Randomized trials of vitamin E in the treatment and prevention of cardiovascular disease. *Archives of Internal Medicine*, *164*(14), 1552–1556. doi:10.1001/archinte.164.14.1552 PMID:15277288

Engelhard, Y. N., Gazer, B., & Paran, E. (2006). Natural antioxidants from tomato extract reduce blood pressure in patients with grade-1 hypertension: A double-blind, placebo-controlled pilot study. *American Heart Journal*, *151*(1), 100. doi:10.1016/j.ahj.2005.05.008 PMID:16368299

Erkkilä, A. T., & Lichtenstein, A. H. (2006). Fiber and cardiovascular disease risk: How strong is the evidence? *The Journal of Cardiovascular Nursing*, *21*(1), 3–8. doi:10.1097/00005082-200601000-00003 PMID:16407729

European Cardiovascular Disease Statistics 2017 - EHN - European Heart Network. (n.d.). Retrieved April 13, 2017, from http://www.ehnheart.org/cvd-statistics.html

European Society of Hypertension-European Society of Cardiology guidelines for the management of arterial hypertension. (2003). Retrieved April 13, 2017, from https://www.ncbi.nlm.nih.gov/pubmed/12777938

Expert Panel on Detection, Evaluation, and Treatment of High Blood Cholesterol in Adults. (2001). Executive Summary of the Third Report of The National Cholesterol Education Program (NCEP) Expert Panel on Detection, Evaluation, And Treatment of High Blood Cholesterol In Adults (Adult Treatment Panel III). *Journal of the American Medical Association*, *285*(19), 2486–2497. doi:10.1001/jama.285.19.2486 PMID:11368702

Fa, G., & A, M. (2007). Inflammation in high blood pressure: a clinician perspective. *Journal of the American Society of Hypertension: JASH*, *1*(2), 113–119. 10.1016/j.jash.2007.01.004

Fibre in food, D. of H. & H. (2017). *Fibre in food*. Retrieved April 13, 2017, from https://www.betterhealth.vic.gov.au:443/health/healthyliving/fibre-in-food

Foods That Lower Cholesterol. (2007, April 17). Retrieved April 13, 2017, http://health.howstuffworks.com/diseases-conditions/cardiovascular/cholesterol/foods-that-lower-cholesterol.htm

Forman. (2015). *Part D. Ch 2: Dietary Patterns - 2015 Advisory Report - health.gov*. Retrieved April 13, 2017, from https://health.gov/dietaryguidelines/2015-scientific-report/07-chapter-2

Foroughi, M., Akhavanzanjani, M., Maghsoudi, Z., Ghiasvand, R., Khorvash, F., & Askari, G. (2013). Stroke and Nutrition: A Review of Studies. *International Journal of Preventive Medicine*, *4*(Suppl 2), S165–S179. PMID:23776719

Fraser, G. E. (1999). Associations between diet and cancer, ischemic heart disease, and all-cause mortality in non-Hispanic white California Seventh-day Adventists. *The American Journal of Clinical Nutrition*, *70*(3Suppl), 532S–538S. doi:10.1093/ajcn/70.3.532s PMID:10479227

Genser, D. (2008). Food and drug interaction: Consequences for the nutrition/health status. *Annals of Nutrition & Metabolism*, *52*(Suppl 1), 29–32. doi:10.1159/000115345 PMID:18382075

Grassi, D., Lippi, C., Necozione, S., Desideri, G., & Ferri, C. (2005). Short-term administration of dark chocolate is followed by a significant increase in insulin sensitivity and a decrease in blood pressure in healthy persons. *The American Journal of Clinical Nutrition*, *81*(3), 611–614. doi:10.1093/ajcn/81.3.611 PMID:15755830

H, K., Fc, L., & Dn, M. (2009). Role of the immune system in hypertensive target organ damage. *Trends in Cardiovascular Medicine, 19*(7), 242–246. 10.1016/j.tcm.2010.02.004

He, J., Klag, M. J., Whelton, P. K., Chen, J. Y., Qian, M. C., & Het, G. Q. (1995). Dietary macronutrients and blood pressure in southwestern China. *Journal of Hypertension, 13*(11), 1267–1274. doi:10.1097/00004872-199511000-00008 PMID:8984124

He, J., Streiffer, R. H., Muntner, P., Krousel-Wood, M. A., & Whelton, P. K. (2004). Effect of dietary fiber intake on blood pressure: A randomized, double-blind, placebo-controlled trial. *Journal of Hypertension, 22*(1), 73–80. doi:10.1097/00004872-200401000-00015 PMID:15106797

He, K., Merchant, A., Rimm, E. B., Rosner, B. A., Stampfer, M. J., Willett, W. C., & Ascherio, A. (2003). Dietary fat intake and risk of stroke in male US healthcare professionals: 14 year prospective cohort study. *BMJ (Clinical Research Ed.), 327*(7418), 777–782. doi:10.1136/bmj.327.7418.777 PMID:14525873

Health Information. (2017). *Fibre Sources and Fibre Supplements Information.* Retrieved April 13, 2017, from https://patient.info/in/health/fibre-and-fibre-supplements

Herrada, A. A., Campino, C., Amador, C. A., Michea, L. F., Fardella, C. E., & Kalergis, A. M. (2011). Aldosterone as a modulator of immunity: Implications in the organ damage. *Journal of Hypertension, 29*(9), 1684–1692. doi:10.1097/HJH.0b013e32834a4c75 PMID:21826023

High Blood Pressure. (2014). *High Blood Pressure (Hypertension) Information | cdc.gov*. Retrieved April 13, 2017, from https://www.cdc.gov/bloodpressure/index.htm

Hipsley, E. H. (1953). Dietary "Fibre" and Pregnancy Toxaemia. *British Medical Journal, 2*(4833), 420–422. doi:10.1136/bmj.2.4833.420 PMID:13066743

Houston, M. (2014). The role of nutrition and nutraceutical supplements in the treatment of hypertension. *World Journal of Cardiology, 6*(2), 38–66. doi:10.4330/wjc.v6.i2.38 PMID:24575172

Houston, M. C., & Harper, K. J. (2008). Potassium, magnesium, and calcium: Their role in both the cause and treatment of hypertension. *Journal of Clinical Hypertension (Greenwich, Conn.), 10*(7Suppl 2), 3–11. doi:10.1111/j.1751-7176.2008.08575.x PMID:18607145

Jackson, R., Lawes, C. M. M., Bennett, D. A., Milne, R. J., & Rodgers, A. (2005). Treatment with drugs to lower blood pressure and blood cholesterol based on an individual's absolute cardiovascular risk. *Lancet (London, England)*, *365*(9457), 434–441. doi:10.1016/S0140-6736(05)70240-3 PMID:15680460

James, P. A., Oparil, S., Carter, B. L., Cushman, W. C., Dennison-Himmelfarb, C., Handler, J., ... Ortiz, E. (2014). 2014 Evidence-Based Guideline for the Management of High Blood Pressure in Adults: Report from the Panel Members Appointed to the Eighth Joint National Committee (JNC 8). *Journal of the American Medical Association*, *311*(5), 507–520. doi:10.1001/jama.2013.284427 PMID:24352797

Jenkins, D. J. A., Kendall, C. W. C., Marchie, A., Faulkner, D. A., Wong, J. M. W., de Souza, R., ... Connelly, P. W. (2005). Direct comparison of a dietary portfolio of cholesterol-lowering foods with a statin in hypercholesterolemic participants. *The American Journal of Clinical Nutrition*, *81*(2), 380–387. doi:10.1093/ajcn.81.2.380 PMID:15699225

Jeppesen, J., Hein, H. O., Suadicani, P., & Gyntelberg, F. (1998). Triglyceride concentration and ischemic heart disease: An eight-year follow-up in the Copenhagen Male Study. *Circulation*, *97*(11), 1029–1036. doi:10.1161/01.CIR.97.11.1029 PMID:9531248

Joseph, T. (2014). *Pharmacotherapy: A Pathophysiologic Approach, Access Pharmacy*. McGraw-Hill Medical. Retrieved April 13, 2017, from http://accesspharmacy.mhmedical.com/book.aspx?bookid=689

Kearney, P. M., Whelton, M., Reynolds, K., Muntner, P., Whelton, P. K., & He, J. (2005). Global burden of hypertension: Analysis of worldwide data. *Lancet*, *365*(9455), 217–223. doi:10.1016/S0140-6736(05)70151-3 PMID:15652604

Kizhakekuttu, T. J., & Widlansky, M. E. (2010). Natural antioxidants and hypertension: Promise and challenges. *Cardiovascular Therapeutics*, *28*(4), e20–e32. doi:10.1111/j.1755-5922.2010.00137.x PMID:20370791

Koçyildiz, Z. C., Birman, H., Olgaç, V., Akgün-Dar, K., Melikoğlu, G., & Meriçli, A. H. (2006). Crataegus tanacetifolia leaf extract prevents L-NAME-induced hypertension in rats: A morphological study. *Phytotherapy Research: PTR*, *20*(1), 66–70. doi:10.1002/ptr.1808 PMID:16397846

Konno, S., Hirooka, Y., Araki, S., Koga, Y., Kishi, T., & Sunagawa, K. (2008). Azelnidipine decreases sympathetic nerve activity via antioxidant effect in the rostral ventrolateral medulla of stroke-prone spontaneously hypertensive rats. *Journal of Cardiovascular Pharmacology*, *52*(6), 555–560. doi:10.1097/FJC.0b013e318192690e PMID:19057394

Krinsky, N. I., & Johnson, E. J. (2005). Carotenoid actions and their relation to health and disease. *Molecular Aspects of Medicine*, *26*(6), 459–516. doi:10.1016/j.mam.2005.10.001 PMID:16309738

Kushi, L. H., Folsom, A. R., Prineas, R. J., Mink, P. J., Wu, Y., & Bostick, R. M. (1996). Dietary antioxidant vitamins and death from coronary heart disease in postmenopausal women. *The New England Journal of Medicine*, *334*(18), 1156–1162. doi:10.1056/NEJM199605023341803 PMID:8602181

Layne, J., Majkova, Z., Smart, E. J., Toborek, M., & Hennig, B. (2011). Caveolae: A regulatory platform for nutritional modulation of inflammatory diseases. *The Journal of Nutritional Biochemistry*, *22*(9), 807–811. doi:10.1016/j.jnutbio.2010.09.013 PMID:21292468

Lehto, S., Rönnemaa, T., Pyörälä, K., & Laakso, M. (2000). Cardiovascular risk factors clustering with endogenous hyperinsulinaemia predict death from coronary heart disease in patients with Type II diabetes. *Diabetologia*, *43*(2), 148–155. doi:10.1007001250050023 PMID:10753035

Lewington, S., Clarke, R., Qizilbash, N., Peto, R., & Collins, R.. (2002). Age-specific relevance of usual blood pressure to vascular mortality: A meta-analysis of individual data for one million adults in 61 prospective studies. *Lancet (London, England)*, *360*(9349), 1903–1913. doi:10.1016/S0140-6736(02)11911-8 PMID:12493255

Lichtenstein, A. H. (1998). Soy Protein, Isoflavones and Cardiovascular Disease Risk. *The Journal of Nutrition*, *128*(10), 1589–1592. doi:10.1093/jn/128.10.1589 PMID:9772121

Ling, B., Aziz, C., Wojnarowicz, C., Olkowski, A., & Alcorn, J. (2010). Timing and Duration of Drug Exposure Affects Outcomes of a Drug-Nutrient Interaction During Ontogeny. *Pharmaceutics*, *2*(4), 321–338. doi:10.3390/pharmaceutics2040321 PMID:27721360

Lipid modification: Cardiovascular risk assessment and the modification of blood lipids for the primary and secondary prevention of cardiovascular disease | Guidance and guidelines | NICE. (n.d.). Retrieved April 12, 2017, from https://www.nice.org.uk

Luft, F. C. (2012). Neural regulation of the immune system modulates hypertension-induced target-organ damage. *Journal of the American Society of Hypertension: JASH*, *6*(1), 23–26. doi:10.1016/j.jash.2011.09.006 PMID:22047671

Lutsey, P. L., Jacobs, D. R., Kori, S., Mayer-Davis, E., Shea, S., Steffen, L. M., ... Tracy, R. (2007). Whole grain intake and its cross-sectional association with obesity, insulin resistance, inflammation, diabetes and subclinical CVD: The MESA Study. *British Journal of Nutrition*, *98*(2), 397–405. doi:10.1017/S0007114507700715 PMID:17391554

Maeda, G., Takara, K., Wada, K., Oki, T., Masuda, M., Ichiba, T., ... Suda, I. (2006). Evaluation of Antioxidant Activity of Vegetables from Okinawa Prefecture and Determination of Some Antioxidative Compounds. *Food Science and Technology Research*, *12*(1), 8–14. doi:10.3136/fstr.12.8

Mancia, G., Fagard, R., Narkiewicz, K., Redón, J., Zanchetti, A., & Böhm, M. (2013). ESH/ESC Guidelines for the management of arterial hypertension: The Task Force for the management of arterial hypertension of the European Society of Hypertension (ESH) and of the European Society of Cardiology (ESC). *Journal of Hypertension*, *31*(7), 1281–1357. doi:10.1097/01.hjh.0000431740.32696.cc PMID:23817082

Mano, R., Ishida, A., Ohya, Y., Todoriki, H., & Takishita, S. (2009). Dietary intervention with Okinawan vegetables increased circulating endothelial progenitor cells in healthy young women. *Atherosclerosis*, *204*(2), 544–548. doi:10.1016/j.atherosclerosis.2008.09.035 PMID:19013573

Mansego, M. L., Solar, G. D. M., Alonso, M. P., Martínez, F., Sáez, G. T., Escudero, J. C. M., ... Chaves, F. J. (2011). Polymorphisms of antioxidant enzymes, blood pressure and risk of hypertension. *Journal of Hypertension*, *29*(3), 492–500. doi:10.1097/HJH.0b013e328341f1b2 PMID:21178785

Marketou, M. E., Kontaraki, J. E., Zacharis, E. A., Kochiadakis, G. E., Giaouzaki, A., Chlouverakis, G., & Vardas, P. E. (2012). TLR2 and TLR4 gene expression in peripheral monocytes in nondiabetic hypertensive patients: The effect of intensive blood pressure-lowering. *Journal of Clinical Hypertension (Greenwich, Conn.)*, *14*(5), 330–335. doi:10.1111/j.1751-7176.2012.00620.x PMID:22533660

Martínez-González, M. Á., Corella, D., Salas-Salvadó, J., Ros, E., Covas, M. I., Fiol, M., ... Estruch, R. (2012). Cohort profile: Design and methods of the PREDIMED study. *International Journal of Epidemiology*, *41*(2), 377–385. doi:10.1093/ije/dyq250 PMID:21172932

Masters, R. C., Liese, A. D., Haffner, S. M., Wagenknecht, L. E., & Hanley, A. J. (2010). Whole and Refined Grain Intakes Are Related to Inflammatory Protein Concentrations in Human Plasma. *The Journal of Nutrition*, *140*(3), 587–594. doi:10.3945/jn.109.116640 PMID:20089789

McGill, H. C. Jr. (1979). The relationship of dietary cholesterol to serum cholesterol concentration and to atherosclerosis in man. *The American Journal of Clinical Nutrition, 32*(12Suppl), 2664–2702. doi:10.1093/ajcn/32.12.2664 PMID:389024

Ministry of health and family, New Delhi, India, (2006). *Home*. Retrieved April 15, 2017, from http://www.fssai.gov.in/home

Moreau, R. A., Whitaker, B. D., & Hicks, K. B. (2002). Phytosterols, phytostanols, and their conjugates in foods: Structural diversity, quantitative analysis, and health-promoting uses. *Progress in Lipid Research, 41*(6), 457–500. doi:10.1016/S0163-7827(02)00006-1 PMID:12169300

Mozaffarian, D. (2008). Fish and n-3 fatty acids for the prevention of fatal coronary heart disease and sudden cardiac death. *The American Journal of Clinical Nutrition, 87*(6), 1991S–1996S. doi:10.1093/ajcn/87.6.1991S PMID:18541600

Muller, D. N., Kvakan, H., & Luft, F. C. (2011). Immune-related effects in hypertension and target-organ damage. *Current Opinion in Nephrology and Hypertension, 20*(2), 113–117. doi:10.1097/MNH.0b013e3283436f88 PMID:21245763

Nair, H. B., Sung, B., Yadav, V. R., Kannappan, R., Chaturvedi, M. M., & Aggarwal, B. B. (2010). Delivery of antiinflammatory nutraceuticals by nanoparticles for the prevention and treatment of cancer. *Biochemical Pharmacology, 80*(12), 1833–1843. doi:10.1016/j.bcp.2010.07.021 PMID:20654584

Nayak, D. U., Karmen, C., Frishman, W. H., & Vakili, B. A. (2001). Antioxidant vitamins and enzymatic and synthetic oxygen-derived free radical scavengers in the prevention and treatment of cardiovascular disease. *Heart Disease (Hagerstown, Md.), 3*(1), 28–45. doi:10.1097/00132580-200101000-00006 PMID:11975768

Nishihara, M., Hirooka, Y., Matsukawa, R., Kishi, T., & Sunagawa, K. (2012). Oxidative stress in the rostral ventrolateral medulla modulates excitatory and inhibitory inputs in spontaneously hypertensive rats. *Journal of Hypertension, 30*(1), 97–106. doi:10.1097/HJH.0b013e32834e1df4 PMID:22157590

Nutraceuticals - opportunities in an emerging market. (n.d.). Retrieved April 14, 2017, from http://www.fimdefelice.org/p2463.html

Ohnishi, N., Kusuhara, M., Yoshioka, M., Kuroda, K., Soga, A., Nishikawa, F., ... Yokoyama, T. (2003). Studies on interactions between functional foods or dietary supplements and medicines. I. Effects of Ginkgo biloba leaf extract on the pharmacokinetics of diltiazem in rats. *Biological & Pharmaceutical Bulletin, 26*(9), 1315–1320. doi:10.1248/bpb.26.1315 PMID:12951478

Olalla, M. T., Medrano, M. J., Sierra, M. J., & Almazán, J. (1999). Time trends, cohort effect and spatial distribution of cerebrovascular disease mortality in Spain. *European Journal of Epidemiology*, *15*(4), 331–339. doi:10.1023/A:1007555000016 PMID:10414373

Overview of hypertension. (2015). Retrieved April 13, 2017, from http://www.uptodate.com/contents/overview-of-hypertension

Pérez-Jiménez, J., & Saura-Calixto, F. (2008). Grape products and cardiovascular disease risk factors. *Nutrition Research Reviews*, *21*(2), 158–173. doi:10.1017/S0954422408125124 PMID:19087369

Quiroz, Y., Johnson, R. J., & Rodríguez-Iturbe, B. (2012). The role of T cells in the pathogenesis of primary hypertension. *Nephrology, Dialysis, Transplantation*, *27*(Suppl 4), iv2–iv5. doi:10.1093/ndt/gfs421 PMID:23036901

Ramaa, C. S., Shirode, A. R., Mundada, A. S., & Kadam, V. J. (2006). Nutraceuticals--an emerging era in the treatment and prevention of cardiovascular diseases. *Current Pharmaceutical Biotechnology*, *7*(1), 15–23. doi:10.2174/138920106775789647 PMID:16472130

Razzouk, L., Muntner, P., Bansilal, S., Kini, A. S., Aneja, A., Mozes, J., ... Farkouh, M. E. (2009). C-reactive protein predicts long-term mortality independently of low-density lipoprotein cholesterol in patients undergoing percutaneous coronary intervention. *American Heart Journal*, *158*(2), 277–283. doi:10.1016/j.ahj.2009.05.026 PMID:19619706

Reedy, J., Wirfält, E., Flood, A., Mitrou, P. N., Krebs-Smith, S. M., Kipnis, V., ... Subar, A. F. (2010). Comparing 3 Dietary Pattern Methods—Cluster Analysis, Factor Analysis, and Index Analysis—With Colorectal Cancer Risk. *American Journal of Epidemiology*, *171*(4), 479–487. doi:10.1093/aje/kwp393 PMID:20026579

Rein, M. J., Renouf, M., Cruz-Hernandez, C., Actis-Goretta, L., Thakkar, S. K., & da Silva Pinto, M. (2013). Bioavailability of bioactive food compounds: A challenging journey to bioefficacy. *British Journal of Clinical Pharmacology*, *75*(3), 588–602. doi:10.1111/j.1365-2125.2012.04425.x PMID:22897361

Review Paleolithic nutrition revisited: A twelve-year retrospective on its nature and implications. (1997). 10.1038/sj.ejcn.1600389

Rodríguez-Iturbe, B., Franco, M., Tapia, E., Quiroz, Y., & Johnson, R. J. (2012). Renal inflammation, autoimmunity and salt-sensitive hypertension. *Clinical and Experimental Pharmacology & Physiology*, *39*(1), 96–103. doi:10.1111/j.1440-1681.2011.05482.x PMID:21251049

Ros, E., Núñez, I., Pérez-Heras, A., Serra, M., Gilabert, R., Casals, E., & Deulofeu, R. (2004). A walnut diet improves endothelial function in hypercholesterolemic subjects: a randomized crossover trial. *Circulation, 109*(13), 1609–1614. .91474. FF10.1161/01.CIR.0000124477

Rosell, M., Appleby, P., Spencer, E., & Key, T. (2006). Weight gain over 5 years in 21 966 meat-eating, fish-eating, vegetarian, and vegan men and women in EPIC-Oxford. *International Journal of Obesity*, *30*(9), 1389–1396. doi:10.1038j.ijo.0803305 PMID:16534521

Sabate, J., & Ang, Y. (2009). Nuts and health outcomes: New epidemiologic evidence. *The American Journal of Clinical Nutrition*, *89*(5), 1643S–1648S. doi:10.3945/ajcn.2009.26736Q PMID:19321572

Savica, V., Bellinghieri, G., & Kopple, J. D. (2010). The effect of nutrition on blood pressure. *Annual Review of Nutrition*, *30*(1), 365–401. doi:10.1146/annurev-nutr-010510-103954 PMID:20645853

Singh, U., Devaraj, S., & Jialal, I. (2005). Vitamin E, Oxidative Stress, and Inflammation. *Annual Review of Nutrition*, *25*(1), 151–174. doi:10.1146/annurev.nutr.24.012003.132446 PMID:16011463

Society, P. (2005). JBS 2: Joint British Societies' guidelines on prevention of cardiovascular disease in clinical practice. *Heart (British Cardiac Society)*, *91*(suppl 5), v1–v52. doi:10.1136/hrt.2005.079988 PMID:16365341

Spencer, E. A., Appleby, P. N., Davey, G. K., & Key, T. J. (2003). Diet and body mass index in 38000 EPIC-Oxford meat-eaters, fish-eaters, vegetarians and vegans. *International Journal of Obesity and Related Metabolic Disorders: Journal of the International Association for the Study of Obesity*, *27*(6), 728–734. doi:10.1038j.ijo.0802300 PMID:12833118

Stampfer, M. J., Hu, F. B., Manson, J. E., Rimm, E. B., & Willett, W. C. (2000). Primary Prevention of Coronary Heart Disease in Women through Diet and Lifestyle. *The New England Journal of Medicine*, *343*(1), 16–22. doi:10.1056/NEJM200007063430103 PMID:10882764

Suekawa, M., Ishige, A., Yuasa, K., Sudo, K., Aburada, M., & Hosoya, E. (1984). Pharmacological studies on ginger. I. Pharmacological actions of pungent constitutents, (6)-gingerol and (6)-shogaol. *Journal of Pharmacobio-Dynamics*, *7*(11), 836–848. doi:10.1248/bpb1978.7.836 PMID:6335723

Sumpio, B. E., Cordova, A. C., Berke-Schlessel, D. W., Qin, F., & Chen, Q. H. (2006). Green tea, the "Asian paradox," and cardiovascular disease. *Journal of the American College of Surgeons*, *202*(5), 813–825. doi:10.1016/j.jamcollsurg.2006.01.018 PMID:16648021

The Nutritional Characteristics of a Contemporary Diet Based Upon Paleolithic Food Groups Abstract 4 I Diet (Nutrition). (n.d.). Retrieved April 13, 2017, from https://www.scribd.com/ document/94643426/The-Nutritional-Characteristics-of-a-Contemporary-Diet-Based-UponPaleolithic-Food-Groups-Abstract-4

Tian, N., Penman, A. D., Manning, R. D. Jr, Flessner, M. F., & Mawson, A. R. (2012). Association between Circulating Specific Leukocyte Types and Incident Chronic Kidney Disease: The Atherosclerosis Risk in Communities (ARIC) Study. *Journal of the American Society of Hypertension*, *6*(2), 100–108. doi:10.1016/j.jash.2011.10.001 PMID:22054781

Touyz, R. M. (2012). New insights into mechanisms of hypertension. *Current Opinion in Nephrology and Hypertension*, *21*(2), 119–121. doi:10.1097/MNH.0b013e328350a50f PMID:22257800

Tse, W. Y., Maxwell, S. R., Thomason, H., Blann, A., Thorpe, G. H., Waite, M., & Holder, R. (1994). Antioxidant status in controlled and uncontrolled hypertension and its relationship to endothelial damage. *Journal of Human Hypertension*, *8*(11), 843–849. PMID:7853328

Tuekpe, M. K.-N., Todoriki, H., Sasaki, S., Zheng, K.-C., & Ariizumi, M. (2006). Potassium excretion in healthy Japanese women was increased by a dietary intervention utilizing home-parcel delivery of Okinawan vegetables. *Hypertension Research: Official Journal of the Japanese Society of Hypertension*, *29*(6), 389–396. doi:10.1291/hypres.29.389 PMID:16940700

Ueeda, M., Doumei, T., Takaya, Y., Shinohata, R., Katayama, Y., Ohnishi, N., ... Kusachi, S. (2008). Serum N-3 polyunsaturated fatty acid levels correlate with the extent of coronary plaques and calcifications in patients with acute myocardial infarction. *Circulation Journal*, *72*(11), 1836–1843. doi:10.1253/circj.CJ-08-0249 PMID:18812674

Vartiainen, E., Laatikainen, T., Peltonen, M., Juolevi, A., Männistö, S., Sundvall, J., ... Puska, P. (2010). Thirty-five-year trends in cardiovascular risk factors in Finland. *International Journal of Epidemiology*, *39*(2), 504–518. doi:10.1093/ije/dyp330 PMID:19959603

Vongpatanasin, W., Thomas, G. D., Schwartz, R., Cassis, L. A., Osborne-Lawrence, S., Hahner, L., ... Shaul, P. W. (2007). C-reactive protein causes downregulation of vascular angiotensin subtype 2 receptors and systolic hypertension in mice. *Circulation, 115*(8), 1020–1028. doi:10.1161/CIRCULATIONAHA.106.664854 PMID:17283257

Walford, R. L., Mock, D., Verdery, R., & MacCallum, T. (2002). Calorie restriction in biosphere 2: Alterations in physiologic, hematologic, hormonal, and biochemical parameters in humans restricted for a 2-year period. *The Journals of Gerontology. Series A, Biological Sciences and Medical Sciences, 57*(6), B211–B224. doi:10.1093/gerona/57.6.B211 PMID:12023257

Whelton, S. P., Hyre, A. D., Pedersen, B., Yi, Y., Whelton, P. K., & He, J. (2005). Effect of dietary fiber intake on blood pressure: A meta-analysis of randomized, controlled clinical trials. *Journal of Hypertension, 23*(3), 475–481. doi:10.1097/01.hjh.0000160199.51158.cf PMID:15716684

Wiseman, H., O'Reilly, J. D., Adlercreutz, H., Mallet, A. I., Bowey, E. A., Rowland, I. R., & Sanders, T. A. (2000). Isoflavone phytoestrogens consumed in soy decrease F(2)-isoprostane concentrations and increase resistance of low-density lipoprotein to oxidation in humans. *The American Journal of Clinical Nutrition, 72*(2), 395–400. doi:10.1093/ajcn/72.2.395 PMID:10919933

Xing, T., Wang, F., Li, J., & Wang, N. (2012). Hypertension: An immunologic disease? *Journal of Hypertension, 30*(12), 2440–2441. doi:10.1097/HJH.0b013e32835953f9 PMID:23151885

Yussif, N. M., Abdul Aziz, M. A., & Abdel Rahman, A. R. (2016). Evaluation of the Anti-Inflammatory Effect of Locally Delivered Vitamin C in the Treatment of Persistent Gingival Inflammation: Clinical and Histopathological Study. *Journal of Nutrition and Metabolism, 2016*, e2978741. doi:10.1155/2016/2978741 PMID:28050280

Zhao, L., Lee, J. Y., & Hwang, D. H. (2011). Inhibition of pattern recognition receptor-mediated inflammation by bioactive phytochemicals: A review of recent research. *Nutrition Reviews, 69*(6), 310–320. doi:10.1111/j.1753-4887.2011.00394.x PMID:21631512

Zierler-Brown, S. (2007). Nutraceuticals: A Guide for Healthcare Professionals. *American Journal of Pharmaceutical Education*, *71*(5). Retrieved from http://www.ncbi.nlm.nih.gov/pmc/articles/ PMC2064899/

Zimmet, P., Alberti, K. G., & Shaw, J. (2001). Global and societal implications of the diabetes epidemic. *Nature*, *414*(6865), 782–787. doi:10.1038/414782a PMID:11742409

Chapter 8
The Protective Role of Nutraceuticals and Functional Food in Hyperlipidemia

Raushan Kumar
University of Allahabad, India

Syed Ibrahim Rizvi
University of Allahabad, India

ABSTRACT

Diets rich in fats and cholesterol are mainly responsible for the production of free radicals which contribute to the incidence of hyperlipidemia and hypercholesterolemia. Both of these are the major factors responsible for CVDs. Hyperlipidemia is characterized by elevated level of total cholesterol (TC), low-density lipoprotein (LDL) and very low-density lipoprotein (VLDL), and reduced level of high-density lipoprotein (HDL) in serum. The main role of diet is to provide ample amount of nutrients to meet the nutritional requirements of an individual. However, there are increasing scientific approaches helping the hypothesis that some food ingredients have beneficial effects over and above the provision of the basic nutrients. So in this chapter, the main focus is food categorized under nutraceutical and functional food and their various protective roles in the case of hyperlipidemia.

INTRODUCTION

Hyperlipidemia is characterized by elevated levels of total cholesterol (TC), low-density lipoprotein (LDL), very- low-density lipoprotein (VLDL), and reduced level of high -density lipoprotein (HDL) in serum (Sissayb.Mecbib, Thierry, Regnier, & Korsten, 2006). Hyperlipidemia is a major contributing factor for the development

DOI: 10.4018/978-1-5225-3267-5.ch008

of atherosclerosis leading to chronic heart disease (CHD) (Defronzoet, 1992). According to current projections, it is estimated that by 2030 about 23.6 million people will die from cardiovascular disease (World Health Organization, 2009). On the other hand, cholesterol-induced oxidative stress is one of the factors that link hypercholesterolemia with atherogenesis and is known to produce vascular atherosclerotic lesion. Recent data show that people from the Indian subcontinent have a genetic predisposition towards hyperlipidemia leading to CVD (Harrison & Griendling, 2003). Diets rich in fats and cholesterol are mainly responsible for the production of free radicals. Among the mechanisms responsible for the development of atherosclerosis, the role of oxidative stress has also been established.

As per World Health Organization (WHO) estimates, approximately 1.5 billion adults are overweight among which, 200 million men and 300 million women are obese. Excess intake of food than required and consequent obesity are some important factors in developing cardiovascular disease, diabetes, atherosclerosis, fatty liver disease various neurodegenerative disease and cancer (Magrone, Perez de Heredia, Jirillo, Morabito, Marcos, & Serafini, 2013). In developing countries, the rate of increase of CVD is almost double in comparison with developed countries (Gaziano, 2005). Cardiovascular disease (CVD) is the main cause of death in India (Mukherjee, 1995) and its contribution to total mortality is increasing.; Deaths due to CVDs are to approximately double between 1985-2015(WHO, 2016).Apart from this, the published data suggest that the death rate in Asian population due to cardiovascular disease is likely to increase 103% in men and 90% in women by 2030 (Mozaffarian, Benjamin, Go, Arnett, Blaha, Cushman, … Turner, 2016). In 2015 CHD has been predicted to rank first among the causes of death in Indian population by (Nag & Ghosh, 2015). A total of nearly 64 million cases of CVD is likely in the year 2015among them nearly 61 million would be CHD cases (the remaining would include stroke, rheumatic heart disease, and congenital heart diseases). The demise of this group of diseases is likely to amount to be a staggering 3.4 million (Global Burden of Disease Cancer Collaboration, 2017). Cardiovascular diseases in India have been generally occurring in urban areas but many vascular deaths also occur in rural regions and this is still where the majority of the population lives. While there is some limited information regarding the causes and management of cardiovascular disease in urban regions, corresponding data for rural regions is negligible (Gupta & Gupta, 1996). It seems reasonable to argue that people with changing lifestyles due to growing urbanization are associated with adverse CVD risk factors irrespective of their habitat (rural vs. urban) (Das, Pal, & Ghosh, 2011).

There are various important factors which are generally responsible for the increasing level of lipids in body and development of cardiovascular disease. Sometimes some people are born with conditions that predispose them to heart disease but most people who are suffering from this disease a combination of factors responsible for it. According to the National Health Service (NHS) of UK, the main risk factors associated with cardiovascular disease are poor diet, lack of physical activity, diabetes, hypertension, hyperlipidemia, drinking too much alcohol, stress, smoking, etc. Atherosclerosis is the main risk factor which occurs due to cardiovascular disease. Atherosclerosis is the narrowing and thickening of arteries. The thickening and narrowing of arteries are due to the deposition of cholesterol and other substances in the walls of blood vessels. The deposits are known as plaques. The main reason behind between stroke or heart attack is the rupture of a plaque.

The main role of diet is to provide ample amount of nutrients to meet the nutritional requirements of an individual, however, there are increasing scientific approaches helping the hypothesis that some food ingredients have beneficial effects over and above the provision of the basic nutrients (Bose & Sarma, 1975). Moreover, the Foods of the plant origin have also been suggested to contain many non-nutritive compounds, which may protect diet-induced diseases, including cardiovascular diseases, diabetes mellitus and cancers (Scalbert, Match, Morand, Rémésy, & Jiménez, 2005a). It is well known that CVD can be prevented by lifestyle changes, including diet (Stampfer, Hu, Manson, Rimm, & Willett, 2000).

Ecological studies and ancient evidence have provided information that there is a direct relationship between diet and CVD (McGill, 1979). It is noted that ingestion of calorie dense, nutritionally poor, highly processed, and rapidly absorbable food can lead to systemic inflammation, reduced insulin sensitivity, and a cluster of metabolic abnormalities, including obesity, hypertension, dyslipidemia, and glucose intolerance (Folsom, Parker, & Harnack, 2007). Currently, the main aim of nutrition research is to understand the effects of whole foods (Aldana, Greenlaw, Salberg, Merrill, Hager, & Jorgensen, 2007). Change in lifestyle, correct food habits and correct pharmacological treatment can reduce the effects of this disease and improve health (Huang & Sumpio, 2008). The survey of the prevalent literature suggests that about 90% of the total population residing in developing countries like India use plants-based products as a traditional medicine for their primary health care need (WHO, 2002). The plant contains a wide variety of secondary metabolites which are mainly responsible for to treatment of CVD (Patil, 2011). There is increasing evidence to show that high supplementation of dietary flavonoids may have a protective effect against several diseases (Riemersma, Rice-Evans, Tyrrell, Clifford, & Lean, 2001).

The current dietary approach is to reduce the risk of CVD includes substituting saturated fat with carbohydrate without changing the protein content. In the USA, the DASH-diet (Dietary Approaches to Stop Hypertension), which is rich in fruits, vegetables, and low-fat dairy products, is recommended to reduce the risk of heart disease. Such high-carbohydrate, low-protein diets are known to reduce blood pressure and low-density lipoprotein (LDL) cholesterol (Appel, Moore, Obarzanek, Vollmer, Svetkey, Sacks, & Karanja, 1997) but also to reduce high-density lipoprotein (HDL) cholesterol levels and to raise fasting triglycerides (Obarzanek, Sacks, Vollmer, Bray, Miller, & Lin, 2001). Previous studies have suggested that an increased consumption of protein, particularly of plant origin, may further lower the risk of hypertension and CVD (Hu, Stampfer, Manson, Rimm, Colditz, Speizer,… Willett, 1999). The human trial conducted by Omni Heart (Optimal Macro-Nutrient Intake to Prevent Heart Disease) indicate that partial replacement of carbohydrate with protein and low saturated fat can help to lower blood pressure, improve lipid profile, and reduce the risk of CVD (Appel, Sacks, Carey, Obarzanek, Swain, & Miller, 2005). Although Ecological studies and various ancient evidence have given information between diet and CVD, there is still considerable scientific uncertainty about the relationship between specific dietary components and cardiovascular risk. Besides these, the previous studies also suggest that intake of higher amount of dietary antioxidant is associated with a lower risk of CVD and death (Appel, 2003). The conflicting results between the apparent protective effects of nutrients as part of dietary intake and the lack of effectiveness of single nutrient supplementation in trials have led to a focus on whole foods or modified diets as protective against CVD (Elliott, 2003). Plants make a huge number of phenolic compounds known as secondary metabolites that may play a vital role in reducing the risk of disease or in improving the health. There are various well-known traditional food products they contain such components which are beneficial for health beyond their basic nutritive value like vegetables, soya, whole grain, fruits, and milk (Watson, Gerald, & Preedy, 2011). Additionally, modern foods are being developed to enhance these valuable components for their health benefits or desirable physiological effects. Rapid changes in food science and technology and great consumer interest in functional foods have increased during the late twentieth century (Scalbert, Manach, Morand, Rémésy, & Jiménez, 2005a).

These foods are basically arisen in Japan and then in Europe, where the concepts of foods were introduced (Arai, 1996). Functional foods are considered as those intended to be consumed as a part of the common diet and the biologically active components offer potential enhancement of health or reduced risk of disease (Kohlmeier, 2015). Specific minerals, fatty acids, vitamins or dietary fibre, foods with added biologically active substances such as phytochemicals or other antioxidants and probiotics with the live beneficial cultures (Cencic & Chingwaru, 2010) all are come under the category of functional food. A huge variety of functional foods has been found to exert a potentially valuable effect in the prevention and treatment of cardiovascular disease (Senftleber, Halline, Veening, & Dayton, 1976). Functional foods administered in ample amounts may result in the decrease of cardiovascular disease risk, at least by several potential mechanisms: improving arterial compliance, reducing low-density lipoprotein oxidation, lowering blood lipid levels, decreasing plaque formation, scavenging free radicals, and inhibiting platelet aggregation

Figure 1. ROS (Reactive Oxygen Species) Induced Lipid Peroxidation and Tissue Damage

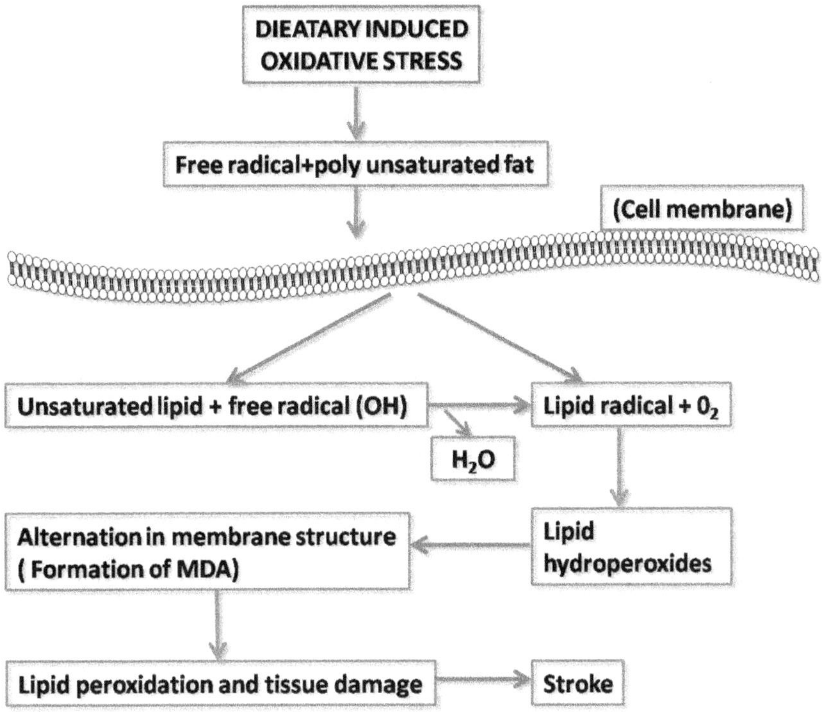

(*Position of the American Dietetic Association,* 1999). So the main objective of this chapter is to understand how the plant-based food materials and functional and Nutraceutical food help us for protecting these diseases.

BACKGROUND

Hyperlipidemia and elevated level of lipid profile is one of the most prominent issues worldwide. Current time people are very aware regarding with their health. The plant-based food materials are very useful for to maintain these elevated parameters. Lots of Nutraceuticals drugs and functional foods are available to present time. The word "Nutraceutical" was coined to incorporate the terms "Nutrition" and "Pharmaceutical" in 1989 by Dr. Stephen DE Felice, Chairman of the Foundation for Innovation in Medicine (Kalra, 2003).Nutraceutical has no exact definition this term is generally used for a nutritional supplement which is a help to prevent or cure the disease. Nutritionist says that nutraceutical is any substance that is a part of food or food and provide medical or health benefits (Kohlmeier, 2015). Such products may range from isolated nutrients, dietary supplements and diets to genetically engineered "designer" foods, herbal products and processed foods such as cereals, soups, and beverages (Wetmur, 1976). Approximately more than 500 nutraceutical and functional food products are available in the market with well-known health benefits (Evans, 1996). The Indian nutraceutical industry has appreciable prospects. Presently a broad range of items has been available, giving an insight into the massive growth. Due to this unhealthy, eating habits coupled with inactive lifestyle have led to increased incidence of diet and its related health issues. On the one hand, there is a growing consciousness on the importance of nutrition and diet for long-term healthy life. In India, these have contributed to convenient market conditions for Nutraceutical industry. India has great advantages like qualified human resources, world-class R & D facilities and various varieties of raw material aspects that give our country a leading edge. While the world market is increasing at a CAGR of7%, the Indian market has been increasing much faster at a CAGR of 18% for the last three years, driven by Beverages and functional food categories The Indian nutraceutical market is controlled mainly by pharmaceuticals and FMCG companies, with very few pure-play nutraceutical companies.

MAIN FOCUS OF THE CHAPTER

The main focus of this chapter is nutraceuticals currently employed against prevention and treatment of CVD due to hyperlipidemia. In this chapter, various types of nutraceutical categories and their differential mode of action are given below.

CATEGORIES OF NUTRACEUTICALS

There are various categories of nutraceuticals products which can either extracted from natural sources (nature like) or manufactured synthetically (man-made), which supplement the diet to provide nutrition over and above regular food and help prevent nutrition-related disorders (Hathcock, 2001).

Nutraceuticals are categorized as follows:

1. On the basis of their chemical constituents (Smith, 2005).
    a. **Nutrients**: Substances with known nutritional functions, like- vitamins, minerals, amino acids and fatty acids.
    b. **Herbals:** Plant products or herbs as concentrates and extracts.

    c. **Dietary Supplement**: Dietary supplements are products administered by mouth that contain a dietary ingredient intended to add something to the foods we eat. Example: Black cohosh for menopausal symptoms, Ginkgo Biloba for memory loss, and glucosamine/chondroitin for arthritis.
2. Traditional and Non-traditional nutraceuticals (Lucas, Blair, Cooper, & Matty, 1975). At the present time, several varieties of nutraceutical foods are present in the market which falls into the category of traditional foods and non-traditional foods.
    a. **Traditional Nutraceuticals**: Traditional nutraceuticals generally contain actual food. It is simply natural, whole foods with new information about their potential health qualities. A large number of fruits, vegetables, grains, fish, dairy, and meat products contain several natural components that deliver benefits beyond basic nutrition, such as lycopene in tomatoes, omega-3 fatty acids in salmon or saponins in soy.
    b. **Non-Traditional Nutraceuticals:** Falling under this is the outcome from agricultural breeding or added nutrients and/or ingredients such as orange juice fortified with calcium, cereals with added vitamins or minerals and flour with added folic acid are nontraditional nutraceutical.

SOME IMPORTANT COMMONLY USED NUTRACEUTICALS

Omega-3-Fatty Acid

These are mainly the polyunsaturated fatty acids (PUFAs) mostly derived from marine sources. In the previous years, various trials have been conducted on Eskimos in Greenland during 1970's to support the finding that omega 3 fatty acid may reduce or inhibit the incidence of death due to CVD. Some well known fatty acid which plays a key role in inhibition of CVDs is Omega-3 eicosapentaenoic acid (EPA) and docosahexaenoic acid (DHA). Moreover, the clinical trials have also highlighted the protective effects of omega-3 fatty acids in reducing the risk of cardiac arrhythmias as well and modestly reduce the incidence of hypertension and atherosclerosis-related plaque formation (Schmoldt, Benthe, & Haberland, 1975). The clinical trial involving 2033 men suffering from post myocardial infarction demonstrated that fish oil supplement intake could decrease mortality rate due to the disease over a period of 2 years (Burr, Fehily, Gilbert, Rogers, Holliday, Sweetnam, … Deadman, 1989). The pharmacological effect shown by this fatty acid is probably due to its ability to maintain membrane fluidity as well as high degree of unsaturation in the host membrane. According to Carroll and Roth, there are various beneficial effects of fatty acid on the prevention of CVDs (Carroll & Roth, 2002). According to various

Table 1. Benefits of Different functional dietary components and nutraceutical

Bioactive Compounds	Sources	Examples	Functional Role
Flavonols	Onion, apple, tea, berries, olives, broccoli, lettuce, red wine, cocoa/chocolate	Quercetin, kaempferol, catechin	↓TC, ↓LDL-C oxidation, ↑HDL-C, AOx, ↓platelet aggregation, ↓eicosanoid synthesis, ↓athero-ELAMs, ↓angiogenesis, ↓MMPs
Flavan-3-ols	Green/black tea, cocoa/ chocolate	Epicatechin, epigallocatechin, epicatechin-3-gallate, epigallocatechin-3-gallate	AOX, ↓apoptosis, ↓LDL-C oxidation, ↓platelet aggregation, ↓athero-ELAMs, ↓angiogenesis, ↓MMPs
Lignans	Flax seed oil, lucerne, clover	Enterolactone, enterodiol	↓LDL-C, AOx, estrogen/ antiestrogen, ↓atherosclerosis *in vivo* but may show adverse CVD effect (pro-oxidant activity with partially defatted flax seed
Isoflavones	Soybeans, legumes	Genistein, daidzein	↓TC and LDL-C, ↓LDL-C oxidation, ↓TG, ↑HDL-C, ↓thrombosis, AOx, estrogen/ antiestrogen, ↓athero-ELAMs, ↓angiogenesis, ↓atherosclerosis *in vivo*, ↓MMPs
Stilbenoids	Grapes, red wine, peanuts	Resveratrol	↓ LDL-C oxidation, ↓ platelet aggregation/thrombosis, ↓ eicosanoid synthesis, AOx, ↓ athero-ELAMs, ↓angiogenesis but promotes angiogenesis in the ischemic heart, ↓ atherosclerosis *in vivo*, ↓MMPs
Carotenoids	Tomatoes, tomato products	Lycopene	↓LDL-C and LDL-C oxidation, Aox, ↓athero-ELAMs, ↓MMPs, but no effects were shown in animal models of ATS and dietary intervention studies using well-defined subjects the population did not provide a clear evidence of lycopene in the prevention of CVD
Soluble Dietary Fibers	Oats, barley, yeast, fruit, vegetables, psyllium seed, fortified cereals and grains	Glucan, pectin, psyllium	↓ atherosclerosis *in vivo*, ↓ MMPs
Monoterpenes	Essential oils of citrus fruit, cherries, mint, herbs	d-Limonene	↓TC and LDL-C, ↓HMGCoAR, ↓angiogenesis
Plant Sterols	Tall oil, soybean oil, rice bran oil	Sitostanol, stigmasterol, Campesterol	↓TC and LDL-C, AOx, ↓cholesterol absorption, ↓carotenoid absorption

continued on following page

Table 1. Continued

Bioactive Compounds	Sources	Examples	Functional Role
ω-3 PUFA	Fish and fish oil, green leaves	DHA, EPA, αLA	↓TC, suppression of cardiac arrhythmias, ↓BP, ↓platelet aggregation, ↓eicosanoid synthesis, ↓athero-ELAMs, ↓angiogenesis, ↓MMPs
Prebiotics	Fruit and vegetable, purified extract from chicory root	Inulin-type fructans	↓TC and ↓TG
Probiotics	Fermented milk products	Selected strains of *Lactobacillus acidophilus, Bifidobacterium bifidum, and Lactobacillus bulgaricus*	↓TC, LDL-C, and BP
Aox- antioxidant activity; BP- blood pressure; CVD- cardiovascular disease; HDL-C- high-density lipoprotein-cholesterol; LDL-C, low-density lipoprotein-cholesterol; TC- total cholesterol; TG- triglycerides; MMPs- metalloproteinases; ELAMs- endothelial leukocyte adhesion molecules.			

clinical trials and epidemiological studies, it is shown that omega 3 fatty acid may reduce death due to the risk of cardiovascular disease by 29% to 52%, the risk of sudden cardiac death by 45% to 81%. Studies show that although omega-3-fatty acids have some adverse effects like bloating and gastrointestinal distress, hyperglycemia, increased the risk of bleeding and sometimes also a slight increase in cholesterol level mainly LDL cholesterol.

Soy

Soy is used as an important nutraceutical product which contains soy proteins and soy isoflavones. Soy isoflavones have been reported to decrease LDL oxidation and improve vascular muscle reactivity (Hasler, 2002). Basically, soy foods are divided into two categories: Unfermented and fermented soy products. Unfermented traditional soy foods basically include fresh green soybeans, whole dry soybeans, soy nuts, soy sprouts, whole-fat soy flour, soymilk and soymilk products, tofu, okara, and yuba. Under the traditional fermented soy foods are included tempeh, miso, soy sauces, natto and fermented tofu and soymilk products (Golbitz, 1995). According to study in Asia, the traditional fermented soy foods are considered to have more health-promoting benefits when consumed in moderate amounts than the super-processed soy products that are consumed in the West (Messina, Persky,

Setchell, & Barnes, 1994). The fermentation process has been reported to increase the observed availability of isoflavones in soy (Hutchins, Slavin, & Lampe, 1995).

Garlic

Garlic has a various well known cardioprotective effect, it mainly reduced the endogenous synthesis of cholesterol. It gives a more favorable HDL: LDL ratio (Banerjee & Maulik, 2002). Garlic contains various constituents such as organosulfur or steroidal saponins. The cholesterol-lowering effects of garlic have been credited not only to its organosulfur constituents but also to a variety of steroidal saponins present in garlic and aged garlic extract (Matsuura, 2001).

Dietary Fibres

Dietary fibres can be defined as they are basically endogenous components of plant part which we include in our diet, and are not digested by enzymes which are produced by humans. On the basis of solubility in bloodstream fibres can be broadly classified into soluble and insoluble fibres. The data presented by National Research Council (US) Committee on Diet and Health, in 1989 suggested that the foods which contain a mixture of complex polysaccharides and isolated polysaccharides are categorized as soluble and insoluble fibre sources respectively. Fibres are important for gastrointestinal health as well as cholesterol-lowering benefits (Weltgesundheits Organization, 2002). Soluble fibres mainly lower blood cholesterol whereas insoluble fibre reduces the rate of colon cancer and diverticulitis, an inflammatory condition of the colon, thus reducing the risk of CHD (Schwencke & De Robichon-Szulmajster, 1976). Wheat, rye, rice all come under the category of insoluble fibre. The main source of soluble fibre is oat barn and fruit pectin. Other sources include psyllium husks and flax seeds. Some fruits and vegetables like legumes, beans, and peas are major sources of both soluble and insoluble fibres.

Study proves that intake of dietary fibres, mainly soluble fibres have been proven to reduce blood cholesterol levels, thus helping to reduce the risk of CHD. Recent findings provide evidence that viscous polysaccharides act in the gastrointestinal tract to reduce blood cholesterol by decreasing absorption of cholesterol or fatty acids and decreasing absorption of biliary cholesterol or bile acids (Bagger, Andersen, Nielsen, & Ryttig, 1996). Fibres may also affect lipid metabolism via altered concentration of hormones in serum either altered the short-chain fatty acids. Glucan, which is abundantly found in oats and barley is a water-soluble fibre, it has been shown to contain an active agent which is responsible for causing the alteration of cholesterol metabolism shown in animal models (Marlett & Slavin, 1997).

According to AHA (American Heart Association), the intakes of 25g to 30 g/day of fibres that come from foods provide an ample amount of nutrient with a minimum level of cholesterol. Mechanisms by which fibres may protect against CHD include lowering blood cholesterol (soluble fibres), attenuating blood triglyceride levels (mostly soluble fibres), decreasing hypertension (all fibres), and normalizing postprandial blood glucose levels (all fibres).

Proteins, Peptides, and Amino Acids

One of the major risk factors associated with CVD is hypertension. Angiotensin-converting enzyme (ACE) inhibitors are the main strategy to control hypertension. Although their use has been associated with several side effects such as hypotension, increased levels of potassium, reduced renal function, cough, angioedema, skin rashes and fetal abnormalities (FitzGerald, Murray, & Walsh, 2004). Proteins such as casein and whey protein are a rich source of ACE inhibitory peptides. There is a very limited number of studies done on a human which show that these peptides have valuable hypotensive effects. It has been hypothesized that excessive milk consumption may have an adverse effect on circulation due to its high calcium content, which promotes calcification and rigidification of large elastic arteries leading to myocardial ischemia (Gellman, Hare, Lowenstein, Gerstenblith, Coombs, Langenberg, … Resar, 2004).

Vegetable proteins are rich sources of arginine. L-arginine is a precursor of nitric oxide synthase which helps in the production of nitric oxide, which acts as a vasodilator thus helping to improve dysfunctional coronary sympathetic responses. Oral supplementation of L-arginine may be therapeutically useful in medically treated hypertensive patients with microvascular angina (Palloshi, Fragasso, Piatti, Monti, Setola, Valsecchi, … Margonato, 2004).

Plant Sterols

Phytosterols, also known as plant sterols are a group of compounds occur naturally in a wide range of plant products including vegetable oils, nuts, grains, seeds, wood pulp, and leaves. Studies on Plant sterols have been shown to reduce LDL cholesterol by 8-15%. Soy, corn and sunflower oil, all are plant-based sterols derived from natural grains. The prevailing studies have proved, the protective role of plant sterols in reducing the risk of CHD (Law, 2000). Studies have demonstrated that consumption of about 2-3gm per day of plant sterols/stanols reduce LDL cholesterol levels between 9%-20% although there is considerable variation amongst individuals (Cater, 2000). Little effect on HDL-Cholesterol or triglyceride levels has been reported. Margarine plant stanol ester has also been shown to be an effective adjunct to hypercholesterolemia treatment using statins and fibrates (Lichtenstein & Deckelbaum, 2001).

Prebiotics

Prebiotics are the nondigestible food component that has been reported to show beneficial effects in the host by selectively stimulating the growth of one or a limited number of bacterial populations in the colon (Gibson & Roberfroid, 1995). They are basically microbial food supplements, which improve the host's intestinal microbial tolerance and thereby have the potential to prevent major diseases like cancer and lower serum cholesterol (Kopp-Hoolihan, 2001). Non-digestible oligosaccharides (prebiotics) stimulates the growth of intestinal microflora (Pogodina, 1975). Inulin-type fructans are the only prebiotics for which sufficient data have been generated to allow their possible role as functional food which includes native inulin, enzymatically hydrolyzed inulin or oligofructose, and synthetic fructooligosaccharides (Roberfroid & Delzenne, 1998). Due to great consumer interest in reducing the heart disease, there is a boom of such nutraceuticals in the market.

Probiotics

Probiotics generally include the live microorganisms that are administered in a significant amount in the host, which confer valuable health benefits on the host. A probiotic may be defined classically as a usable microbial dietary supplement that beneficially affects the host through its effects in the intestinal tract. For human nutrition, the following definition has been proposed: *a live microbial food ingredient that is beneficial to health* (Salminen, Bouley, Boutron-Ruault, Cummings, Franck, Gibson,... Rowland, 1998). The main work of probiotic bacteria is to provide resistance to infection, boost the immune system, inhibit the growth of dangerous bacteria and to promote good digestion. (Smirnov, Reznik, V'iunitskaia, Sorokulova, Samgorodskaia, & Tofan, 1993). Probiotics are widely used in fermentation and dairy industry to prepare fermented dairy products such as yogurt or freeze-dried cultures]. Studied show that role of Probiotics (live organisms) in the form of a fermented milk product exert cholesterol-lowering properties, and non-digestible fermentable carbohydrate prebiotics has been shown to decrease triacylglycerol levels in animal studies.

Flaxseed

Flax seeds have cardioprotective effects in many ways. It prevents the body reabsorbing cholesterol. It's mucilaginous gelatinous texture bulks up the stool and gently pulls toxins, cholesterol and waste out of the body. Lignans which are an example of flaxseed helps to decrease plasma cholesterol (Mel'nikova, Gracheva, Belikov, Blatun, & Shcherbakova, 1993).

Flavonoids

Flavonoids are naturally occurring polyphenol which found in both free states and as glycosides. Polyphenolic compounds like, isoflavones, flavonoid glycosides, catechins, and anthocyanins which suggested playing a dominant role in the prevention of metabolic diseases and heart disease. The protective effect of these flavonoids is due to influence on arachidonic acid metabolism.Flavonoids are a basically potent source of antioxidants found in tea (green and black), wine, fruits, and vegetables. These antioxidants reduce platelet activation, but their role in the reduction in CHD is still unclear (Rimm, Katan, Ascherio, Stampfer, & Willett, 1996). Flavonols and flavones are subgroups of flavonoids. Since these compounds bear antioxidant properties, the intake of these dietary compounds is associated with a lower risk of fatal and nonfatal CHD. The wine polyphenol, resveratrol prevents the platelet aggregation via main inhibition of cyclooxygenase 1(COX) activity, this cyclooxygenase activity is mainly responsible for the synthesis of thromboxane A2, an inducer of the platelet aggregation and vasoconstrictor (Demrow, Slane, & Folts, 1995). The ability to stimulate Ca++- activated K+ channels and to enhance nitric oxide signaling in the endothelium are other pathways by which resveratrol exerts vasorelaxant activity (Schächinger, Britten, & Zeiher, 2000). The direct relation between cardiovascular diseases (CVDs) and oxidation of LDL is now well established. LDL oxidation is a hallmark of coronary heart diseases and myocardial infarctions. Experimental Studies have shown that resveratrol potentially inhibits the oxidation of the LDL particles via chelating copper or by direct scavenging of the free radicals. The well- known health benefits of tea is due to its polyphenolic metabolites which mainly help to protect from diabetes and another cardiovascular disease. (Rizvi & Zaid, 2009; Ankolekar, Terry, Johnson, Johnson, Barbosa, & Shetty, 2011). Due to its health beneficial properties, it is the most popular beverage in this globe and has to gain more and more attention. Tea based polyphenols which include theaflavins and catechins show multifunctional properties and is known to be effective in the prevention or treatment of various cancers, cardiovascular disease, chronic inflammation, obesity, metabolic syndrome, and neurodegenerative diseases. catechins. (−) epicatechin (EC), (−)-epigallocatechin (EGC), (−)-epicatechin-3-

gallate (ECG), and (−)-epigallocatechin-3-gallate (EGCG) are the biologically active components of green tea catechin.

Green tea has a various protective mechanism like- lowering lipid levels, reducing oxidative stress, inhibiting platelet aggregation, and decreasing apolipoprotein B levels and increasing the ratio of ApoA-1/ApoB. It was revealed that green tea consumption of ≥5 cups/d had a lower risk of CVD mortality as compared with those consumed <1 cup/day. Thus, concluded that green tea consumption is associated with reduced mortality due to cardiovascular disease. The effect on total and LDL cholesterol appear moderate but size on systolic blood pressure is small. Longer-term separate clinical trials evaluating the effects of green tea are still awaited.

Nuts

Nut contains various active compounds like unsaturated fats, plant fibers, and arginine. Unsaturated fats and plant fiber both have the capacity to reduce the level of LDL. Arginine is a precursor of nitric acid which is made in the walls of the blood vessel. It relaxes the blood vessels and prevents clotting. Nuts, especially walnuts contain alpha-linolenic acid. Alpha-linolenic acid is a precursor to omega-3 fatty acid, which helps protect against CVD. red yeast rice Chinese Monacolin K a natural food obtained after fermenting rice with. In red yeast rice major active compounds are Monacolin K and its related substances and they chemically resemble cholesterol-lowering drugs, statins, as effective HMGR inhibitors (Heber, 1999). Another component in red yeast rice, such as unsaturated fatty acids, phytosterols, flavonoids, and threonine derivatives may also contribute to the hypocholesterolemic effects.

ISSUES, SOLUTIONS, AND RECOMMENDATIONS

The relationship between dietary components and their health benefits is now being understood. Scientific regulatory and business frameworks must be in place to evaluate the vast data available in public domain for efficacy and safety of these novel food products. The improvements of corresponding new functional components should also be taken care of in the regulatory oversight. Herbal products are increasingly being used and are mostly available over the counter. In needs to be emphasized that there is no blanket proof that all herbal products are safe. Thus the regulatory oversight should also be for the food industry.

FUTURE RESEARCH DIRECTIONS

Currently, the functional foods present in the market represent a small fraction of products. The role of existing nutrients, advancement in the identification of bioactive compounds and health benefits of these compounds, as well as the intersection of genomics and nutrition science, grows almost daily with new insight. In spite of having much knowledge, additional research is needed in these areas to ensure that this emerging science continues to be valid for the benefit of society. There is an urgent need for a continuous supply of scientific hypotheses, to support the entire effort.

CONCLUSION

Hyperlipidemia is a prime cause of death worldwide. It seems reasonable to argue that changing lifestyles due to growing urbanization, unhealthy dietary habits coupled with sedentary nature of work are the major contributing factors towards an upsurge of CVD worldwide. Ecological studies and ancient evidence provide compelling evidence of a direct relationship between diet and hyperlipidemia. There is an increasing scientific awareness leading to the hypothesis that some food ingredients have beneficial effects over and above the provision of basic nutrients. Foods which are mainly of the plant origin contain many active compounds which may protect age-related diseases, such as cardiovascular, diabetes or cancers. Nutritional supplements may thus help to reduce the growing incidence of High lipid profile.

REFERENCES

Aldana, S. G., Greenlaw, R., Salberg, A., Merrill, R. M., Hager, R., & Jorgensen, R. B. (2007). The effects of an intensive lifestyle modification program on carotid artery intima-media thickness: A randomized trial. *American Journal of Health Promotion: AJHP*, *21*(6), 510–516. doi:10.4278/0890-1171-21.6.510 PMID:17674638

Ankolekar, C., Terry, T., Johnson, K., Johnson, D., Barbosa, A. C. L., & Shetty, K. (2011). Anti-hyperglycemia properties of Tea (Camellia sinensis) bioactives using in vitro assay models and influence of extraction time. *Journal of Medicinal Food*, *14*(10), 1190–1197. doi:10.1089/jmf.2010.0291 PMID:21859352

Appel, L. J. (2003). The effects of protein intake on blood pressure and cardiovascular disease. *Current Opinion in Lipidology*, *14*(1), 55–59. doi:10.1097/00041433-200302000-00010 PMID:12544662

Appel, L. J., Moore, T. J., Obarzanek, E., Vollmer, W. M., Svetkey, L. P., Sacks, F. M., & Karanja, N. (1997). A clinical trial of the effects of dietary patterns on blood pressure. DASH Collaborative Research Group. *The New England Journal of Medicine*, *336*(16), 1117–1124. doi:10.1056/NEJM199704173361601 PMID:9099655

Appel, L. J., Sacks, F. M., Carey, V. J., Obarzanek, E., Swain, J. F., Miller, E. R., ... OmniHeart Collaborative Research Group. (2005). Effects of protein, monounsaturated fat, and carbohydrate intake on blood pressure and serum lipids: Results of the OmniHeart randomized trial. *Journal of the American Medical Association*, *294*(19), 2455–2464. doi:10.1001/jama.294.19.2455 PMID:16287956

Arai, S. (1996). Studies on functional foods in Japan--state of the art. *Bioscience, Biotechnology, and Biochemistry*, *60*(1), 9–15. doi:10.1271/bbb.60.9 PMID:8824819

Bagger, M., Andersen, O., Nielsen, J. B., & Ryttig, K. R. (1996). Dietary fibres reduce blood pressure, serum total cholesterol and platelet aggregation in rats. *British Journal of Nutrition*, *75*(3), 483–493. doi:10.1079/BJN19960149 PMID:8785220

Banerjee, S. K., & Maulik, S. K. (2002). Effect of garlic on cardiovascular disorders: A review. *Nutrition Journal*, *1*(1), 4. doi:10.1186/1475-2891-1-4 PMID:12537594

Bose, K. S., & Sarma, R. H. (1975). Delineation of the intimate details of the backbone conformation of pyridine nucleotide coenzymes in aqueous solution. *Biochemical and Biophysical Research Communications*, *66*(4), 1173–1179. doi:10.1016/0006-291X(75)90482-9 PMID:2

Burr, M. L., Fehily, A. M., Gilbert, J. F., Rogers, S., Holliday, R. M., Sweetnam, P. M., ... Deadman, N. M. (1989). Effects of changes in fat, fish, and fibre intakes on death and myocardial reinfarction: Diet and reinfarction trial (DART). *Lancet (London, England)*, *2*(8666), 757–761. doi:10.1016/S0140-6736(89)90828-3 PMID:2571009

Carroll, D. N., & Roth, M. T. (2002). Evidence for the cardioprotective effects of omega-3 Fatty acids. *The Annals of Pharmacotherapy*, *36*(12), 1950–1956. doi:10.1345/aph.1A314 PMID:12452760

Cater, N. B. (2000). Plant stanol ester: Review of cholesterol-lowering efficacy and implications for coronary heart disease risk reduction. *Preventive Cardiology*, *3*(3), 121–130. doi:10.1111/j.1520-037X.2000.80370.x PMID:11834929

Cencic, A., & Chingwaru, W. (2010). The Role of Functional Foods, Nutraceuticals, and Food Supplements in Intestinal Health. *Nutrients*, *2*(6), 611–625. doi:10.3390/nu2060611 PMID:22254045

Defronzo, R. A. (1992). Insulin resistance, hyperinsulimemia and coronary artery disease a complex metabolic. *Journal of Cardiovascular Pharmacology*. PMID:1284137

Demrow, H. S., Slane, P. R., & Folts, J. D. (1995). Administration of wine and grape juice inhibits in vivo platelet activity and thrombosis in stenosed canine coronary arteries. *Circulation*, *91*(4), 1182–1188. doi:10.1161/01.CIR.91.4.1182 PMID:7850957

Elliott, P. (2003). Protein intake and blood pressure in cardiovascular disease. *The Proceedings of the Nutrition Society*, *62*(2), 495–504. doi:10.1079/PNS2003266 PMID:14506897

Evans, W. C. (1996). Trease and Evans' pharmacognosy (14th ed.). London: WB Saunders.

FitzGerald, R. J., Murray, B. A., & Walsh, D. J. (2004). Hypotensive peptides from milk proteins. *The Journal of Nutrition*, *134*(4), 980S–988S. doi:10.1093/jn/134.4.980S PMID:15051858

Folsom, A. R., Parker, E. D., & Harnack, L. J. (2007). Degree of concordance with DASH diet guidelines and incidence of hypertension and fatal cardiovascular disease. *American Journal of Hypertension*, *20*(3), 225–232. doi:10.1016/j.amjhyper.2006.09.003 PMID:17324731

Gaziano, T. A. (2005). Cardiovascular disease in the developing world and its cost-effective management. *Circulation*, *112*(23), 3547–3553. doi:10.1161/CIRCULATIONAHA.105.591792 PMID:16330695

Gellman, J., Hare, J. M., Lowenstein, C. J., Gerstenblith, G., Coombs, V., Langenberg, P., ... Resar, J. R. (2004). L-arginine ameliorates the abnormal sympathetic response of the dysfunctional human coronary microvasculature. *Angiology*, *55*(1), 1–8. doi:10.1177/000331970405500101 PMID:14759083

Gibson, G. R., & Roberfroid, M. B. (1995). Dietary modulation of the human colonic microbiota: Introducing the concept of prebiotics. *The Journal of Nutrition*, *125*(6), 1401–1412. PMID:7782892

Fitzmaurice, C., Allen, C., Barber, R. M., Barregard, L., Bhutta, Z. A., ... Naghavi, M. (2017). Global, Regional, and National Cancer Incidence, Mortality, Years of Life Lost, Years Lived With Disability, and Disability-Adjusted Life-years for 32 Cancer Groups, 1990 to 2015: A Systematic Analysis for the Global Burden of Disease Study. *JAMA Oncology*, *3*(4), 524–548. doi:10.1001/jamaoncol.2016.5688 PMID:27918777

Golbitz, P. (1995). Traditional soyfoods: Processing and products. *The Journal of Nutrition, 125*(3Suppl), 570S–572S. PMID:7884535

Hasler, C. M. (2002). The cardiovascular effects of soy products. *The Journal of Cardiovascular Nursing, 16*(4), 50–63, quiz 75–76. doi:10.1097/00005082-200207000-00006 PMID:12597262

Hathcock, J. (2001). Dietary supplements: How they are used and regulated. *The Journal of Nutrition, 131*(33s), 1114S–1117S. doi:10.1093/jn/131.3.1114S PMID:11238828

Heber, D. (1999). Dietary supplement or drug? The case for cholestin. *The American Journal of Clinical Nutrition, 70*(1), 106–108. doi:10.1093/ajcn/70.1.106 PMID:10393149

Hu, F. B., Stampfer, M. J., Manson, J. E., Rimm, E., Colditz, G. A., Speizer, F. E., ... Willett, W. C. (1999). Dietary protein and risk of ischemic heart disease in women. *The American Journal of Clinical Nutrition, 70*(2), 221–227. doi:10.1093/ajcn.70.2.221 PMID:10426698

Huang, C. L., & Sumpio, B. E. (2008). Olive oil, the mediterranean diet, and cardiovascular health. *Journal of the American College of Surgeons, 207*(3), 407–416. doi:10.1016/j.jamcollsurg.2008.02.018 PMID:18722947

Hutchins, A. M., Slavin, J. L., & Lampe, J. W. (1995). Urinary isoflavonoid phytoestrogen and lignan excretion after consumption of fermented and unfermented soy products. *Journal of the American Dietetic Association, 95*(5), 545–551. doi:10.1016/S0002-8223(95)00149-2 PMID:7722188

Kalra, E. K. (2003). Nutraceutical--definition and introduction. *AAPS PharmSci, 5*(3), E25. doi:10.1208/ps050325 PMID:14621960

Kohlmeier, M. (2015). *Nutrient metabolism: structures, functions, and genes*. Retrieved from http://alltitles.ebrary.com/Doc?id=11055728

Kopp-Hoolihan, L. (2001). Prophylactic and therapeutic uses of probiotics: A review. *Journal of the American Dietetic Association, 101*(2), 229–238, quiz 239–241. doi:10.1016/S0002-8223(01)00060-8 PMID:11271697

Law, M. (2000). Plant sterol and stanol margarines and health. *BMJ (Clinical Research Ed.), 320*(7238), 861–864. doi:10.1136/bmj.320.7238.861 PMID:10731187

Lichtenstein, A. H., & Deckelbaum, R. J. (2001). AHA Science Advisory. Stanol/sterol ester-containing foods and blood cholesterol levels. A statement for healthcare professionals from the Nutrition Committee of the Council on Nutrition, Physical Activity, and Metabolism of the American Heart Association. *Circulation*, *103*(8), 1177–1179. doi:10.1161/01.CIR.103.8.1177 PMID:11222485

Lopez, A. D., & Murray, C. C. (1998). The global burden of disease, 1990-2020. *Nature Medicine*, *4*(11), 1241–1243. doi:10.1038/3218 PMID:9809543

Lucas, M. L., Blair, J. A., Cooper, B., & Matty, A. J. (1975). Further investigations with pH microelectrodes into the jejunal microclimate in rat and man. *Gut*, *16*(10), 844. PMID:1331

Magrone, T., Perez de Heredia, F., Jirillo, E., Morabito, G., Marcos, A., & Serafini, M. (2013). Functional foods and nutraceuticals as therapeutic tools for the treatment of diet-related diseases [1]. *Canadian Journal of Physiology and Pharmacology*, *91*(6), 387–396. doi:10.1139/cjpp-2012-0307 PMID:23745830

Marlett, J. A., & Slavin, J. L. (1997). Position of the American Dietetic Association. *Journal of the American Dietetic Association*, *97*(10), 1157–1159. doi:10.1016/S0002-8223(97)00279-4 PMID:9336564

Matsuura, H. (2001). Saponins in garlic as modifiers of the risk of cardiovascular disease. *The Journal of Nutrition*, *131*(33s), 1000S–1005S. doi:10.1093/jn/131.3.1000S PMID:11238805

McGill, H. C. Jr. (1979). The relationship of dietary cholesterol to serum cholesterol concentration and to atherosclerosis in man. *The American Journal of Clinical Nutrition*, *32*(12Suppl), 2664–2702. doi:10.1093/ajcn/32.12.2664 PMID:389024

Mel'nikova, V. M., Gracheva, N. M., Belikov, G. P., Blatun, L. A., & Shcherbakova, E. G. (1993). The chemoprophylaxis and chemotherapy of opportunistic infections. *Antibiotiki I Khimioterapiia*, *38*(10–11), 44–48.

Messina, M. J., Persky, V., Setchell, K. D., & Barnes, S. (1994). Soy intake and cancer risk: A review of the in vitro and in vivo data. *Nutrition and Cancer*, *21*(2), 113–131. doi:10.1080/01635589409514310 PMID:8058523

Mozaffarian, D., Benjamin, E. J., Go, A. S., Arnett, D. K., Blaha, M. J., Cushman, M., ... Turner, M. B. (2016). Heart Disease and Stroke Statistics—2016 Update: A Report From the American Heart Association. *Circulation*, *133*(4), e38–e360. doi:10.1161/CIR.0000000000000350 PMID:26673558

Mukherjee, A. K. (1995). India's health - today and tomorrow. *Journal of the Indian Medical Association*, *93*(8), 312–315. PMID:8713248

Nag, T., & Ghosh, A. (2015). Prevalence of cardiovascular disease risk factors in a rural community in West Bengal, India. *International Journal of Medicine and Public Health*, *5*(4), 259. doi:10.4103/2230-8598.165941

Obarzanek, E., Sacks, F. M., Vollmer, W. M., Bray, G. A., Miller, E. R. III, Lin, P. H., ... Proschan, M. A. (2001). Effects on blood lipids of a blood pressure-lowering diet: The Dietary Approaches to Stop Hypertension (DASH) Trial. *The American Journal of Clinical Nutrition*, *74*(1), 80–89. doi:10.1093/ajcn/74.1.80 PMID:11451721

Palloshi, A., Fragasso, G., Piatti, P., Monti, L. D., Setola, E., Valsecchi, G., ... Margonato, A. (2004). Effect of oral L-arginine on blood pressure and symptoms and endothelial function in patients with systemic hypertension, positive exercise tests, and normal coronary arteries. *The American Journal of Cardiology*, *93*(7), 933–935. doi:10.1016/j.amjcard.2003.12.040 PMID:15050504

Patil, S. P. D. (2011). Speech by her Excellency, the President of India, Shrimati Pratibha Devisingh Patil at the presentation of the National Florence Nightingale Awards for nursing personnel. *Nursing Journal of India*, *102*(7), 146–147. PMID:22482305

Pogodina, V. V. (1975). Elizaveta Nilolaevna Levkovich-75th birthday. *Acta Virologica. English Ed.*, *19*(6), 509. PMID:2002

Position of the American Dietetic Association. (1999). Position of the American Dietetic Association. *Journal of the American Dietetic Association*, *99*(10), 1278–1285. doi:10.1016/S0002-8223(99)00314-4 PMID:10524397

Reddy, K. S. (1993). Cardiovascular diseases in India. *World Health Statistics Quarterly. Rapport Trimestriel De Statistiques Sanitaires Mondiales*, *46*(2), 101–107. PMID:8303903

Riemersma, R. A., Rice-Evans, C. A., Tyrrell, R. M., Clifford, M. N., & Lean, M. E. (2001). Tea flavonoids and cardiovascular health. *QJM: Monthly Journal of the Association of Physicians*, *94*(5), 277–282. doi:10.1093/qjmed/94.5.277 PMID:11353103

Rizvi, S. I., & Zaid, M. A. (2009). Effect of tea catechins on erythrocyte Ca^{++} -pump in type 2 diabetes mellitus. *Pharmaceutical Biology*, *47*(5), 440–443. doi:10.1080/13880200902822588

Roberfroid, M. B., & Delzenne, N. M. (1998). Dietary fructans. *Annual Review of Nutrition, 18*(1), 117–143. doi:10.1146/annurev.nutr.18.1.117 PMID:9706221

Salminen, S., Bouley, C., Boutron-Ruault, M. C., Cummings, J. H., Franck, A., Gibson, G. R., ... Rowland, I. (1998). Functional food science and gastrointestinal physiology and function. *British Journal of Nutrition, 80*(S1Suppl 1), S147–S171. doi:10.1079/BJN19980108 PMID:9849357

Scalbert, A., Manach, C., Morand, C., Rémésy, C., & Jiménez, L. (2005). Dietary polyphenols and the prevention of diseases. *Critical Reviews in Food Science and Nutrition, 45*(4), 287–306. doi:10.1080/1040869059096 PMID:16047496

Schächinger, V., Britten, M. B., & Zeiher, A. M. (2000). Prognostic impact of coronary vasodilator dysfunction on adverse long-term outcome of coronary heart disease. *Circulation, 101*(16), 1899–1906. doi:10.1161/01.CIR.101.16.1899 PMID:10779454

Schmoldt, A., Benthe, H. F., & Haberland, G. (1975). Digitoxin metabolism by rat liver microsomes. *Biochemical Pharmacology, 24*(17), 1639–1641. doi:10.1016/0006-2952(75)90094-5 PMID:10

Schwencke, J., & De Robichon-Szulmajster, H. (1976). The transport of S-adenosyl-L-methionine in isolated yeast vacuoles and spheroplasts. *European Journal of Biochemistry, 65*(1), 49–60. doi:10.1111/j.1432-1033.1976.tb10388.x PMID:6283

Senftleber, F. C., Halline, A. G., Veening, H., & Dayton, D. A. (1976). Reversed-phase liquid-chromatographic analysis of hemodialysate from uremic patients. *Clinical Chemistry, 22*(9), 1522–1527. PMID:8223

Sissayb, Thierry, Regnier, & Lise. (2006). Citrus sinensisdisease survey: knowledge, attitude and management practices in Ethiopia. *Tropical Research Journal*, (4), 1-9.

Smirnov, V. V., Reznik, S. R., V'iunitskaia, V. A., Sorokulova, I. B., Samgorodskaia, N. V., & Tofan, A. V. (1993). The current concepts of the mechanisms of the therapeutic-prophylactic action of probiotics from bacteria in the genus Bacillus. *Mikrobiolohichnyi Zhurnal (Kiev, Ukraine: 1993), 55*(4), 92–112.

Smith, R. (2005). Medical Journals Are an Extension of the Marketing Arm of Pharmaceutical Companies. *PLoS Medicine, 2*(5), e138. doi:10.1371/journal.pmed.0020138 PMID:15916457

Stampfer, M. J., Hu, F. B., Manson, J. E., Rimm, E. B., & Willett, W. C. (2000). Primary Prevention of Coronary Heart Disease in Women through Diet and Lifestyle. *The New England Journal of Medicine, 343*(1), 16–22. doi:10.1056/NEJM200007063430103 PMID:10882764

Watson, R. R., Gerald, J. K., & Preedy, V. R. (Eds.). (2011). *Nutrients, dietary supplements, and nutriceuticals: cost analysis versus clinical benefits*. New York: Humana Press.

Weltgesundheitsorganisation (Ed.). (2002). *Reducing risks, promoting healthy life*. Geneva: World Health Organization.

Wetmur, J. G. (1976). Hybridization and renaturation kinetics of nucleic acids. *Annual Review of Biophysics and Bioengineering*, *5*(1), 337–361. doi:10.1146/annurev.bb.05.060176.002005 PMID:7992

World Health Organization. (2009). *Cardiovascular disease; Fact sheet N°317. Geneva,473*. World Health Organization.

Section 5

Brain and Neurodegenerative Disorders

Chapter 9
Role of Diet, Functional Foods, and Nutraceuticals in Brain Disorders

Vandana Bharat Patravale
Institute of Chemical Technology, India

Shivraj Vasantrao Naik
Institute of Chemical Technology, India

Shrikant Ninaji Dhage
Institute of Chemical Technology, India

ABSTRACT

This chapter presents an overview of various complementary nutritional approaches for the management of brain disorders. Numerous epidemiological studies emphasize the growing burden of brain disorders worldwide. Due to the complex pathophysiology, lack of precise diagnostic and therapeutic options, there is growing need to have alternative approaches. One important strategy for the prevention and treatment of brain impairment is based on dietary supplements, functional foods, and nutraceuticals. The current chapter illustrates various aspects of available nutritional products for the brain disorder. Considering the recent surge in the nutritional products and as it destined to play an important role in future, existing regulatory framework is explained here which ensures purity, safety, and efficacy of the marketed products.

DOI: 10.4018/978-1-5225-3267-5.ch009

OVERVIEW OF BRAIN DISORDERS

Brain disorders are part of neurological disorders, which are described by WHO as diseases of the central and peripheral nervous system. These disorders include Alzheimer disease and other dementias, Parkinson's disease, traumatic disorders of the nervous system due to head trauma, brain tumors, epilepsy, cerebrovascular diseases including stroke, migraine and other headache disorders, multiple sclerosis, neuroinfections, and neurological disorders due to malnutrition. Symptoms and severity of brain disorders vary greatly.

Many bacterial, viral, fungal and parasitic infections can affect the nervous system. Brain disorders may be caused by aging, illness, genetics, or traumatic injury. Furthermore, the extension of life expectancy and the aging of the general populations in both developed and developing countries are likely to increase the occurrence of many chronic and progressive physical and mental conditions including neurological disorders. Harvard School of Public Health, World Health Organization (WHO) and the World Bank conducted a collaborative study called 'The Global Burden of Disease (GBD) study' which states that the neurological disorders were seriously underestimated by traditional epidemiological and health statistical methods that take into account only mortality rates but not disability rates (Murray, Lopez, WHO, World Bank, & Harvard School of Public Health, 1996). Based on these results, World Federation of Neurology (WFN) and WHO conducted an international Survey of Country Resources for Neurological Disorders including 109 countries and covering over 90% of the world's population. The findings show that there is a lack of resources for patients with neurological disorders in most of the parts of the world; they highlight inequalities in the access to neurological care across different populations, especially in those living in low-income countries and in the developing regions of the world (Janca, Aarli, Prilipko, Dua, Saxena, & Saraceno, 2006). Gooch et al. (2017) reported the United States alone carries a substantial fiscal burden resulting from the nearly 100 million Americans with a neurological disease which is nearly 800 billion dollars and is rapidly rising due to the aging of the U.S. (Gooch, Pracht, & Borenstein, 2017). There are various risk factors associated with the brain disorders. Older age and family history are the most significant factors for the neurodegenerative diseases. Brain tumors can affect people at any age. The personal risk of the brain disorders depends on the genetics and exposure to environmental risk factors like radiation. The risk of brain disorders is higher if the patient has stressful life experiences or a traumatic brain injury.

Diagnosis of Brain Disorders

Diagnostic tests and procedures are important tools that facilitate physicians to ensure or rule out the presence of a brain disorder or different medical condition. In the previous century, an autopsy of the dead patient was the only way to make a diagnosis of the neurological disorder. Due to the extensive research made regarding the characteristics of the illness, and advancement in the diagnostic techniques permit scientists and physicians to envision within the living brain and monitor neurological activity. This has given physicians a powerful tool for the diagnosis of the brain disorders at early stages. Evaluation and diagnosis of brain disorders are very complicated and complex process as similar symptoms appear in different disorders and also some brain disorders do not have definite causes, biomarkers or tests. Various diagnostic imaging techniques and biochemical tests are used for the detection and treatment of neurological disorders. The results of these tests help in planning an appropriate treatment.

Limitations of Current Treatment Approaches

The pharmaceutical industry has shown promising progress in the diagnosis and treatment of a number of diseases; however, it is lagging behind in the area of brain disorders. There is definite medical therapy for some brain disorders; for example, millions of people with mental disorders live normal lives whereas other disorders, like neurodegenerative diseases and some traumatic brain injuries, have no promising cure. Patients with these conditions significantly face permanent changes in their behavior and mental abilities. In such cases, treatment focuses on supporting people in learning to live with the disorder and retain as much independence as possible. Drug approvals for the treatment of various brain disorders are significantly fewer compared to other diseases. The factors affecting for this failure includes incomplete understanding of both disease pathophysiology and drug delivery systems to the brain, the complicated chemical reactions driving human consciousness, higher risk of clinical failure, extended drug development time and cost (Pardridge, 2002b). The outlook depends on the type and severity of the brain disorder. For example, receptor modifying drugs are used successfully in the treatment of Schizophrenia and depression; however, an incomplete understanding of the functionality of these receptors, in combination with the basic genetic differences between patients, has resulted in the variable therapeutic efficacy and substantial side effects. Additionally, lack of truly representative animal models to study brain disorders complicates the treatment process. Though several symptoms have been reproduced in animals, there will always be differences between the species which limits the prediction of treatment efficacy (Rockenstein, Crews, & Masliah, 2007). Central nervous system is protected by the blood–brain barrier (BBB) which is a homeostatic defense mechanism designed for the protection against pathogens and toxins by regulating solute entry via the transcellular route; however, this also limits the ability to deliver therapeutically beneficial compounds as well. Still small lipophilic molecules of size less than 400 Da can pass BBB and proves to be the effective treatment modality in various brain disorders but many biotechnologically derived products such as monoclonal antibodies, enzymes and engineered proteins having larger molecular size fails to pass through BBB and thus making them unsuitable candidates for the effective treatment (Fischer, Gottschlich, & Seelig, 1998; Pardridge, 2007). Currently, there is increasing interest of the researchers in the development of successful delivery systems using the principles of both biotechnology and nanotechnology. BBB permeability of many novel compounds has been improved significantly by using molecular engineering approach of biotechnology to develop complex therapeutic moieties with various functional ligands, such as monoclonal antibodies or receptor binding functionalities. Nanotechnology has been utilized to develop drug delivery systems capable of delivering high doses of the drug *in vitro* and *in vivo*. Efficacy of treatment of brain disorders has been enhanced successfully by combining these two technologies(Pardridge, 2002a).

Nano Systems Targeting the Blood Brain Barrier

Silva defined nanotechnology as the development of a system or device having a functional organization in at least one dimension on the nanometer scale (Silva, 2007). Nanoparticles have been used extensively in drug delivery systems as they offer various advantages over conventional delivery systems such as bioavailability enhancement, site-targeted drug delivery specifically to the CNS and for medical imaging (Kabanov & Gendelman, 2007; Kreuter, 2007). Nanoparticles have a solid core-shell structure of less than 1000 nm in diameter and preferably less than 100 nm for delivery to the CNS. Formulation of nanoparticles generally utilizes biocompatible materials to provide a small size, high surface materials capable of penetrating a number of biological tissues. The performance of nanoparticles *in vivo* is affected by various factors such as particle size, surface charge, and composition. Nanoparticles are rapidly cleared by the reticuloendothelial system (RES) which limits the *in vivo* residence time. Nanoparticles have been explored to enhance BBB penetration. To demonstrate the effect of nanoparticle properties on *in vivo* performance, Jallouli et al. (2007) studied the binding, uptake, and transcytosis of 60-nm highly porous maltodextrin nanoparticles based on surface charge and inner composition. They proved that differences in surface charge affect the mechanism of transport of nanoparticles across CNS (Jallouli, Paillard, Chang, Sevin, & Betbeder, 2007). Kuo et al. (2007) showed that nanoparticle composition and the carrier selection affects on the BBB penetration. In this study, they evaluated the *in vitro* performance of nanoparticles prepared separately by using solid lipids, methylmethacrylate-sulfopropylmethylacrylate, and poly butyl cyanoacrylate. They found that there was a synergistic effect of the carrier material with drug loading to affect BBB permeation (Kuo & Su, 2007). Trojan horse technologies can be used to enhance the delivery and targeting of nanoparticles. Liposomes have been explored extensively for CNS targeting. In contrast with the nanoparticles, liposomes have a lipid bilayer encapsulating the contents which are typically in liquid form. Schmidt et al. (2003) have successfully explored the use of PEGylated liposomes for the delivery of glucocorticosteroids in the treatment of multiple sclerosis. They used prednisolone as a model drug and proved that the PEGylated liposome formulation showed 5 fold higher therapeutic efficacy (Schmidt, Metselaar, Wauben, Toyka, Storm, & Gold, 2003). From the above examples, it is evident that various nanotechnology approaches have proven to be excellent drug delivery strategies for targeting CNS with higher drug loading.

NUTRITIONAL INTERVENTION IN BRAIN DISORDERS

The concept of having food which is enriched in therapeutically beneficial actives is largely based on the principle, *Let food be thy medicine, and medicine be thy food* advocated by Hippocrates (460–377 BC), the well-recognized father of modern medicine, emphasize the association between nutrition and human health, and conceptualized the relationship between the use of appropriate foods for health and their therapeutic benefits (da Costa, 2017; Katan, 2002). 'Nutraceuticals', 'dietary supplements' and 'functional foods', as well as other terms, are all used interchangeably, though these have significant differences – albeit not always evident (Hardy, 2000). Dietary supplements contain nutrients derived from food products and are commonly concentrated in capsule, powder, liquid or pill form. Kalra described 'functional food' as a product containing the necessary nutrients – including vitamins – for survival, while 'nutraceuticals', as per definitions, not only are complementary to the diet, but also aid in the prevention and/or treatment of disease and/or health disorder(s) (Kalra, 2003; da Costa, 2017).

DIETARY SUPPLEMENTS

Dietary supplements include a wide range of products, including vitamins and minerals, herbal products and botanical agents, and extracts from organs or glands (DeAngelis & Fontanarosa, 2003). The Dietary Supplement Health and Education Act (DSHEA) defines the term, 'dietary supplement', as 'a product (other than tobacco) that is intended to supplement the diet which contains one or more of the following dietary ingredients: a vitamin, a mineral, an herb or other botanical, an amino acid, a dietary substance for use by man to supplement the diet by increasing the total daily intake or a concentrate, metabolite, constituent, extract, or combination of any ingredient described above'. The law further states that dietary supplements in part as products taken orally that contain a 'dietary ingredient' mentioned above. Dietary supplements are provided in various forms such as tablets, capsules, powders, and liquids. Also according to DSHEA, the product should be labeled as a 'dietary supplement' and it is not represented for use as a conventional food or as a sole item of a meal or the diet (Kalra, 2003). Currently marketed dietary supplement products includes vitamin and mineral products, botanical or herbal products, amino acid products, enzyme supplements etc.

People use dietary supplements for a wide variety of reasons such as to compensate the conditions that limit the intake of essential vitamins and nutrients like improper diets, medical conditions, or eating habits. Postmenopausal women take dietary supplements to counter a rapid drop in estrogen levels (USFDA, 2016).

Understanding Dietary Supplements

FDA suggests that consumer must refer to the health care professionals prior the use of dietary supplements, though they are often claimed as safe and natural. Dietary supplements contain the components with strong biological effects. Hence, they cannot be taken blindly as there may be a risk for those who are suffering from any health-related problem. There is certain advice to be considered while taking the dietary supplements as discussed below:

1. Dietary supplements are the complementary health approaches and not proposed to treat, diagnose, or improve the disease condition and they should not be seen as a replacement for the drugs. However, FDA has approved various supplements that are useful in reducing the risk of certain diseases and are authorized to make label claims accordingly. For example, folic acid supplements may make a claim about reducing the risk of birth defects related to brain and spinal cord.

2. Many dietary supplements from the herbal origin contain a number of potent compounds with diverse biological activities. Taking a combination of supplements or using these products together with medicine can lead to untoward results.
3. Many dietary supplements are not advisable in certain conditions such as pregnancy, nursing mothers, or children. Similarly, these supplements are not tested for the possible unwanted effects before, during, or after surgery. For example, supplements containing garlic, ginkgo biloba, ginseng, and Vitamin E has bleeding as a potential side effect. Also, the supplements having kava and valerian act as sedatives which can synergies anesthetics activity during surgery (USFDA, 2015).

Dietary Supplements in Brain Disorders

It is well-established fact that relative abundance or deficiency of any specific nutrients can affect the normal cognitive functions. Dietary factors were shown to have effects on neuronal function and synaptic plasticity and its influences vital mechanisms that are responsible for the effects of diet on brain health and mental function. Several gut hormones that are produced in the brain itself are known to influence the cognitive ability. In addition, well-established regulators of synaptic plasticity, such as brain-derived neurotrophic factor, can function as metabolic modulators, responding to peripheral signals such as food intake. To understand how diet can affect or promote mental fitness, it is necessary to know molecular basis of the effects of food on cognition.

CURRENTLY USED DIETARY SUPPLEMENTS

Here, we will discuss various dietary supplements which are proven to be beneficial for improving various brain conditions. Various dietary supplements for brain disorders are summarized in Table 1.

Polyunsaturated Fatty Acids (PUFA's)

Saturated and monounsaturated fatty acids can be synthesized de novo within the brain, but PUFAs are mainly supplied by the food. The PUFAs linoleic acid (LNA) and α-linolenic acid (ALA) are obtained through the diet and act as precursors of arachidonic acid (ARA) and docosahexaenoic acid (DHA), which are also PUFA (Bazinet & Layé, 2014). Omega-3 fatty acids (e.g. alpha-linolenic acid) and omega-6 fatty acids (e.g. linoleic acid) are the key players among various families

Table 1. Dietary supplements for brain disorders

Dietary Supplements	Mechanism	References
Polyunsaturated Fatty Acids	Neuroprotective under conditions of reduced GST activity, diminished SAM, increased accumulation of SAH, and deprived folate	Panza et al., (2009)
Multivitamin and Mineral Supplements	During periconception promote lower incidence of ASD children Improve sleep, reduce autistic symptoms and ameliorate biomarkers of energy production and oxidative stress, improving mitochondrial function	Adams et al., (2011)
Vitamin B	Inhibit tau hyper-phosphorylation and accumulation in hippocampus and cortex	Wei et al., (2011)
Grape Seed Extract	Reduces Aβ levels and microgliosis in the brain and serum of the mice.	Y.-J. Wang et al., (2009)
Ginkgo Biloba Extract	Antioxidant elicits neuro recovery of damaged midbrain DA neurones, improves locomotion	(Rojas, Montes, Rojas, Serrano-García, & Rojas-Castañeda, 2012)
Rhinacanthus Nasutus	Glutamate and Amyloid-β Neurotoxicity	(Brimson, Brimson, Brimson, Rakkhitawatthana, & Tencomnao, 2012)

of polyunsaturated fatty acids. The human body is unable to synthesize linoleic acid hence it must be supplied as a dietary supplement. All other members of the omega–6 group are derivatives of linoleic acid while the parent compound of the omega–3 group is alpha-linolenic acid (ALA) (Yehuda, 2003). The human brain is highly augmented with fatty acids. In the brain, PUFA's are present in the form of esterified to the phospholipid cell membrane. PUFA's performs many vital biological functions such as signal transduction, regulate several processes within the brain, such as neurotransmission, cell survival, and neuroinflammation, and thereby mood and cognition. PUFA levels and the signaling pathways are altered in various neurological disorders, including Alzheimer's disease and major depression. PUFAs as dietary supplements open as a new array of complementary health approach for the prevention and treatment of brain disorders (Bazinet & Layé, 2014).

Trace Elements

Adequate levels of various trace elements in the human body are essential for the brain to carry out its normal functions. Trace elements work as cofactors for the stabilization of proteins and transcription materials, catalysis of enzymes, and cellular transport (Parker, Koistinaho, White, & Kanninen, 2013). Enzymatic antioxidants such as superoxide dismutase (SOD), catalase (CAT), and glutathione peroxidase

(Gpx) act as a defense system against reactive oxygen species. Trace elements form the basic components of the enzymatic defense system. Their role in many diseases including neurological and psychiatric disorders have been examined by many researchers (Vural, Demirin, Kara, Eren, & Delibas, 2010) whereas their imbalance is associated with number of neurological conditions such as Alzheimer's disease, Parkinson's disease, Huntington's disease, and amyotrophic lateral sclerosis (ALS) (Parker, Koistinaho, White, & Kanninen, 2013).

1. **Zinc:** Brain has the highest concentration of Zinc (Zn) as compared with the other organ systems and it is almost 10 times more than blood plasma level (Mocchegiani, Bertoni-Freddari, Marcellini, & Malavolta, 2005). Zn metabolism plays a central role in the synthesis and degradation of carbohydrates, lipids, proteins, nucleic acids and other micronutrients (Chasapis, Loutsidou, Spiliopoulou, & Stefanidou, 2012). The role of zinc in various brain disorders including behavior and cognitive functioning has been studied in relation to dietary zinc deficiency and catalysis of enzymes for a large number of cellular processes (Bitanihirwe & Cunningham, 2009). Zinc is essential in many important events such as neurogenesis, neuronal migration and synaptogenesis and its deficiency could interfere with neurotransmission and subsequent neuropsychological behavior (Bhatnagar & Taneja, 2001). Thus, an appropriate amount of zinc must be provided as dietary supplements for healthy brain functioning.
2. **Magnesium:** Magnesium (Mg) is one of the most important cofactors playing a crucial role in a number of metabolic events in the body including protein synthesis, production and storage of cellular energy, DNA and RNA synthesis, nerve transmission, muscular contraction, blood pressure, glucose, and insulin metabolism. In the case of brain disorders, Mg levels in plasma were found to be low in a study of patients with Alzheimer's disease (Vural, Demirin, Kara, Eren, & Delibas, 2010). In a study, it is demonstrated that patients suffering from Alzheimer's disease showed better improvement in the symptoms after receiving Mg with Memantine. Mg as dietary supplements has shown to improve the conditions of mental depressions with fewer side effects (Ozturk & Cillier, 2006).
3. **Selenium:** It is a well-known fact that the oxidative stress is responsible for the generation of reactive oxygen species (ROS) which is the major cause of many brain disorders (Wang & Michaelis, 2010). Selenium (Se) shows a promising neuroprotective effect against ROS-induced cell injury. Se has a crucial role in the brain disorders; not only due to its antioxidant property, but also through its involvement in the modulation of neurogenesis, regulating mitochondrial

dynamics, redox balance, and maintenance of calcium channels (Cardoso, Roberts, Bush, & Hare, 2015). Thus, various neurological disorders caused by the deficiency of Se can be prevented and treated by supplementing it via diet.

4. **Iron:** In the brain, iron is important for the oxygen transport, neurotransmitter synthesis, electron transfer, and myelin production (Stankiewicz, Panter, Neema, Arora, Batt, & Bakshi, 2007). Both the iron deficiency and iron excess is responsible for certain brain disorders. Various studies have shown that neurotransmitters and the associated receptors are altered due to reduced oxygen supply in case of iron deficiency leading to a number of brain disorders (Agarwal, 2001). On the other hand, high concentrations of reactive iron can enhance oxidative-stress-induced neuronal susceptibility (Zecca, Youdim, Riederer, Connor, & Crichton, 2004). Diet rich in iron can easily treat such complications of brain disorders.
5. **Copper:** Copper (Cu) is a vital trace element essential for a variety of enzymatic activities, proper neurodevelopment and neurological function (Desai & Kaler, 2008). It is involved in the generation of toxic ROS due to its redox activity which is responsible for mitochondrial damage, DNA breakage, and neuronal injury (Scheiber, Mercer, & Dringen, 2014). Impaired copper metabolism is additionally inferred in an increasing variety of different neurologic conditions (Bandmann, Weiss, & Kaler, 2015).

In conclusion, deficiency in some of these trace elements in the body can lead to various brain disorders characterized by progressive and permanent damage to the brain. Trace element deficiencies are caused majorly due to improper eating habits and diseases related with them can sometimes cause serious public health issues. It is possible to treat or stop the progression of these diseases through the early detection of deficiency and replacement of deficient trace elements with dietary interventions.

Botanical or Herbal Products

1. Ginkgo Biloba

Ginkgo tree extracts are widely used as complementary products which have its origin in traditional Chinese and Japanese medicine. Biologically active components are Ginkgo flavonoids, obtained from leaf extracts; however, these constituents differ as per its botanical source. Ginkgo biloba has shown promise in various brain disorders by modulating excitotoxic glutamatergic neurotransmission, reduction of amyloid-β aggregation and free radical scavenging activity which reduces the damage to cell membranes causing malfunction and cell death in the brain. EGb

761®, is the widely studied Ginkgo biloba extract which is available on the market containing ginkgolides, bilobalide, and flavonoids (Nash & Shah, 2015). Ginkgold® and Ginkoba® are manufactured by Dr. Willmar Schwabe GmbH & Co. in Germany and are marketed in the United States by Nature's Way Products, Inc. and Pharmaton Natural Health Products, respectively (Tatli, 2015).

2. Bacopa Monnieri

Bacopa monnieri (L.) Wettst. (family, Plantaginaceae) known commonly as Brahmi, is a perennial, creeping herb native to India which has been explored medicinally for thousands of years by Ayurvedic physicians in India. Numerous ancient Indian Ayurvedic texts including the Charaka Samhita (2500 B.C.) and the Sushruta Samhita (2300 B.C.) exhibits clear reference to its action on the central nervous system (Nemetchek, Stierle, Stierle, & Lurie, 2017). The active components of Brahmi are a mixture of saponins including bacoside A, bacopasides I and II, and bacopasaponin C. Number of studies shows Brahmi's neuroprotective effect both in *vitro* and *in vivo* Alzheimer's disease models. Similarly, Brahmi also has the ability to regulate neuroinflammation (Chauhan & Mehla, 2014).

Vitamins

Various vitamins have reported being effective in the clinical management of neurological disorders, out of which vitamin D and vitamin B plays a crucial role.

1. Vitamin D

Vitamin D is involved in neuroprotection, modulation of pro-inflammatory cytokine-induced cognitive dysfunction, and synthesis of calcium-binding proteins as well as acetylcholine which is a well-known neurotransmitter. Alzheimer's disease is associated with low serum vitamin D concentrations which can be treated effectively by providing dietary supplementation of vitamin D (Annweiler, Llewellyn, & Beauchet, 2013). Vitamin D also regulates signal transduction and gene expression. It shows promise in the prevention and treatment of brain disorders through the regulation of calcium-sensing receptor expression, increasing the clearance of amyloid β peptides, and modulating inflammatory cytokine expression (Annweiler, Rolland, Schott, Blain, Vellas, Herrmann, & Beauchet, 2012). Calciterol (1,25-dihydroxyvitamin D3) is the most effective supplementation form of vitamin D in treating the progression of Alzheimer's disease and Parkinson's disease (Suzuki, Yoshioka, Hashimoto, Murakami, Noya, Takahashi, & Urashima, 2013; Peterson, Murchison, Zabetian, Leverenz, Watson, Montine, & Quinn, 2013).

2. Vitamin B

Parkinson's disease is characterized with the higher plasma homocysteine levels damaging dopaminergic nerves. Some studies have demonstrated increased risk of Parkinson's disease with decreased intake of vitamin B, as vitamin B9 (folate) and B12 plays a fundamental role in the metabolism of homocysteine thus halting the disease progression (Shen, 2015).

FUNCTIONAL FOODS

The term 'functional food' was originated in Japan. Apart from normal nutrition, functional foods offer various health benefits. These are different from medical foods and dietary supplements, but they may overlap with those foods which are developed for special dietary uses and fortified foods. Japan is the first country which has made certain regulatory legislation i.e. FOSHU (Foods of Specified Health Use) legislation and market the functional foods. There is no agreement between Europe and the USA regarding a concrete definition of functional foods, leading to a series of different terms: nutraceutical, designer food, pharma-food, etc., which has contributed to increasing the confusion among professionals and consumers.

It is important to highlight that functional food must be a food, not a drug. Functional foods must exhibit beneficial effects after consuming normal amounts within the normal diet. The ultimate goal of the food industry should be to develop functional foods for improving life quality of the general population. The 'American dietetic association' has given a glossary containing major basic definitions for functional foods. They are:

- **Functional Food:** Any food or modified ingredient that can make a beneficial effect beyond that provided by common nutrients;
- **Chemopreventive Agent:** Food compound nutrient or otherwise that has been scientifically investigated as a potential inhibitor of carcinogenesis;
- **Designer Food:** Processed foods that are supplemented with food ingredients, naturally rich in substances that prevent diseases involving genetic engineering of foods;
- **Pharma-Food:** Food or nutrient with potential health or medical use, including prevention and treatment of diseases;
- **Phytochemical:** Substances found in fruits and vegetables that can be ingested daily (in grams) and those that exhibit a potential to modulate human metabolism by favoring prevention of cancer and other diseases;

- **Nutraceutical:** Substance considered as food or a part of it that offers health or medical benefits, including prevention and treatment of diseases.

Due to the increasing demand from the population for foods that promote health, functional foods are one of the fastest growing sectors of the food industry (Mollet & Lacroix, 2007). In 2015 the global functional foods market size was USD 129.39 billion which is expected to reach USD 255.10 billion by 2024 (Grand View Research, 2016). Functional foods must generally be provided to people with good organoleptic properties and in the usual daily dietary pattern (Augustin, 2001; Kwak & Jukes, 2001). Extensive research has been done in the development of functional foods for improving the health of the general public. New functional food products launched in the global food market have followed the route of fortification or addition of desirable nutrients and bioactive including vitamins, minerals, antioxidants, plant extracts, prebiotics, probiotics, and fiber augmentations. Many of these ingredients to be added are susceptible to degradation and can interact with other components of the food matrix which may lead towards a loss in quality of the functional food products.

To overcome issues related to fortification, the additional bioactive ingredient ought to be isolated from environments that promote degradation or undesirable interactions (Smith & Charter, 2010). Though certain natural foods such as strawberries or onions are claimed as functional foods, but only those foods which are submitted to certain methodologies such as addition or removal of a component, modification of the food processing, genetic engineering, etc., to develop new products with additional value are considered as functional foods. The most important components that can be added to food are:

- **Probiotics**: Certain living microorganisms (for example bacteria like Lactobacilli and Bifidobacteria) which when ingested in certain amounts, have a positive impact on host health, which offers additional nutritional effects (Isolauri, 2001). They can be given with fermented foods such as yogurt, fermented vegetables or meats.
- **Prebiotics**: These are the short-chain carbohydrates that may be fermented in a large bowl which provides beneficial health effects on the microflora on the host, such as fiber, inulin, lactulose, sugar alcohols.
- **Synbiotics:** A mixture of prebiotics and probiotics.
- **Nutrients**: Minerals, vitamins, fatty acids or dietary fiber, for example, that are specific and have a targeted action (Lopez-Varela, Gonzalez-Gross, & Marcos, 2002).

Health Effects of Functional Foods

Regular consumption of functional foods reduces the risk for several chronic diseases, such as neurological disorders, cardiovascular disease, cancer, diabetes, hypertension, and osteoporosis (Lopez-Varela, Gonzalez-Gross, & Marcos, 2002). Generally, all foods may be claimed as functional, as they provide some nutritive health effects, taste, or flavor. The term functional serves different meaning when applied to foods as providing an additional health benefit beyond that of basic nutritional needs. Functional food science has been originated from the joint collaborative venture of food sciences and the public need. It is the combination of food science, nutrition, and medicine as it produces nourishment that crosses between food and pharmaceuticals. Specifically, researchers study food components and their beneficial health effects. Functional food scientists determine the health effects and safe dosages of functional foods. Despite the extensive research, universal definition of functional foods is not available leading to numerous global consequences. Due to the ambiguity about the concept of 'functional food' between various regulatory bodies, the sense of overall mistrust about the health benefits claims prevail. While 'functional food' has generated billions of dollars in sales worldwide, the lack of a standard definition has prevented functional food scientists from delivering functional food to chronically ill populations (Martirosyan & Singh, 2015). There are various steps involved in the designing and development of functional foods as shown in Figure 1 (GEN, 2005).

Functional Foods in Brain Disorder

There is marked increase in the development of the functional foods due to the growing burden of chronic diseases such as neurological disorders and population aging. Alzheimer's disease is another important health problem that remains without cure so far. Functional foods have shown promise where drugs have failed to be efficacious. Functional foods containing antioxidants plays a crucial role in the treatment of neurodegenerative diseases by maintaining the integrity of neurons through suppression of apoptosis and necrosis. Alzheimer's disease is the most common form of dementia and which may be fatal at later stages. Accumulation of amyloid β proteins, mitochondrial dysfunction, and release of iron and copper are the most frequent causes of the disease progression. Quercetin proves to be helpful in the disease management by chelating these metals which could reduce the pathological severity. Tocopherol and ascorbic acid are used as promising nutritional therapy. Carotenoids have been explored successfully in the treatment of dementia. Caffeic acid and catechins inhibit peroxynitrite-induced dopamine oxidation thus exhibiting

Figure 1. Steps for the designing and development of functional foods

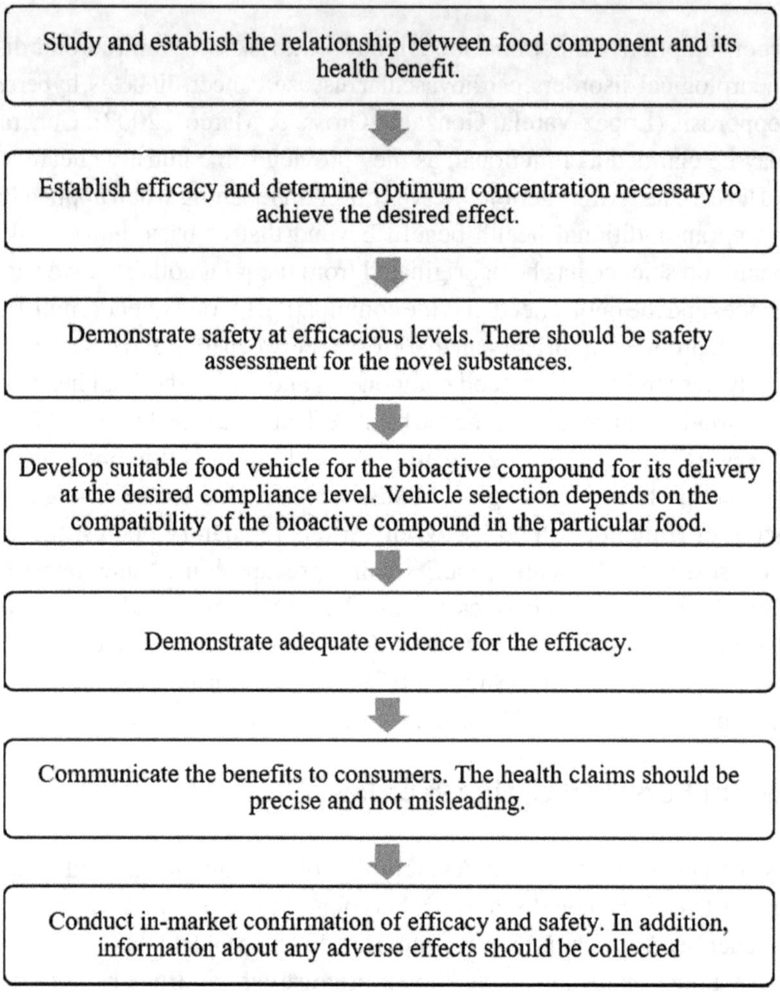

prominent anti-Alzheimer's activity (Ferrari & Torres, 2003). These all are the natural foods which are efficacious in the management of various brain disorders. There are three functional foods which are developed and marketed having regulatory approval that claims to offer symptomatic benefits in the treatment of Alzheimer's disease *viz.* Axona®, Souvenaid®, and CerefolinNAC®. Axona® provides ketone bodies as alternative energy source to the neurons, Souvenaid® provides precursors thought to enhance synaptic function and CerefolinNAC® minimizes the role of oxidative stress related to memory loss (Thaipisuttikul & Galvin, 2012).

Axona

It is a functional food developed by Accera, Inc., indicated for the clinical management of the impairment of metabolic processes associated with mild to moderate Alzheimer's disease. It contains caprylic triglyceride, a medium-chain triglyceride and it is Generally Recognised As Safe (GRAS) by the FDA which is obtained from fractionation of coconut oil. In Alzheimer's disease brain's ability to use glucose as a normal energy source gets impaired. During the digestion of Axona, the triglycerides get broken down into medium-chain fatty acids which rapidly pass to the liver where they undergo oxidation to form the ketone bodies which serves as alternative energy source to the brain. Axona was formulated for oral administration and was first sold in March 2009. Axona was being administered to about 30,000 patients in the US by 2012. Nestlé has been investing heavily in the area of medical nutrition and nutrition-based solutions designed to tackle neurodegenerative diseases. In July 2012, Nestlé acquired a stake in U.S.-based Accera, maker of Axona (Axona, 2017).

NUTRACEUTICALS

The industrialized world of this century forced to deal with new challenges such as excess healthcare costs, longer life expectancy and changes in a living manner. Nutritionists have enthusiastically accepted the idea of 'optimal nutrition', which focuses on optimizing daily diet quality in terms of its nutraceutical value for the proper health. As a result, development of nutraceuticals comes into play. The term 'Nutraceuticals' was coined by Stephen DeFelice, who defined it as a "foods (or part of a food) that provide medical or health benefits, including the prevention and/or treatment of a disease" (DeFelice, 1995). Due to the close resemblance of the term, 'Nutraceuticals' with 'dietary supplements' and 'functional foods', it is often used as interchangeably for later and vice versa. Similarly due to the lack of clear definition from regulatory bodies added to the confusion. So it is necessary to have a clear sharply defined and quantifiable concept, which will eventually help for effective regulatory implementation and will avoid conflicts. After studying the number of available definition in public domain, Palthur et al. comes up with the working definition which says 'A nutraceutical is a food or a part of a food for oral administration with demonstrated safety and health benefits beyond the basic nutritional functions to supplement diet, presented in a nonfood matrix or nonconventional food formats, in such a quantity that exceeds those that could be obtained from normal foods and with such frequency as required to realize such properties', and is labeled as a 'nutraceutical' (Palthur, Palthur, & Chitta, 2010).

Insights Into the Actions of Nutraceuticals

Here, we will discuss various nutraceuticals reported for assisting in the prevention and treatment of brain diseases by reducing doses of drugs or alleviating side effects. Traditional medicinal knowledge or tribal practices offer nutritious agents that serve as a basis for understanding their molecular actions that cure diseases. In recent years, there has been increasing evidence that shows that these nutraceuticals can act as effective neuroprotective agents. The goal then is to elucidate how these bioactive molecules make the brain healthier. Underlined mechanisms of neuroprotection at the cellular, biochemical, and molecular levels are often been due to a direct antioxidant effect and/or to an anti-inflammatory action (Kelsey, Wilkins, & Linseman, 2010; Costa, Garrick, Roque, & Pellacani, 2016).

Nutraceuticals in Brain Disorders

In past numerous attempts have been made to categories the nutraceuticals based on origin, form, in terms of their effects on the body etc., however classification based on their chemical nature and/or active ingredients remains the most accepted one (Espín, García-Conesa, & Tomás-Barberán, 2007; da Costa, 2017). Numerous studies have demonstrated the role of nutraceuticals in the prevention and treatment of neurological disorders. Various nutraceuticals explored for brain disorders are summarized in Table 2.

Polyphenols

Polyphenols are the rich source of antioxidants of our diet and are widely spread components of various fruits, vegetables, cereals, dry legumes, chocolates, and beverages. Many nutritionists attracted towards dietary polyphenols because of their promising health effects.

Antioxidant Activity of Polyphenols as Neuro Nutraceuticals

Antioxidant activity is the most explored effect of polyphenols (Shefa, Yeo, Kim, Song, Jung, Jeong, & Huh, 2017; Cilla, Alegría, Attanzio, Garcia-Llatas, Tesoriere, & Livrea, 2017). Among the major pathological reasons for neurodegenerative disorders are oxidative damage to neuronal molecules, accumulation of iron ion species in the brain, and decreased cellular reserve antioxidant pool. Polyphenols exert their antioxidant effects through different mechanisms like the interaction with the HIF-1 alpha pathway, regulation of reactive oxygen species by interacting with

Table 2. Nutraceuticals for brain disorders

Nutraceuticals	Mechanism	References
Blueberry Polyphenols	Augment the increased IGF-1 expression and antagonizes LPS, DA- Aβ (42)-induced deficits in CAR in primary hippocampus neuronal cells	(Shukitt-Hale, Lau, Carey, Galli, Spangler, Ingram, & Joseph, 2013; Joseph, Shukitt-Hale, Brewer, Weikel, Kalt, & Fisher, 2010)
Curcumin	Reduces Aβ levels in the brain and serum of mice	Y.-J. Wang et al., (2009)
Dihydroguaiaretic Acid	Inhibits Aβ fibril (f Aβ) formation and extension from Aβ (1–40) and Aβ (1–42)	(Ono, Hasegawa, Naiki, & Yamada, 2004)
(-) Epigallocatechin -3-Gallate (EGCG)	Inhibits in vitro fibril formation by RCM kappa-CN	(Hudson, Ecroyd, Dehle, Musgrave, & Carver, 2009)
Ellagic Acid	Inhibits beta-secretase (BACE1) activity	H.-M. Kwak et al., (2005)
Green Tea Polyphenol (*Camelia Sinensis*)	Ameliorates deleterious effects of d-galactose and Aβ (25–35) And improves animal's learning and memory	(Lü, Guo, & Yang, 2006)
Resveratrol	Inhibits Aβ polymerization	(Rivière, Richard, Quentin, Krisa, Mérillon, & Monti, 2007)
Genistein	Elicit neuroprotection from Aβ protein exposure, inhibits AChE, modulates estrogenic activity, Antioxidative activity, inhibit Aβ aggregation and exhibit metal chelating properties	(Lee, Lee, & Sohn, 2005; Qiang, Sang, Yuan, Li, Liu, Bai, Deng, 2014)
Luteolin	improve ASD symptoms by targeting JAK2/STAT3 signaling	Parker-Athill et al., (2009)
Sulforaphane	Activate Nrf2/ARE pathway, promoting the upregulation of GSH Antioxidant potential upon exposure to Aβ25–35, upregulate antioxidant enzymes via activation of Nrf2, prevent Aβ-mediated apoptosis	Tarozzi et al., (2013)
Myricetin	Reduces apoptotic changes and caspase-3 activation Decreases Aβ 1–40 and Aβ 1–42 levels in culture media Activates and up-regulates alpha-secretase (ADAM10) protein levels	(Shimmyo, Kihara, Akaike, Niidome, & Sugimoto, 2008)
Morin, Mangiferin	Inhibit glutamate-induced activation of calpains, normalize the levels of phosphorylated Akt kinase and Erk1/2, as well as of cytosolic Bax, inhibit AIF release from mitochondria, and regulate the nuclear translocation of NF-kappaB	(Campos-Esparza, Sánchez-Gómez, & Matute, 2009)

oxidative pathways and scavenging metal ions as pathogenic free radicals (Ebrahimi & Schluesener, 2012; Kelsey, Wilkins, & Linseman, 2010).

Anti-Acetylcholinesterase Activity of Polyphenols

Neurodegenerative diseases are characterized by the impairment of cholinergic system which ultimately leads to the cognitive decline due to reduction in Acetylcholine (Ach) synthesis, choline uptake, cholinergic neuronal and axonal abnormalities, and degeneration of cholinergic (Bohnen, Kaufer, Hendrickson, Ivanco, Lopresti, Davis, & DeKosky, 2005; Fisher, 2008). One of the promising approach in the treatment of neurodegenerative diseases lies in the use of Acetylcholinesterase inhibitors, which exert their efficacy through stimulation of both muscarinic and nicotinic acetylcholine receptors. Several natural polyphenols have shown to exert anti-cholinesterase activity which was accompanied by improvement of cognitive functions, like learning and memory (Zhang, Cao, Wen, & Xu, 2009). Several polyphenols such as Epigallocatechin gallate (EGCG) have been shown their effectiveness in affecting cholinergic system by regulating nAChR signaling pathway through down-regulation of α9-nAChR expression as well as inhibition of (3H)-Nic/ α 9- nAChR binding activity (Tu, Ku, Ho, Chen, Huang, Lee, & Ho, 2011), whereas resveratrol blocks acetylcholine release from adrenal chromaffin cells (Chang-Mu, Jen-Kun, Shing-Hwa, & Shoei-Yn, 2010).

Polyphenol Activity Against NMDA Neurotoxicity

NMDA neurotoxicity and glutamate excitotoxicity play a significant role in progressions of neurodegenerative diseases and cognitive impairment associated with aging (Choi, Monyer, Giffard, Goldberg, & Christine, 1990). Excessive activation of NMDA receptors is associated with the formation of free radicals (e.g., NO and ROS) and other enzymatic processes that result in neuronal damage and cell death. Therefore, NMDA receptor inhibitors have been explored for cognitive impairment not only in neurodegenerative diseases but also in psychiatric disorders with cognitive dysfunction (Lipton, 2007; Shim, Hammonds, & Kee, 2008). There is strong evidence of protective effects of several natural polyphenols against NMDA neurotoxicity (Ebrahimi & Schluesener, 2012).

Quercetin

Quercetin is a potent polyphenolic antioxidant, exerts its activity through redox regulation of proteins, transcription factors and a broad range of kinase-dependent signaling cascades, some of which are linked to cellular survival mechanisms. Oral intake of quercetin associated with erratic absorption followed by metabolic steps. The nutraceutical additive actions of quercetin will be best served by its pharmaceutical formulation to expedite optimal delivery and such a preparation effectively produced recovery of brain activity with improved breathing, motor and feeding behavior in perinatal hypoxia (Blasina, Vaamonde, Silvera, Tedesco, & Dajas, 2015).

Alkaloids

Huperzine A

Huperzine A, is an alkaloid, obtained from the moss, *Huperzia Serrata*, and was a part of traditional Chinese medicines for centuries to treat various ailments such as fever and inflammation. Various research studies indicated that huperzine A could be a potent neuroprotective agent against the impairment of cholinergic neurons. Huperzine A has been proven to be efficacious in the treatment of multi-infarct dementia and for patients with short-term and long-term memory loss caused by cerebral arteriosclerosis. In addition, the latest research on the efficacy of huperzine, including its effects on Alzheimer's disease, proves the effectiveness and safety of this substance in human participants (McDougall, Austin-Wells, & Zimmerman, 2005).

REGULATORY ASPECTS

1. **Dietary Supplements:** Dietary supplements are defined by the Dietary Supplement Health and Education Act (DSHEA) in 1994, as a food category which cannot contain anything that may have *a significant or unreasonable risk of illness or injury* when it is used as directed on the label, or with normal use if there are no directions on the label. DSHEA gives the roadmap for the registration of the dietary supplement for the marketing purpose. A dietary supplement is considered as "new" if it contains an ingredient which is not documented as a food substance unless it was sold as a supplement before October, 1994. As per the guidelines provided by DSHEA, FDA can stop a company from making a dietary supplement only when they can prove that the product shows a significant risk that means they are found unsafe only after they cause harm. This is in contrast to the practice of how prescription and non-prescription drugs are handled. Dietary supplements are usually self-prescribed, so there's no controlled system for reporting bad reactions and side effects. Doctors and patients can report problems but are not required to do so.

2. **Functional Foods:** Development and regulatory oversight of functional foods began in Japan in the early eighties with advances in the chemical identification of bioactive compounds, processing, and formulation of functional foods. In Japan, Functional foods had been registered under 'foods for specified health use' (FOSHU) policy. Since 1991 over 600 FOSHU products has been registered. According to International Food Information Council (IFIC), the functional foods are dietary components with a health benefit beyond basic nutrition. On the other hand, International Life Sciences Institute of North America (ILSI) also defines functional foods as physiologically active food components which provide health benefits. Another definition by Health Canada described the functional food which is capable of reducing the risk of chronic diseases. USA, European Union, and Canada, all of which now have various regulatory bodies to govern the manufacture and marketing of health-promoting food products.
3. **Nutraceuticals:** Despite the growth and need of nutraceuticals by global market there are no apparent regulatory definitions and approval process pathways available. There is a need for the development of regulatory guidelines for the rapidly expanding global nutraceutical industry. Although regulations in the United States, the United Kingdom, and Europe are efficient and have become favorable in the development of various nutraceutical products (Ray, Joshi, & Gulati, 2016).

CONCLUSION

Brain disorders encompass a broad category which varies significantly in symptoms and severity including brain injuries, brain tumors, neurodegenerative diseases and mental disorders. Currently, most of the pharmaceutical industries engaged in the development of new drugs have come up with very few novel drug discoveries. Additionally, there is scarcity in the new drug development for the neurological disorders due to the complexity of the disease pathophysiology and lack of precise diagnostic tools. The hunt for new remedies is now focusing in various similar areas which include nutraceuticals, dietary supplements, and various herbal products. Many of the dietary supplements, functional foods and nutraceuticals have shown promising results in the prevention and treatment of various brain disorders. Currently, diet, in particular, has become the object of research in relation to cognitive function and neurodegenerative disease. One important strategy to prevent brain impairment is based on dietary supplements, functional foods, and nutraceuticals. Since brain disorders are often associated with tissue damage or neurodegeneration, regular consumption of these nutrients may help repair these damages and limit the risk of brain disorders. Specific nutrients are essential for promoting healthy brain development of infants and children and preserving the cognitive function of elders. Despite the usefulness of these diet, nutraceuticals and functional food and the ever-growing research, these products are not approved officially by the concerned regulatory authorities throughout the world. To date, Japan is the only country that has established a specific regulatory approval process for functional foods known as Foods for Specified Health Use (FOSHU). Along with nutrient deficiencies, the aspects of nutrient toxicities have to be considered. Thus, dietary supplements, functional foods, and nutraceuticals play an important role in the prevention and treatment of various brain disorders.

REFERENCES

Adams, J. B., Audhya, T., McDonough-Means, S., Rubin, R. A., Quig, D., Geis, E., & Lee, W. (2011). Effect of a vitamin/mineral supplement on children and adults with autism. *BMC Pediatrics*, *11*(1), 111. doi:10.1186/1471-2431-11-111 PMID:22151477

Agarwal, K. N. (2001). Iron and the brain: Neurotransmitter receptors and magnetic resonance spectroscopy. *British Journal of Nutrition*, *85*(S2), S147. doi:10.1079/BJN2000307 PMID:11509103

Annweiler, C., Llewellyn, D. J., & Beauchet, O. (2013). Low serum vitamin D concentrations in Alzheimer's disease: A systematic review and meta-analysis. *Journal of Alzheimer's Disease*, *33*(3), 659–674. PMID:23042216

Annweiler, C., Rolland, Y., Schott, A. M., Blain, H., Vellas, B., Herrmann, F. R., & Beauchet, O. (2012). Higher vitamin D dietary intake is associated with lower risk of alzheimer's disease: A 7-year follow-up. *The Journals of Gerontology. Series A, Biological Sciences and Medical Sciences*, *67*(11), 1205–1211. doi:10.1093/gerona/gls107 PMID:22503994

Augustin, M. A. (2001). Functional foods : An adventure in food formulation. *Food Australia*, *53*(10), 428–432.

Axona. (2017, March 13). In *Wikipedia*. Retrieved from https://en.wikipedia.org/w/index.php?title=Axona&oldid=770058091

Bandmann, O., Weiss, K. H., & Kaler, S. G. (2015). Wilson's disease and other neurological copper disorders. *Lancet Neurology*, *14*(1), 103–113. doi:10.1016/S1474-4422(14)70190-5 PMID:25496901

Bazinet, R. P., & Layé, S. (2014). Polyunsaturated fatty acids and their metabolites in brain function and disease. *Nature Reviews. Neuroscience*, *15*(12), 771–785. doi:10.1038/nrn3820 PMID:25387473

Bhatnagar, S., & Taneja, S. (2001). Zinc and cognitive development. *British Journal of Nutrition*, *85*(S2Suppl2), S139–S145. doi:10.1079/BJN2000306 PMID:11509102

Bitanihirwe, B. K. Y., & Cunningham, M. G. (2009). Zinc: The brain's dark horse. *Synapse (New York, N.Y.)*, *63*(11), 1029–1049. doi:10.1002yn.20683 PMID:19623531

Blasina, F., Vaamonde, L., Silvera, F., Tedesco, A. C., & Dajas, F. (2015). Intravenous nanosomes of quercetin improve brain function and hemodynamic instability after severe hypoxia in newborn piglets. *Neurochemistry International*, *89*, 149–156. doi:10.1016/j.neuint.2015.08.007 PMID:26297982

Bohnen, N. I., Kaufer, D. I., Hendrickson, R., Ivanco, L. S., Lopresti, B., Davis, J. G., & DeKosky, S. T. (2005). Cognitive correlates of alterations in acetylcholinesterase in Alzheimer's disease. *Neuroscience Letters*, *380*(1–2), 127–132. doi:10.1016/j.neulet.2005.01.031 PMID:15854764

Brimson, J. M., Brimson, S. J., Brimson, C. A., Rakkhitawatthana, V., & Tencomnao, T. (2012). Rhinacanthus nasutus Extracts Prevent Glutamate and Amyloid-β Neurotoxicity in HT-22 Mouse Hippocampal Cells: Possible Active Compounds Include Lupeol, Stigmasterol and β-Sitosterol. *International Journal of Molecular Sciences*, *13*(4), 5074–5097. doi:10.3390/ijms13045074 PMID:22606031

Campos-Esparza, M. R., Sánchez-Gómez, M. V., & Matute, C. (2009). Molecular mechanisms of neuroprotection by two natural antioxidant polyphenols. *Cell Calcium*, *45*(4), 358–368. doi:10.1016/j.ceca.2008.12.007 PMID:19201465

Cardoso, B. R., Roberts, B. R., Bush, A. I., & Hare, D. J. (2015). Selenium, selenoproteins and neurodegenerative diseases. *Metallomics*, *7*(8), 1213–1228. doi:10.1039/C5MT00075K PMID:25996565

Chang-Mu, C., Jen-Kun, L., Shing-Hwa, L., & Shoei-Yn, L.-S. (2010). Characterization of neurotoxic effects of NMDA and the novel neuroprotection by phytopolyphenols in mice. *Behavioral Neuroscience*, *124*(4), 541–553. doi:10.1037/a0020050 PMID:20695653

Chasapis, C. T., Loutsidou, A. C., Spiliopoulou, C. A., & Stefanidou, M. E. (2012). Zinc and human health: An update. *Archives of Toxicology*, *86*(4), 521–534. doi:10.100700204-011-0775-1 PMID:22071549

Chauhan, N. B., & Mehla, J. (2014). Ameliorative Effects of Nutraceuticals in Neurological Disorders. Elsevier Inc.

Choi, D. W., Monyer, H., Giffard, R. G., Goldberg, M. P., & Christine, C. W. (1990). Acute brain injury, NMDA receptors, and hydrogen ions: Observations in cortical cell cultures. *Advances in Experimental Medicine and Biology*, *268*, 501–504. doi:10.1007/978-1-4684-5769-8_55 PMID:2150160

Cilla, A., Alegría, A., Attanzio, A., Garcia-Llatas, G., Tesoriere, L., & Livrea, M. A. (2017). Dietary phytochemicals in the protection against oxysterol-induced damage. *Chemistry and Physics of Lipids*, *207*, 192–205. doi:10.1016/j.chemphyslip.2017.03.001 PMID:28267434

Costa, L. G., Garrick, J., Roque, P. J., & Pellacani, C. (2016). Nutraceuticals in CNS Diseases: Potential Mechanisms of Neuroprotection. In R. C. Gupta (Ed.), *Nutraceuticals* (pp. 3–13). Boston: Academic Press. doi:10.1016/B978-0-12-802147-7.00001-2

Da Costa, J. P. (2017). A current look at nutraceuticals – Key concepts and future prospects. *Trends in Food Science & Technology*, *62*, 68–78. doi:10.1016/j.tifs.2017.02.010

DeAngelis, C. D., & Fontanarosa, P. B. (2003). Drugs Alias Dietary Supplements. *Journal of the American Medical Association*, *290*(11), 1519–1520. doi:10.1001/jama.290.11.1519 PMID:13129996

DeFelice, S. L. (1995). The nutraceutical revolution: Its impact on food industry R&D. *Trends in Food Science & Technology*, *6*(2), 59–61. doi:10.1016/S0924-2244(00)88944-X

Desai, V., & Kaler, S. G. (2008). Role of copper in human neurological disorders. *The American Journal of Clinical Nutrition*, *88*(3), 855S–858S. doi:10.1093/ajcn/88.3.855S PMID:18779308

Ebrahimi, A., & Schluesener, H. (2012). Natural polyphenols against neurodegenerative disorders: Potentials and pitfalls. *Ageing Research Reviews*, *11*(2), 329–345. doi:10.1016/j.arr.2012.01.006 PMID:22336470

Espín, J. C., García-Conesa, M. T., & Tomás-Barberán, F. A. (2007). Nutraceuticals: Facts and fiction. *Phytochemistry*, *68*(22–24), 2986–3008. doi:10.1016/j.phytochem.2007.09.014 PMID:17976666

Ferrari, C. K. B., & Torres, E. A. F. S. (2003). Biochemical pharmacology of functional foods and prevention of chronic diseases of aging. *Biomedicine and Pharmacotherapy*, *57*(5–6), 251–260. doi:10.1016/S0753-3322(03)00032-5 PMID:12888262

Fischer, H., Gottschlich, R., & Seelig, A. (1998). Blood-Brain Barrier Permeation: Molecular Parameters Governing Passive Diffusion. *The Journal of Membrane Biology*, *165*(3), 201–211. doi:10.1007002329900434 PMID:9767674

Fisher, A. (2008). Cholinergic treatments with emphasis on m1 muscarinic agonists as potential disease-modifying agents for Alzheimer's disease. *Neurotherapeutics; the Journal of the American Society for Experimental NeuroTherapeutics*, *5*(3), 433–442. doi:10.1016/j.nurt.2008.05.002 PMID:18625455

GEN. (2005). *GEN, 25*(9). Retrieved from http://www.genengnews.com/gen-articles/opportunities-and-challenges-for-developing-functional-foods/361

Gooch, C. L., Pracht, E., & Borenstein, A. R. (2017). The burden of neurological disease in the United States: A summary report and call to action: Burden of Neurological Disease. *Annals of Neurology*, *81*(4), 479–484. doi:10.1002/ana.24897 PMID:28198092

Grand View Research. (2016, November 17). *Functional Foods Market Is Expected To Reach $255.10 Billion By 2024*. Grand View Research, Inc. Retrieved April 14, 2017, from http://www.prnewswire.com/news-releases/functional-foods-market-is-expected-to-reach-25510-billion-by-2024-grand-view-research-inc-601642985.html

Hardy, G. (2000). Nutraceuticals and functional foods: Introduction and meaning. *Nutrition (Burbank, Los Angeles County, Calif.)*, *16*(7), 688–689. doi:10.1016/S0899-9007(00)00332-4 PMID:10906598

Hudson, S. A., Ecroyd, H., Dehle, F. C., Musgrave, I. F., & Carver, J. A. (2009). (-)-epigallocatechin-3-gallate (EGCG) maintains kappa-casein in its pre-fibrillar state without redirecting its aggregation pathway. *Journal of Molecular Biology*, *392*(3), 689–700. doi:10.1016/j.jmb.2009.07.031 PMID:19616561

Isolauri, E. (2001). Probiotics in human disease. *The American Journal of Clinical Nutrition*, *73*(6), 1142S–1146S. doi:10.1093/ajcn/73.6.1142S PMID:11393192

Jallouli, Y., Paillard, A., Chang, J., Sevin, E., & Betbeder, D. (2007). Influence of surface charge and inner composition of porous nanoparticles to cross blood–brain barrier in vitro. *International Journal of Pharmaceutics*, *344*(1–2), 103–109. doi:10.1016/j.ijpharm.2007.06.023 PMID:17651930

Janca, A., Aarli, J. A., Prilipko, L., Dua, T., Saxena, S., & Saraceno, B. (2006). WHO/WFN Survey of neurological services: A worldwide perspective. *Journal of the Neurological Sciences*, *247*(1), 29–34. doi:10.1016/j.jns.2006.03.003 PMID:16624322

Joseph, J. A., Shukitt-Hale, B., Brewer, G. J., Weikel, K. A., Kalt, W., & Fisher, D. R. (2010). Differential protection among fractionated blueberry polyphenolic families against DA-, Aβ42 and LPS-induced decrements in Ca2+ buffering in primary hippocampal cells. *Journal of Agricultural and Food Chemistry*, *58*(14), 8196–8204. doi:10.1021/jf100144y PMID:20597478

Kabanov, A. V., & Gendelman, H. E. (2007). Nanomedicine in the diagnosis and therapy of neurodegenerative disorders. *Progress in Polymer Science*, *32*(8–9), 1054–1082. doi:10.1016/j.progpolymsci.2007.05.014 PMID:20234846

Kalra, E. K. (2003). Nutraceutical-definition and introduction. *The AAPS Journal*, *5*(3), 27–28. doi:10.1208/ps050325

Katan, M. B. (2002). Nutrition in the Prevention and Treatment of Disease. *The New England Journal of Medicine*, *346*(22), 1754–1754. doi:10.1056/NEJM200205303462221

Kelsey, N. A., Wilkins, H. M., & Linseman, D. A. (2010). Nutraceutical antioxidants as novel neuroprotective agents. *Molecules (Basel, Switzerland)*, *15*(11), 7792–7814. doi:10.3390/molecules15117792 PMID:21060289

Kreuter, J. (2007). Nanoparticles-a historical perspective. *International Journal of Pharmaceutics*, *331*(1), 1–10. doi:10.1016/j.ijpharm.2006.10.021 PMID:17110063

Kuo, Y.-C., & Su, F.-L. (2007). Transport of stavudine, delavirdine, and saquinavir across the blood–brain barrier by polybutylcyanoacrylate, methylmethacrylate-sulfopropylmethacrylate, and solid lipid nanoparticles. *International Journal of Pharmaceutics*, *340*(1–2), 143–152. doi:10.1016/j.ijpharm.2007.03.012 PMID:17418986

Kwak, H.-M., Jeon, S.-Y., Sohng, B.-H., Kim, J.-G., Lee, J.-M., Lee, K.-B., & Song, K.-S. (2005). beta-Secretase (BACE1) inhibitors from pomegranate (Punica granatum) husk. *Archives of Pharmacal Research*, *28*(12), 1328–1332. doi:10.1007/BF02977896 PMID:16392663

Kwak, N.-S., & Jukes, D. J. (2001). Functional foods. Part 2: The impact on current regulatory terminology. *Food Control, 12*(2).

Lee, Y.-B., Lee, H. J., & Sohn, H. S. (2005). Soy isoflavones and cognitive function. *The Journal of Nutritional Biochemistry, 16*(11), 641–649. doi:10.1016/j.jnutbio.2005.06.010 PMID:16169201

Lipton, S. A. (2007). Pathologically-Activated Therapeutics for Neuroprotection: Mechanism of NMDA Receptor Block by Memantine and S-Nitrosylation. *Current Drug Targets, 8*(5), 621–632. doi:10.2174/138945007780618472 PMID:17504105

Lopez-Varela, S., Gonzalez-Gross, M., & Marcos, A. (2002). Functional foods and the immune system: A review. *European Journal of Clinical Nutrition, 56*(S3), S29–S33. doi:10.1038j.ejcn.1601481 PMID:12142958

Lü, J.-H., Guo, J., & Yang, W.-H. (2006). Effects of green tea polyphenol on the behaviour of Alzheimer' s disease like mice induced by D-galactose and Abeta25-35. *Zhong Yao Cai, 29*(4), 352–354. PMID:16913491

Martirosyan, D. M., & Singh, J. (2015). A new definition of functional food by FFC: What makes a new definition unique? *Functional Foods in Health and Disease, 5*(6), 209–223.

McDougall, G. J., Austin-Wells, V., & Zimmerman, T. (2005). Utility of Nutraceutical Products Marketed for Cognitive and Memory Enhancement. *Journal of Holistic Nursing : Official Journal of the American Holistic Nurses'. Association, 23*(4), 415–433.

Mocchegiani, E., Bertoni-Freddari, C., Marcellini, F., & Malavolta, M. (2005). Brain, aging and neurodegeneration: Role of zinc ion availability. *Progress in Neurobiology, 75*(6), 367–390. doi:10.1016/j.pneurobio.2005.04.005 PMID:15927345

Mollet, B., & Lacroix, C. (2007). Where biology and technology meet for better nutrition and health. *Current Opinion in Biotechnology, 18*(2), 154–155. doi:10.1016/j.copbio.2007.03.003

Murray, C. J. L., & Lopez, A. D. (1996). T*he Global burden of disease : a comprehensive assessment of mortality and disability from diseases, injuries, and risk factors in 1990 and projected to 2020 : summary*. WHO. Retrieved from http://www.who.int/iris/handle/10665/41864

Nash, K. M., & Shah, Z. A. (2015). Current Perspectives on the Beneficial Role of Ginkgo biloba in Neurological and Cerebrovascular Disorders. *Integrative Medicine Insights*, *10*, 1–9. doi:10.4137/IMI.S25054 PMID:26604665

Nemetchek, M. D., Stierle, A. A., Stierle, D. B., & Lurie, D. I. (2017). The Ayurvedic plant Bacopa monnieri inhibits inflammatory pathways in the brain. *Journal of Ethnopharmacology*, *197*, 92–100. doi:10.1016/j.jep.2016.07.073 PMID:27473605

Ono, K., Hasegawa, K., Naiki, H., & Yamada, M. (2004). Anti-amyloidogenic activity of tannic acid and its activity to destabilize Alzheimer's beta-amyloid fibrils in vitro. *Biochimica et Biophysica Acta*, *1690*(3), 193–202. doi:10.1016/j.bbadis.2004.06.008 PMID:15511626

Ozturk, S., & Cillier, A. E. (2006). Magnesium supplementation in the treatment of dementia patients. *Medical Hypotheses*, *67*(5), 1223–1225. doi:10.1016/j.mehy.2006.04.047 PMID:16790324

Palthur, P., Palthur, S., & Chitta, S. K. (2010). *Nutraceuticals: a conceptual definition*. Academic Press.

Panza, F., Frisardi, V., Capurso, C., D'Introno, A., Colacicco, A. M., Di Palo, A., & Solfrizzi, V. (2009). Polyunsaturated Fatty Acid and S-Adenosylmethionine Supplementation in Predementia Syndromes and Alzheimer's Disease: A Review. *The Scientific World Journal*, *9*, 373–389. doi:10.1100/tsw.2009.48 PMID:19468660

Pardridge, W. M. (2002a). Targeting Neurotherapeutic Agents Through the Blood-Brain Barrier. *Archives of Neurology*, *59*(1), 35. doi:10.1001/archneur.59.1.35 PMID:11790228

Pardridge, W. M. (2002b). Why is the global CNS pharmaceutical market so under-penetrated? *Drug Discovery Today*, *7*(1), 5–7. doi:10.1016/S1359-6446(01)02082-7 PMID:11790589

Pardridge, W. M. (2007). Brain Drug Development and Brain Drug Targeting. *Pharmaceutical Research*, *24*(9), 1729–1732. doi:10.100711095-007-9387-0 PMID:17629776

Parker, S. J., Koistinaho, J., White, A. R., & Kanninen, K. M. (2013). Biometals in rare neurodegenerative disorders of childhood. *Frontiers in Aging Neuroscience*, 5. PMID:23531702

Parker-Athill, E., Luo, D., Bailey, A., Giunta, B., Tian, J., Shytle, R. D., & Tan, J. (2009). Flavonoids, a prenatal prophylaxis via targeting JAK2/STAT3 signaling to oppose IL-6/MIA associated autism. *Journal of Neuroimmunology*, *217*(1–2), 20–27. doi:10.1016/j.jneuroim.2009.08.012 PMID:19766327

Peterson, A. L., Murchison, C., Zabetian, C., Leverenz, J. B., Watson, G. S., Montine, T., & Quinn, J. F. (2013). Memory, Mood, and Vitamin D in Persons with Parkinson's Disease. *Journal of Parkinson's Disease*, *3*(4), 547–555. PMID:24081441

Qiang, X., Sang, Z., Yuan, W., Li, Y., Liu, Q., Bai, P., & Deng, Y. (2014). Design, synthesis and evaluation of genistein-O-alkylbenzylamines as potential multifunctional agents for the treatment of Alzheimer's disease. *European Journal of Medicinal Chemistry*, *76*, 314–331. doi:10.1016/j.ejmech.2014.02.045 PMID:24589487

Ray, A., Joshi, J., & Gulati, K. (2016). Regulatory Aspects of Nutraceuticals. In Nutraceuticals (pp. 941–946). Elsevier. doi:10.1016/B978-0-12-802147-7.00066-8

Rivière, C., Richard, T., Quentin, L., Krisa, S., Mérillon, J.-M., & Monti, J.-P. (2007). Inhibitory activity of stilbenes on Alzheimer's beta-amyloid fibrils in vitro. *Bioorganic & Medicinal Chemistry*, *15*(2), 1160–1167. doi:10.1016/j.bmc.2006.09.069 PMID:17049256

Rockenstein, E., Crews, L., & Masliah, E. (2007). Transgenic animal models of neurodegenerative diseases and their application to treatment development. *Advanced Drug Delivery Reviews*, *59*(11), 1093–1102. doi:10.1016/j.addr.2007.08.013 PMID:17869376

Rojas, P., Montes, P., Rojas, C., Serrano-García, N., & Rojas-Castañeda, J. C. (2012). Effect of a phytopharmaceutical medicine, Ginko biloba extract 761, in an animal model of Parkinson's disease: Therapeutic perspectives. *Nutrition (Burbank, Los Angeles County, Calif.)*, *28*(11–12), 1081–1088. doi:10.1016/j.nut.2012.03.007 PMID:22817828

Scheiber, I. F., Mercer, J. F. B., & Dringen, R. (2014). Metabolism and functions of copper in brain. *Progress in Neurobiology*, *116*, 33–57. doi:10.1016/j.pneurobio.2014.01.002 PMID:24440710

Schmidt, J., Metselaar, J. M., Wauben, M. H. M., Toyka, K. V., Storm, G., & Gold, R. (2003). Drug targeting by long-circulating liposomal glucocorticosteroids increases therapeutic efficacy in a model of multiple sclerosis. *Brain*, *126*(Pt 8), 1895–1904. doi:10.1093/brain/awg176 PMID:12805101

Shefa, U., Yeo, S. G., Kim, M.-S., Song, I. O., Jung, J., Jeong, N. Y., & Huh, Y. (2017). Role of Gasotransmitters in Oxidative Stresses, Neuroinflammation, and Neuronal Repair. *BioMed Research International*, *2017*, 1–15. doi:10.1155/2017/1689341 PMID:28386548

Shen, L. (2015). Associations between B Vitamins and Parkinson's Disease. *Nutrients*, *7*(9), 7197–7208. doi:10.3390/nu7095333 PMID:26343714

Shim, S. S., Hammonds, M. D., & Kee, B. S. (2008). Potentiation of the NMDA receptor in the treatment of schizophrenia: Focused on the glycine site. *European Archives of Psychiatry and Clinical Neuroscience*, *258*(1), 16–27. doi:10.100700406-007-0757-8 PMID:17901997

Shimmyo, Y., Kihara, T., Akaike, A., Niidome, T., & Sugimoto, H. (2008). Multifunction of myricetin on A beta: Neuroprotection via a conformational change of A beta and reduction of A beta via the interference of secretases. *Journal of Neuroscience Research*, *86*(2), 368–377. doi:10.1002/jnr.21476 PMID:17722071

Shukitt-Hale, B., Lau, F. C., Carey, A. N., Galli, R. L., Spangler, E. L., Ingram, D. K., & Joseph, J. A. (2013). Blueberry polyphenols attenuate kainic acid-induced decrements in cognition and alter inflammatory gene expression in rat hippocampus. *Nutritional Neuroscience*. PMID:18681986

Silva, G. A. (2007). Nanotechnology approaches for drug and small molecule delivery across the blood brain barrier. *Surgical Neurology*, *67*(2), 113–116. doi:10.1016/j.surneu.2006.08.033 PMID:17254859

Smith, J., & Charter, E. (Eds.). (2010). *Functional food product development*. Chichester, UK: Wiley-Blackwell. doi:10.1002/9781444323351

Stankiewicz, J., Panter, S. S., Neema, M., Arora, A., Batt, C. E., & Bakshi, R. (2007). Iron in Chronic Brain Disorders: Imaging and Neurotherapeutic Implications. *Neurotherapeutics; the Journal of the American Society for Experimental NeuroTherapeutics*, *4*(3), 371–386. doi:10.1016/j.nurt.2007.05.006 PMID:17599703

Suzuki, M., Yoshioka, M., Hashimoto, M., Murakami, M., Noya, M., Takahashi, D., & Urashima, M. (2013). Randomized, double-blind, placebo-controlled trial of vitamin D supplementation in Parkinson disease. *The American Journal of Clinical Nutrition*, *97*(5), 1004–1013. doi:10.3945/ajcn.112.051664 PMID:23485413

Tarozzi, A., Angeloni, C., Malaguti, M., Morroni, F., Hrelia, S., & Hrelia, P. (2013). Sulforaphane as a Potential Protective Phytochemical against Neurodegenerative Diseases. *Oxidative Medicine and Cellular Longevity*, *2013*, e415078. doi:10.1155/2013/415078 PMID:23983898

Tatli, I. I. (2015). Ginkgo biloba Extracts in Neurological Disorders Therapy: Clinical Trials. In R. R. Watson & V. R. Preedy (Eds.), *Bioactive Nutraceuticals and Dietary Supplements in Neurological and Brain Disease* (pp. 113–124). San Diego, CA: Academic Press. doi:10.1016/B978-0-12-411462-3.00012-6

Thaipisuttikul, P., & Galvin, J. E. (2012). Use of medical foods and nutritional approaches in the treatment of Alzheimer's disease. *Clinical Practice (London, England)*, *9*(2), 199–209. doi:10.2217/cpr.12.3 PMID:23362453

Tu, S.-H., Ku, C.-Y., Ho, C.-T., Chen, C.-S., Huang, C.-S., Lee, C.-H., & Ho, Y.-S. (2011). Tea polyphenol (-)-epigallocatechin-3-gallate inhibits nicotine- and estrogen-induced α9-nicotinic acetylcholine receptor upregulation in human breast cancer cells. *Molecular Nutrition & Food Research*, *55*(3), 455–466. doi:10.1002/mnfr.201000254 PMID:21370452

USFDA. (2015, July 25). *Consumer Updates - FDA 101: Dietary Supplements*. Retrieved April 14, 2017, from https://www.fda.gov/ForConsumers/ConsumerUpdates/ucm050803.htm

USFDA. (2016, July 26). *Dietary Supplement Products & Ingredients*. Retrieved March 17, 2017, from https://www.fda.gov/Food/DietarySupplements/ProductsIngredients/

Vural, H., Demirin, H., Kara, Y., Eren, I., & Delibas, N. (2010). Alterations of plasma magnesium, copper, zinc, iron and selenium concentrations and some related erythrocyte antioxidant enzyme activities in patients with Alzheimer's disease. *Journal of Trace Elements in Medicine and Biology*, *24*(3), 169–173. doi:10.1016/j.jtemb.2010.02.002 PMID:20569929

Wang, X., & Michaelis, E. K. (2010). Selective neuronal vulnerability to oxidative stress in the brain. *Frontiers in Aging Neuroscience*, *2*, 12. PMID:20552050

Wang, Y.-J., Thomas, P., Zhong, J.-H., Bi, F.-F., Kosaraju, S., Pollard, A., & Zhou, X.-F. (2009). Consumption of grape seed extract prevents amyloid-beta deposition and attenuates inflammation in brain of an Alzheimer's disease mouse. *Neurotoxicity Research*, *15*(1), 3–14. doi:10.100712640-009-9000-x PMID:19384583

Wei, W., Liu, Y.-H., Zhang, C.-E., Wang, Q., Wei, Z., Mousseau, D. D., & Liu, G.-P. (2011). Folate/vitamin-B12 prevents chronic hyperhomocysteinemia-induced tau hyperphosphorylation and memory deficits in aged rats. *Journal of Alzheimer's Disease. JAD*, *27*(3), 639–650. PMID:21860088

Yehuda, S. (2003). Omega-6/omega-3 ratio and brain-related functions. *World Review of Nutrition and Dietetics*, *92*, 37–56. doi:10.1159/000073791 PMID:14579682

Zecca, L., Youdim, M. B. H., Riederer, P., Connor, J. R., & Crichton, R. R. (2004). Iron, brain ageing and neurodegenerative disorders. *Nature Reviews. Neuroscience*, *5*(11), 863–873. doi:10.1038/nrn1537 PMID:15496864

Zhang, L., Cao, H., Wen, J., & Xu, M. (2009). Green tea polyphenol (-)-epigallocatechin-3-gallate enhances the inhibitory effect of huperzine A on acetylcholinesterase by increasing the affinity with serum albumin. *Nutritional Neuroscience*, *12*(4), 142–148. doi:10.1179/147683009X423283 PMID:19622237

Chapter 10
Nutraceuticals Role in Stress, Aging, and Neurodegenerative Disorders

Manisha Choudhary
Nims University Rajasthan, India

Sandeep Tripathi
Nims University Rajasthan, India

Rajesh Kumar Kesharwani
Nims University Rajasthan, India

ABSTRACT

Nutraceuticals and functional foods have attracted considerable interest recently because of their well-known safety and potential nutritional and therapeutic effects. Nutraceuticals include food supplements, dietary supplements, value-added processed foods, as well as non-food supplements such as tablets, soft gels, and capsules etc. which are packed with bioactive components. Life expectancy continues to rise and along with a rise in the lifestyle diseases (i.e., obesity, diabetes, hypertension, cardiovascular diseases, and neurodegenerative disorders). Functional foods and nutraceuticals constitute a great promise to improve health, neurodegenerative disorders, and aging-related chronic diseases. A collective effort by the academia, industry, government, and research organization must keep on promoting nutraceutical and functional food to contain the menace of lifestyle diseases.

DOI: 10.4018/978-1-5225-3267-5.ch010

INTRODUCTION

The new term known as "Nutraceuticals" was coined two words from "nutrition" (nourishing food or food component) and "pharmaceutical" (medical drug), by Stephen DeFelice founder and chairman of the Foundation for Innovation in Medicine (FIM), in 1989 (Das, Bhaumik, Raychaudhuri, & Chakraborty, 2012). Nutraceutical can be defined as is a food or food product that provides health and medical benefits, including the prevention and treatment of disease. Phytochemicals and antioxidants are two specific types of nutraceuticals (Keservani, Kesharwani, Sharma, Vyas, & Chadoker, 2010a). Research has proved that the combination of food ingredients or phytochemicals provide protection from many life-threatening diseases including cancer, diabetes, heart disease, hypertension, and neurodegenerative disorders (Keservani, Kesharwani, Vyas, Jain, Raghuvanshi, & Sharma, 2010b). Over the last 20 years, numbers of Nutraceuticals are available for self-medication or for sale. Nutraceuticals a lot of widespread in the modern society due to the belief of reduced chances of adverse effects, being natural, the ease of self-medication and the positive effects on the aging population (Pathak, 2010).

CATEGORIES OF NUTRACEUTICALS

Nutraceuticals are non-specific biological therapies used for the prevention in many diseases are categorized on the basis of their sources or origin, pharmacology as well as chemical component (Dureja, Kaushik, & Kumar, 2003; Hathcock, 2001; Chauhan, Kumar, Kalam, & Ansari, 2013) (Figure 1):

1. Dietary Supplements
2. Functional Food
3. Medicinal Food
4. Pharmaceuticals

Dietary Supplements

A dietary supplement is a product that contains nutrients derived from food products. The "dietary ingredients" present in these products are: metabolites, vitamins, minerals, herbs, and amino acids.

Functional Foods

Functional foods are designed foods which provide enriched foods close to their natural state to consumer, rather than manufactured dietary supplements in liquid or capsule form. A process of making enriched food is called Nutrification. Functional foods provide required amount of vitamins, fat, carbohydrate, amino acid etc to body. Established requirement that functional food should possess are (Singh, Kesharwani, & Keservani, 2018; Aluko, 2012):

1. Functional foods should be in their naturally-occurring form,
2. Functional foods should be an essential part of our daily diet,
3. Functional foods should regulate a biological process in hopes of preventing or controlling disease.

Medicinal Foods

Transgenic cows and lactoferrin for immune enhancement, transgenic plants for oral vaccination against infectious diseases and health bars with added medications. If you want to try medicinal foods, it must be under the guidance and supervision of a trained and experienced medical professional (Salak-Johnson, & McGlone, 2007).

Nutrients: Substances which have established Nutritional functions e.g. Vitamins, Minerals, Amino Acids, Fatty acids, etc. Minerals and Vitamins or in combination of both together with other antioxidants are most common Nutrients used or supplemented for wellness of human being (Keservani, Sharma, & Kesharwani, 2016).

Pharmaceuticals

Pharmaceuticals are medically valuable components produced from modified agricultural crops or animals. The term is a combining of the words "farm" and "pharmaceuticals". Proponents of this concept are convinced that using crops (and possibly even animals) as pharmaceutical factories is much more cost effective than conventional methods, with higher revenue for agricultural producers (Zilberman, Yarkin, & Heiman, 1997).

SOURCES OF NUTRACEUTICALS

The most of nutraceuticals are natural products and obtained from plants and animals. Example-lycopene extracted from plant, carnitine, creatine and carotenoids produced by fermentation for example-coenzyme Q10 and Sadenosyl glycoside (Lockwood, 2007).

1. A number of nutraceuticals have GRAS ("generally recognized as safe") status as defined by FDA, and increasingly manufacturers gain GRAS certification for product. A list of GRAS is published on the internet (Chaturvedi, Sharma, Garg, & Bansal, 2011).
2. For the process of identification and quantification of nutraceuticals and pharmaceuticals, same analytical procedure are used.

FUNCTIONS OF NUTRACEUTICALS

Benefits of Nutraceuticals in Health

Many years' nutraceuticals have considerable interest due to their potential nutritional, safety and therapeutic effects. They have a role in a plethora of biological processes, including antioxidant defenses, cell proliferation, gene expression, and safeguarding of mitochondrial integrity. Therefore nutraceuticals are used to improve

Table 1. Nutraceuticals and their sources

Nutraceuticals	Source	Extraction/Fermentation/ Manufacturer
Glucosamine	Bovine trachea, Shellfish	Chitin acid hydrolysis, Fish shell enzymes hydrolysis (Barrow & Shahidi, 2007)
Methylesulfonylmethane	Meat, milk	Peroxide oxidation of DMSO (Kim, Axelrod, Howard, Buratovich, & Waters, 2006)
Coenzyme Q10	Common food	NaOH digest of hearts/livers after H2S treatment, fermentation (Chaturvedi, Sharma, Garg, & Bansal, 2011)
Carnitine	Heart, skeletal Muscles	Chiral synthesis from butyrolactone (Wang & Hollingsworth, 1999)
Flax Lignans	Linumusitatissimum	Supercritical extraction Co_2 (Comin, Temelli, & Saldaña, 2011)
Resveratrol	Red wine,polygonum,ca psidatum root	Mid polarity solvent extraction (Dai & Mumper, 2010)
Grape Seed	Vitisvinifera	Water/ethanol extraction (Bagchi, Bagchi, Stohs, Das, Ray, Kuszynski, ... & Pruess, 2000)
Lycopene	Foods including tomato, green algae	Tamato extraction, chemical synthesis (Upadhyay, Kesharwani, & Misra, 2009; Story, Kopec, Schwartz, & Harris, 2010)

Figure 1. Concepts of nutraceuticals

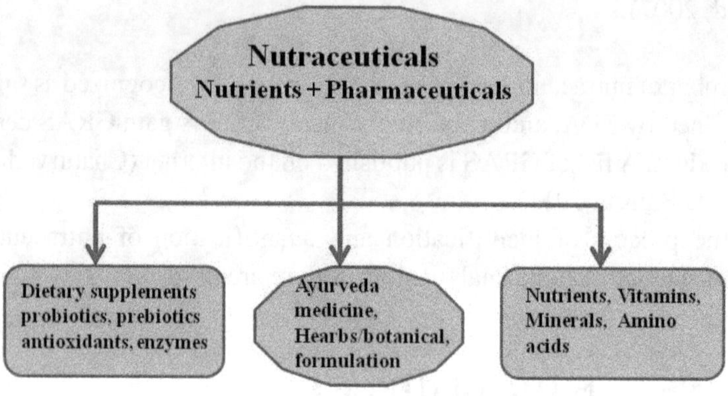

health, prevent chronic diseases, postpone the aging process (and in turn increase life expectancy), or just support functions and integrity of the body (Wildman, 2016). They are considered to be healthy sources for prevention of life threatening diseases such as diabetes, renal and gastrointestinal disorders, as well as different infections. A wide variety of nutraceuticals have shown to impose important roles in immunity and susceptibility to certain disease status. They also exhibit diseases modifying indications related to oxidative stress including allergy, Alzheimer's disease, cardiovascular diseases, cancer, eye conditions, Parkinson's diseases and obesity (Jiang, Sun, & Chen, 2016) (Figure 2).

NUTRACEUTICALS USED AS A THERAPEUTIC AGENT

The majority of the nutraceuticals do possess multiple therapeutic benefits and have been claimed to have physiological benefits (Kumar & Kumar, 2015) or provide

Figure 2. Classification of nutraceuticals (Scicchitano, Cameli, Maiello, Modesti, Muiesan, Novo, ... & di Studio Ipertensione, 2014)

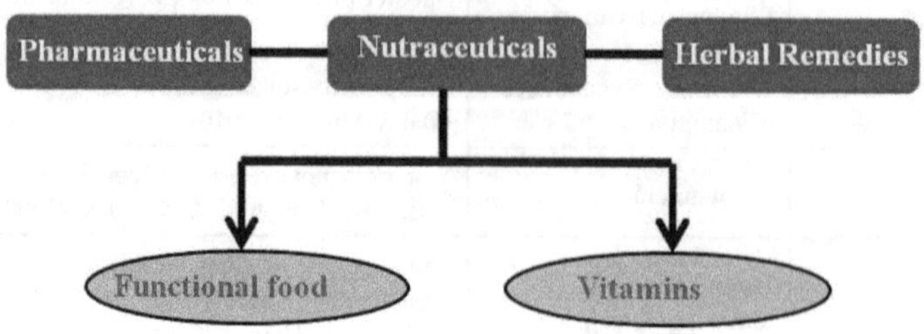

protection against various diseases as the following products: Cardiovascular agents, Anti-obese agents, Anti-diabetic agents, Anti-cancer agents, Immune boosters, Substances that manage chronic inflammatory disorders and Formulations to cure degenerative diseases (Rajasekaran, Sivagnanam, & Xavier, 2008) (Table 1).

The Role of Nutraceuticals in Brain Disorders (AD)

Alzheimer's disease (AD), also called senile dementia of the Alzheimer type (SDAT), primary degenerative dementia of the Alzheimer's type (PDDAT), or simply Alzheimer's, is the most common form of dementia. The various Nutraceuticals, which are used to cure Alzheimer's disease are (Keservani, Sharma, & Kesharwani, 2016):

Antioxidants

Antioxidants are playing important role in the modern medicinal system and among that vitamin C and vitamin Eare mostly prescribed by the medical practitioners all over the world, and also helps in the rapid treatment of almost all diseases. The logic behind the supplementation of antioxidants because oxidative stress is very important factor in most of chronic diseases like in case of neurodegenerative diseases e.g. Alzheimer's disease (AD), Parkinson's disease (PD), and Huntington's disease (HD) (Traber & Stevens, 2011).

Nutraceuticals which are having antioxidant properties are necessary to be part of daily diet in the sufficient amount during aging and lack of such contents accelerate the aging in early life with the increase of oxidative stress. Scientist all over the world have already proven by ample amount of rigorous study on association between high dietary antioxidant intake and a decreased risk of AD which is very imperative because preventing a disease is significantly easier than treating it (Fatima, Kesharwani, Misra, & Rizvi, 2013) (Figure 3).

Alpha-Lipoic Acid

Alpha-lipoic acid (ALA) also plays a responsibility in brain function. Oxidative stress and energy diminutions are biochemical characteristics and brand of AD. Alpha lipoic acid is potent antioxidant, which also progress glucose metabolism and consumption in the brain. Hager et al (2001) gave 600 mg ALA day by day to nine patients with AD and related dementia, who were already getting standard acetyl cholinesterase inhibitors, in an open study lasting about 337 days. Results showed that those receiving the ALA had a stabilization of cognitive function demonstrated by stable scores on

Table 2. Health Benefits of different common nutraceuticals

Nutraceuticals		Health Benefits
Fat Soluble Vitamins	Vitamin A	Act as antioxidant, essential for growth and development, healthy vision, skin and mucous membranes, prevention and treatment of certain cancers and certain skin disorders (Nieves, 2013)
	Vitamin D	Essential for formation of bones and teeth and helps the body to absorb and use calcium (Semo, Kesselman, Danino, & Livney, 2007)
	Vitamin E	Antioxidant, helps of blood cells and boosts immune system (Ajjawi,& Shintani, 2004)
	Vitamin K	Essential for blood clotting (Velikov & Pelan, 2008)
Water Soluble Vitamins	Vitamin C	Antioxidant, healthy bones, gums, teeth and skin helps in wound healing, prevent from common cold (Dillard & German, 2000)
	Vitamin B 1	Helps in carbohydrate metabolism and essential for neurological function (Houston, 2005)
	Vitamin B 2	Energy metabolism, maintain healthy eye, skin and nerve function (Lee, Koo, N., & Min, 2004)
	Vitamin B 3	Energy metabolism and brain function(Depeint, Bruce, Shangari, Mehta, & O'Brien, 2006; Lee, Koo, N., & Min, 2004)
	Vitamin B 6	Helps to produce essential proteins, convert proteins to energy (Lee, Koo, N., & Min, 2004)
	Vitamin B 12	Producing genetic material, formation of RBC, maintenance of CNS, synthesis of amino acids, involved in metabolism of protein, fat and carbohydrate (Lee, Koo, N., & Min, 2004)
	Folic acid	Formation of RBC, genetic material of cell and more essential during pregnancy (Lee, et al., 2004)
	Pantothenic acid	Synthesis of cholesterol, steroids, fatty acids, crucial for intraneuronal synthesis of acetylcholine (Lee, Koo, N., & Min, 2004)
Vitamins Like Compounds (Das,Bhaumik, Raychaudhuri, & Chakraborty, 2012)	L- Carnitine	Helps in oxidation of fatty acids and role in oxidative phosphorylation
	Choline	Lipotropic agent, treat fatty liver and disturbed fat metabolism
	Inositol	Amino acid transport and movement of potassium and sodium
	Taurine	Helps in retinal photoreceptor activity, bile acid conjugation, WBC antioxidant activity, CNS neuromodulation, platelet aggregation, cardiac contractibility, sperm motility, insuline activity,
Minerals (Houston, 2005)	Calcium	Bone and teeth, maintaining bone strength, nerve, muscle and glandular function, blood clotting
	Iron	Energy production, Hb, oxygen transport
	Magnesium	Healthy nerve and muscle function and bone formation
	Phosphorous	Energy production, phosphorylation process, bone and teeth, genetic material
	Cobalt	Component of Vit. B 12 and B 12 coenzymes
	Copper	Hb and collagen production, function of heart, energy production, Absorption of Iron
	Iodine	Proper function of thyroid gland
	Chromium	With insulin it helps in conversion of carbohydrate and fat into energy, treatment of diabetes
	Selenium	Antioxidant, functioning of heart muscle, part of GPX enzyme
	Zinc	Cell reproduction, development in Neonates, wound healing, production of sperm and testosterone hormone

the MMSE scale and AD assessment scales. Phosphatidylserine is a very interesting complex. Phosphatidlyserine is the key phospholipids in the brain and it makes up the basic configuration of the cell membrane. Membrane phosphatidlyserine and phospholipids play a vital role in cell-to-cell announcement and transfer of biochemical letters to the cell. Phosphatidylserine boost cellular metabolism and communication, and oral supplemental outcomes neuronal membranes, cell metabolism and specific neurotransmitters: acetylcholine, norepinephrine, serotonin, and dopamine (Vance, 008). Numerous double-blind placebo-controlled studies have been carried out on phopatidlyserine and they show that it can lead to very noteworthy improvements in early dementia, early AD, and age-related cognitive decline (Ballard, Margallo-Lana, Juszczak, Douglas, Swann, Thomas, ... & Lee, 2015).

Parkinson's disease is a brain disorder that results from nerve damage in certain regions of the brain causing muscle rigidity, shaking, and difficult walking (Singleton, Farrer, Johnson, Singleton, Hague, Kachergus,... & Lincoln, 2003) usually occurring in mid to late adult life. Canadian researchers indicated that vitamin E in food may be protective against Parkinson's disease (Yang, Wolk, Håkansson, Pedersen, & Wirdefeldt, 2017). Creatine appeared to modify Parkinson's disease features as measured by a decline in the clinical signs. Researchers have also studied glutathione to determine its effect on nerve and its power as an antioxidant. The appropriate long-term dosing, side-effects and the most effective method of administration are not yet clear. Nutritional supplements have shown some promising results in preliminary studies, it is important to remember that there is not sufficient scientific data to recommend them for Parkinson's disease at present. The patients should be cautioned that over-the counter medications do have side effects and interactions with other drugs and are also expensive (Singleton, Farrer, Johnson, Singleton, Hague, Kachergus,... & Lincoln, 2003).

Figure 3. Broad Sources of nutraceuticals (Chadha, 2015; Dillard & German, 2000)

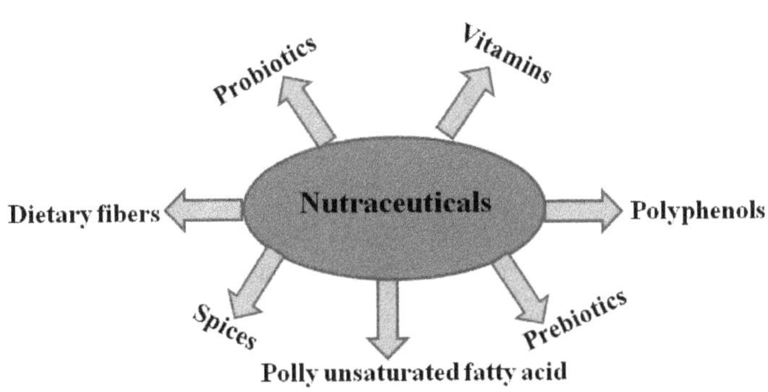

Nutraceuticals Used Against Alzheimer's Disease (AD)

Alzheimer"s disease (AD), also called senile dementia of the Alzheimer type (SDAT), primary degenerative dementia of the Alzheimer's type (PDDAT), or simply Alzheimer's, is the most common form of dementia. The various Nutraceuticals, which are used to cure Alzheimer's disease are:

1. **Anti-Oxidants:** Antioxidants like vitamin E and vitamin C (Boothby & Doering, 2005; Coppen & Bolander-Gouaille, 2005; Zee,1991).
2. **Gingko Biloba:** Ginkgo biloba is perhaps the most studied herbs with reference to memory, cognition, overall brain performance and certainly AD.
3. **Huperzine Alpha:** Huperzine alpha or huperzine A is a very appealing plant compound that is extracted from club moss or Huperziaserrata (Pohanka, 2014).

Current Research in Nutraceuticals

A great deal of current research is focused on traditional herbal extracts. Investigators are examining claims linking these extracts with health enhancement and prevention of chronic diseases. At least in part, this represents an effort to legitimize homeopathic remedies and Eastern medicine. Additionally, it seeks to provide patients and physicians with much-needed safety and efficacy data. The urgent demand of bioactive materials for nutraceuticals and functional foods is being driven by mostly cited health concerns:

1. Cardiovascular disease
2. Breast, skin, colorectal and brain cancers
3. Female health concerns
4. CNS disorders
5. Metabolism management
6. Gastrointestinal disorders
7. Immunomodulation

A significant problem with the use of nutraceuticals in treating diseases is the lack of serious studies published with clear clinical evidence. The latest scientific research and clinical trials continue to boost and add impetus to this industry.

Types of Brain Disorders

Neurodegenerative disorders are among the most serious health issue for our society, causing untold human suffering. They are also among the most mysterious of all diseases, and our ignorance of the underlying disease mechanisms is a major obstacle to the development of better treatments. It can affect anyone, but your risk factors are different for different types of brain disorders.

There are many types of brain disorders, including:

1. Alzheimer's disease (AD)
2. Dementia
3. Epilepsy
4. Multiple sclerosis
5. Parkinson's disease
6. Migraines
7. Strokes
8. Depression
9. Schizophrenia
10. Anxiety

In the Treatment of Diet-Related Diseases

The scientific research showed that the incidence of diet related diseases are progressively in increasing order due to their hypercaloric food intake and life style. Obesity, diabetes, atherosclerosis and neurodegeneration are major diet-related pathologies that share a common pathogenic denominator of low-grade inflammation. Nutraceuticals and functional foods may represent a novel therapeutic approach for the attenuation or prevention of diet-related disease such as inflammatory disease. In particular, activation of intestinal regulatory cells and homeostatic regulation of the gut microbiota have the potential to reduce low-grade inflammation in diet-related diseases.

Functional Foods

The term functional foods was first introduced in Japan in the mid1980s and refers to foods and their components that may provide a health benefit beyond basic nutrition (Cencic, & Chingwaru, 2010). Functional foods are similar in appearance

Table 3. Types of functional food in brain

Components		Sources	Benefits
Carotenoids	Beta-Carotene	Carrots, Various fruits	Neutralizes free radicals which may damage cells; bolsters cellular antioxidant defences (Noviendri, Hasrini, & Octavianti, 2013)
Fatty Acids	Polly unsaturated fatty acids(PUFAS) omega-3 fatty acid (ALA)	Walt nut, Flaxseed	Maintenance mental disorders (Wildman, 2016)
	Polly unsaturated fatty acid (PUFA)- omega-3 fatty acids- DHA/EPA	Salmon, Tuna, Marine and other fish oils	Maintenance mental disease (Lobo, Patil, Phatak, & Chandra, 2010)
Flavonoids	Anthocyanidins	Berries, Cherries, Red grapes	Bolster cellular antioxidant defenses, may contribute to maintenance of brain functions (Tapas, Sakarkar, & Kakde, 2008)
	Flavnones	Citrus foods	Neutralize free radicals which may damage cells; bolster cellular antioxidatant defenses (Tapas, Sakarkar, & Kakde, 2008)
	Flavonols	Onions, Apples, Tea, Broccoli	Neutralize free radicals which may damage cells; bolster cellular antioxidatant defenses (Georgiev, Ananga & Tsolova, 2014)
Isothiocyanats	Sulfoophane	Cauliflower, Broccoli, Brussels sprouts, Cabbage Kale, Horseradish	Bolster cellular antioxidant defences (Moreno, Carvajal, López-Berenguer, & García-Viguera, 2006)
Phenols	Caffieic acid, Ferulic acid	Apple, Pears, Citrus fruits, Some vegetables	Bolster cellular antioxidant defences (Lin & Zhao, 2007)

to conventional foods; the former being consumed as part of the normal diet also can play a role in reducing the risk of disease and promoting good health. All foods have a function when consumed in proper balance as part of an overall healthy diet. Those foods that have been fortified, enriched, or enhanced with nutrients, phytochemicals, or botanicals, as well as dietary supplements, also fall within the realm of functional foods. Thus, functional food provides the body with the required amount of vitamins, fats, proteins, carbohydrates, etc., needed for its healthy survival. Recently food science and technology, an aging population, the rapid rise in health care costs, have increased the amount of omega-3 in the eggs they sell (Cencic, & Chingwaru, 2010).

Figure 4. Future of nutraceuticals

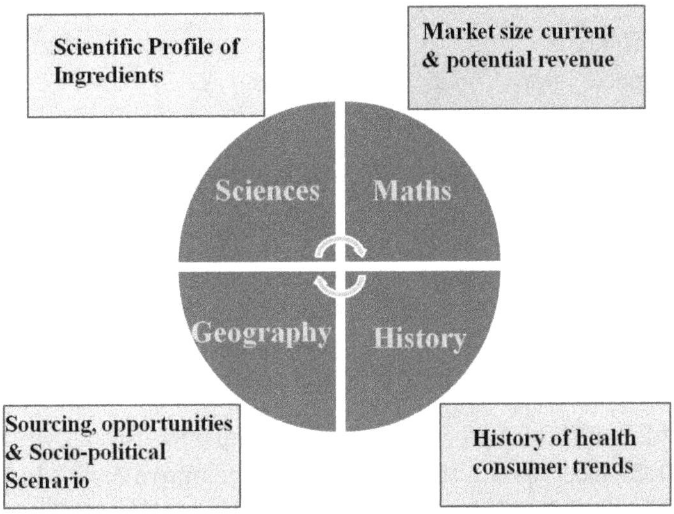

CONCLUSION AND FUTURE PROSPECTS

In the view of increasing number of cases of neurodegenerative disorders, the role of nutraceuticals and functional food are very crucial and important. The proper mechanism through which nutraceuticals prevent such chronic diseases has not been fully elucidated. Many of these phytochemicals have been found to alter antioxidant defence of cells through the induction of DNA repair processes or enzymatic antioxidant defence at the gene level. It has been suggested that they may also affect cell cycle progression cell communication (Hwang & Bowen, 2004; Stahl & Sies, 2000) hormone and growth factor signaling and apoptosis (Zhang, Xuan, Bouxsein, von Stechow, Akeno, Faugere, ... & Clemens, 2002). Therefore, any health benefits attributed to functional foods should be based on sound and accurate scientific criteria, including rigorous studies of safety and efficacy. Interactions with other dietary components and potential adverse interactions with pharmaceutical agents must be clearly imparted. Consumers must realize that functional foods are not a ——wonder food or a panacea for poor health habits. Nutraceuticals have great potential, as an alternative to substance obtained by plant. Yet, some time they also cause harmful effect as seen with ephedrine, a widely used botanical ingredient in weight-loss products. Now days peoples are more conscious about their health and these products offer the promised health benefits. The proper diet and together with life style, functional foods may very effective to maximize health and reduce neurodegenerative disorder risk. Nutraceuticals in Nutrition and Pharmaceuticals, indeed will be positively sustain better future in therapeutics (Figure 4).

REFERENCES

Ajjawi, I., & Shintani, D. (2004). Engineered plants with elevated vitamin E: A nutraceutical success story. *Trends in Biotechnology*, *22*(3), 104–107. doi:10.1016/j.tibtech.2004.01.008 PMID:15043044

Aluko, R. E. (2012). *Functional foods and nutraceuticals*. New York: Springer. doi:10.1007/978-1-4614-3480-1

Bagchi, D., Bagchi, M., Stohs, S. J., Das, D. K., Ray, S. D., Kuszynski, C. A., ... Pruess, H. G. (2000). Free radicals and grape seed proanthocyanidin extract: Importance in human health and disease prevention. *Toxicology*, *148*(2), 187–197. doi:10.1016/S0300-483X(00)00210-9 PMID:10962138

Ballard, C., Margallo-Lana, M., Juszczak, E., Douglas, S., Swann, A., Thomas, A., ... Lee, L. (2005). Quetiapine and rivastigmine and cognitive decline in Alzheimer9s disease: Randomised double blind placebo controlled trial. *BMJ (Clinical Research Ed.)*, *330*(7496), 874. doi:10.1136/bmj.38369.459988.8F PMID:15722369

Barrow, C., & Shahidi, F. (Eds.). (2007). *Marine nutraceuticals and functional foods*. CRC Press.

Boothby, L. A., & Doering, P. L. (2005). Vitamin C and vitamin E for Alzheimer's disase. *The Annals of Pharmacotherapy*, *39*(12), 2073–2080. doi:10.1345/aph.1E495 PMID:16227450

Cencic, A., & Chingwaru, W. (2010). The role of functional foods, nutraceuticals, and food supplements in intestinal health. *Nutrients*, *2*(6), 611–625. doi:10.3390/nu2060611 PMID:22254045

Chadha, R., Bhalla, Y., Vashisht, M. K., & Chadha, K. (2015). Cocrystallization in Nutraceuticals. In *Recrystallization in Materials Processing*. InTech. doi:10.5772/59365

Chaturvedi, S., Sharma, P. K., Garg, V. K., & Bansal, M. (2011). Role of nutraceuticals in health promotion. *Health, 4*, 5.

Chauhan, B., Kumar, G., Kalam, N., & Ansari, S. H. (2013). Current concepts and prospects of herbal nutraceutical: A review. *Journal of Advanced Pharmaceutical Technology & Research*, *4*(1), 4. doi:10.4103/2231-4040.107494 PMID:23662276

Comin, L. M., Temelli, F., & Saldaña, M. A. (2011). Supercritical CO2 extraction of flax lignans. *Journal of the American Oil Chemists' Society*, *88*(5), 707–715. doi:10.100711746-010-1704-9

Coppen, A., & Bolander-Gouaille, C. (2005). Treatment of depression: Time to consider folic acid and vitamin B12. *Journal of Psychopharmacology (Oxford, England), 19*(1), 59–65. doi:10.1177/0269881105048899 PMID:15671130

Dai, J., & Mumper, R. J. (2010). Plant phenolics: Extraction, analysis and their antioxidant and anticancer properties. *Molecules (Basel, Switzerland), 15*(10), 7313–7352. doi:10.3390/molecules15107313 PMID:20966876

Das, L., Bhaumik, E., Raychaudhuri, U., & Chakraborty, R. (2012). Role of nutraceuticals in human health. *Journal of Food Science and Technology, 49*(2), 173–183. doi:10.100713197-011-0269-4 PMID:23572839

Das, L., Bhaumik, E., Raychaudhuri, U., & Chakraborty, R. (2012, April). Role of nutraceuticals in human health. *Journal of Food Science and Technology, 49*(2), 173–183. doi:10.100713197-011-0269-4 PMID:23572839

Depeint, F., Bruce, W. R., Shangari, N., Mehta, R., & O'Brien, P. J. (2006). Mitochondrial function and toxicity: Role of the B vitamin family on mitochondrial energy metabolism. *Chemico-Biological Interactions, 163*(1), 94–112. doi:10.1016/j.cbi.2006.04.014 PMID:16765926

Dillard, C. J., & German, J. B. (2000). Phytochemicals: Nutraceuticals and human health. *Journal of the Science of Food and Agriculture, 80*(12), 1744–1756. doi:10.1002/1097-0010(20000915)80:12<1744::AID-JSFA7253.0.CO;2-W

Dureja, H., Kaushik, D., & Kumar, V. (2003). Developments in nutraceuticals. *Indian Journal of Pharmacology, 35*(6), 363–372.

Fatima, M., Kesharwani, R. K., Misra, K., & Rizvi, S. I. (2013). Protective effect of theaflavin on erythrocytes subjected to in vitro oxidative stress. *Biochemistry Research International*. PMID:24455262

Georgiev, V., Ananga, A., & Tsolova, V. (2014). Recent advances and uses of grape flavonoids as nutraceuticals. *Nutrients, 6*(1), 391–415. doi:10.3390/nu6010391 PMID:24451310

Hager, K., Marahrens, A., Kenklies, M., Riederer, P., & Münch, G. (2001). Alpha-lipoic acid as a new treatment option for Azheimer type dementia. *Archives of Gerontology and Geriatrics, 32*(3), 275–282. doi:10.1016/S0167-4943(01)00104-2 PMID:11395173

Hathcock, J. (2001). Dietary supplements: How they are used and regulated. *The Journal of Nutrition, 131*(3), 1114S–1117S. doi:10.1093/jn/131.3.1114S PMID:11238828

Hernández-Díaz, S., Werler, M. M., Walker, A. M., & Mitchell, A. A. (2000). Folic acid antagonists during pregnancy and the risk of birth defects. *The New England Journal of Medicine*, *343*(22), 1608–1614. doi:10.1056/NEJM200011303432204 PMID:11096168

Houston, M. C. (2005). Nutraceuticals, vitamins, antioxidants, and minerals in the prevention and treatment of hypertension. *Progress in Cardiovascular Diseases*, *47*(6), 396–449. doi:10.1016/j.pcad.2005.01.004 PMID:16115519

Hwang, E. S., & Bowen, P. E. (2004). Cell cycle arrest and induction of apoptosis by lycopene in LNCaP human prostate cancer cells. *Journal of Medicinal Food*, *7*(3), 284–289. doi:10.1089/jmf.2004.7.284 PMID:15383220

Jiang, T., Sun, Q., & Chen, S. (2016). Oxidative stress: A major pathogenesis and potential therapeutic target of antioxidative agents in Parkinson's disease and Alzheimer's disease. *Progress in Neurobiology*, *147*, 1–19. doi:10.1016/j.pneurobio.2016.07.005 PMID:27769868

Keservani, R. K., Kesharwani, R. K., Sharma, A. K., Vyas, N., & Chadoker, A. (2010a). Nutritional supplements: An overview. *Int J Curr Pharm Rev Res*, *1*, 59–75.

Keservani, R. K., Kesharwani, R. K., Vyas, N., Jain, S., Raghuvanshi, R., & Sharma, A. K. (2010b). Nutraceutical and functional food as future food: A review. *Der Pharmacia Lett*, *2*, 106–116.

Keservani, R. K., Sharma, A. K., & Kesharwani, R. K. (2016). Medicinal effect of nutraceutical fruits for the cognition and brain health. *Scientifica*. PMID:26966612

Kim, L. S., Axelrod, L. J., Howard, P., Buratovich, N., & Waters, R. F. (2006). Efficacy of methylsulfonylmethane (MSM) in osteoarthritis pain of the knee: A pilot clinical trial. *Osteoarthritis and Cartilage*, *14*(3), 286–294. doi:10.1016/j.joca.2005.10.003 PMID:16309928

Kumar, K., & Kumar, S. (2015). Role of nutraceuticals in health and disease prevention: A review. *South Asian J Food Technol Environ*, *1*, 116–121.

Lee, J., Koo, N., & Min, D. B. (2004). Reactive oxygen species, aging, and antioxidative nutraceuticals. *Comprehensive Reviews in Food Science and Food Safety*, *3*(1), 21–33. doi:10.1111/j.1541-4337.2004.tb00058.x

Lin, D., & Zhao, Y. (2007). Innovations in the development and application of edible coatings for fresh and minimally processed fruits and vegetables. *Comprehensive Reviews in Food Science and Food Safety*, *6*(3), 60–75. doi:10.1111/j.1541-4337.2007.00018.x

Lobo, V., Patil, A., Phatak, A., & Chandra, N. (2010). Free radicals, antioxidants and functional foods: Impact on human health. *Pharmacognosy Reviews*, *4*(8), 118. doi:10.4103/0973-7847.70902 PMID:22228951

Lockwood, B. (2007). *Nutraceuticals: a guide for healthcare professionals*. Pharmaceutical Press.

Moreno, D. A., Carvajal, M., López-Berenguer, C., & García-Viguera, C. (2006). Chemical and biological characterisation of nutraceutical compounds of broccoli. *Journal of Pharmaceutical and Biomedical Analysis*, *41*(5), 1508–1522. doi:10.1016/j.jpba.2006.04.003 PMID:16713696

Nieves, J. W. (2013). Skeletal effects of nutrients and nutraceuticals, beyond calcium and vitamin D. *Osteoporosis International*, *24*(3), 771–786. doi:10.100700198-012-2214-4 PMID:23152094

Noviendri, D., Hasrini, R. F., & Octavianti, F. (2011). Carotenoids: Sources, medicinal properties and their application in food and nutraceutical industry. *Journal of Medicinal Plants Research*, *5*(33), 7119–7131.

O'connor, T. (2017). Developing New Functional Food and Nutraceutical Products. *Journal of Nutrition Education and Behavior*, *49*(9), 793. doi:10.1016/j.jneb.2017.05.356

Olesen, J., Gustavsson, A., Svensson, M., Wittchen, H. U., & Jönsson, B. (2012). The economic cost of brain disorders in Europe. *European Journal of Neurology*, *19*(1), 155–162. doi:10.1111/j.1468-1331.2011.03590.x PMID:22175760

Over the Counter & Complementary Therapies. (2017). Parkinson's Foundation. Retrieved from www.parkinson.org/Understanding-Parkinsons/Treatment/Over-the-Counter-and-Complementary-Therapies

Pathak, Y. V. (Ed.). (2010). Handbook of Nutraceuticals: Vol. 1. Ingredients, Formulations, and Applications. CRC Press.

Perera, T., & Thevathasan, W. (2014). *An Introduction to Parkinson's Disease*. Academic Press.

Pohanka, M. (2014). Alzheimer s disease and oxidative stress: A review. *Current Medicinal Chemistry*, *21*(3), 356–364. doi:10.2174/09298673113206660258 PMID:24059239

Rajasekaran, A., Sivagnanam, G., & Xavier, R. (2008). Nutraceuticals as therapeutic agents: A Review. *Res J Pharm Tech*, *1*(4), 328–340.

Riggs, K. M., Spiro, A. I. I. III, Tucker, K., & Rush, D. (1996). Relations of vitamin B-12, vitamin B-6, folate, and homocysteine to cognitive performance in the Normative Aging Study. *The American Journal of Clinical Nutrition*, *63*(3), 306–314. doi:10.1093/ajcn/63.3.306 PMID:8602585

Rimm, E. B., Willett, W. C., Hu, F. B., Sampson, L., Colditz, G. A., Manson, J. E., ... Stampfer, M. J. (1998). Folate and vitamin B6 from diet and supplements in relation to risk of coronary heart disease among women. *Journal of the American Medical Association*, *279*(5), 359–364. doi:10.1001/jama.279.5.359 PMID:9459468

Salak-Johnson, J. L., & McGlone, J. J. (2007). Making sense of apparently conflicting data: Stress and immunity in swine and cattle. *Journal of Animal Science, 85*(13_suppl), E81-E88.

Schloss, J. M., Colosimo, M., Airey, C., Masci, P. P., Linnane, A. W., & Vitetta, L. (2013). Nutraceuticals and chemotherapy induced peripheral neuropathy (CIPN): A systematic review. *Clinical Nutrition (Edinburgh, Lothian)*, *32*(6), 888–893. doi:10.1016/j.clnu.2013.04.007 PMID:23647723

Scicchitano, P., Cameli, M., Maiello, M., Modesti, P. A., Muiesan, M. L., Novo, S., ... di Studio Ipertensione, G. (2014). Nutraceuticals and dyslipidaemia: Beyond the common therapeutics. *Journal of Functional Foods*, *6*, 11–32. doi:10.1016/j.jff.2013.12.006

Semo, E., Kesselman, E., Danino, D., & Livney, Y. D. (2007). Casein micelle as a natural nano-capsular vehicle for nutraceuticals. *Food Hydrocolloids*, *21*(5), 936–942. doi:10.1016/j.foodhyd.2006.09.006

Singh, P., Kesharwani, R. K., & Keservani, R. K. (2018). Antioxidants and Vitamins: Roles in Cellular Function and Metabolism. In Sustained Energy for Enhanced Human Functions and Activity (pp. 385-407). Academic Press.

Singh, U., & Jialal, I. (2008). Retracted: Alpha-lipoic acid supplementation and diabetes. *Nutrition Reviews*, *66*(11), 646–657. doi:10.1111/j.1753-4887.2008.00118.x PMID:19019027

Singleton, A. B., Farrer, M., Johnson, J., Singleton, A., Hague, S., Kachergus, J., ... Lincoln, S. (2003). α-Synuclein locus triplication causes Parkinson's disease. *Science*, *302*(5646), 841–841. doi:10.1126cience.1090278 PMID:14593171

Skeggs, H. R., & Wright, L. D. (1944). The use of Lactobacillus arabinosus in the microbiological determination of pantothenic acid. *The Journal of Biological Chemistry*, *156*, 21–26.

Stahl, W., & Sies, H. (2003). Antioxidant activity of carotenoids. *Molecular Aspects of Medicine*, *24*(6), 345–351. doi:10.1016/S0098-2997(03)00030-X PMID:14585305

Story, E. N., Kopec, R. E., Schwartz, S. J., & Harris, G. K. (2010). An update on the health effects of tomato lycopene. *Annual Review of Food Science and Technology*, *1*(1), 189–210. doi:10.1146/annurev.food.102308.124120 PMID:22129335

Sunitha, Nandha Kishore Chary, & Hemalatha, & Unissa. (2016). A Review on Nutraceuticals. *International Journal of Pharmaceutical Research And Bio-Science.*, *5*(1), 123–135.

Tapas, A. R., Sakarkar, D. M., & Kakde, R. B. (2008). Flavonoids as nutraceuticals: A review. *Tropical Journal of Pharmaceutical Research*, *7*(3), 1089–1099. doi:10.4314/tjpr.v7i3.14693

Traber, M. G., & Stevens, J. F. (2011). Vitamins C and E: Beneficial effects from a mechanistic perspective. *Free Radical Biology & Medicine*, *51*(5), 1000–1013. doi:10.1016/j.freeradbiomed.2011.05.017 PMID:21664268

Upadhyay, J., Kesharwani, R. K., & Misra, K. (2009). Comparative study of antioxidants as cancer preventives through inhibition of HIF-1 alpha activity. *Bioinformation*, *4*(6), 233–236. doi:10.6026/97320630004233 PMID:20975915

Vance, J. E. (2008). Thematic Review Series: Glycerolipids. Phosphatidylserine and phosphatidylethanolamine in mammalian cells: two metabolically related aminophospholipids. *Journal of Lipid Research*, *49*(7), 1377–1387. doi:10.1194/jlr.R700020-JLR200 PMID:18204094

Velikov, K. P., & Pelan, E. (2008). Colloidal delivery systems for micronutrients and nutraceuticals. *Soft Matter*, *4*(10), 1964–1980. doi:10.1039/b804863k

Wang, G., & Hollingsworth, R. I. (1999). Synthetic routes to L-carnitine and L-gamma-amino-beta-hydroxybutyric acid from (S)-3-hydroxybutyrolactone by functional group priority switching. *Tetrahedron, Asymmetry*, *10*(10), 1895–1901. doi:10.1016/S0957-4166(99)00169-X

Ward, S., Chackalamannil, S., & Rotella, D. (2017). Comprehensive. *Medicinal Chemistry (Shariqah, United Arab Emirates)*, III. PMID:28724914

Wildman, R. E. (Ed.). (2016). *Handbook of nutraceuticals and functional foods.* CRC press.

Yang, F., Wolk, A., Håkansson, N., Pedersen, N. L., & Wirdefeldt, K. (2017). Dietary antioxidants and risk of Parkinson's disease in two population-based cohorts. *Movement Disorders*, *32*(11), 1631–1636. doi:10.1002/mds.27120 PMID:28881039

Zee, J., Carmichael, L., Codère, D., Poirier, D., & Fournier, M. (1991). Effect of storage conditions on the stability of vitamin C in various fruits and vegetables produced and consumed in Quebec. *Journal of Food Composition and Analysis*, *4*(1), 77–86. doi:10.1016/0889-1575(91)90050-G

Zhang, M., Xuan, S., Bouxsein, M. L., von Stechow, D., Akeno, N., Faugere, M. C., ... Clemens, T. L. (2002). Osteoblast-specific knockout of the insulin-like growth factor (IGF) receptor gene reveals an essential role of IGF signaling in bone matrix mineralization. *The Journal of Biological Chemistry*, *277*(46), 44005–44012. doi:10.1074/jbc.M208265200 PMID:12215457

Zilberman, D., Yarkin, C., & Heiman, A. (1997, August). *Agricultural biotechnology: economic and international implications*. Invited paper presented at the International Agricultural Economics Association meeting, Sacramento, CA.

Section 6
Anemia

Chapter 11
Nutraceutical and Functional Foods in Treatment of Anemia

Vandana B. Patravale
Institute of Chemical Technology, India

Namrata A. Kadwadkar
Institute of Chemical Technology, India

Shalaka R. Patki
Tatyasaheb Kore College of Pharmacy, India

John Intru DiSouza
Tatyasaheb Kore College of Pharmacy, India

ABSTRACT

WHO database mentions that the global anemia-affected population is 24.8%. To name a few conditions in which compromisation of the red blood corpuscles and hemoglobin occurs are iron deficiency anemia, gestational anemia, anemia due to malaria and parasitism, hemolytic anemia, sickle cell anemia. The line of treatment in case of anemia involves administration of iron supplements, plasmapheresis, steroids, blood transfusion at regular intervals, and lifestyle changes. The systematic approach applied for the pharmaceutical molecules should be equally inculcated in the case of nutraceuticals. The traditional system when woven carefully with the novel drug delivery system will give effective nutrient delivery. Functional foods have inherent nutritional value. Nutraceuticals and functional food cannot cure the anemic condition, but help the patient lead life almost like a normal individual.

DOI: 10.4018/978-1-5225-3267-5.ch011

INTRODUCTION

Overview of Anemia

Anemia is a well-known public health problem majorly in gestational women and young children. The factors can be either being decreased red blood cell production or increased red blood cell destruction. The Figure 1 gives frame-diagram of anemia for understanding causes of anemia. A daily requirement of 20 to 30 mg of iron is required by the body for erythropoiesis and other biological processes. A lack of this supply of this iron or its absorption due to varied causes leads to anemia (Greenburg, 1996). WHO 2011 gives us a look at the worldwide prevalence of anemia; same is given in Table 1. Figure 2 gives us an insight about the prevalence of the anemia on the global level in infants and children.

Causes of Anemia

Out of abundant elemental iron available, only a small part of dietary iron is available to the human body, out which 20% is stocked in the storage compartment and 1 and 2mg of iron is lost each day. The total body iron in adult male is 3000 to 4000mg as opposed to 2000mg to 3000mg in adult female. This itself reflects the reason for smaller reserves of iron in female, hence the lower hemoglobin. *Figure 3* explains the physiological turnover of iron in male and female body.

Figure 1. Frame-diagram of anemia for understanding causes of anemia

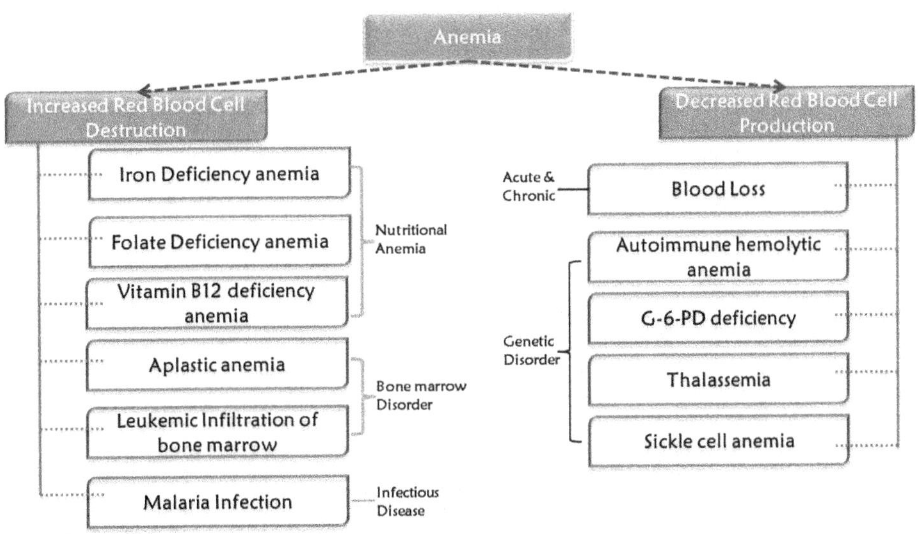

Table 1. Global and WHO regional mean blood hemoglobin concentration and prevalence of anemia by population group for 2011 (WHO, 2011, used with permission)

WHO Region	Mean (95% CI) Blood Hemoglobin Concentration (g/l)	Percentage (95% CI) of Population With Anemia[a]	Number (95% CI) of People With Anemia (Millions)[b]	Percentage (95% CI) of Population With Severe Anemia[c]	Number (95% CI) of People With Severe Anemia (Millions)[c]
Children Aged 6-59 Months					
African Region	104 (103 to 105)	62.3 (59.6 to 64.8)	84.5 (81 to 87.9)	3.6 (2.9 to 4.4)	4.9 (4.0 to 6.0)
Region of the Americas	119 (117 to 121)	22.3 (17.7 to 27.9)	17.1 (13.5 to 21.3)	0.2 (0.1 to 0.5)	0.18 (0.1 to 0.4)
South-east Asia Region	107 (104 to 112)	53.8 (39.9 to 63.9)	96.7 (71.7 to 115.0)	1.5 (0.4 to 3.7)	2.7 (0.8 to 6.6)
European Region	119 (115 to 122)	22.9 (14.9 to 32.8)	12.7 (8.2 to 18.1)	0.3 (0.1 to 0.8)	0.2 (0.0 to 0.5)
Eastern Mediterranean Region	109 (106 to 112)	48.6 (40.4 to 57.0)	35.8 (29.7 to 41.9)	2.0 (1.0 to 3.1)	1.5 (0.7 to 2.3)
Western Pacific Region	120 (114 to 125)	21.9 (12 to 36.9)	25.7 (14.2 to 43.4)	0.2 (0.0 to 0.6)	0.2 (0.0 to 0.7)
Global	111 (110 to 113)	42.6 (37.7 to 47.4)	273.2 (241.8 to 303.7)	1.5 (1.0 to 2.2)	9.6 (6.9 to 14.1)
Non-Pregnant Women Aged 15-49 Years					
African Region	124 (121 to 126)	37.8 (31.8 to 43.7)	69.9 (58.8 to 80.7)	1.8 (1.3 to 2.7)	3.3 (2.4 to 5.1)
Region of the Americas	131 (128 to 134)	16.5 (12.2 to 23.7)	38.1 (28.1 to 54.7)	0.5 (0.3 to 1.1)	1.3 (0.7 to 2.6)
South-east Asia Region	121 (117 to 126)	41.5 (28.7 to 52.6)	190.6 (131.7 to 241.3)	1.9 (0.7 to 3.8)	8.6 (3.4 to 17.5)
European Region	128 (126 to 130)	22.5 (16.4 to 30.1)	48.4 (35.2 to 64.7)	0.6 (0.3 to 1.2)	1.3 (0.7 to 2.6)
Eastern Mediterranean Region	123 (120 to 126)	37.7 (30.7 to 45.6)	55.2 (44.9 to 66.8)	1.8 (1.1 to 2.6)	2.6 (1.6 to 3.8)
Western Pacific Region	129 (124 to 134)	19.8 (10.9 to 36.6)	92.6 (50.8 to 170.9)	0.5 (0.2 to 1.3)	2.2 (0.8 to 6.0)
Global	126 (124 to 128)	29.0 (23.9 to 34.8)	496.3 (409.3 to 595.1)	1.1 (0.7 to 1.7)	19.4 (12.7 to 29.4)

continued on following page

Table 1. Continued

WHO Region	Mean (95% CI) Blood Hemoglobin Concentration (g/l)	Percentage (95% CI) of Population With Anemia[a]	Number (95% CI) of People With Anemia (Millions)[b]	Percentage (95% CI) of Population With Severe Anemia[c]	Number (95% CI) of People With Severe Anemia (Millions)[c]
Pregnant Women Aged 15-49 Years					
African Region	111 (110 to 114)	46.3 (40.6 to 51.0)	9.2 (8.13 to 10.1)	1.5 (1.0 to 2.3)	0.3 (0.2 to 0.5)
Region of the Americas	119 (116 to 122)	24.9 (19.0 to 32.5)	2.4 (1.8 to 3.1)	0.3 (0.1 to 0.6)	0.0 (0.0 to 0.1)
South-east Asia Region	110 (106 to 114)	48.7 (36.1 to 58.9)	11.5 (8.5 to 13.9)	1.1 (0.5 to 2.2)	0.3 (0.1 to 0.5)
European Region	118 (115 to 121)	25.8 (19.8 to 33.6)	1.8 (1.4 to 2.3)	0.3 (0.1 to 0.6)	0.0 (0.0 to 0.0)
Eastern Mediterranean Region	113 (111 to 116)	38.9 (32.7 to 46.3)	3.9 (3.3 to 4.6)	1.1 (0.6 to 1.6)	0.1 (0.1 to 0.2)
Western Pacific Region	119 (114 to 124)	24.3 (15.1 to 37.7)	3.6 (2.2 to 5.5)	0.4 (0.1 to 0.9)	0.1 (0.0 to 0.1)
Global	114 (112 to 116)	38.2 (33.5 to 42.6)	32.4 (28.41 to 36.2)	0.9 (0.6 to 1.3)	0.8 (0.5 to 1.1)
All Women of Reproductive Age (15-49 Years)					
African Region	123 (120 to 125)	38.6 (32.9 to 44.2)	79.1 (67.3 to 90.5)	1.8 (1.3 to 2.7)	3.6 (2.6 to 5.5)
Region of the Americas	131 (128 to 133)	16.8 (12.6 to 23.8)	40.5 (30.2 to 57.3)	0.5 (0.3 to 1.1)	1.3 (0.7 to 2.7)
South-east Asia Region	121 (117 to 125)	41.9 (29.4 to 52.7)	202.0 (141.8 to 254.3)	1.8 (0.7 to 3.8)	8.9 (3.5 to 18.1)
European Region	128 (125 to 130)	22.6 (16.6 to 29.9)	50.2 (36.8 to 66.5)	0.6 (0.3 to 1.2)	1.4 (0.7 to 2.7)
Eastern Mediterranean Region	122 (120 to 125)	37.8 (31.0 to 45.5)	59.1 (48.4 to 71.2)	1.8 (1.1 to 2.5)	2.7 (1.7 to 3.9)
Western Pacific Region	129 (124 to 134)	19.9 (11.1 to 36.3)	96.2 (53.5 to 175.3)	0.5 (0.2 to 1.3)	2.3 (0.8 to 6.1)
Global	125 (124 to 127)	29.4 (24.5 to 35.0)	528.7 (440.3 to 629.4)	1.1 (0.7 to 1.7)	20.2 (13.3 to 30.5)

CI: confidence interval

a. Anemia is defined as blood hemoglobin concentration < 110g/L for children and pregnant women and <120 g/L for non-pregnant women

b. Estimates of the number of children affected correspond to the age range 0-59 months

c. Severe anemia is defined as blood hemoglobin concentration <70 g/L for children and pregnant women and <80 g/L for non-pregnant women

Figure 2. Global estimates of the prevalence of anemia in infants and children aged 6–59 months, 2011 Source: WHO, 2011

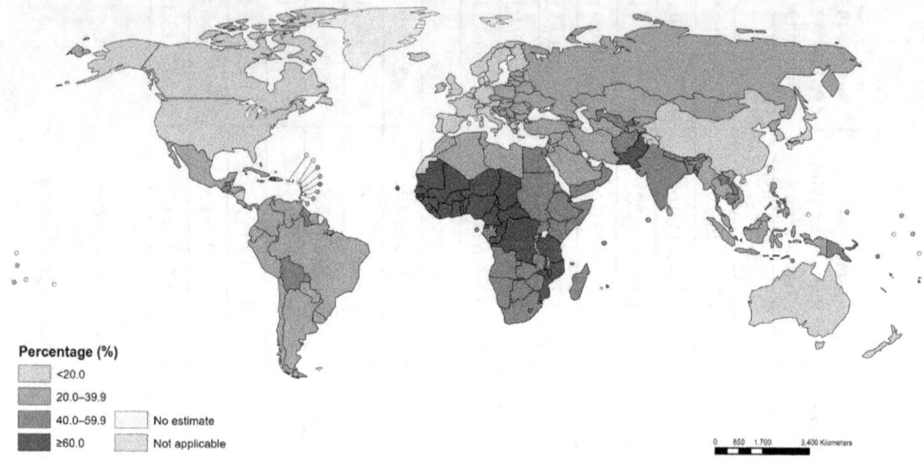

Figure 3. The physiological turn-over of iron in male and female body

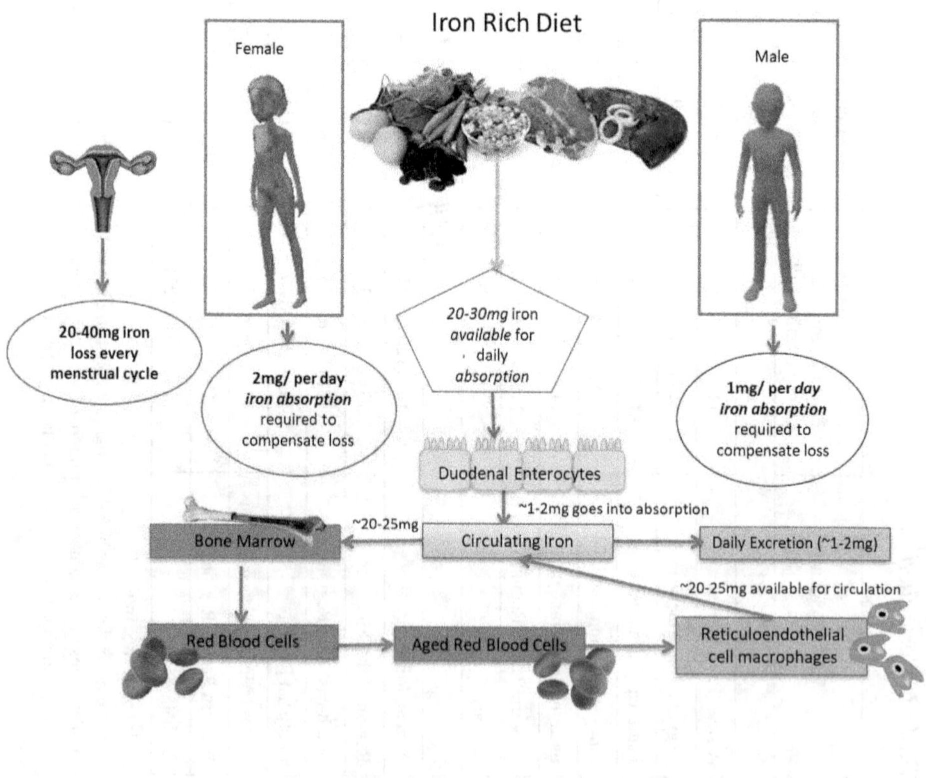

Understanding Types Anemia and Its Causes

Anemia is a condition in which there is a deficiency of red cells or of hemoglobin in the blood, resulting in paleness and fatigue. Anemic condition can be temporarily caused to due increased body needs or due to medications used for treating other ailments. A permanent type of anemia is the one which occurs due to genetic deformation. Let us understand both the types and its causes in detail in this subsection.

Iron deficiency anemia is a case of temporary anemia. It is majorly observed in adolescents in the higher amounts as compared to adults due to the increased iron needs in the growing and developing body. The adolescent females have higher iron demand as compared to adolescent males as the female body is subject to blood loss during menstruation (Dallman, 1992).

The chronic consumption of alcohol makes the person susceptible to anemia. The chronic alcoholism results in occult bleeding causing iron deficiency, also the inadequate balanced diet results in folate deficiency by decreased renal reabsorption of folic acid and the deficiency of pyridoxine due to metabolic disorder contributes to anemia.(Ballard, 1997; Caballero, Finglas, & Toldrá, 2015; Halsted, Villanueva, Devlin, & Chandler, 2002; Latvala, Parkkila, & Niemelä, 2004). Patients who are exposed to large amounts of Aluminum via dialysis fluids or aluminum phosphate binders are subjected to microcytic hypochromic anemia; in this case the red blood cell integrity is impaired, reduced iron absorption occurs and delivery to cells to follows(Wills & Savory,1989).

Gestational anemia is the most talked and highly addressed type of anemia, as this type of anemia can be treated and cured with appropriate dietary measures with few food supplements like nutraceuticals (Allen, De Benoist, Dary, Hurrell, & World Health Organization, 2006). Gestational anemia or anemia caused due to pregnancy occurs as consequence of hormonal changes and the demand to supply ration of the iron for producing new red blood cells due to increased blood volume and the account of blood loss during delivery (Bothwell & Charlton, 1981).

Anemia is also caused due to the effects of the malarial parasites; these cause vascular hemolysis and also trigger suppression of erythropoietin through the immune response (Kasili, 1999; Loban, Polozok, Efimov, & Khorin, 1987; Spielman, 2001). Another parasite that is responsible for iron deficiency anemia are the hookworms, they reside in the intestinal tract of an individual where they feed on the blood passing through the villi thus reducing the ability to preserve stores in the affected individuals (van den Broek, 1996)

Permanent Anemia is that type of anemia which is not curable using medications, but dietary changes and food supplements help the individual lead almost a normal life. Genetic anemia and bone marrow disorders are the ones which fall in this category. Thalassemia, autoimmune-hemolytic anemia, Glucose-6-phosphatase deficiency anemia, sickle cell anemia, aplastic anemia, and leukemia infiltration of bone marrow are the examples of this category.

Thalassemia occurs as a genetic defect in production of hemoglobin. The hemoglobin is composed of heme unit and globin unit. In case of thalassemia either the defect is present in alpha globin unit or beta globin unit causing α-thalassemia or β-thalassemia respectively (Muncie & Campbell, 2009). Furthermore effect of the defect is depending on the affected globin chains. Typically the alpha globin is made up of 4 chains; in this case one or more of the four alpha globin chain genes has the defect and hence fails to function. When one or two alpha genes are non-functional or dysfunctional, these patients are carriers and lead a normal life apart from the production of microcytic red blood cells which can be detected in normal laboratory testing. Three alpha globin genes being dysfunctional leads to the disease called hemoglobin H disease, in this case the patient produces abnormal hemoglobin due to the disturbance of balance of alpha and beta chains in the red blood cells. These patients develop severe anemia and require regular blood transfusions. Hemoglobin Barts disease develops when all the four alpha globin chains are dysfunctional, this causes the abnormal type of hemoglobin HbBarts to be retained in the red blood cells and thus gets accumulated. The HbBarts has high affinity towards oxygen thus zero oxygen reaches the tissue causing necrosis and death of the tissue. Those affected do not survive and die the condition being called hydropfetalis, death of the fetus in the uterus. When one beta globin chain is dysfunctional the patient produces RBCs that are small, microcyctic. The severity of anemia is mild and no symptoms are observed, as the other beta globin chain is active and functional thus the alpha-beta combination is running and the anemic condition is mild. When both the beta globin chains are dysfunctional it causes life threatening disorder for the ones who are affected.

Regular blood transfusion is a must for these patients as they suffer from severe anemia (Figueiredo, 2015; Rund, & Rachmilewitz, 2001; Schrier, 1994).

Autoimmune hemolytic anemias (AIHA) are of varied types depending on the nature of the auto-antibodies activity against the red blood cells, as a result the reduction of survival of RBCs, causing hemolytic anemia. When the auto-antibodies are active below 30°C it causes cold agglutinin disease (CAD) and paroxysmal cold hemoglobinuria (PCH) both are the AIHA-cold type. IgM autoantibodies are responsible for CAD while PCH is caused by an IgG immunoglobulin. Auto-antibodies those are active between the temperatures of 37-40°C are the ones which cause AIHA-warm type. IgG alone or with complement C3 are responsible for AIHA-warm type. When nocuous effects are seen in a patient at either body temperature or lower temperatures, they might be suffering from AIHA-mixed type in which IgG with complement C3 and IgM agglutinins are found significant. Drug induced AIHA occurs as a result of involvement of certain drugs like cephalosporins (cefotetan and ceftriaxone), levodopa, methyldopa, penicillin and its derivatives, quinidine and some NSAIDs (Michel, 2014; Schrier, 1994; Semple & Freedman, 2005).

Glucose-6-phosphate dehydrogenase deficiency (G-6-PD) leads to hereditary hemolytic anemia. The cause for G-6-PD is the defect in the G-6-PD enzyme which leads to flawed production of nicotinamide adenine dinucleotide phosphate and sustainment of the redox state of erythrocytes. The G-6-PD deficiency is X-linked, human RBCs G-6-PD is composed of 515 amino acids and numerous mutations in these amino acids results in a varied G-6-PD deficiency in different populations (Cappellini & Fiorelli, 2008).

Sickle cell anemia is an inherited blood disorder that affects red blood cells. Hemoglobin S is the predominant in people with sickle cell disease, HbS, an abnormal type of hemoglobin. Hemoglobin S and hemoglobin C are abnormal types of hemoglobin. In case of SCA variant, the hydrophobic amino acid valine replaces the hydrophilic glutamic acid at the sixth amino acid position of the HBB polypeptide chain. This substitution creates a hydrophobic spot on the outside of the protein structure that sticks to the hydrophobic region of an adjacent hemoglobin molecule's beta chain. Sickling of red blood cells occurs to the clumping together (polymerization) of HbS molecules into rigid fibres. The RBCs containing mostly hemoglobin S do not live as long as normal red blood cells (normally about 16-20days). They also become sickled in shape, have difficulty in passing through the body's capillary network. There are several types of sickle cell disease. The most common being Sickle Cell Anemia (SS), Sickle-Hemoglobin C Disease (SC), Sickle Beta-Plus Thalassemia and Sickle Beta-Zero Thalassemia. Sickle Cell trait (AS) is an inherited condition in which both hemoglobin A and S are produced in the red blood cells, always more A than S. Sickle cell trait is not a type of sickle cell disease. People with sickle cell trait are generally healthy, a regular iron rich diet or iron supplementation helps them lead a normal life. Aplastic anemia is caused as the result of stem cell defect, immune mediated inhibition of hemopoesis (Lang, Roll, Myssina, Schittenhelm, Scheel-Walter, Kanz, & Wieder, 2002; Quirolo & Vichinsky, 2016; Serjeant, 1992). Aplastic anemia is an autoimmune disease; this can be either genetic or acquired resulting in the body to react to its own immune system. When the stem cells are destroyed due to some reason aplastic anemia occurs. A few causes of stem cell destruction being chemotherapy treatment, this causes the destruction of cancer cells along with healthy cells and in some cases stem cells, thus causing aplastic anemia. Viral infections affecting the bone marrow can also cause aplastic anemia. Viral infections such as Epstein Barr's virus, hepatitis, parovirus B19, HIV show its harmful effects on the bone marrow. In few cases pregnancy can also result in aplastic anemia, as the immune system starts attacking the bone marrow. A few patients also suffer from idiopathic aplastic anemia, in which the cause is unknown. (Bacigalupo, 2007; Mishra, Malhotra, Ratho, Singh, Varma, & Varma, 2005).

Prevalence of Anemia

While hemoglobin is the most common indicator of anemia, fluctuations in the same do not conclude anemia or cause of anemia and its prevalence. For understanding the anemia and its prevalence WHO carried out study and data analysis to give global estimates of anemia. They included the study in which the population was provided with iron supplements to rule out iron-deficiency anemia contributing as the major factor of anemia. The classification of anemia as public health problem is as follows <5%, no public health problem; 5–19.9%, mild public health problem; 20–39.9%, moderate public health problem; ≥40%, severe public health problem. The results of the same are portrayed in *Figure 4*, *Figure 5*, *Figure 6* gives an insight of the prevalence of anemia on global level in case of reproductive women from ages of 15years to 49 years (WHO, 2011).

Global prevalence of anemia in the pregnant women, non-pregnant women and children below 3 years is 41.8%, 30.2%, and 47.4% respectively. Gestational anemia is prevalent in lower income group in developed countries, an approximate of 30% women in the US in third trimester are anemic. In India prevalence of anemia is the highest in the world especially in the pregnant women and children. About 87% of pregnant women are found to be anemic in India.

Figure 4. Global estimates of the prevalence of anemia in women of reproductive age, 15–49 years, 2011 .Prevalence of anemia, all women aged 15–49 years, 2011 Source: WHO, 2011

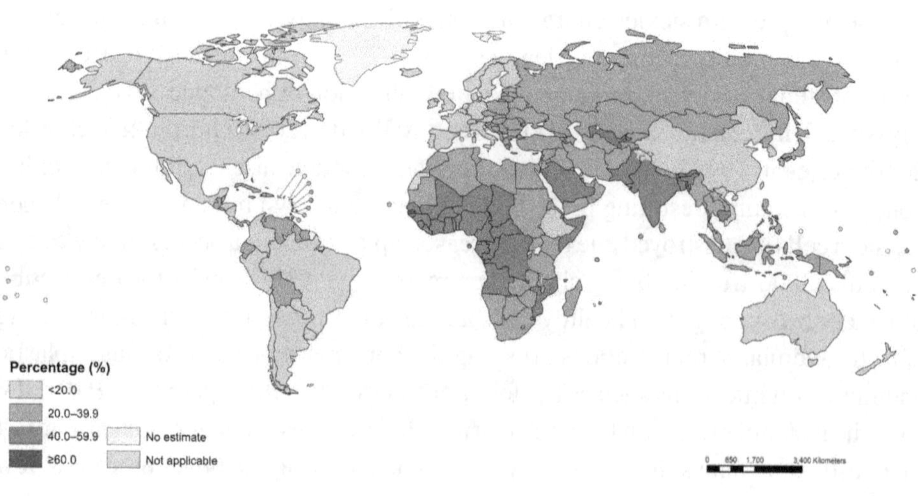

Figure 5. Global estimates of Prevalence of anemia, pregnant women aged 15–49 years, 2011 Source: WHO, 2011

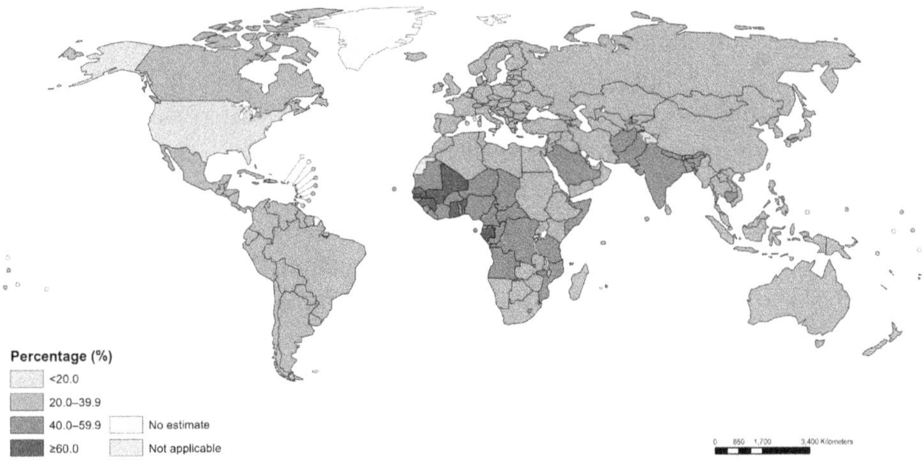

Figure 6. Global estimates of Prevalence of anemia, non-pregnant women aged 15–49 years, 2011 Source: WHO, 2011

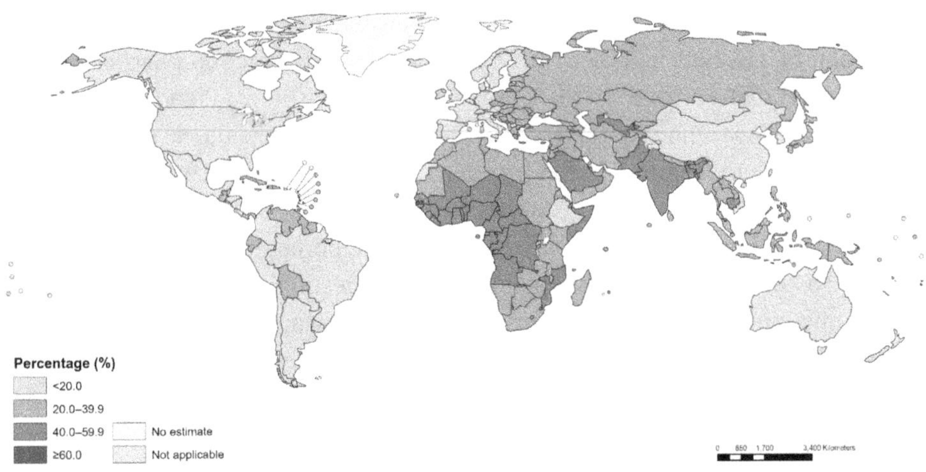

Cold agglutinin disease (CAD) is more common in people over the age of 55 years, while paroxysmal cold hemoglobinuria (PCH) typically presents in young children. Drug-induced AIHA is more common in adults as opposed to children, still a few fatal cases have been reported in cases of children. The drug induced-AIHA is rare; annual incidence is estimated at about 1 in 10 lakhs. The American Journal of Hematology states that 0.7 to 4.1 out of every one million people each year are affected by Aplastic anemia thus it is rare.

Round about 2.34 per one million people are affected each year and is given in a report by the journal Haematologica. National Institute of Diabetes and Digestive and Kidney Diseases gave an estimate that the disorder affects men and women equally, and most frequently develops in adults between ages 20 and 25, as well as those over 60. Sickle cell anemia survey shows that HbS allele is present in the Middle East and India, the African continent and is localized in Mediterranean regions.

Folate malabsorption also leads to anemia; USA, Canada, Israel, Chile, Saudi Arabia are the few countries where Folate food fortification is mandatory.

Food fortification is helping reduce the diet associated causes of anemia. Food fortification with essential nutrients like folic acid, vitamin B_{12}, iron, iron absorbing aiding foods is the key to reduce the incidences of anemia. Nutraceuticals and functional foods can help achieve this task with wider spread to masses with ease of acceptability.

PRELUDE TO NUTRACEUTICALS AND FUNCTIONAL FOODS

History of Nutraceuticals and Functional Foods

Nutraceutical is the term coined by founder, chairman of Foundation of Innovation, Dr. Stephen L. DeFelice. The term literally means nutrition and pharmaceutical. Nutraceutical can be food or food product, food constituent, food part, dietary supplements. The technology and research has further broadened the nutraceuticals to isolated nutrient, engineered food products like cereals, beverages, cellular level nutrient supplementation. The history of nutraceuticals dates back to a stage where the patients with extreme short bowel syndrome required nutrients in its simplest form for absorption being the key point, without digestion as the rate limiting step. Such simple nutrients are amino acids, fatty acids, sugars, essential vitamins and minerals these were formulated as medical foods, nutraceuticals or pharma foods and administered to patients. The foods which showed improved physiological functions are called physiological foods, these food not only benefit the patient but also impart an improved healthy life. The functional foods have been in use in last 2000 years. Hippokrates was the one who used the line *let thy food be your medicine*. He also did not distinguish between food and drugs. His method as a practitioner included the vigilant choice of food.

Polyunsaturated fatty acids (PUFAs) belong to class of nutraceuticals which have been good cardio-protective, fish oil, garlic oil have been the ones which have been used since a long time for the same. Arginine is the non-essential amino acid and is used for inhibiting the thrombocyte aggregation and adhesion in cases of anemia.

Also, arginine has also been used for improving the immune system by improving the T cell response.

'Food of Gods' is quoted by Romans for abundantly used functional food mushrooms, these have the medicinal property of improving the host resistance against infections caused by viruses, bacteria, parasites. The neurodevelopment in infants with anemia is improvised with fortified milk enriched with flaxseeds. Teff is naturally occurring and bioavailable helping prevent iron deficiency anemia in pregnancy.

Maintenance of nutritional well-being of a patient providing nourishment with sufficient quantities is the foremost important task of nutraceuticals and functional foods. The maintenance of nutrition is being done since ages through foods. Research has helped give a thorough understanding of nutrients. Further, technology is helping develop designer foods for getting nutritionally complete products, disease-specific products, products engineered to increase certain nutrients or micronutrients or metabolites to gain specific results.

Depending on the recognition of nutraceuticals it is classified and the same is addressed in the next section.

Classification of Nutraceuticals

General Classification of nutraceuticals is given Figure 7. Traditional nutraceuticals are absolutely natural occurring foods with no processing or alternations made into it. Food contains several natural components that not only delivers basic nutrition but also benefits beyond. Listing a few traditional nutraceuticals are lycopene in tomatoes, omega-3 fatty acids in salmon or saponins in soy.

Figure 7. Classification of Nutraceutical

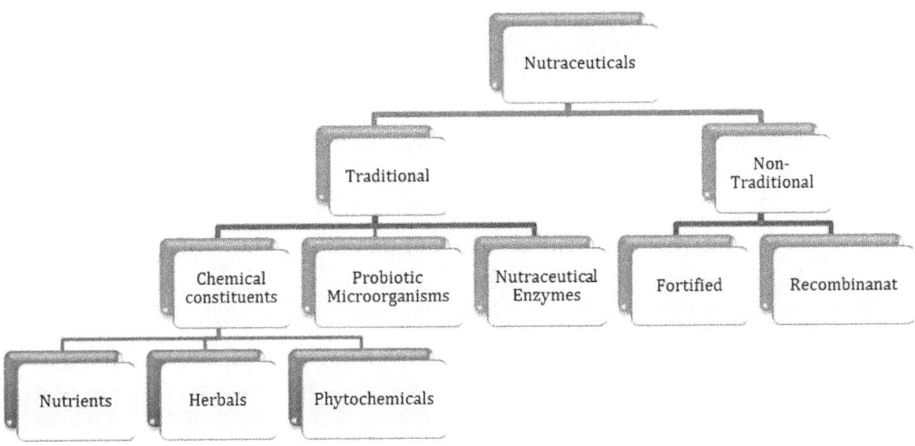

Classification of Nutraceuticals is well established; in this section a relationship with reference to nutraceuticals for anemia is specified.

- The traditional nutraceutical category includes chemical constituents which is further subdivided as follows:
  - **Nutrients:** Foodstuffs such as vitamins, minerals, amino acids and fatty acids with recognized nutritional utility are termed as nutrients. Most vegetables, wholegrain cereals, dairy products, fruits and animal products such as meat, poultry, contain peptides, organic acids, which help solubilize the non-heme in intestine and aid absorption of iron, thus retention of the erythrocyte membrane occurs and help manage the anemia. Minerals found in plant, animal and dairy products are useful in, anemia. Flax seed and salmon contain fatty acids omega-3 PUFAs, which yield in short chain fatty acids these are small organic molecules absorbed by diffusion or ion exchange, thus creating an environment for iron absorption. Parmigiano-Reggiano and Grana Padano aids mineral absorption, improves iron status and reduces anemia (Addeo, Chianese, Salzano, Sacchi, Cappuccio, Ferranti, & Malorni, 1992; Pellegrino, Battelli, Resmini, Ferranti, Barone, &Addeo, 1997).
  - **Herbals:** A plant or plant part or an extract or mixture of these used in preparations to maintain health and to prevent, alleviate, or cure disease is an herbal preparation. Nutraceuticals obtained from herbals exhibit a huge assurance in betterment of health and prevent chronic diseases. Some examples, which help maintain blood flow and improve oxygen carrying capacity so that no agglutination of clotting occurs are *Vitisvinifera, Zingberofficiale, Solanum lycopersicum, Chicory* (cichoriumintybus), Nettle (*Urticadioica*), Niprisan®, *Khaya senegalensis, Allium sativum contains* 31.2 g /100g of vitamin C, thus aiding the absorption process of iron (Fall, Vanhaelen-Fastré, Vanhaelen, Lo, Toppet, Ferster, & Fondu, 1999; Obodozie, Ameh, Afolabi, Oyedele, Ache, Onanuga, & Inyang, 2010).
  - **Phytochemicals:** Also called phytonutrient is a bioactive chemical compounds found in plants, as antioxidants, considered to be beneficial to human health. There are phytochemicals which show effects of anti-clotting, anti-sickling and antioxidation. Each of these activities helps manage different types of anemia by a varied action. Examples *Careyaarborea* contains terpenoids, flavonoids which have property to prolong the clotting time, *Fagopyrum esculentum* contain flavonoids, major one being rutin, this has property that prevents platelets from clotting unreasonably thus maintain the blood flow. *Entandrophragma*

utile, Chenopodium ambrosioides, and *Petriveria alliacea, Capsicum annuum* contains vitamin C, helping absorption of iron (Ameh, Tarfa, & Ebeshi, 2012).

- **Probiotic Microorganisms:** Probiotics are defined as live microorganisms, which when consumed in sufficient quantity, bestow health & fitness on the host. These are traditional nutraceuticals which are affable bacteria that encourage healthy digestion and absorption of some nutrients. Only the bacteria that can survive through the acidic conditions of stomach can colonize in the intestinal walls and benefit the host. To name a few probiotic microorganisms which are considered healthy are *Lactobacillus acidophilus, Bifidobacterium bifidum, Lactococcuslactis.* These probiotics act as a vehicle for absorption of other nutrients. To cite a few examples of probiotics include Yoghurt, Kefir, and Yakult® (Shimakawa, Matsubara, Yuki, Ikeda, & Ishikawa, 2003).
- **Nutraceutical Enzymes:** Enzymes are a vital element of life, devoid of which our body would stop to function. Those people who are suffering from medical conditions such as hypoglycemia, blood sugar disorders, digestive problems and obesity, eliminate the symptoms by enzyme supplements to their diet. These enzymes are derived from microbial, plant and animal sources. Examples of marketed nutraceutical enzymes include NattoSEB (Nattokinase), DairySEB (multienzyme blend). Cheddar Cheese phosphopeptide improves mineral absorption, reduces anemia (Ong, Henriksson, & Shah, 2007; Singh, Fox, & Healy, 1997).
- Non-traditional nutraceuticals are simulated foods manufactured by using biotechnology. These are food products specially processed to amalgamate bioactives into food for human well-being and health. The non-traditional nutraceuticals can be further sub divided into:
    - **Fortified Nutraceuticals:** It comprises fortified foodstuff from agricultural produce or added nutrients and/or ingredients. e.g. orange juice fortified with calcium, cereals with added vitamins or minerals and flour with added folic acid. Some examples are fortified milk, Teff bread fortified with iron.
    - **Recombinant Nutraceuticals:** Foodstuffs which are source of energy and vigor like bread, alcohol, fermented starch, yogurt, cheese, vinegar, and others are produced using various biotechnological processes, Sprinkles ® microencapsulated micronutrients in a sachet. Combats iron deficiency anemia. IntraMAX® vitamin E supplement IntraLINE nutraceuticals, helps treat vitamin E induced anemia. Lactoferrin and lysozyme proteins are on a higher side in genetically modified

rice thus improving diet source of heme iron and its absorption. (Humphrey & Kalsing, 2002) VeganSafe B-12®methylcobalamin and adenosylcobalamin helps combat the anemia due to lack of Vitamin B complex in daily diet.

Differences Between Nutraceuticals and Pharmaceuticals

The drugs and supplements are out looked by the Food and Drug Administration (FDA) differently. Under the Dietary Supplement Health and Education Act (DSHEA), the FDA essentially treats supplements as if they were foods. DSHEA defines nutritional supplements as products taken by mouth that contain an ingredient intended to supplement the diet.

An upfront demarcation among supplements and pharmaceuticals is that supplements supply the deficient nutrient, or provides a benefit by consumption of additional amounts. On the other hand, pharmaceuticals treat an illness by intervening in normal or disease-state metabolism. In other words supplements are the ones which correct imbalances and pharmaceuticals are the ones which treats symptoms. Those ingredients could include vitamins, minerals, or natural biological substances which may include enzymes. They can be made available in a variety of forms, including extracts and concentrates, and as tablets, capsules, powders, or liquids. Drugs are legally defined as substances intended to diagnose, treat, or prevent disease.

Pharmaceuticals are synthetic chemicals that impact physiological functions. The chemicals resulting from plants or proteins have an eccentricity of being called as nutraceuticals. The key differentiation is that pharmaceuticals are intended exclusively for medical use under a physician's supervision, and are subject to Food and Drugs Administration approval. Health supplements (including nutraceuticals, food or dietary supplements) may not need medical supervision, or Food and Drugs Control Administration approval. *Table 2* gives the regulations needs for nutraceuticals and functional foods in few countries and thus its management.

Table 2. Regulation requirements for Nutraceuticals and Functional Foods

Country	Regulation Needs
USA	Companies must register their manufacturing facilities. Dietary supplements do not require approval by USFDA.
Japan	All and any functional food has been given supplied/administered/sold in their naturally occurring form. No functional food should be in tablet, capsule, or powder type of dosage form. Functional food to consume as part of diet for prevention or control disease condition.
Europe	General Food Law Regulations are applicable which include food safety, traceability, recall and notifications
Australia	A dedicated Council, Complementary Healthcare Council of Australia, regulates the rules for manufacture and supply of nutraceuticals

The crux is pharmaceutical as per the rules of FDA mandates a prescription or recommendation from a certified medical practitioner for procurement. Examples, ferric carboxymaltose, hydroxyurea, chloroquine, atovaquone etc. Health supplements are put up for sale devoid of limitations at health food stores, grocery stores, drug stores, national discount chains, mail-order and Internet. To name a few Cosamin DS (glucosamine), Coenzyme Q10 (ubiquinone), Ciklavit (extract of *Cajanuscajan*) (Akinsulie, Temiye, Akanmu, Lesi, & Whyte, 2005).

POTENTIAL OF NUTRACEUTICALS AND FUNCTIONAL FOODS

Current Therapies for Anemia

Nutrition based anemia can be corrected with appropriate iron supplements. Anemia caused as a consequence of some other physiological or pathological malice can be treated depending on its severity and the age at which anemia occurs.

The primary line of treatment in case of iron deficiency anemia involves administration of Iron supplements, ferrous sulphate, ferrous fumarate, ferrous gluconate, folic acid, ferric carboxymaltose (intravenous delivery). Therapy for IDA can be designed by general practitioner for pregnant women and children. Practitioners also introduce iron absorption enhancers like ascorbic acid, erythrobic acid. In case of severe, hemolytic, genetic anemias; treatment involves plasmapheresis, bone marrow stem cell transplants, steroids, blood transfusion at regular intervals, and life style changes.

In case of known family history, early diagnosis, preferably in the newborn period can help aid the health maintenance for patients with sickle cell disease. This includes starting with penicillin prophylaxis, vaccination against *Pneumococcus bacteria* and folic acid supplementation. Psychosocial support is an important key when the treatment includes complications and often antibiotics, pain management, intravenous fluids, blood transfusion and surgery. Like all patients with chronic disease, patients are best managed in a comprehensive multi-disciplinary program of care. Recurrent pain crises, risk of stroke and other complications are reduced when regular intermittent blood transfusions are done along with drug therapy. Because red blood cells contain iron, and there is no natural way for the body to eliminate it, patients who receive repeated blood transfusions can accumulate iron in the body until it reaches toxic levels.

Iron toxicity may occur due to accumulation of excess iron in heart, liver, and other organs and may lead to organ damage. Treatments are available to eliminate iron overload. Patients frequently experience a vicious circle of events called a "Sickle cell disease crisis", in which low oxygen tension in tissue causes sickling, which leads to ruptured RBC and further leads to a serious decrease in RBC count and more sickling which often causes death. The medication in circulation and showing benefit for SCA patients is hydroxyurea along with essential nutrients.

A treatment regimen with essential nutrients deficiency includes supplements of the essential nutrients like folic acid, Vitamin B_{12}, copper, zinc. Anemias due to infections like malaria, helminthiasis and so on have mandatory use of the drugs for curing the critical infection along with iron supplementation.

The major concern with the short coming of the treatment for nutritional type of anemia is detection of anemia at an initial stage, keeping a vigilant watch on reoccurrence of anemia and titer the dosage regimen accordingly. Another reason for downfall of current treatment is an insufficient reach of medicines to the rural population and to the population below poverty line.

Functional foods and nutraceuticals can reach the masses and thus help improve the statistics of anemia globally. The prototype example is fortification of common table salt with iodine and provision of the same across the globe. This has not only reduced the cases of goiter, but also has improved the health of patients globally.

Diet Affecting the Iron Absorption

Iron absorption can be broadly divided on basis of heme component and non heme component. In human beings the heme component is easily absorbed as opposed to the non-heme component. Iron absorption occurs in the upper intestinal tract majorily duodenum and upper jejunm. A transporter comes in role for uptake of Ferrtin which is stored in the enterocyte. When required the ferritin is converted to $Fe3+$ by transferrin and used. An individual utilizes approximately 20mg of iron each day for production of new RBCs, most of the iron comes from old RBCs (McKie, Barrow, Latunde-Dada, Rolfs, Sager, Mudaly, & Peters, 2001).

In order to improve the bioavailability of dietary iron, it is necessary that promoters of heme absorption (functional foods) are consumed. Degermed corn flour, legumes, dates, salmon, tuna, haddock, help in absorption of the heme component as opposed to the non-heme component. Diet containing phytates, tannins inhibit the iron absorption as opposed to diet containing ascorbic acid, citric acid, amino acids which facilitate the iron absorption. There are also competitors for the iron uptake which are lead, cobalt, zinc, manganese.

Daily an adult human carries approximately 4g or body iron most of which is circulating as hemoglobin within the red blood cells. Body stores roughly 1g as ferritin and hemosiderin. Approximately 0.3g goes into myoglobin and respiratory enzymes. The human body absorbs only 1mg daily from diet when the diet is iron rich with 10-20mg of iron. Red blood cells have a life span of 120days and hence 0.8% of circulating red blood cells are replaced daily.

There are various factors for absorption of iron, the most important being availability of absorbable iron. Heme iron is always 20% absorbed irrespective of meal iron being 4 folds say, whether it was a 1.5mg or 6mg iron. In contrast, the non heme iron absorption dropped from 18% to 6% when the meal iron was increased four folds. *Table 3* gives details of food with high iron content which is absorbable.

Role of Nutraceuticals and Functional Foods in Anemia

Functional Food is the one which is beneficial to the human body by targeting one or more biochemical and physiological functions in the body. This is achieved when the functional food can improve well-being of the person and also reduces or eliminates risk from the body; as the functional food gives more nutrition and nutrients to target the specific functions. Functional food can be natural food, food which is engineered to provide one of the nutrients in high quantities or engineered in a tactically to remove the deleterious component and engineered food which is a carrier of modified nutrients.

Minerals are vital in forming blood, building bones, maintaining a healthy immune system and most importantly for electrolyte balance. Minerals like copper, zinc, iron and their absorption is limited due to presence of phytic acid in whole grains. This can be overcome by introducing phytases through foods like Milk. *Lactobacillus helveticus* fermented milk helps binding essential minerals by producing proteases. *Mitsuokella jalaludinii* in form of probiotic helps release phytases thus improve mineral bioavailability. Caseinophosphopeptides (CPP) are product enzymatic hydrolysis of casein (milk protein) which yields phosphorylated peptides. Milk is fortified with

Table 3. Iron rich foods

Food (Iron in 100g)	Iron Content
Tofu	2.7mg
Dark Chocolate and Cocoa Powder	17mg
Green Leafy Vegetables (Spinach)	3.6mg
Whole Grains	1.5mg
Beans and Pulses	3.7mg
Beef and Lamb	3.8mg
Nuts (Cashew, Hazelnut, almond)	6.1mg
Seafood (Oysters, Mussels, Clams)	9.2mg
Liver(Chicken)	13mg
Squash and Pumpkin Seeds	15mg

calcium and iron in presence of CPP this helps improve the bioavailability of calcium and iron and anemia (Bouhallab & Bougle, 2004). Fortified bread with iron, wheat flour fortified with iron, help reduce anemia in low income group. Also, fortification of common table salt with iron has shown improved bioavailability of iron.

Iron absorption promoter foods which contain ascorbic acid should be consumed by anemic patients on routine basis. Foods like fruits, juices, potatoes, and tubers, green leafy vegetables, cauliflower, and sprouted pulses. The heme iron in meat, poultry, fish, and seafood has a high bioavailability. Target specific fortification of food helps supply optimal quantities of iron to the target group. Example, infant formula fortification of milk, fortification of salts, wheat flour, legumes, fish sauce, soy sauce in case of menstruating and pregnant women. Iron compounds used for fortification of food are ferrous sulphate, ferrous fumarate, electrolytic iron, ferric pyrophosphate, NaFeEDTA, ferrous biglycinate, ferric ammonium citrate. These compounds aid in improving the daily requirement of iron in populations with anemia due to varied reasons including infection based anemia. These compounds are used in bread, whole maize, brown rice, soy bean, infant cereal, white wheat flour.

The above mentioned iron compounds selected for fortification are preferred considering the aspects of solubility of free iron, elemental iron, poor bioavailability of inorganic iron used as supplements, stability of iron when in food (iron is susceptible to oxidation). Fortification of dairy products is done using iron citrate, casein, ascorbic acid, ferrous sulphate. While fortifying dairy products the key aspect that is tackled is improving the oxidative stability of lipids. Table 4 gives an overview of products that are fortified, and the doses at which these fortified products are useful.

Phytochemicals like *Allium sativum, Terminalia catappa leaves, Carica papaya* leaf and unripe fruit extracts have been used in managing SCD over decades. But excess of any of these can cause toxicity. Excess of garlic can lead to hemolytic anemia. Vitamin E can help counter the effects of garlic. Vitamin E prevents reduction of glutathione thus providing erythrocyte membrane protection.

Biofortification is explored by introducing gene which will improve iron load thus potentially giving high amount of absorbable iron from plant and better absorption in humans. Example, incorporation of ferretin gene from soy or *Phaseolus vulgaris* in rice increase iron content by two- three folds; introduction of ferric reductase gene in plant root system will improve uptake of elemental iron from soils into plants.

Functional Foods have the potential to have an impact on greater population because of its ease of availability and cost effectiveness. In this context few examples are cite cauliflower (has iron content of 1.1g and anthocyanins which aid the absorption process of the same, it is also rich source of vitamin C), strawberries (iron content 1g, and source of vitamin helps absorb the non heme component).

Functional Foods are easily available in all the geographies of the globe. Hence geography specific functional foods can be supplied to the populations of the

Table 4. Fortification iron in various food products

Food	Fortifier	Doses	References
Bread	Ferrous Sulphate	10,20,30,40mg	Muhammad Ilyas, et.al
Whole maize	Ferrous bisglycinate	-	Bovell-Benjamin, et.al, (1999) Bovell-Benjamin, et.al, (2000)
Maize	NaFeEDTA	30, 60mg/kg	Bovell-Benjamin, Frankel et.al, (1999)
Infant whole milk powder	Microencapsulated ferrous sulphate	-	Martinez et.al, (2002)
Cheese	Iron casein and ferric chloride	-	Martinez et.al, (2002)
Yoghurt	Ferric chloride	10mg Fe/100ml	Hekmat, (1997)
Milk	Ferrous Sulphate	15mg/l	Uicich et al., (1999)
Whole wheat, peanuts, jaggery Cereal products, salt, sugar, condiments	NaFeEDTA	Hb: 5g/100g	Martinez et.al, (2002)
Sugar	FeNaEDTA	1g	Viteri et al., (1995)

anemic deficient region. Example: molasses are produced/ generated in 45 tropical countries; molasses have high iron content approximately 15g, with presence of natural folates, vitamin B. Wheat bran contains 14.9g of iron content along with low glycemic index, hence they do not have acids interfering with iron absorption in the intestine; round about 75% of production is done in China, India, USA, the Russia Federation, France, Turkey and Pakistan.

With the time, the technology for developing formulation systems has taken a leap and same knowledge can be applied in nutraceuticals. The next section deals with the new delivery systems and its need for application in nutraceuticals.

DRUG DELIVERY SYSTEMS

Types of Drug Delivery Systems

Pharmaceuticals have approved well-established drug delivery systems which are being utilized to administer nutraceuticals since a decade. The drug delivery system is broadly classified into conventional drug delivery system and nano-drug delivery system. Conventional drug delivery systems include tablet, capsules, powders, syrups etc. With detailed study modified drug release systems like controlled release, extended release systems came as a boon in assisting drug delivery. Examples of Conventional and modified release nutraceuticals are ferrous fumarate tablets, ferrocontin controlled released tablets, lycopene tablets, Omacor® capsules, NutreStore® Powder Sachets, alpha-lipoic acid capsules and tablets, ferrous sulphateheptahydrate drops, ascorbic acid extended release tablets, Ciklavit® and so on.

These all products are available over the counter and have shown an immense improvement in managing anemia.

With time and technology, newer methods have emerged in drug delivery systems which can carry the phytochemical of interest and release at the site of absorption without changing or affecting the form of the nutraceutical.

Need of Nanodrug Delivery Systems in Anemia

The predicament with the conventional nutraceuticals can be overcome with the aid of Novel Drug Delivery systems (NDDS). NDDS helps enhance stability, tissue and biodistribution thus improving the pharmacological activity. An approach for sustained, extended nutrient delivery can be achieved using NDDS. The technology for the development of NDDS-formulations has been well established and available for exploring its application on nutraceutical and naturally derived molecules. Novel Drug Delivery Systems such as phytosomes, solid lipid nanoparticles, self-emulsifying drug delivery systems, nanolipid carriers help the delivery of the nutrients at a low dose with efficacy and desired therapeutic effect.

Nanodrug delivery will benefit delivery of nutraceutical and phytochemical. It will help protect the nutraceutical or phytochemical in the gastric pH, thus avoiding the worry of gastrointestinal compatibility. Further the nano drug delivery will be able to extend and display a predictable delivery of the nutraceutical where it reaches the maximum absorption site. Enhance bioavailability and efficacy of the nutraceutical.

Applications of Nanosystems for Delivery of Nutraceuticals

One of the major applications of nanosystems is enhancing the oral bioavailability of nutraceuticals for anemia. The major concern in treating anemia is making iron bioavailable for uptake and absorption. There are categories of compounds which helps iron uptake, which interfere with iron absorption, which compete with iron uptake. *Table 5* gives an insight about tried and test novel nanosystems for improving iron absorption.

Types of Nanodelivery systems applied for nutraceuticals in a nut shell are as follows, examples for the same are as follows:

Table 5. Type of compounds and its effect on iron absorption

Type of Compound	Example
Inhibitor	Phytates, tannins, soil clay, laundry starch, iron overload, antacids
Competitors	Lead, cobalt, strontium, manganese, zinc
Facilitators	Ascorbate, citrate, amino acids.

- Liposomes are spherical microscopic lipid vesicles formed from phospholipids, delivery vehicle for both hydrophilic and lipophilic compounds. Liposomes have been investigated to enhance the oral bioavailability of varying of nutraceuticals. Successful inclusion of resveratrol a rich source of vitamin c and other minerals in liposomal carrier system has shown improvements in stability, biological activity and efficacy (Amri, Chaumeil, Sfar, & Charrueau, 2012). Fortification and synergistic antioxidant action of ascorbic acid and α tocopherol together was achieved by incorporating the two in liposomes (Marsanasco, Márquez, Wagner, Alonso, & Chiaramoni, 2011).
- Phytosomes these are structurally related to liposomes, but the phytochemical encapsulated in liposome is not bound to the phospholipid carried system. Phytosomes show 3-6 fold increase in bioavailability when compared to plain solutions of the phytoconstituent. Phytosome complex of curcumin shows better bioavailability to only curcumin solutions. This complex is said to show improved anti parasitic effect caused due to *H.pylori* resulting in destruction of RBCs (Gupta, Patchva, & Aggarwal, 2013).
- Nanoemulsion, these are emulsions in the scale of <100nm, these are two immiscible liquids stabilized using a surfactant. These require energy to be stabilized as opposed to microemulsion system. Sunflower nanoemulsion when incorporated in steaks, reduced its microbial, improved its shelf life and retained the iron contents (Salminen et.al, 2013). Nanoemulsions are used to deliver omega-3 fatty acids, flavonoids and other nutraceuticals.
- Solid lipid Nanoparticles (SLN) are submicron emulsions which comprise of solid lipid and semi solid lipid/ liquid lipid as the core. These are difficult to break down in Gastric fluids hence port the phytoconstituent safely to intestines for absorption. SLN of β carotene is used for food fortification which aid in iron absorption (Huynh, 2012).

Application of nanosystem is vast and still to be explored in depth. While designing the optimum delivery system for nutraceuticals following key points should be considered:

Table 6. Precise insight of nanosystems applied for iron compounds

Compound	Nanosystem	Notable Effect	Reference
Ferrous Sulphate	Liposomes	1.4.1.1 Fortification of Milk with these liposomes increased iron concentration to 15mg/L 1.4.1.2 Stable liposomes on heat treatment to 100°C for 30mins 1.4.1.3 Stable for a duration of 1 week at the storage condition of 4°C	Xia and Xu, 2005
Iron and Zinc	Nanoparticles	1. Product with surface area of 190m^2/g, which showed almost no change in color of food when compared to elemental iron addition. 2. Bioavailability of nanoparticle Iron was equivalent to the ferrous salt of Iron. 3. No excess detectable iron in the gut wall or other lymphatic tissue, so no detrimental effects of excessive iron.	Hiltyet, al., (2010)
Fe(III) poly oxo-hydroxide	Nanoparticles combined with dietary tartaric acid and succinic acid	1. Iron Absorption efficiency was found to be 3times more than ferric chloride salt. 2. Adherance and uptake of Nanoparticles by the epithelial cells was higher than solubility in the gastric fluid. 3. No toxic effect was observed with soluble ferrous iron, as the nanoparticle formulation concentration is 7times lower when considered toxic effect with 1mM concentration	Pereira et.al, (2014)

- Protection of labile compounds
- Improvement of intestinal adherence time
- Controlled/Delayed release
- Intestinal permeability enhancement
- Modulation of metabolites

Once the nanosytems formulation is made the critical part is its characterization for confirming its activity, safety and efficacy. The next subsection highlights the characterization of nutraceuticals.

REGULATORY CHARACTERIZATION OF NUTRACEUTICALS

Superiority of a finished food creation is mainly an imperative indicator of quality to the consumer. Finished products have to accomplish each and every prerequisite on quality. They should have the suitable nutritive value, distinctive sensory properties, and more than all, fulfill the entire set of necessities from a safety position. That is why the quality control of finished products is the critical point of the entire quality control string.

The perception of functional foods is inclined by diverse interpretations that are referred to their characteristics, their active components, or their regulatory outline

The major confront of nutraceuticals is standardization of quality policies in assessment of nutraceuticals. For the mainstream, the quality testing of botanical substances has been recognized by individual corporations, and numerous of these processes are proprietary and invalidated, making it rigid to ascertain a consistent modus operandi, for marker compounds, and reference standards. Nutraceutical providers ought to oversee the variations in raw materials and finished products to guarantee the quality and safety of the product.

Health claims are different from structure/function claims, which also may appear on conventional food or dietary supplement labels. Unlike health claims, structure/function claims do not deal with disease-risk reduction. When the manufacturer uses a structure/function claim, the company is responsible for making sure the claim is truthful and not misleading.

Many academic, scientific and regulatory organizations are considering ways to establish the scientific basis to support claims (other than health claims) for the functional components of nutraceuticals. These are the five types of health-related statements allowed on food and dietary supplement labels:

- Nutrient-content claims indicate the presence of a specific nutrient at a certain level.
- Structure and function claims describe the effect of dietary components on the normal structure or function of the body.
- Dietary-guidance claims describe the health benefits of broad categories of foods.
- Qualified health claims convey a developing relationship between components in the diet and risk of disease, supported by the weight of credible scientific evidence available.
- Health claims confirm a relationship between components in the diet and risk of disease or health condition, supported by significant scientific agreement.

PERSPECTIVE OF NUTRACEUTICALS

A regulatory body which can put forth strict rules can help take the nutraceuticals to a peak use in the health industry. One such regulatory body includes International Alliance of Dietary Food Supplements Association (IADSA), a body which works across six continents. The major focus of IADSA is coordinating strategy and action on global regulatory issues, particularly in relation with Codex Alimentarus Committee (CAC) [created by UN organizations FAO and WHO in 1962]. The CAC goal is "international mechanism for promotion of health and economic interests of consumers while encouraging fair international trade in food." Further, the new body Codex Committee on Nutrition and Foods for Special Dietary Uses (CCNFSDU) addresses guidelines for safety, purity and bioavailability of sources of minerals and vitamins. Dietary Supplement Health and Education Act (DSHEA) of the US Food and Drug Administration (FDA) clearly mentions regulations for specific claims like nutrient content claims, high potency claims and health claims. The DSHEA benefits the US consumers by making a wide range of dietary supplements available to them.

Striking a balance between risk and access to consumer helps the entry of product into the market. The entry of the product in the market is dependent on the regulatory infrastructure and framework within a given country like India, South East Asian Nations, European Union, United States. These countries regulate the product as food-like category, which includes registration or notification based system unlike the drug-like category which requires pre-market approval system. When the product is treated in food like category, the regulation body has positive list of allowable ingredients in the product, especially from botanical sources. In cases of registration detailed information in form of registration dossier is required, which would be reviewed by regulators. The nutraceutical industry is not as regulated as the health care industry, but the responsible approach by using cGMP for the best benefit to the consumer will enable a boost in the nutraceutical industry. A platform of knowledge is well established for the pharmaceutical industry, utilization of the knowledge will improve the compliance, reduce the rate of rejection, number of withdrawals from market, and this will in turn increase the profit for the nutraceutical industry.

An overview of the guidelines recommended in diverse continents crossways suggests a vague outline. The reason behind maybe that, Nutraceuticals is a developing conception with changeable definitions across the globe. Some of the developed countries have implemented legislations as early as in 2004. In Canada, nutraceuticals are named 'Natural Health Products'.

They are known as "Dietary Supplements" in the US and Japan calls them 'Foods for Special Health Use' (FOSHU). In US, Canada and in EU there are distinct definitions and guidelines for dietary supplements and functional foods where as in Japan they are governed under same set of rules. In Canada, raditional and herbal medicines form a part of the definition of dietary supplements, but same is not the case in Japan. In US, Herbs and botanicals find place in nutraceuticals.

The Indian definition (as per Food Safety and Security Act passed in 2006, yet to be implemented) enlists the ingredients a nutraceutical product must possess and its general properties. A traditional medicine is not a part of nutraceuticals. Foods for special dietary use are specifically processed or formulated to suit exact dietary necessities which exist for the reason that a physical or physiological condition or specific disease. These are presented as such, where in the composition of these foodstuffs ought to vary considerably from the Indian Standard (IS) composition of ordinary foods of equivalent nature, if such usual food exists and possibly contains one or more of the subsequent ingredients, to be precise:

- Plants or botanicals or their parts in the form of powder, concentrate or extract in water, ethyl alcohol or hydro alcoholic extract, single or combination.
- Minerals or vitamins or proteins or metals or their compounds or amino acids (in amounts not exceeding the Recommended Daily Allowance (RDA) for Indians) or enzymes with permissible limits
- Substances of animal origin
- Dietary substances for use by human beings to supplement the diet by increasing the total dietary intake.

FUTURE TRENDS

Application of nutraceutical for managing anemia across globe only emerges recently on commercial scale since the concept of functional food and nutraceutical has been introduced to the world merely a decade ago. Nutraceuticals and functional foods used in treatment of anemia are liable to instabilities due to its natural source of origin. Hence, utilization of drug delivery systems and nanosystems; its vast knowledge, its successful application in pharmaceuticals should be put to use and test for nutraceuticals equally. Pharmaceuticals have already laid down platform technologies and methods, appropriate application will take nutraceuticals to next level with improved bioavailability. A mountain of work still needs to be done in the area of formulation for nutraceuticals, mainly aiming the safety, efficacy and regulation before it can go out to the global masses. Certainly regulation has caught up with some areas, especially when the product is going to reach the masses/ consumer on global level. But still a clear law, protocols and harmonization methods should be established across the globe for benefiting the science and consumer together. Nutraceuticals and especially with nanosystems have a long way to go. These will need to provide clarity and legal certainty to manufacturers, policy makers, health-care providers, enforcement authorities, and the consumers.

REFERENCES

Addeo, F., Chianese, L., Salzano, A., Sacchi, R., Cappuccio, U., Ferranti, P., & Malorni, A. (1992). Characterization of the 12% trichloroacetic acid-insoluble oligopeptides of Parmigiano-Reggiano cheese. *The Journal of Dairy Research*, *59*(03), 401–411. doi:10.1017/S0022029900030673

Akinsulie, A. O., Temiye, E. O., Akanmu, A. S., Lesi, F. E. A., & Whyte, C. O. (2005). Clinical evaluation of extract of Cajanuscajan (Ciklavit®) in sickle cell anemia. *Journal of Tropical Pediatrics*, *51*(4), 200–205. doi:10.1093/tropej/fmh097 PMID:15917266

Allen, L. H., De Benoist, B., Dary, O., & Hurrell, R. (2006). *Guidelines on food fortification with micronutrients*. WHO.

Ameh, S. J., Tarfa, F. D., & Ebeshi, B. U. (2012). Traditional herbal management of sickle cell anemia: Lessons from Nigeria. *Anemia*. PMID:23198140

Amri, A., Chaumeil, J. C., Sfar, S., & Charrueau, C. (2012). Administration of resveratrol: What formulation solutions to bioavailability limitations? *Journal of Controlled Release*, *158*(2), 182–193. doi:10.1016/j.jconrel.2011.09.083 PMID:21978644

Appendino, G., Belcaro, G., Cornelli, U., Luzzi, R., Togni, S., Dugall, M., ... Pellegrini, L. (2011). Potential role of curcumin phytosome (Meriva) in controlling the evolution of diabetic microangiopathy.A pilot study. *Panminerva Medica*, *53*(3Suppl 1), 43–49. PMID:22108476

Bacigalupo, A. (2007). Aplastic anemia: Pathogenesis and treatment. *Hematology*, *2007*(1), 23–28. doi:10.1182/asheducation-2007.1.23 PMID:18024605

Ballard, H. S. (1997). The hematological complications of alcoholism. *Alcohol Health and Research World*, *21*, 42–52. PMID:15706762

Bothwell, T. H., & Charlton, R. W. (1981). *Iron deficiency in women: a report of the International Nutritional Anemia Consultative Group (INACG)*. New York: The Nutrition Foundation.

Bouhallab, S., & Bouglé, D. (2004). Biopeptides of milk: Caseinophosphopeptides and mineral bioavailability. *Reproduction, Nutrition, Development*, *44*(5), 493–498. doi:10.1051/rnd:2004053 PMID:15636166

Bovell-Benjamin, A. C., Allen, L. H., Frankel, E. N., & Guinard, J. X. (1999). Sensory quality and lipid oxidation of maize porridge as affected by iron amino acid chelates and EDTA. *Journal of Food Science*, *64*(2), 371–376. doi:10.1111/j.1365-2621.1999.tb15903.x

Bovell-Benjamin, A. C., Allen, L. H., & Guinard, J. X. (1999). Toddlers' acceptance of whole maize meal porridge fortified with ferrous bisglycinate. *Food Quality and Preference*, *10*(2), 123–128. doi:10.1016/S0950-3293(98)00058-5

Bovell-Benjamin, A. C., Viteri, F. E., & Allen, L. H. (2000). Iron absorption from ferrous bisglycinate and ferric trisglycinate in whole maize is regulated by iron status. *The American Journal of Clinical Nutrition*, *71*(6), 1563–1569. doi:10.1093/ajcn/71.6.1563 PMID:10837299

Caballero, B., Finglas, P., & Toldrá, F. (2015). *Encyclopedia of food and health*. Oxford, UK: Academic Press.

Cappellini, M. D., & Fiorelli, G. (2008). Glucose-6-phosphate dehydrogenase deficiency. *Lancet*, *371*(9606), 64–74. doi:10.1016/S0140-6736(08)60073-2 PMID:18177777

Dallman, P. R. (1992). Changing iron needs from birth through adolescence. Nestle nutrition workshop series (USA).

Fall, A. B., Vanhaelen-Fastré, R., Vanhaelen, M., Lo, I., Toppet, M., Ferster, A., & Fondu, P. (1999). In vitro antisickling activity of a rearranged limonoid isolated from Khayasenegalensis. *Planta Medica*, *65*(03), 209–212. doi:10.1055-1999-14083 PMID:10232063

Figueiredo, M. S. (2015). The compound state: Hb S/beta-thalassemia. *Revista Brasileira de Hematologia e Hemoterapia*, *37*(3), 150–152. doi:10.1016/j.bjhh.2015.02.008 PMID:26041415

Gault, P. M., Allen, K. R., & Newton, K. E. (2005). Plasma aluminium: A redundant test for patients on dialysis? *Annals of Clinical Biochemistry*, *42*(1), 51–54. doi:10.1258/0004563053026862 PMID:15802033

Greenburg, A. G. (1996). Pathophysiology of anemia. *The American Journal of Medicine*, *101*(2), 7S–11S. doi:10.1016/S0002-9343(96)00161-1 PMID:8831424

Gupta, S. C., Patchva, S., & Aggarwal, B. B. (2013). Therapeutic roles of curcumin: Lessons learned from clinical trials. *The AAPS Journal*, *15*(1), 195–218. doi:10.120812248-012-9432-8 PMID:23143785

Hallberg, L., Hôgdahl, A. M., Nilsson, L., & Rybo, G. (1966). Menstrual blood loss–a population study. *Acta Obstetricia et Gynecologica Scandinavica*, *45*(3), 320–351. doi:10.3109/00016346609158455 PMID:5922481

Halsted, C. H., Villanueva, J. A., Devlin, A. M., & Chandler, C. J. (2002). Metabolic interactions of alcohol and folate. *The Journal of Nutrition*, *132*(8), 2367S–2372S. doi:10.1093/jn/132.8.2367S PMID:12163694

Hekmat, S., & McMahon, D. J. (1997). Manufacture and quality of iron-fortified yogurt. *Journal of Dairy Science*, *80*(12), 3114–3122. doi:10.3168/jds.S0022-0302(97)76282-9 PMID:9436092

Hilty, F. M., Arnold, M., Hilbe, M., Teleki, A., Knijnenburg, J. T., Ehrensperger, F., & Zimmermann, M. B. (2010). Iron from nanocompounds containing iron and zinc is highly bioavailable in rats without tissue accumulation. *Nature Nanotechnology*, *5*(5), 374–380. doi:10.1038/nnano.2010.79 PMID:20418865

Humphrey, B. D., Huang, N., & Klasing, K. C. (2002). Rice expressing lactoferrin and lysozyme has antibiotic-like properties when fed to chicks. *The Journal of Nutrition*, *132*(6), 1214–1218. doi:10.1093/jn/132.6.1214 PMID:12042436

Kasili, E. G. (1989). Malnutrition and infections as causes of childhood anemia in tropical Africa. *The American Journal of Pediatric Hematology/Oncology*, *12*(3), 375–377. doi:10.1097/00043426-199023000-00023 PMID:2122763

Lang, K. S., Roll, B., Myssina, S., Schittenhelm, M., Scheel-Walter, H. G., Kanz, L., & Wieder, T. (2002). Enhanced erythrocyte apoptosis in sickle cell anemia, thalassemia and glucose-6-phosphate dehydrogenase deficiency. *Cellular Physiology and Biochemistry*, *12*(5-6), 365–372. doi:10.1159/000067907 PMID:12438773

Latvala, J., Parkkila, S., & Niemelä, O. (2004). Excess alcohol consumption is common in patients with cytopenia: Studies in blood and bone marrow cells. *Alcoholism, Clinical and Experimental Research*, *28*(4), 619–624. doi:10.1097/01.ALC.0000122766.54544.3B PMID:15100613

Loban, K. M., Polozok, E. S., Efimov, L. S., & Khorin, A. T. (1987). Treatment of imported tropical malaria caused by chloroquine-resistant strains of P. falciparum. *Terapevticheskii Arkhiv*, *59*(1), 69–72. PMID:3551176

Marsanasco, M., Márquez, A. L., Wagner, J. R., Alonso, S. D. V., & Chiaramoni, N. S. (2011). Liposomes as vehicles for vitamins E and C: An alternative to fortify orange juice and offer vitamin C protection after heat treatment. *Food Research International*, *44*(9), 3039–3046. doi:10.1016/j.foodres.2011.07.025

Martınez-Navarrete, N., Camacho, M. M., Martınez-Lahuerta, J., Martınez-Monzó, J., & Fito, P. (2002). Iron deficiency and iron fortified foods—a review. *Food Research International, 35*(2), 225–231. doi:10.1016/S0963-9969(01)00189-2

McKie, A. T., Barrow, D., Latunde-Dada, G. O., Rolfs, A., Sager, G., Mudaly, E., & Peters, T. J. (2001). An iron-regulated ferric reductase associated with the absorption of dietary iron. *Science, 291*(5509), 1755–1759. doi:10.1126cience.1057206 PMID:11230685

Michel, M. (2014). Warm autoimmune hemolytic anemia: Advances in pathophysiology and treatment. *La Presse Medicale, 43*(4), e97–e104. doi:10.1016/j.lpm.2014.02.009 PMID:24680421

Mishra, B., Malhotra, P., Ratho, R. K., Singh, M. P., Varma, S., & Varma, N. (2005). Human parvovirus B19 in patients with aplastic anemia. *American Journal of Hematology, 79*(2), 166–167. doi:10.1002/ajh.20347 PMID:15929106

Muncie, H. L. Jr, & Campbell, J. (2009). Alpha and beta thalassemia. *American Family Physician, 80*(4), 339–344. PMID:19678601

Obodozie, O. O., Ameh, S. J., Afolabi, E. K., Oyedele, E. O., Ache, T. A., Onanuga, C. E., & Inyang, U. S. (2010). A normative study of the components of niprisan—an herbal medicine for sickle cell anemia. *Journal of Dietary Supplements, 7*(1), 21–30. doi:10.3109/19390210903534988 PMID:22435571

Ong, L., Henriksson, A., & Shah, N. P. (2007). Angiotensin converting enzyme-inhibitory activity in Cheddar cheeses made with the addition of probiotic Lactobacillus casei sp. *Le Lait, 87*(2), 149–165. doi:10.1051/lait:2007004

Pellegrino, L., Battelli, G., Resmini, P., Ferranti, P., Barone, F., & Addeo, F. (1997). Effects of heat load gradient occurring in moulding on characterization and ripening of Grana Padano. *Le Lait, 77*(2), 217–228. doi:10.1051/lait:1997215

Pereira, D. I., Bruggraber, S. F., Faria, N., Poots, L. K., Tagmount, M. A., Aslam, M. F., & Powell, J. J. (2014). Nanoparticulate iron (III) oxo-hydroxide delivers safe iron that is well absorbed and utilised in humans. *Nanomedicine; Nanotechnology, Biology, and Medicine, 10*(8), 1877–1886. doi:10.1016/j.nano.2014.06.012 PMID:24983890

Quirolo, K., & Vichinsky, E. (2016). Sickle cell anemia, thalassemia, and congenital hemolytic anemias. *Rossi's Principles of Transfusion Medicine*, 126-143.

Rund, D., & Rachmilewitz, E. (2001, October). Pathophysiology of α-and β-thalassemia: Therapeutic implications. *Seminars in Hematology*, *38*(4), 343–349. doi:10.1016/S0037-1963(01)90028-9 PMID:11605169

Salminen, H., Herrmann, K., & Weiss, J. (2013). Oil-in-water emulsions as a delivery system for n-3 fatty acids in meat products. *Meat Science*, *93*(3), 659–667. doi:10.1016/j.meatsci.2012.11.035 PMID:23273478

Schrier, S. L. (1994). Thalassemia: Pathophysiology of red cell changes. *Annual Review of Medicine*, *45*(1), 211–218. doi:10.1146/annurev.med.45.1.211 PMID:8198378

Semple, J. W., & Freedman, J. (2005, July). Autoimmune pathogenesis and autoimmune hemolytic anemia. *Seminars in Hematology*, *42*(3), 122–130. doi:10.1053/j.seminhematol.2005.04.002 PMID:16041661

Serjeant, G. R., & Serjeant, B. E. (1992). *Sickle cell disease* (Vol. 3). New York: Oxford university press.

Shimakawa, Y., Matsubara, S., Yuki, N., Ikeda, M., & Ishikawa, F. (2003). Evaluation of Bifidobacterium breve strain Yakult-fermented soymilk as a probiotic food. *International Journal of Food Microbiology*, *81*(2), 131–136. doi:10.1016/S0168-1605(02)00224-6 PMID:12457587

Singh, T. K., Fox, P. F., & Healy, Á. (1997). Isolation and identification of further peptides in the diafiltrationretentate of the water-soluble fraction of Cheddar cheese. *The Journal of Dairy Research*, *64*(03), 433–443. doi:10.1017/S0022029997002227 PMID:9275258

Spielman, A., Pollack, R. J., Kiszewski, A. E., & Telford, S. R. III. (2001). Issues in public health entomology. *Vector Borne and Zoonotic Diseases (Larchmont, N.Y.)*, *1*(1), 3–19. doi:10.1089/153036601750137606 PMID:12653132

Ting, Y., Jiang, Y., Ho, C. T., & Huang, Q. (2014). Common delivery systems for enhancing in vivo bioavailability and biological efficacy of nutraceuticals. *Journal of Functional Foods*, *7*, 112–128. doi:10.1016/j.jff.2013.12.010

Uicich, R., Pizarro, F., Almeida, C., Díaz, M., Boccio, J., Zubillaga, M., & O'Donnell, A. (1999). Bioavailability of microencapsulated ferrous sulfate in fluid cow's milk. Studies in human beings. *Nutrition Research (New York, N.Y.)*, *19*(6), 893–897. doi:10.1016/S0271-5317(99)00049-4 van den Broek, N. (1996). The aetiology of anemia in pregnancy in West Africa. *Tropical Doctor*, *26*(1), 5–7. doi:10.1177/004947559602600103 PMID:8693577

Viteri, F. E., Álvarez, E., Batres, R., Torun, B., Pineda, O., Mejía, L. A., & Sylvi, J. (1995). Fortification of sugar with iron sodium ethylenediaminotetraacetate (FeNaEDTA) improves iron status in semirural Guatemalan populations. *The American Journal of Clinical Nutrition*, *61*(5), 1153–1163. doi:10.1093/ajcn/61.5.1153 PMID:7733042

Wills, M. R., & Savory, J. (1989). Aluminum and chronic renal failure: Sources, absorption, transport, and toxicity. *Critical Reviews in Clinical Laboratory Sciences*, *27*(1), 59–107. doi:10.3109/10408368909106590 PMID:2647415

World Health Organization. (2015). *The global prevalence of anemia in 2011*. WHO.

Xia, S., & Xu, S. (2005). Ferrous sulfate liposomes: Preparation, stability and application in fluid milk. *Food Research International*, *38*(3), 289–296. doi:10.1016/j.foodres.2004.04.010

Young, N. S., Bacigalupo, A., & Marsh, J. C. (2010). Aplastic anemia: Pathophysiology and treatment. *Biology of Blood and Marrow Transplantation*, *16*(1), S119–S125.

Section 7
Cancer

Chapter 12
Nutraceutical and Functional Foods in Cancer Management and Therapy

Sakshi Bajaj
Delhi Institute of Pharmaceutical Sciences and Research, India

Satish Manchanda
Delhi Institute of Pharmaceutical Sciences and Research, India

ABSTRACT

Cancer is an insidious disease affecting mankind in every country. The progression of cancer cells from one part of the body to another (metastasis) is one of the biggest problems in curing cancer. The present study brings new hope of future therapies to fight cancer. Designing an appropriate food to maintain proper health has become a necessity worldwide. Due to this, the food industries in many countries are modifying their products as a response to consumer demands. In recent years, many of the natural products are gaining popularity as nutraceuticals.

INTRODUCTION

Active substances whichever way extracted from plants (phytocomplexes) or of animal origin extracted, concentrated and administered in an appropriate pharmaceutical form, can make an exceptionally encouraging toolbox helpful to forestall and bolster the therapy of some pathologic conditions given their demonstrated clinical adequacy. It is overall perceived that diet and lifestyle are fundamental to advance and keep up prosperity and decent being state, other than help to forestall ailments

DOI: 10.4018/978-1-5225-3267-5.ch012

conceivable beginning. Both non-correct dietary habits and lifestyle can, indeed, determine pathological conditions.

Prevention is the key methodology for an effective proactive medicine, in which endeavors are routed to prevention and, consequently, to bring down the risk associated with lifestyle-related diseases diminishing, in the meantime, any National Health Systems cost expected to ensure the correct restorative approach given pharmaceuticals. Nutraceuticals use in counteractive action is a proactive switch approach tool to pre-clinical health conditions. They can be adequately utilized, by including in the daily diet, in a region which shades in the range "past the diet, before drugs," since they join both dietary and helpful healthy properties of food extracts with the mending properties of specific active compounds.

Nutraceuticals characterize another classification which shades the outskirts between drugs and food. Nutraceutical, a portmanteau of the words "nutrient" and "pharmaceutical", was coined by Stephen DeFelice, who defined nutraceuticals is "foods (or part of a food) that provide medical or health benefits in addition to its nutritional content, including the prevention and/or treatment of a disease" (DeFelice, 1995). Nutraceuticals are 'natural' substances isolated or purified from food substances and used in a medicinal fashion. Several naturally derived food substances have been studied in cancer in an attempt to identify natural preventative therapies for this disease. Vitamin E, selenium, vitamin D, green tea, soy, and lycopene have all been examined in human studies. Other potential nutraceuticals that lack human data, most notably pomegranate, might also have a preventative role in this disease. Recently, nutraceuticals have gained much attention in the area of cancer research because of their pleiotropic effects and relatively non-toxic behavior (Nair, Sung, Yadav, Kannappan, Chaturvedi, & Aggarwal, 2010).

Otherwise, the boundary between nutraceuticals and functional foods is not always clear being the main difference the format in which they are consumed: nutraceuticals are consumed as capsules, pills, tablets, etc. while functional foods are always consumed as ordinary foods. Thus, when a phytochemical is included in a food formulation is considered a functional food. If the same phytochemical is included in a capsule it will constitute a nutraceutical. The capacity of some plant-derived foods to reduce the risk of chronic diseases has been associated, at least in part, to the occurrence of secondary metabolites (phytochemicals) that have been shown to exert a wide range of biological activities. In general, these metabolites have low potency as bioactive compounds when compared to pharmaceutical drugs, but since they are ingested regularly and in significant amounts as part of the diet, they may have a noticeable long-term physiological effect (Espín, García-Conesa, & Tomás-Barberán, 2007).

Cancer is regarded as one of the most fatal diseases and characterized by the uncontrolled growth of abnormal cells (Pérez-Herrero & Fernández-Medarde, 2015) is a multistage process by which a normal cell is transformed into a cancerous cell. It interplays between genes and the environment, and multiple cumulative genetic changes are required for the transformation of normal cells into fully malignant cells. Essentially, self-sufficiency in growth signals, insensitivity to growth inhibitory (antigrowth) signals, evasion of programmed cell death (apoptosis), limitless replicative potential, sustained angiogenesis, and tissue invasion and metastasis are the main characteristics of tumourigenesis (Deorukhkar, Krishnan, Sethi, & Aggarwal, 2007).

Chemopreventive molecules target each of these steps including anti-initiation strategies (e.g DNA repair, detoxification, free-radical scavenging and carcinogen metabolism) and antipromotional strategies (e.g. Free-radical scavenging, proliferation, suppression, differentiation induction, immunity enhancement, inflammation reduction, increase in apoptosis, altered gene expression and decreases in angiogenesis (Balunas & Kinghorn, 2005; Tsao, Kim, & Hong 2004). From initial development of a single cell, to invasion, angiogenesis, proliferation and metastasis, there are many cellular mediators involved to be manipulated. Although predisposing of cancer cannot be signaled out by a single factor, a panel of factors places some people at a higher risk. Most of the high-risk cases may have a genetic background, but dietary choices could dictate the outcome of health (Pericleous, Mandair, & Caplin, 2013). Bioactive components of dietary phytochemicals with chemopreventive proparties include curcumin, genistein, resveratrol, diallyl sulphide, S-allyl cysteine, allicin, lycopene, capsaicin, diosgenin, (6)-gingerol, ellagic acid, ursolic acid, catechins, eugenol, isoeugenol, carotene, lucopene, isoflavones and flavonoid (Aggarwal & Shishodia, 2006a). Etiology (Figure 1) and the pathogenesis of cancer can be explained with the help of 6 hallmarks of cancer (Pecorino, 2008).

Colourful vegetables such as spinach, beets, winter squash, asparagus, tomatoes, carrots and sweet potatoes contain carotenoids, which have a preferred lower glycemic index, are loaded with fibre and have cancer-fighting properties. Colorful berries contain a powerful agent ellagic acid, which triggers apoptosis in prostate cancer cells. This "self-destruction" mechanism is found in raspberries, strawberries, dark cherries, blueberries, cranberries and blackberries. These powerfully pigmented vegetables also act as antioxidants, protecting healthy cells from chemotherapy and radiation. Cruciferous vegetables such as cabbage, broccoli, sprouts, and cauliflower are also known for their cancer-fighting phytochemicals. This group of plant food also helps detoxifying the body.

Green tea has shown potential to prevent and prolong remission in cancer patients. Studies show that drinking green tea daily inhibits cell division and metastasis. The polyphenolic compounds found in green tea such as catechin and epicatechin have been found to act as antioxidants and immune stimulants. Decaffeinated tea does not appear to have the same cancer fighting abilities. All cells in the body, even

Figure 1. Etiology and the pathogenesis of cancer can be explained with the help of 6 hallmarks of cancer

Growth signal autonomy

- For the purpose of division normal cells need external signals from growth factors.
- Acquired mutations short-circuit growth factor pathway leading to unregulated growth.

⇩

Evasion of growth inhibitory cells

- In order to maintain homeostasis normal cells respond to inhibitory signals.
- Acquired mutations thereby interfere with the inhibitory pathways.

⇩

Evasion of apoptosis

- Apoptosis results in removal of normal cells in response to DNA damage.
- Cancer cells evade apoptotic signals.

⇩

Unlimited replicative potential

- There is an autonomous counting device in normal cells that defines a finite number of cell doubling after which they become senescent. The cellular counting device is represented in form of shortening of chromosomal ends, telomeres that occurs during every round of DNA replication. But there's no variation in length of telomeres of cancer cells.
- Altered regulation of telomere maintainance results in unlimited replicative potential.

⇩

Angiogenesis

- For the purpose of growth of tumor cells angiogenesis is induced by cancer cells.
- Angiogenesis is activated by altered balance between angiogenic inducers and inhibitors.

⇩

Invasion of metastasis

- Mutation alters the activity of enzymes involved in invasion and alter molecules involved in cell- cell and cellular- extracellular adhesion.
- Thus, migration of cancer cells unlike normal cells to other body parts is the major cause of death.

immune cells, need healthy fats and oils. Fat is the preferred fuel of muscle and it is a critical component of cell membranes. Fish oil, olive oil, flax oil and even real butter in moderation are recommended. All these prospects make nutraceuticals potentially useful in deadly chronic diseases like cancer. They are non-specific biological therapies used to promote wellness, prevent malignant processes and control symptoms. A large number of studies have demonstrated that dietary habit is one of the most important determinants of chronic diseases such as cardiovascular disease, diabetes, gallstones, neurodegenerative diseases, cataract and several types of cancer (Smith-Warner et al., 2000). Such an association between dietary habit and disease shows that food has a direct impact on health.

Functional Foods

The term "functional food" was first used in 1984 in Japan as a result of a study on the relationships between nutrition, sensory satisfaction, fortification and modulation of physiological systems in order to define those food products fortified with special constituents that possess advantageous physiological effects (Hardy 2000; Kwak & Jukes, 2001). It can be any ordinary food that has components or ingredients added to give it a specific medical or physiological benefit, other than a purely nutritional effect.

Functional foods' objectives are manifold: they improve the general conditions of the body (e.g., pre- and probiotics), decrease the risk of some diseases (e.g., cholesterol-lowering products), and could be used for curing some illnesses (Mark-Herbert, 2004; Menrad, 2003). Functional foods are those that exert a scientifically proven specific health benefit (health claim) beyond their nutritional properties but the consumption of its specific formulation is not essential for human life. The format of presentation of functional foods is a food or derivative such as fortified beverages, juices, milk, yoghurts, margarines, cereals, etc.

Functional foods have been developed almost in all food categories, even if they are not homogeneously distributed over all segments of the food industry. As a consequence, consumer preferences may vary between markets. Among all the food markets, functional foods have been mainly launched in the dairy-, confectionery, soft-drinks, bakery and baby-food market (Kotilainen, Rajalahti, Ragasa, & Pehu, 2006; Menrad, 2003). The extant literature proposes different classification of functional foods. From a product point of view, (Kotilainen, Rajalahti, Ragasa, & Pehu, 2006; Spence, 2006), have proposed the following classification:

- Food fortified with additional supplements (marked invigorated items), such as natural product juices braced with vitamin C, vitamin E, folic acid, zinc and calcium.

- Food with extra new supplements or components not regularly found in a specific food (marked enhanced items), like probiotics or prebiotics.
- Food from which a deleterious component has been removed, or replaced by another with beneficial effects (labeled altered products), for example fibers as fat releasers in meat or dessert.
- Food in which one of the components have been normally improved (marked improved wares), e.g., eggs with expanded omega-3 content.

Dietary bioactive food components that interact with the immune response have considerable potential to reduce the risk of cancer. The reduction of chronic inflammation or its downstream consequences may represent a key mechanism whose effects can be reduced by targeting signal transduction or through antioxidant effects. Some of the most important immunomodulators are phytochemicals such as the polyphenols, epigallocatechin gallate (EGCG) and curcumin (Ferguson & Philpott, 2007; Shukla & Gupta, 2005). Oxidative stress and associated mechanisms involving inflammation, aberrant signalling pathways, and gap junction intercellualar communications is increasingly associated with the pathogenesis of various chronic degenerative disorders such as atherosclerosis, neurodegeneration and cancer (Soobrattee, Bahorun, & Aruoma, 2006). The consumption of fresh fruits, vegetables and teas has the capacity to reduce the risk of cancer.

BACKGROUND

Designing an appropriate food to maintain proper health has become a necessity worldwide. Due to this, the food industries in many countries are modifying their products as a response to consumer demands. In recent years, many of the natural products are gaining popularity as nutraceuticals. They are the natural bioactive products with food values including dietary supplements and fortified foods that are marketed in a medicinal format such as a Tablet, Capsule or powder in a prescribed dose and show promising therapeutic properties in several diseases. More rigorously, it is a designer food containing phytochemicals, biologically active compounds with a medical health benefit, including the prevention and treatment of chronic disease. They are mostly phytochemicals derived from dietary or medicinal plants. Natural products may be included either singly or in combination in the nutraceutical products for various purposes. They may be used to reduce the risk of various cancers. The potential of using nutraceuticals as chemopreventive agents has prompted a surge of in-vitro studies on of their biological effects in cultured human cells. So there is an urgent need to search for better medicines for cancer. Chemoprevention is the use of small molecules, including dietary or herbal chemicals, to prevent cancers, as opposed to chemotherapeutics, where chemicals, mostly synthetic, are used to remove or alleviate cancer symptoms.

MARKET SCENARIO OF NUTRACEUTICALS

Globally, the US and Japan are the most developed markets for nutraceuticals, due to the consumer acceptability achieved in these regions. India, China and Brazil are developing nations which show huge potential for the nutraceuticals market. India and china have emerged as a key sourcing destination for natural ingredients. The global market for nutraceuticals is projected to reach US$250 billion by 2018, driven primarily by the growing affinity among the general populace towards adopting a healthy lifestyle. Nutraceutical foods were the largest market segment in 2007, worth $39.9 billion. This is expected to increase $56.7 billion in 2013. Nutraceutical supplements have the second largest market share, generating $39.0 billion in 2007. This segment should reach $48.8 billion in 2013.The nutraceutical beverages segment represents the fastest growing segment and is expected to have the largest share of the market by 2013. This segment was worth $38.4 billion in 2007 and is expected to increase to and $71.3 billion in 2013 (Frost & Sullivan, 2011).

REGULATORY CONCEPTS

Nutraceuticals have received considerable interest because of their presumed safety and potential nutritional and therapeutic effects (Ray, Joshi, & Gulati, 2016). There is a need of regulating or categorizing these food products under specific definitions and according to food laws. The primary regulatory obligations of manufacturers and marketers of nutraceuticals include product safety and accuracy of the labeling that describes product identity and composition. As foods and/or food ingredients, these substances are regulated by the FDA under the authority of the Federal Food, Drug, and Cosmetic Act (Anon, 1938), though they are not specifically defined by law. In fact, the only legally-defined term is that of "dietary supplements" (Finley, 2016). Because, according to the FDA, no drug may enter the food market and food is defined as *used for food or drink (or) components of any such article* (John Weldon Finley, Finley, Ellwood, & Hoadley, 2014), this has complex implications not only in the creation and development of new products with (potential) health benefits, but also in their marketing claims. These restrictive definitions also bolster some evident contradictions. FDA defines "drug", among other, as *a substance intended for use in the diagnosis, cure, mitigation, treatment, or prevention of disease* which certainly includes Vitamin C, present and often added in foodstuffs and key in the prevention of scurvy (Carpenter, 1988). It should also be mentioned that it is necessary to define what a "claim" is. Within such context, a claim refers to "health" and/or "structure/function" claims. These may be defined as claims describing an established relationship between a *food substance and reduced risk of a disease or health-related condition* or "the effects that a substance has on the structure or function of the body", respectively (Borchers, Keen, & Gershwin, 2016).

Different countries have different nutraceutical terminologies and their regulations which are as follows (Table 1).

Table 1.

Country	Body Known as	Body Governed by	Definition Covers
Canada	Natural health products in 2004	FDA	Vitamins, mineral, homeopathic, Chinese medicine, amino acids, essential fatty acids
EU	Food supplements in 2002	Food safety authority	Concentrated sources of nutrients, substances with nutritional or physiological effects
Russia	Biologically active food in 1997	Ministry of health and social development	Vitamins, aminoacids, dietary fibers, para-pharmeceuticals (bioflavonoid, polysaccharides)
USA	Dietary supplement in 1994	FDA	Vitamins, minerals, botanicals, amino acids, herbal extracts
Australia	Complementary medicines in 1991	Department of health and ageing	Herbal medicines, Vitamins, minerals, nutritional supplements.
Japan	Foods for specific health Use in 1991	Japan health and nutritional food association	Functional foods that can have three functions: nutrition, sensory, satisfaction, physiological improvement
India	Foods for special dietary use in 2005	Food safety and standards act passes in 2006 yet to be implemented	Vitamins, minerals, botanicals, herbal extracts
China	Health food	State food and drug administration (SFDA) in 2003	Any finished product or raw material intended for people to eat or drink, as well as any product that has traditionally served as both food and medication, with the exception of products used solely for medical purposes.

NUTRACEUTICALS IN PREVENTION OF CANCER

In the last two decades, much evidence has emerged indicating that, at the molecular level, most chronic diseases, including cancer, are caused by a dysregulated inflammatory response. Inflammation is often linked to neoplastic development and acts as a driving force in premalignant and malignant transformation of cells (Philip, Rowley, & Schreiber, 2004). There is now growing evidence supporting the notion that chronic inflammation may lead tomalignancies of different organs including the skin, stomach, colon, breast, prostate, and pancreas (Li, Withoff, & Verma, 2005; Marx, 2004; Michael Karin & Greten, 2005). One of the most important links between inflammation and cancer is proinflammatory transcription factor nuclear factor-kappa B (NF-B) (Karin, 2009). NF-B is a ubiquitous and evolutionarily conserved transcription factor that regulates the expression of genes involved in the transformation, survival, proliferation, invasion, angiogenesis, and metastasis of cancer cells. Many nutraceuticals are shown to exert chemopreventive/anticancer activity by suppressing the NF-B signaling pathway (Shishir Shishodia & Aggarwal, 2004; Siddiqui, Shukla, Adhami, Sarfaraz, Asim, Hafeez, Bin, & Mukhtar, 2008; Roy, Madan, Kalra, Nigam, George, Ray… Shukla, 2009). Humans are unknowingly exposed to environmental insults such as pesticides, fumes, automobile exhaust, ionizing, ultraviolet radiation, etc., which cause the formation of oxidants bymetabolic activity within cells. When in excess, these oxidants can cause an imbalance, leading to production of reactive oxygen species (ROS) or oxidative stress (Galli, Piroddi, Annetti, Aisa, Floridi, & Floridi, 2005).

Normally, there is equilibrium between ROS generation and antioxidant defense systems, and any imbalance between them can lead to oxidative stress. Oxidative stress can alter the structure of cellular components such as DNA, proteins, and lipids, which, when left unrepaired, can induce cell death or cancer development through various mechanisms (Ames, Shigenaga, & Gold, 1993). Imbalance of oxidative stress has been shown to be able to trigger the activation of multiple signaling pathways, including the activation of various transcription factors (e.g.,NF-B) and phosphorylation cascades of mitogen-activated protein kinases (MAPKs) (Thannickal & Fanburg, 2000). Thus, cancer control can be achieved by decreasing the rate of oxidative stress and enhancing antioxidant defense mechanisms. The potential role of dietary antioxidants present in nutraceuticals in reducing the risk of cancer by suppressing the state of oxidative stress has been well documented in the literature (Chu, Sun, Wu, & Liu, 2002; Dragsted, Strube, & Larsen, 1993). Another major cause of neoplastic development is the dysregulation of body homeostasis, a fundamental characteristic of living beings. The balance between cell proliferation and apoptosis is a critical step in the maintenance of homeostasis (Green, 2000; Meier, Finch, & Evan, 2000).

The dysregulation of apoptosis is a hallmark of cancer and is critical for cancer development and tumor cell survival (Hanahan & Weinberg, 2000). Cancer cells can invade apoptosis mainly through two signaling pathways: extrinsic (receptor mediated) and intrinsic (mitochondria mediated). The extrinsic pathway is triggered by a complex set of antiapoptotic and proapototic proteins, including caspase family proteins, Bax, B cell lymphoma (Bcl)-2 family proteins, cytochrome c, apoptotic protease activating factor (Apaf)-1, and death receptors (APO-1/TRAIL). The intrinsic pathway is initiated by cellular developmental signals or as a result of severe cellular stress, including DNA damage. Some antiapoptotic proteins, such as Bcl-2 and Bcl-2 extra large (Bcl-xL) (S. Wang, Yang, & Lippman, 2003), are overexpressed in many cancer types. Therefore, selective downregulation of antiapoptotic proteins and upregulation of proapoptotic proteins in cancer cells offer promising therapeutic interventions for cancer treatment. A number of nutraceuticals, mostly phytochemicals derived from dietary or medicinal plants, have shown potential to reduce cancer incidence by inducing apoptosis with the use of various mechanisms in multiple types of cancer cells (Gosslau & Chen, 2004).

HERBAL PRODUCTS AS HIDDEN MEDICAL WEAPONS

Although modern medicines have become more powerful and more specific for treating various conditions, there is a growing emphasis on the importance of diet, nutrition

Figure 2. Classification of nutraceuticals and functional foods

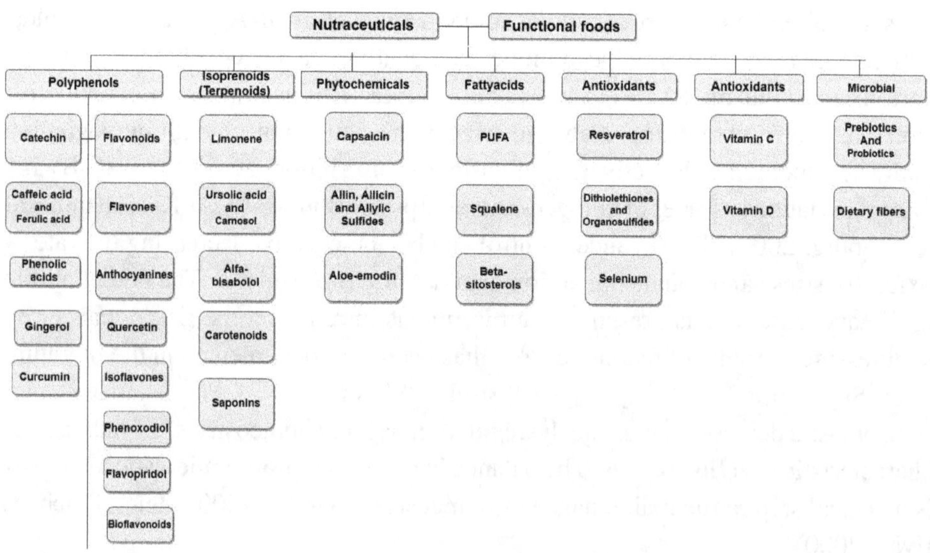

and lifestyle in preventing health problem and promoting wellbeing. Herbal products were mankind's first medicine and they have served that function for centuries. In fact, most of the world's population is still treated with herbal medicines. Several herbs and herbal compounds are believed to suppress the transformative, hyperproliferative and inflammatory process that initiates carcinogenesis and dramatically inhibit the vascular endothelial growth factor (VEGF), whose production is considered essential for the migration of cancer cell and for angiogenesis. Herbs may be included either singly or in combination in the nutraceutical products to reduce the risk of cancer.

TRADITIONAL HERBS AND PLANTS WITH ANTI CARCINOGENIC POTENTIAL

Polyphenols

Under the denomination "phenolic compounds" there are more than 4000 compounds divided in 12 subclasses. Vegetables, fruits, fungi and some bacteria produce, as part of their secondary metabolism, a wide variety of phenolic compounds. In the early 1960s, phenolic compounds were widely viewed as metabolic waste products that were stored in the plant vacuole. Whilst there was interest at that time in their function as flower colorants, and in their distribution between plant taxa, the earliest investigations of their biosynthesis had just begun (Quideau, 2006). Among the most interesting nutraceutical candidates to act as anti-inflammatory, polyphenols are another outstanding example Some of them are highly important for their physiological functions, some others are used to defend themselves from stress situations or to attract or repeal other organisms.

The benefits of using polyphenols are mainly associated with their high antioxidant capacity that slows down the oxidative stress rate. They are a class of vegetal natural origin substances which are able to modulate human cellular signaling and gene expression. These compounds include phenolic acids, flavonoids, catechins, hydroxycinnamates, coumarins, anthocyanins, ellagic acid, lignans, ellagitannins and isoflavones. In a similar way to amides and carotenoids, polyphenols predominantly act as antioxidants, by scavenging free radicals and chelating metalions. Some polyphenols also increase the levels of glutathione and the expression of antioxidant enzymes such as glutathione peroxidase, catalase, and superoxide dismutase. The beneficial effects of nutraceuticals and functional foods had been ascribed to their high content of polyphenolic flavonoids. These compounds have been shown to possess antioxidant/radical scavenging activity and increase the capacity of endogenous antioxidant defenses, thus, modulating the cellular redox state. All are able to reduce the oxidative stress, which has been associated to the occurrence of chronic diseases and is believed to promote cell proliferation and causing, among others, malfunctions in heart disease, diabetes, and autoimmune disease (Rosa, Alvarez-Parrilla, González-Aguilar, & Wiley InterScience (Online Service, 2010). Recent evidence indicates that besides their well-established antioxidant and iron chelating properties, polyphenol catechins have a profound effect on cell survival/death genes and signal transduction pathways (Schroeter, Boyd, Spencer, Williams, Cadenas, & Rice-Evans, 2002; Mandel, Avramovich-Tirosh, Reznichenko, Zheng, Weinreb, Amit, & Youdim, 2005). Flavones and isoflavones are perhaps the most studied active ingredients of nutraceuticals and functional foods. They have been hailed as highly anti-inflammatory, antioxidant, anticarcinogenic and anti-metastatic agents (yung sheng Huang, 2010; Kasala, Bodduluru, Barua, & Gogoi, 2016; Venkatachalam, Nayak, & Jayashree, 2012; Yang, Yang, Kuo, Chang, Chu, & Hsieh, 2008), and have also been described to exhibit radioprotective and immunomodulatory activityes (Hillman, Singh-Gupta, Hoogstra, Abernathy, Rakowski, Yunker, … Joiner, 2013; Zhou, Lin, Ge, Niu, Wang, Wang, … Tan, 2015). Poly phenols are receiving considerable attention for the potential implications in cancer therapy, particularly resveratrol (grapes), quercetin (Broccoli, onions and tea), Curcumin (Turmeric), genistein (Soy), epigallocatechin (green tea) and their sources.

Catechin

The term catechins are also commonly used to refer to the related family of flavonoids and the subgroup flavan-3-ols (or simply flavanols). Found in apples, berries, black and green tea, chocolate, grapes and wine. Potential benefits include increased immune function; decreased cholesterol production. Catechins are a powerful form of antioxidant that acts as a powerful inhibitor of cancer growth. In fact, catechins are 100 times more powerful than vitamin C and 25 times more powerful than vitamin E in their antioxidant/growth inhibitor powers. The flavonoids and catechins together have proven ability to protect cells from x-ray damage, block the progression of the cell cycle, and inhibit mutations. Studies suggest that a particular catechin found in green tea, epigallocatechin gallate (EGCG), may be good for the prostate by suppressing growth of tumors as well as inhibiting enzymes that are involved in the spread of cancer cells) (Figure 3) (Yang, Yang, Kuo, Chang, Chu, & Hsieh, 2008). It has been shown to inhibit a variety of processes involved in cancer cell growth, survival and metastasis (Khan, Afaq, Saleem, Ahmad, & Mukhtar, 2006). EGCG has been most extensively investigated because of its relative abundance and strong cancer-preventive properties, particularly in the chemoprevention of breast cancer (Pan, Lin, Lin, & Chen, 2007).

Figure 3. [(2R, 3R)-5,7-dihydroxy-2-(3,4,5-trihydroxyphenyl)chroman-3-yl]3,4,5-trihydroxybenzoate

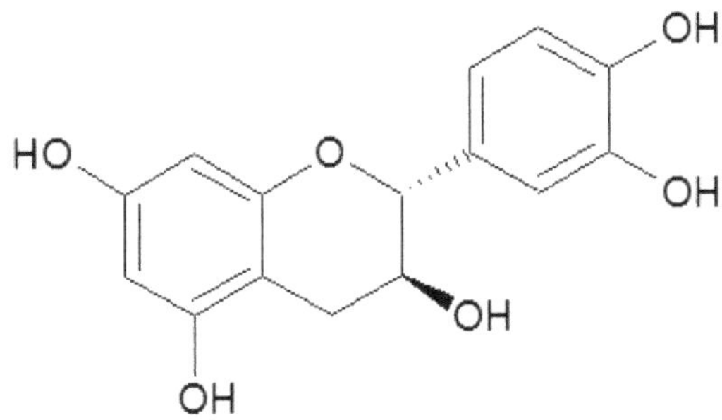

Caffeic Acid and Ferulic Acid

Caffeic acid is a naturally occurring compound. It is found in apples, asparagus, cabbage, grains, spinach, and tomatoes which are sources of cancer fighting agents. Caffeic acid phenethyl ester, an active phenolic component extracted from honey bee propolis, blocks tumorigenesis in a two stage model of mouse skin cancer (Figure 4a). Caffeic acid phenethyl ester has been reported induce apoptosis in HL-60 leukemic cells and mouse epidermal JB6 Cl 41 cells. Caffeic acid (CA) and its derivative, Caffeic acid phenethyl ester (CAPE) have shown tumor-shrinking properties. When CA and CAPE were administered orally and sub cutaneously it showed a significant reduction in liver metastasis. These results confirmed and laid the base for the therapeutic potential of the compound. This also established the anti-metastatic and anti-tumor effects of CA and CAPE are mediated through the selective suppression of MMP-9 (Matrix Metallopeptidase 9) enzyme activity and transcriptional down-regulation by the dual inhibition of NF-κB (Nuclear factor Kappa B) as well as MMP-9 catalytic activity (Chung, Moon, Chang, Ko, Lee, Cho, … Kim, 2004).

Ferulic Acid (FA), which is a phenolic phytochemical found in plant's cell-wall such as arabinoxylans as covalent side chains. It possesess antitumor - promoter, anti inflammatory, anti-viral and arteriodilator properties (Figure 4b). Ferulic acid may have direct antitumor activity against breast cancer and liver cancer as suggested by *invitro* and animal studies (Ghasemzadeh & Jaafar, 2013). Ferulic acid is effective in preventing cancer induced by exposure to the carcinogenic compounds benzopyrene and 4-nitroquinoline-1-oxide. Further alkyl ferulate, ferulic acid derivative has anti-carcinogenic property. Another derivative of FA in which geranyl group is attached to the phenolic hydroxyl group of ethyl ferulate, exhibits anti-colon carcinogenesis (Srinivasan, Sudheer, & Menon, 2007).

Figure 4. (a) 3-(3, 4-Dihydroxyphenyl)-2-propenoic acid, (b): 3-(4-hydroxy-3-methoxy- phenyl) prop-2-enoic acid

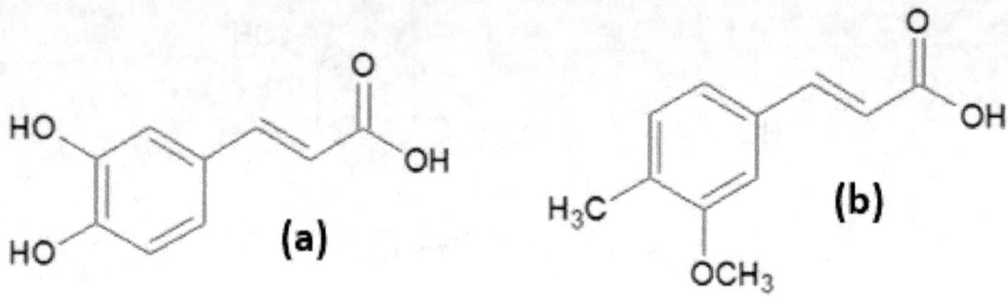

Phenolic Acid

Phenolic acid is found in cruciferous vegetable, eggplant, peppers, tomatoes, celery, parsley, soya, flaxseed, citrus, whole grains, cherries and berries. It Fights cancer through nitrosamine formation. The possible oncoprotective nechanisms of phenolic acids include antioxidant effects, steroid receptor binding, direct interaction with intracellular elements and signaling systems and aryl hydrocarbon receptor (AhR) binding and modification of subsequent signaling pathways (Bonnesen, Eggleston, & Hayes, 2001).

Ginger

Gingerol or (6) gingerol, the phenolic substance responsible for the spicy taste of fresh ginger (Zingiber officinale), has diverse pharmacological effects, such as being antioxidant, anti-apoptotic and anti-inflammatory (Figure 5). Though it was used dates back 2500 years, its anticancer and chemopreventive properties came to light only recently (Shukla & Singh, 2007). Inhibition of COX2 expression has been co-related as a molecular basis for its antitumour effects (Kim, Chun, Kundu, & Surh, 2004). Ginger has demonstrated effectiveness with chemotheraphy-induced nausea in meta-analysis of randomized clinical trials (Boon & Wong, 2004). Important adaptogens to consider in oncology include *Eleutherococcus senticosus, Panax ginseng, Rhodiola rosea, Schisandra chinensis, Rhaponticum carthamoides* and *aralia manchurica*. Extensive studies using various cytotoxic therapies in animal and human models with tumours have demonstrated that these adaptogens reduced chemotherapic drug toxicity, in combination with cytotoxic agents, particularly in bone marrow restoration, and they enhanced antitumour and antimetastatic effects (Panossian, Wikman, & Wagner, 1999).

Figure 5. 5-hydroxy-1-(4-hydroxy-3-methoxyphenyl)-3-decanone

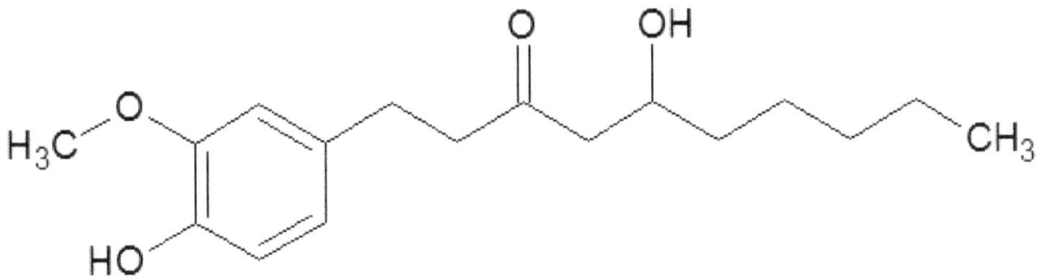

Curcumin

Curcumin (Diferuloylmethane) is a polyphenolic compound present in rhizomes of curcuma longa. Curcumin is derived from turmeric, the powdered rhizome of the medicinal plant *curcuma longa Linn.*, which is widely used as a spice in southeast Asian and middle eastern cooking (Figure 6). Turmeric is thought to have numerous therapeutic properties; it is utilized as a disinfectant foot cuts, burns, and wounds and utilized as an antibacterial agent. In Asian countries, curcumin can also help with stomach problems and other ailments. Although the broad curative properties of curcumin have been known for centuries, its potential anticancer and chemopreventive properties have been established only recently (Aggarwal, Surh, & Shishodia, 2007). Curcumin induces apoptosis in colon carcinoma cells, leukemic cells, prostate cancer cells, melanoma cells, and breast cancer cells.

The anticancer potential of curcumin has been demonstrated in various invitro and in vivo models. Curcumin has been shown to block transformation, tumor initiation, tumor promotion, invasion, angiogenesis, and metastasis. In *In-vivo* studies, Curcumin suppressed carcinogenesis of the skin, forestomach, colon, and liver in mice. Curcumin has been shown to inhibit proliferation of a wide variety of tumor cells, including B-cell and T- cell leukemias (Kuo, Huang, & Lin, 1996; Ranjan, Johnston, Reddy, Wu, Bondada, & Chen, 1999; Piwocka, Zabłocki, Wieckowski, Skierski, Feiga, Szopa, … Sikora, 1999; Han, Chung, Robertson, Ranjan, & Bondada, 1999), colon carcinoma, (Chen, Davis, Bissonnette, Scaglione-Sewell, & Brasitus, 1999), epidermoid carcinoma (Korutla & Kumar, 1994), head and neck squamous cell carcinoma (Aggarwal, Takada, Singh, Myers, & Aggarwal, 2004), multiple myeloma (Bharti, Donato, & Aggarwal, 2003) and mantle cell lymphoma. It has also been shown to suppress proliferation of various breast carcinoma cell lines in culture (Mehta, Pantazis, McQueen, & Aggarwal, 1997; Ramachandran & You, 1999; Simon, Allais, Duroux, Basly, Durand-Fontanier, & Delage, 1998). Young-Joon Surh (College of Pharmacy, Seoul National University, Seoul, South Korea) found that Curcumin, a yellow coloring agent contained in turmeric (*Curcuma longa L.*, Zingiberaceae) inhibits expression of COX-2 in mouse skin treated with the tumor promoter 12-O-tetradecanoylphorbol- 13-acetate (TPA) through inactivation of the eukaryotic transcription factor NF-nB (Surh, 2002). Curcumin has been shown to suppress carcinogenesis in other organs such as the oral cavity, skin, liver, lung, colon, stomach and breast to lower blood cholesterol, to promote wound healing, to prevent skin wrinkling, to inhibit inflammation, to suppress rheumatoid arthritis and to inhibit HIV replication. Curcumin mediates this wide variety of therapeutic effects through the regulation of the transcription factors NF-nB and signal transducer and activator of transcription 3(STAT-3), and suppression of InB kinase (Shishodia, Potdar, Gairola, & Aggarwal, 2003). He also reported that combination of two subeffective low concentrations of celecobix and curcumin, such that each per se does not have biological effect, resulted in blockade of NF-nB activation.

Anthocyanins (Bilberry, Cranberry, Elderberry, Raspberry Seed)

Several preclinical animal studies have been conducted that demonstrate the remarkable chemopreventive activity of flavonoids such as green tea catechins, curcumin, anthocyanins, quercetin or silibinin. Anthocyanins are water-soluble vacuolar pigments that may appear red, purple, or blue according to pH. They belong to a parent class of molecules called flavonoids. Blueberries, blackberries, elderberries, strawberries, grapes, purple grapes and black currants are rich sources of anthocyanin .These phytochemicals help reduce cancer risk for breast, pancreas, esophageal, skin, colon and prostate cells. When anthocyanin-rich extracts (AREs) of commercially prepared grape (*Vitis vinifera*), bilberry (*Vaccinium myrtillus* L.), and chokeberry (Aronia meloncarpa E.) were investigated for their anti-carcinogenic activity against colon cancer, the results had shown that all extracts inhibited the growth of colon-cancer-derived HT-29cells and indicated that chokeberry is the most

Figure 6. (1E, 6E)-1, 7-bis(4-hydroxy-3-methoxyphenyl)–1, 6-heptadiene-3, 5-dione

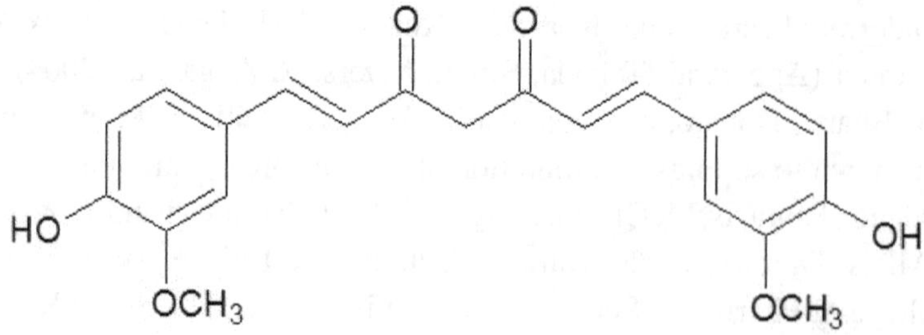

potent inhibitor (Zhao, Giusti, Malik, Moyer, & Magnuson, 2004). Gary Stoner et al. showed that freeze-dried black raspberry, strawberry and blackberry powders at concentrations of 5% and 10% fed to Fischer-344 rats before, during and after treatment with the esophageal carcinogen, N-nitrosomethylbenzylamine (NMBA), inhibit the number of esophageal tumors by 40–60% relative to NMBA controls (Kresty, Morse, Morgan, Carlton, Lu, Gupta, ... Stoner, 2001). This inhibition correlated with a reduction in DNA damage. Chemoprevention by berries was also reported in oral cavity cancers. Oral cavity cancers represent 2.5% of the cancer incidences in the United States and are ranked sixth worldwide, said Dr. Christopher Weghorst. An extract of lyophilized black raspberries dramatically inhibits the in vitro proliferation of cells derived from a human oral squamous cell carcinoma (SCC-83), in a dose dependent manner and to a maximum of 40%, suggesting that the chemoprevention of human oral cancer by raspberry extract components is possible (Casto, Kresty, Kraly, & Pearl, 2004). Mechanistic studies indicate that berries inhibit the growth of premalignant esophageal cells, in part, through down-regulation of cyclooxygenase-2 (COX-2) and down-regulation of the transcription activators, AP-1 and NF-nB in JB-6 mouse epidermal cells (Huang, Huang, Li, & Hu, 2002).

Anthocyanins also exhibit antioxidant properties which are credited to their phenolic structure. Demonstration of the antioxidant effects of anthocyanins were carried out *invitro* using several cell culture systems including colon, endothelial, liver, breast and leukemic cells and keratinocytes. This demonstration indicated that anthocyanins have shown various hostile to lethal and against cancer-causing effects such as: directly scavenging reactive oxygen species (ROS), expanding the oxygen-radical engrossing limit of cells, empowering the expression of Phase II detoxification enzymes, reducing the formation of oxidative adducts in DNA, decreasing lipid peroxidation, inhibiting mutagenesis by environmental toxins and carcinogens, and reducing cellular proliferation by modulating signal transduction pathways (Wang & Stoner, 2008).

Quercetin

Quercetin is a plant-derived flavonoid (Flavanol), used as a nutritional supplement, found in apple skins, berries, brassica vegetables, broccoli, brussel sprouts, cereals, cherries, and cauliflower, grape juice, kohlrabi, oregano, pears, peppers, red and yellow onions, tea, tomatoes leaves, and wine (Figure 7). Quercetin, like parsely can also help retard activity of the enzymes that cause cancer growth and spread. It is the strongest of nature's anti-inflammatory drugs (Hirpara, Aggarwal, Mukherjee, Joshi, & Burman, 2009). Quercetin strongly inhibited in a time and dose-dependent the expression of the mutated p53 protein in breast cancer (Avila, Velasco, Cansado, & Notario, 1994). Quercetin also shows anti-tumour properties. Studies have shown that when treated with a combination of quercetin and ultrasound at 20 kHz for 1 minute term, skin and prostate diseases indicate 90% mortality inside 48 hours with no unmistakable mortality of typical cells (Paliwal, Sundaram, & Mitragotri, 2005). Also quercetin aglycone has been shown to interact with some receptors, particularly an aryl hydrocarbon receptor, which is involved in the development of cancers induced by certain chemicals. Quercetin aglycone has also been shown to modulate several signal transduction pathways involving MEK/ERK and Nrf2/keap1, which are associated with the processes of inflammation and carcinogenesis (Murakami, Ashida, & Terao, 2008).

Isoflavones

Isoflavones are a type of naturally occurring isoflavonoid. Some isoflavones and isoflavone-rich foods possess activity against certain types of breast and prostate cancer. These are generously found in soyabeans. Soya isoflavones have been regarded as dietary components having an important role in reducing the incidence of breast and prostate cancers. Genistein (Figure 8), an isoflavonoid found with a large number

Figure 7. 2-(3, 4- dihydroxyphenyl)- 3,5,7- trihydroxy- 4H- chromen- 4-one

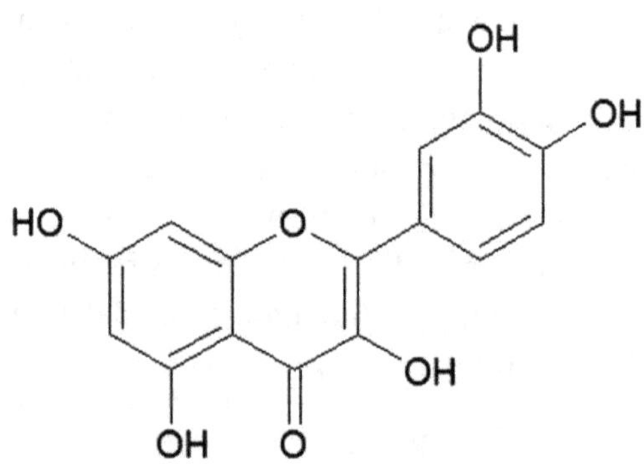

Figure 8. 5, 7-Dihydroxy-3-(4-hydroxyphenyl) chromen-4-one

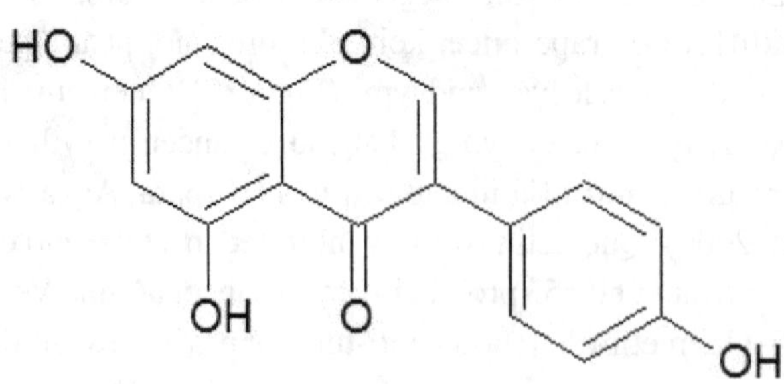

of other isoflavonoids in several members of the family fabaceae, particularly in Glycine max, has been established as a prostate cancer chemopreventive agent (Dixon & Sumner, 2003). Genistein is the predominant isoflavone in soya, inhibits the growth of blood vessels. Tumors need to stimulate the growth of blood vessels to receive oxygen and nutrients. Without these new blood vessels tumors can't grow. Recent preliminary data suggest that soya may inhibit the growth of blood vessels in humans. Thus, isoflavones may actually be useful in the treatment of existing tumors. In addition, it has been demonstrated that genistein represses the initiation of NF-kappa B and Akt signaling pathways, both of which are known to maintain a homeostatic balance between cell survival and apoptosis. Furthermore, genistein has been found to show potent inhibitor of angiogenesis and metastasis. Soya contains at least eight known classes of anti-cancer and cell anti-proliferation components. These include protease inhibitors, phytosterols, saponins, phenolic acids, omega-3 fatty acids, phospholipids (lecithin) and isoflavones (Sarkar & Li, 2003).

Phenoxodiol

Phenoxodiol (Figure 9), a synthetic analogue of diadzein, an isoflavone present in members of the family fabaceae (Pueraria tuberosa, Glycine max), is being developed for the treatment of cervical, ovarian, prostate,, renal and vaginal cancers and induces apoptosis through inhibition of antiapoptopic proteins (Kamsteeg, Rutherford, Sapi, Hanczaruk, Shahabi, Flick, … Mor, 2003).

Flavopiridol

Flavopiridol is a semisynthetic flavonoid and has been shown to be a potent inhibitor of cyclin-dependent kinases (Figure 10). Flavopiridol also induces apoptosis, suppresses inflammation and modulates the immune response (Deorukhkar, Krishnan, Sethi, & Aggarwal, 2007).

Figure 9. 7, 4'-Dihydroxyisoflav-3-ene

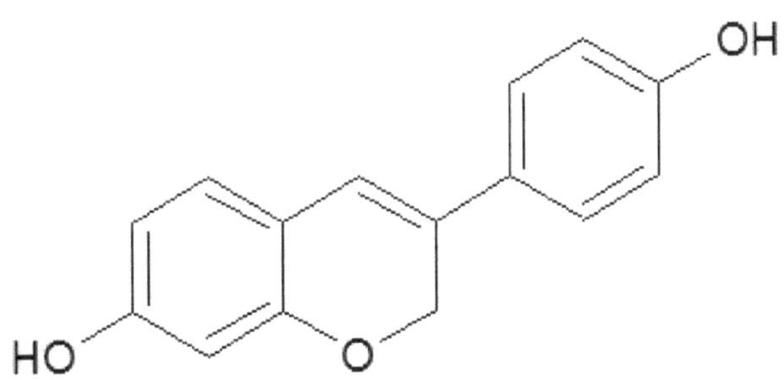

Figure 10. 2-(2-chlorophenyl)-5, 7-dihydroxy-8-[(3S,4 R)-3-hydroxy-1-methylpiperidin-4- yl]chromen-4-one

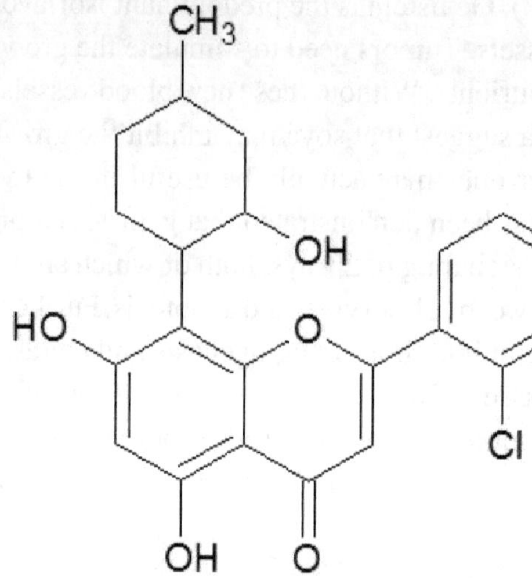

Bioflavonoids

Flavonoids (or bioflavonoids), also collectively known as Vitamin P and citrin. These are richly found in orange, tangerine, peach, pear, yellow pepper, grapefruit, pineapple, lemon, apricot, papaya and yellow raisin. They work with vitamin C to help reduce the risk of cancer, strengthen bones and teeth, heal wounds, keep skin healthy and lower the risk of heart attacks. Physiological processing of unwanted flavonoid compounds induces so-called Phase II enzymes that also help to eliminate mutagens and carcinogens, and therefore may be of value in cancer prevention. Flavonoids could also induce mechanisms that may kill cancer cells and inhibit tumor invasion. It has been found that study participants who ate foods containing certain flavonoids, such as catechins found in strawberries, green and black teas; kaempferol from brussel sprouts and apples; and quercetin from beans, onions and apples, have reduced risk of lung cancer (Rice-Evans & Miller, 1996).

Terpenes and Especially Triterpenes

Terpenes, which could be also named as isoprenoids, constitute the largest and most diverse class of natural products.

A majority of these compounds are found only in plants, but some of the larger and more complex terpenes occur in animals. Squalene, which is a natural complex terpene produced by all plants and animals, has been proposed to be an important ingredient of the Mediterranean diet as it may be a chemopreventive substance that protects against cancer. Terpenes and terpenoids are the primary constituents of the essential oils of many types of plants and flowers (Ha, Ko, Lee, Kim, Chung, Kim, … Kim, 2006; Golmakani & Rezaei, 2008; Prieto, Iacopini, Cioni, & Chericoni, 2007) or cereals (Pérez-Fons, Aranda, Guillén, Villalaín, & Micol, 2006) and they have shown antibacterial and antioxidant activity among other beneficial effects for human health. Terpenes, and especially triterpenes, due to their broad spectrum of biological activity, are studied by many researchers since there is growing interest in the evaluation of triterpenoid extracts for cancer treatment (Melnick, 2006). Several triterpene compounds that have recently appeared in the literature in preclinical studies suggest potential therapeutic opportunities. Betullinic acid, boswellic acid, squalene, ursolic acid, oleanolic acid and triterpenoid saponins are among the growing number of compounds evaluated in preclinical and some clinical studies (Sporn & Suh, 2000).

Limonene

Limonene is a colourless liquid hydrocarbon classified as a cyclic terpene possessing a strong smell of oranges. Lemon and orange oils contain limonene and geraniol also found in cumin. Limonene is derived from the essential oils of citrus fruits, mints, caraway, dill, lemongrass and other plants (Figure 11). These components of lemon and orange oils have been shown to inhibit tumor growth. Although the exact mechanism of action is unknown, D-Limonene and its metabolites, perillic acid, dihydroperillic acid, uroterpenol, and limonene1,2-diol, may inhibit tumor growth via inhibition of p21-dependent signaling and apoptosis resulting from induction of the transforming growth factor beta-signaling pathway (Kaji Tatsuta, Iishi, Baba, Inoue, & Kasugai, 2001). Animal studies show activity of D-limonene against pancreatic, stomach, colon, skin, and liver cancers. Data also indicate that D-limonene slows the promotion/progression stage of carcinogen-induced tumors in rats (Uedo, Tatsuta, Iishi, Baba, Sakai, Yano, & Otani, 1999). Because these oils are contained only in the peels of the fruit, researchers are looking at ways to include rind in filtered juices.

Ursolic Acid and Carnosol

Ursolic acid is a pentacyclic triterpene acid, used in cosmetics (Figure 12a). It is found in Rosemary and sage. Ursolic acid also capable of inhibiting various types of cancer cells by inhibiting the STAT3 activation pathway and human fibrosarcoma cells by reducing the expression of matrix metalloproteinase-9 by acting through

Figure 11. 1-methyl-4-(prop-1-en-2-yl)-cyclohexenes)

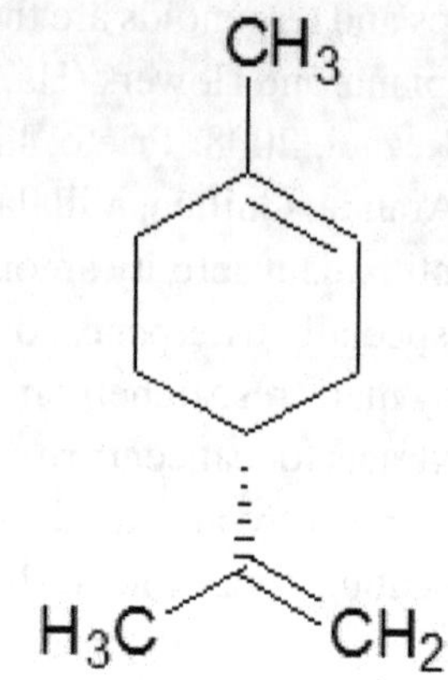

the glucocorticoid receptor (Pathak, Bhutani, Nair, Ahn, Chakraborty, Kadara, … Aggarwal, 2007).

Ursolic acid and carnosol are potent antioxidants that possess anti-tumor activity. Rosemary is a rich source of carnosol, a compound with antioxidant, anti-inflammatory and anti-carcinogenic activity (Figure 12b). Studies suggest that carnosol detoxifies substances than can initiate the breast cancer process. It may also protect against Prostate, Breast, colon, skin and lung cancers (Johnson, 2011). The carnosol found in rosemary has demonstrated potent anticancer properties in animal studies. It increases the production of an enzyme that protects cellular DNA from being damaged, and in one test appeared to have some success in offsetting the effects of a carcinogen known to cause breast cancer (Huang, Ho, Wang, & Conney, 1994).

Figure 12. (a) 3beta-Hydroxyurs-12-en-28-oic acid, (b) Hexahydrophenanthrene-4a- carboxylic acid

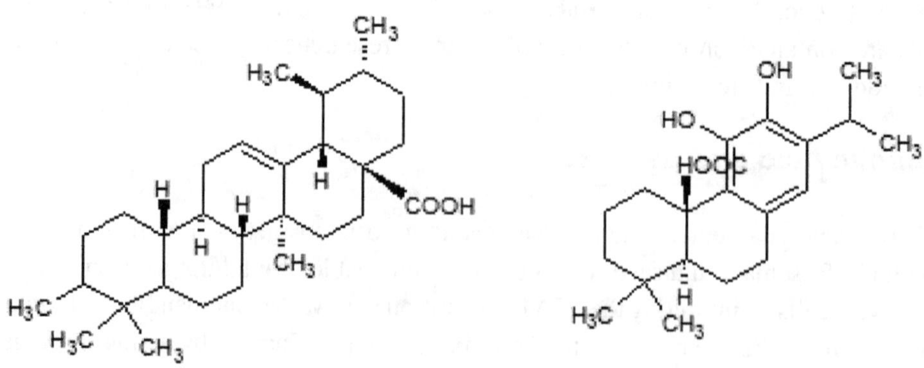

Alfa-Bisabolol

Alfa-bisabolol is a sesquiterpene alcohol present in the essential oil of chamomile and other plants which exerts, according to (Cavalieri, Mariotto, Fabrizi, de Prati, & Gottardo, 2004), a strong time and dose-dependent cytotoxic action against human pancreatic cell line (Figure 13). However, it failed to affect the viability of human fibroblasts. Based on these results, alfa-bisabolol should be considered a novel promising compound for inhibiting the growth and survival of transformed cells with high malignancy.

Carotenoids

Carotenoids are a class of more than 600 naturally occurring pigments synthesized by plants, algae, yeast, fungi and photosynthetic bacteria. They are prominent for their distribution, structural diversity and various functions. Fruits and vegetables provide most of the carotenoids in the human diet. Carotenoids can be broadly classified into two classes, carotenes (-carotene, -carotene or lycopene) and xanthophylls (cryptoxanthin, lutein or zeaxanthin). It is found in carrots, sweet potatoes, tomatoes and. Lycopene is increasingly gaining ground as the most powerful antioxidant in the carotenoids family, particularly in relation to prostate and breast cancer. Two carotenoids found in the eye, lutein and zeaxanthinwatermelons. These powerfully pigmented vegetables also act as antioxidants, protecting healthy cells from chemotherapy and radiation. Carotenoids are fat soluble, so more will be absorbed when eaten with a meal or snack containing some healthy fat. In population studies, alpha carotene is related to reduce risk of lung cancer (Figure 14a). It may slow down the proliferation of cancer cells. Carotenoids appear to play an anticancer role and enhance immunity, are believed to protect against the leading cause of

Figure 13. 3-Cyclohexene-1-methanol

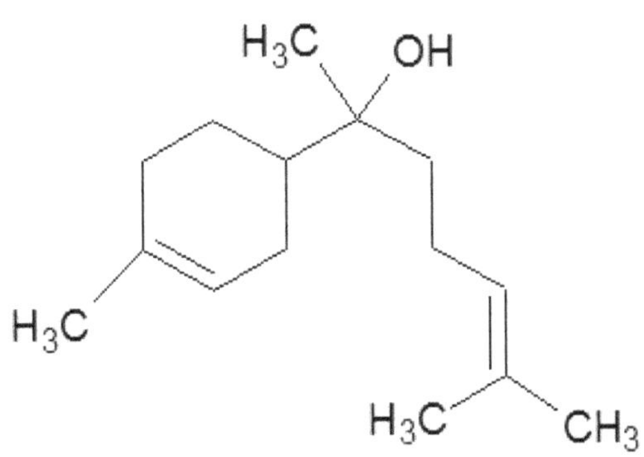

Figure 14. (a) (1E, 3E, 5E, 7E, 9E, 11E, 13E, 15E, 17E)-3, 7, 12, 16-tetramethyl-1-(2, 6, 6-trimethyl-1-cyclohexenyl) - 18-(2, 6, 6-trimethyl-1-cyclohex-2-enyl) octadeca-1, 3, 5, 7, 9, 11, 13, 15, 17-nonaene and (b) 1, 1'-(3, 7, 12, 16-Tetramethyl-1, 3, 5, 7, 9, 11, 13, 15, 17-octadecanonaene-1, 18-diyl) bis [2, 6, 6-trimethylcyclohexene]

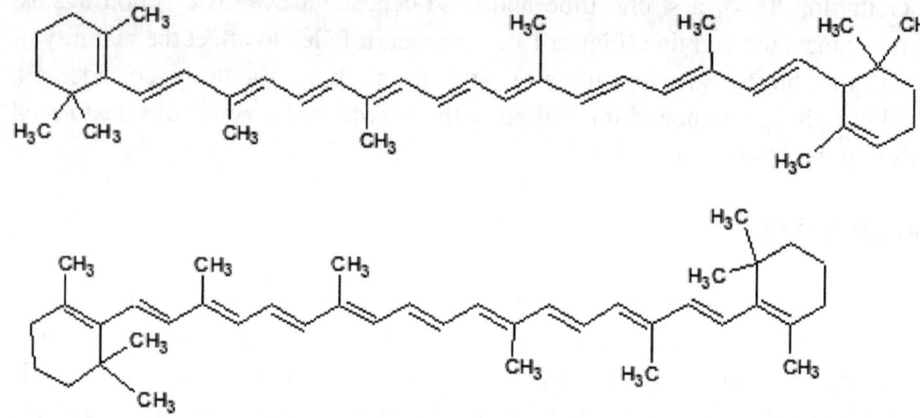

blindness in people over 65. Carotenoids also play a role in heart health; In LDL oxidation, antioxidants are consumed in a sequence that begins with vitamin E; lycopene is next, followed by beta carotene. Although carotenoids appear to be heat resistant, sunlight breaks them down in the presence of oxygen, so don't cut up vegetables and leave them out on the counter for a long time before using them. β-Carotene is an organic compound and classified as a terpenoid. It is a strongly-coloured red-orange pigment abundant in plants and fruits. As a carotene with beta-rings at both ends, it is the most common form of carotene (Figure 14b). It is a precursor (inactive form) of vitamin A. As a naturally occurring phytonutrient, some of the richest food sources of beta carotene are green, yellow, orange and red fruits and vegetables such as asparagus, broccoli, carrot, pumpkin, spinach, sweet potato, and watermelon. Beta Carotenes' possible benefits include reduced risk of cataract, coronary artery disease, and breast cancer and enhancing immunity for the elderly patients. Studies show that people who eat a diet rich in carotenoids, had a much lower risk of breast, colon cancer and lung cancer. One way that carotenoids fight cancer is through their antioxidant capacity. Another way that they help is to keep body cells in proper communication, an effective preventive measure against the growth of cancer cells. Studies suggest that consuming beta-carotene may be effective in reducing the risk of prostate cancer in men who have low blood levels of beta-carotene (Omenn, Goodman, Thornquist, Balmes, Cullen, Glass, … Hammar, 1996; Russell & Mayer, 2002).

Cooking foods lightly makes their carotenoids more readily available· These compounds show antioxidant and inmunomodulation activities, and they can prevent degenerative diseases, such as cardiovascular diseases, diabetes, and several types of cancer especially prostate and digestive-tract tumors. Algae and microalgae are also important sources of carotenoids as astaxanthin, -carotene, lutein, cantaxanthin, violaxanthin, lutein and neoxanthin, being HPLC the analytical tool most frequently employed to identify these compounds. Some carotenoids, like -carotene, and lycopene, which presents antioxidant, inmunomodulation and anti-cancer properties have been determined by HPLC-UV/Vis or DAD in Thai fruits (Charoensiri, Kongkachuichai, Suknicom, & Sungpuag, 2009), chesnut (de Vasconcelos do, Bennett, Quideau, Jacquet, Rosa, & Ferreira-Cardoso, 2010) and tea seed oils (Fazel, Sahari, & Barzegar, 2008).

Lycopene

Recent epidemiologic studies have shown good correlation between dietary intake of carotenoids and reduced risk of cancer and cardiovascular diseases. Tomato is rich in various carotenoids. Lycopene is the precursor of β-carotene in tomato, which accumulates after the lycopene cyclase gene is down regulated during ripening (Figure 15). Lycopene and β-carotene can induce apoptosis in prostate cancer cells and malignant lymphoblast cells.

Saponins

Saponins are natural glycosides of steroid or triterpene which exhibit many different biological and pharmacological actions: e.g. immunomodulatory, antitumor, antiinflammatory, molluscicidal, antiviral, antifungal, hypoglycemic, hypocholesterolemic found in beans and legumes. The plant biochemicals that produce suds in root beer are also effective antimicrobial, cholesterol-lowering, and anticancer phytochemicals. Some saponins, such as digitalis, are also used as heart

Figure 15. (6E, 8E, 10E, 12E, 14E, 16E, 18E, 20E,22E,24E,26E)-2,6,10,14,19,23,27,31-octamethyldotriaconta-2,6,8,10,12,14,16,18,20,22,24,26,30-tridecaene

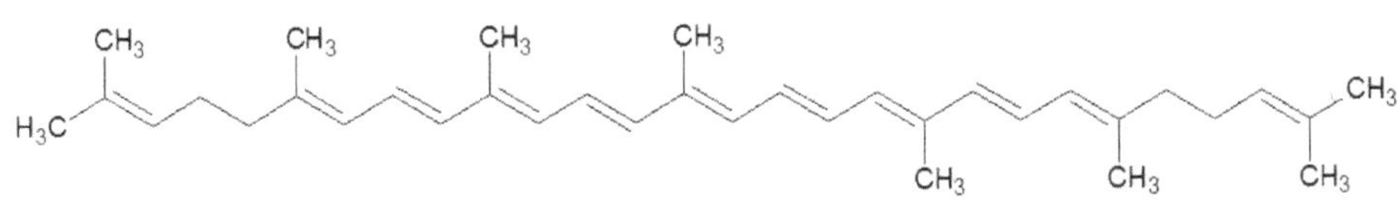

medications. Saponins may prevent cancer cells from multiplying by influencing the DNA in the cells 137 (Sun, Xie, & Ye, 2009)[(123)].

Phytochemicals

Capsaicin

Capsaicin (8-methyl-N-vanillyl-6-nonenamide) is the major pungent ingredient for the piquancy of chilli pepper (Capsicum annum). In experimental animals, it is suspected to acts reduces risk of colon, gastric and rectal cancers; inhibits tumor growth; destroys cancer causing substances. It is also a digestive aid, a topical painkiller, and a potential cancer-fighting compound (Figure 16). Capsaicin is able to kill prostate cancer cells by causing them to undergo apoptosis as reported by American Association for Cancer Research .The studies were performed on tumors formed by human prostate cancer cell cultures grown in mouse models, and showed tumors treated with capsaicin were about one-fifth the size of the untreated tumors. There have been several clinical studies conducted in Japan and China that showed natural capsaicin directly inhibits the growth of leukemic cells (Ito, Nakazato, Yamato, Miyakawa, Yamada, Hozumi, … Kizaki, 2004). Capsaicin blocks the translocation of nuclear factor kappa B (NF-kB), activator protein 1 (AP-1), and signal transducer and activator of transcription (STAT3) signaling pathways that are required for carcinogenesis (Oyagbemi, Saba, & Azeez, 2010).

Allin, Allicin and Allylic Sulfides

Found in Garlic and Allium vegetables and onions (*Allium cepa*) contain a number of compounds that have been associated with anti carcinogenic effect. The positive effect appears to be related to the presence of both oil- and water-soluble organo-sulfur compounds, primarily allyl derivatives such as allicin. Garlic is one of the oldest natural medicines known to mankind and can easily be included in recipes or

Figure 16. 8-Methyl-N-vanillyl-6-nonenamide

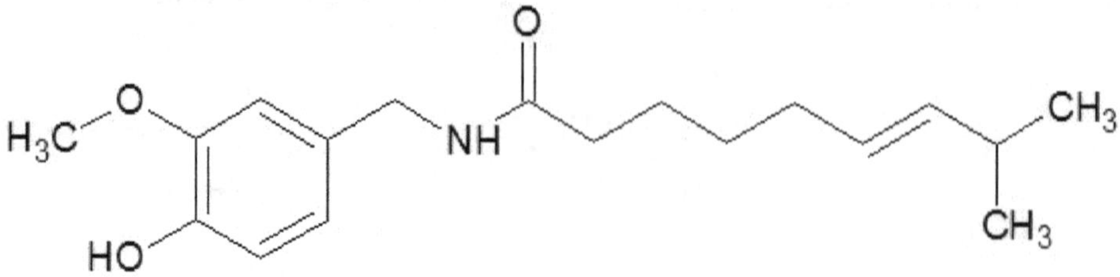

taken as a tablet supplement. The active sulfur compounds may inhibit development of prostate tumors. Onions and garlic are powerhouses that contain substances like quercetin, allicin, S-allyl cysteine and selenium. The use of garlic as anticancer agent has long been established. Components of garlic has likewise been found to inhibit the activity of diverse chemical carcinogen during both the start and advancement phases of carcinogenesis (Lau, Tadi, & Tosk, 1990). Diallylsulfide and diallyldisulfide induce apoptosis in non-small cell lung cancer cells and in prostate cancer and breast cancer cells. They lower the incidence of esophageal, prostate, laryngeal, oral cavity, pharynx, breast, ovarian, prostate, renal, gastric and colorectal cancers. Garlic protects against certain cancers by halting cell cycle progression and inducing apoptosis of cancer cells as well as by decreasing angiogenesis and influencing carcinogen metabolism (Powolny & Singh, 2008).

Aloe-Emodin

Aloe-emodin, a hydroxyanthraquinone from aloe vera and other plants, has been indicated as a new antiangiogenic compound with a remarkable photocytotoxic effect on tumour cells (Cardenas, Quesada, & Medina 2006). Emodin has been reported to be non-toxic for normal cells while possessing specific toxicity for neuroectodermal tumour cells (Pecere, Gazzola, Mucignat, Parolin, Vecchia, Cavaggioni, … Palù, 2000).

FATTY ACIDS

Polyunsaturatted Fatty Acids (PUFA) Omega-3-Fatty Acids

Poly unsaturated fatty acids (PUFs) are fatty acids that contain more than one double bond in their backbone. This class includes many important compounds, such as essential fatty acids. Essential fatty acids, or EFAs, are fatty acids that humans and other animals must ingest for good health because the body requires them but can't make them from other food components.

Only two EFAs are known for humans: Alpha-linolenic acid (an omega-6 fatty acids), lauric acid (a saturated fatty acids), and palmitoleic acid (a monounsaturated fatty acids). Essential fatty acids have an impact in numerous metabolic processes, and there is proof to recommend that low levels of EFA, or the wrong balance of sorts among the EFA, might be a factor in various sicknesses, including osteoporosis.

Fatty acids, especially omega-3 polyunsaturated fatty acids (PUFAs) such as alpha-linoleic, eicosapentaenoic acid (EPA), docosapentaenoic acid (DPA), and docosahexaenoic acid (DHA) are found in high levels in some fishes and to a lesser extent in walnuts and vegetable oils. Omega-3 PUFAs have been widely evaluated in epidemiological studies. The intake of omega-3- enriched foods has been correlated with health benefits including cardio-protective effects such as anti-arrhythmic, anti-thrombotic, anti-inflammatory, anti-hypertensive, and anti-hyperlipidemia effects (Buhr & Bales, 2010). EFSA has authorized a number of health claims dealing with omega-3 PUFAs as essential nutrient, including the contribution to maintenance of normal cardiac function, normal blood pressure, as well as maintenance of normal (fasting) blood concentrations of triglycerides Reduces symptoms of BPH such as painful and frequent urgency to urinate; may also improve blood flow to the penis; possibly may help to prevent prostate cancer. Omega-3 fatty acids reduce prostate tumor growth, slow down histopathological progression, and increase survival (Berquin, Min, Wu, Wu, Perry, Cline,… Chen, 2007). High levels of docosahexaenoic acid, the most abundant n-3 poly unsaturated fatty acid [omega-3] in erythrocyte membranes, are associated with a reduced risk of breast cancer (Pala, Krogh, Muti, Chajès, Riboli, Micheli, … Berrino, 2001).

Squalene

Squalene is a characteristic natural compound originally acquired for commercial purposes principally from shark liver oil, however plant sources (essentially vegetable oils) are utilized too, including amaranth seed, rice grain, wheat germ, and olives (Figure 17). All plants and animals produce squalene, and are also found in Olive oil. Experimental studies have shown that squalene can effectively inhibit chemically-induced colon, lung and skin tumour genesis in rodents. The protective effect is observed when squalene is given before and/or during carcinogen treatment. The mechanism for the chemopreventive action of squalene may incorporate hindrance of Ras farnesylation, modulation of cancer-causing agent enactment and hostile to oxidative activities (Sotiroudis & Kyrtopoulos, 2008).

Figure 17. (6E, 10E, 14E, 18E)-2,6,10,15,19,23-hexamethyltetracosa-2,6,10,14,18,22-hexaene

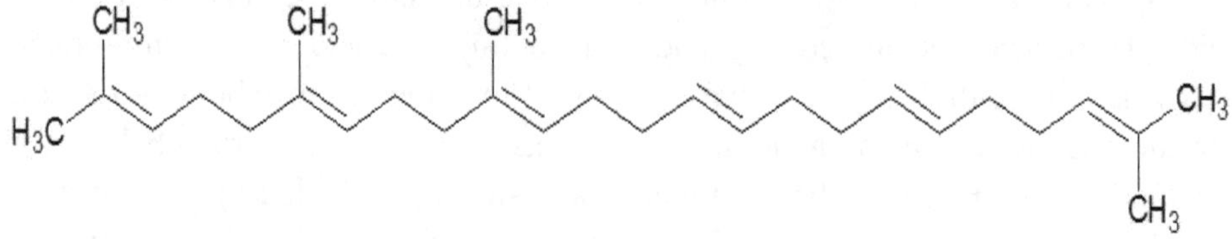

Beta-Sitosterol

β-Sitosterol is one of several phytosterols (plant sterols) with similar structure to that of cholesterol (Figure 18). Sitosterols are white, waxy powders with a characteristic odor. They are hydrophobic and soluble in alcohols. They are abundantly found in beans, corn oil, nuts, peas, seeds, soybeans, wheat germ and whole grains. It is also used for boosting the immune system and for preventing colon cancer, as well as for HIV/AIDS, cervical cancer, fibromyalgia. A study using the prostate cancer cell line LNCaP (an androgen-dependent tumor) showed that beta-sitosterol decreased cancer cell growth by 24% and induced apoptosis (programmed cell death) fourfold (Awad, Chen, Fink, & Hennessey, 1996).

Antioxidants

Reactive oxygen species (ROS) including superoxide radicals, hydroxyl radicals, singlet oxygen and hydrogen peroxide are often generated as byproducts of biological reaction or from exogenous factors. In vivo, some of these ROS assume an imperative part in cell metabolism including energy production, phagocytosis and intercellular signaling. However, these ROS produced by sunlight, ultraviolet light, ionizing radiation, chemical reactions and metabolic processes have a wide variety of pathological effects such as cell membrane disintegration, protein, lipid, and deoxyribose nucleic acid (DNA) damage which can further initiate or propagate the development of many chronic and degenerative diseases DNA damage, carcinogenesis

Figure 18. (5-Ethyl-6-methylheptan-2-yl)-10, 13-dimethyl-2, 3, 4, 7, 8, 9, 11, 12, 14, 15, 16, 17-dodecahydro-1H-cyclopenta[a]phenanthren-3-ol

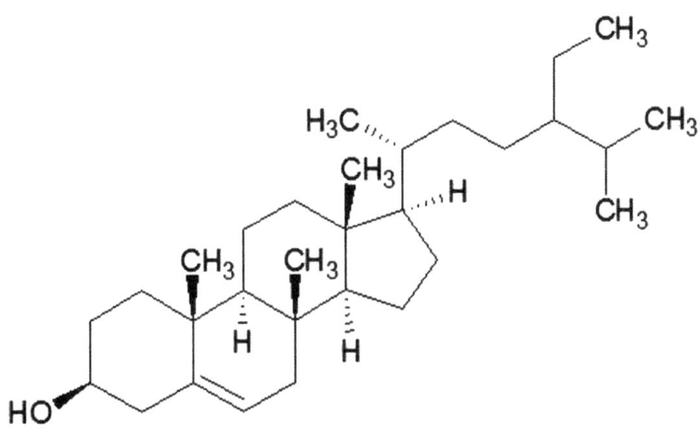

and various degenerative disorders such as cardiovascular diseases, aging and neuro-degenerative diseases. Oxidative stress, arising as a result of imbalance between free radical generation and key endogenous antioxidant defence in tissues, plays a key role in the initiation and progression of almost all these conditions (Halliwell & Gutteridge, 1985). Normal cells have a low level of ROS. Increased ROS, for example, due to inflammation or environmental factors, are generally thought to increase mutations in DNA and thereby risk of cancer. In any case, the expanded level of ROS in malignancy cells is adjusted by an expanded defense against ROS so the cell does not exceed the ROS edge for cell demise. The increase in ROS leads to activation of signaling pathways that favor cell growth, migration, and proliferation. Besides, numerous disease treatments (e.g., radiation, chemotherapy) prompt enormous measures of ROS that surpass the ROS edge and actuate growth cell demise (Trachootham, Alexandre, & Huang, 2009). Thus, although antioxidants may theoretically prevent transformation of normal cells to cancerous cells, they may theoretically also lower the efficacy of cancer treatment.

Resveratrol

Resveratrol (3, 5, 4'-trihydroxystilbene) is an oligomeric polyphenol, is present in black grapes and its preparations like red wine. It is found as dimer, trimer and tetramer in the families vitaceae, Dipterocarpaceae, cyperaceae, Gnetaceae and Leguminosae (Figure 19). Resveratrol is implicated in the prevention of cardiovascular diseases in vasoprotection and neuro protection (Ramawat & Merillon, 2007). Apart from its cardioprotective effects, resveratrol exhibits anticancer properties as demonstrated by its ability to suppress proliferation of a wide variety of neoplasms, including

Figure 19. 3, 5, 4'-trihydroxystilbene

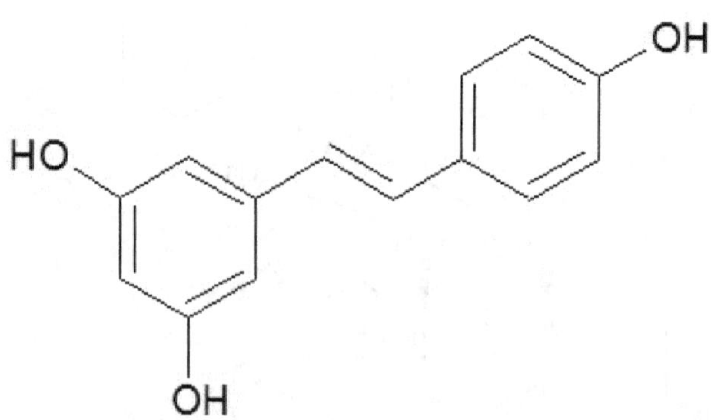

lymphoid and myeloid cancers, multiple myeloma, and cancer of the breast, prostate, colon, stomach and pancreas (Aggarwal & Shishodia, 2006b) .

Dithiolethiones and Organosulfides

Dithiolethiones are a well-known class of cancer chemopreventive agents, found in cruciferous vegetables. Increased consumption of cruciferous vegetables such as broccoli, cabbage and brussels sprouts may reduce the risk of certain cancers, particularly breast cancer. Cruciferous vegetables contain indoles - a unique class of phytonutrients that have been scientifically shown to balance hormone levels, detoxify the intestines and liver and reinforce the body's immune system. They reduce risk of gastric, colon, and lung cancers, enhance immune system, inhibit tumor promotion, and reduce cholesterol, lower blood pressure. The chemopreventive effects of dithiolethione compounds are attributed to their activation of antioxidant response elements (AREs) by reacting with the Nrf2/Keap1 [Nuclear factor (erythroid derived 2)] protein complex. Dithiolethione compound ACS-1 exerts antiproliferative effects in human cancer cell lines (A549 and MDA-MB-231)) by increasing the activity of the tumor suppressor protein phosphatase 2A (PP2A) (Switzer, Ridnour, Cheng, Sparatore, Soldato, Del, Moody, … Wink, 2009). In a study by a group of researchers reported a novel anticarcinogenic activity of an organosulfur compound from garlic, diallyl disulfide (DADS).Rodent demonstrations indicated significant inhibition of growth of H-rasoncogene transformed tumour (Singh, Mohan, Agarwal, Benson, Hu, Rudy, … Zaren, 1996).

Selenium

Selenium, an essential dietary trace mineral, is an important component of antioxidant systems such as glutathione peroxidase that neutralize and protect against damage caused by free radicals and reactive oxygen species. It is present in nuts, grains, poultry, pumpkin seeds, and seafood. Protects against benign prostatic hyperplasia (BPH) as well as heart disease; may prevent oxidative damage to lipids, vitamins, hormones, and enzymes involved in normal prostate functioning; preliminary studies have shown that pumpkin seeds (high in selenium) may reduce hormonal damage to prostate cells, thus possibly reducing the risk of developing prostate cancer. Data suggest its benefits in preventing gastrointestinal and lung cancer (Facompre & El-Bayoumy, 2009; Klein, Thompson, Lippman, Goodman, Albanes, Taylor, & Coltman, 2000).

VITAMINS

Vitamin C

It is found in broccoli, cabbage, citrus fruits (grapefruit, lemons, oranges), cranberries, leafy green vegetables (kale, spinach), melons, peppers, potatoes, strawberries, and tomatoes. Vitamin C help to prevent cancer growth by taking up volatile oxygen free radical molecules and prevent the damage they are known to do to our delicate DN.

Vitamin D

Vitamin D is a group of fat-dissolvable secosteroids, the two noteworthy physiologically significant types of which are vitamin D2 (ergocalciferol) and vitamin D3 (cholecalciferol). Vitamin D helps promote production of enzymes called phosphotases, which help de-activate other enzymes called kinases, essential to growth and reproduction of cancer cells. Polymorphisms of the vitamin D receptor (VDR) gene have been associated with an increased risk of breast cancer. Women with mutations in the VDR gene had an increased risk of breast cancer (Buyru, Tezol, Yosunkaya-Fenerci, & Dalay, 2003). Breast cancer disease progression and bone metastases are also associated with low levels of vit D (Garland, Garland, Gorham, Lipkin, Newmark, Mohr, & Holick, 2006).

MICROBIALS

Prebiotics and Probiotics

Another type of compounds commonly referred to as "nutraceuticals" which also present a nutritional value are pre- and probiotics (Burgain, Gaiani, Linder, & Scher, 2011; Douglas & Sanders, 2008). Both helpfully influence the host by "specifically stimulating the growth or activity of one or a set number of microbes" in the digestive tract, in this way enhancing the host's health (Gibson & Roberfroid, 1995). Prebiotics are non- digestible food ingredients that stimulate the growth and/or activity of bacteria in the digestive system in ways claimed to be beneficial to health. Traditional dietary sources of prebiotics include soybeans, inulin sources, raw oats, unrefined wheat, unrefined barley, and yacon. Some of the oligosaccharides that naturally occur in breast milk are believed to play an important role in the development of a healthy immune system in infants. Probiotics are live microorganisms which when administered in adequate amounts confer a health benefit on the host. Lactic acid bacteria (LAB) and bifidobacteria are the most common types of microbes used as probiotics; but certain yeasts and bacilli may also be used. Probiotics are regularly devoured as a part of fermented food with specially added active live cultures; for example, in yogurt, soy yogurt, or as dietary supplements.

Probiotics are live microorganisms that when ingested in sufficient sums present a medical advantage on the host. The majority of probiotic bacteria used in nutraceuticals belong to the genera Lactobacillusand Bifidobacterium, which are Gram-positive, lacticacid- producing bacteria present in some foodstuffs and constitute a major part of the normal intestinal microbiota. In addition, some yeasts such as Saccharomyces boulardii and Saccharomyces cerevisiae found in some foods as bread, beer, wine, mangosteen fruit, etc. are also included within probiotics (de Vrese & Schrezenmeir, 2008). Numerous studies have shown that probiotics exert beneficial effects in the host by modulating the gut microbiota, maintaining the integrity of the gut barrier and avoiding bacterial translocation, as well as modulating the gut-associated immune system (Kotzampassi & Giamarellos-Bourboulis, 2012). It should be noted that some studies have observed the reduction of these healthy bacteria as well as the increase of potentially pathogenic species in the gut microbiota of elderly people. For this reason, there is a growing interest to evaluate the effect of some probiotics to maintain the health of elderly people (Malaguarnera, Leggio, Vacante, Motta, Giordano, Bondi, ... Salmeri, 2012). Prebiotics and probiotics differ in the fact that the former refers to non-digestible, fiber compounds. These pass undigested and act as a substrate for the growth of beneficial bacteria, with concomitant positive health contributions that may range from energy balance, bowel function and immunologic function to sensory perception, pressure regulation and glycemic control (Delzenne, Neyrinck, Bäckhed, & Cani, 2011). It should also be noted that, in the specific case of prebiotics, the term does not apply only to the effects on the gut microbiome, but also on that of other areas of the body, such as skin, as it has been shown that certain moisturizers can actively contribute to the improvement of the skin microbiome (Schloss, 2014). These, however, are a group of diverse ingredients that are still not fully understood in regard to their modes of action, effects and required dosages for measurable health benefits (Douglas & Sanders, 2008). The majority of clinical or epidemiological studies have been conducted with probiotic-enriched foods (functional foods), usually lactobacilli and bifidobacteria, evidencing beneficial activities on prevention of antibiotic-associated diarrhea and enteric infections, functional bowel problems (constipation and irritable bowel syndrome), inflammatory bowel diseases, stimulation of the immune system and prevention of cancer (Ritchie & Romanuk, 2012). In addition, a meta-analysis of clinical trials reported that diets rich in probiotics decrease total cholesterol and LDL-cholesterol concentration in plasma (Guo, Liu, & Zhang, 2011).

Dietary Fibres

Dietary fiber is a heterogeneous group of substances which are resistant to hydrolysis by human alimentary enzymes in the small bowel. The most important fibers are cellulose, hemicellulose, pectin, inulin, glucan, digestion-resistant starch, etc. and they are present in varying amounts in plant foods. Fibers play an essential role in the physiology of the gastrointestinal tract such as modifying the absorption of nutrients (particularly carbohydrates and lipids), improving the gut transit as well as being the main nutritional source for the colonic microbiota. Epidemiological investigations have suggested that higher fiber intake is associated with lower overall mortality, in particular from cardiovascular and digestive tract diseases (Lattimer & Haub, 2010). Dietary fiber (roughage or ruffage) is the indigestible portion of plant foods having two main components: Dissolvable (might be prebiotic and/or gooey) fiber that is promptly aged in the colon into gases and physiologically dynamic results, and insoluble fiber (might be metabolically dormant and give building or metabolically aged in the digestive organ as a prebiotic fiber).

Bulking fibers absorb water as they move through the digestive system, easing defecation. Fermentable insoluble fibers mildly promote regularity, although not to the extent that bulking fibers do, but they can be readily fermented in the colon into gases and physiologically active byproducts.

FUTURE PROSPECTS

Globalization of the nutraceuticals and functional food industries presents noteworthy difficulties, not the minimum of which is the regulatory divergence between countries dynamic in the marketplace. Next issue is that the claims of medicinal advantages of the product should require to be consented by company. Knowledge on quality assembling strategies, cGMP and standardized analytical techniques with respect to safety, efficacy and quality testing and marketing authorisation methodology ought to be explored.

CONCLUSION

The therapeutic potential of herbs has been well recognized by various indigenous systems of medicine. Besides their therapeutic use, herbs are disease preventers and also used as cosmetics, dietary supplements and for reducing obesity. The priority of developed countries is different from that of developing countries in relation to medicinal plants. Cancer is a deadly disease and complexities of disease are such that no single available anticancer agent can satisfactory combat the multiple disorders of the disease. Therefore, there is an urgent need to search for better medicines for cancer. Cancer represents one of the most severe health problems worldwide, and the search for more effective anticancer agents continues. Cancer alone caused over six million deaths in 2000, affecting over ten million people worldwide. In this context, nutraceuticals are promising candidates to treat cancer. Most of the plants and herbs as mentioned are used in remote villages and tribal pockets as folk medicine and are not known to the mainstream population. Nutraceuticals, an entirely new segment of the health industry has been predicted to be the next financial blockbuster. Nutraceuticals are the next generation of food supplements that bridge the gap between supplements and pharmaceuticals .Undoubtedly, nutraceuticals have provided useful drugs to mankind for their health care and other needs. The effort to combat the diseases, for which there is no satisfactory solution as yet, should be continued relentlessly. Hopefully, plant kingdom i.e. miraculous herbs or so called *sanjivini bootis* of today will help us in the discovery of new drug products useful for the alleviation of deadly human diseases like cancer. The traditional use of plants provides a lead for cancer chemopreventive molecules. The development of new derivatives from bioactive compounds of food origin has been a viable way to reduce toxicity and increase their effectiveness against cancer.

REFERENCES

Aggarwal, B. B., & Shishodia, S. (2006a). Molecular targets of dietary agents for prevention and therapy of cancer. *Biochemical Pharmacology*, *71*(10), 1397–1421. doi:10.1016/j.bcp.2006.02.009 PMID:16563357

Aggarwal, B. B., & Shishodia, S. (2006b). *Resveratrol in health and disease*. CRC Taylor & Francis.

Aggarwal, B. B., Surh, Y.-J., & Shishodia, S. (Eds.). (2007). *The Molecular Targets and Therapeutic Uses of Curcumin in Health and Disease* (Vol. 595). Boston, MA: Springer US. doi:10.1007/978-0-387-46401-5_1

Aggarwal, S., Takada, Y., Singh, S., Myers, J. N., & Aggarwal, B. B. (2004). Inhibition of growth and survival of human head and neck squamous cell carcinoma cells by curcumin via modulation of nuclear factor B signaling. *International Journal of Cancer*, *111*(5), 679–692. doi:10.1002/ijc.20333 PMID:15252836

Ames, B. N., Shigenaga, M. K., & Gold, L. S. (1993). DNA lesions, inducible DNA repair, and cell division: three key factors in mutagenesis and carcinogenesis. *Environmental Health Perspectives, 101*(Suppl 5), 35–44.

Avila, M. A., Velasco, J. A., Cansado, J., & Notario, V. (1994). Quercetin mediates the down-regulation of mutant p53 in the human breast cancer cell line MDA-MB468. *Cancer Research, 54*(9), 2424–2428. PMID:8162591

Awad, A. B., Chen, Y. C., Fink, C. S., & Hennessey, T. (n.d.). beta-Sitosterol inhibits HT-29 human colon cancer cell growth and alters membrane lipids. *Anticancer Research, 16*(5A), 2797–804.

Balunas, M. J., & Kinghorn, A. D. (2005). Drug discovery from medicinal plants. *Life Sciences, 78*(5), 431–441. doi:10.1016/j.lfs.2005.09.012 PMID:16198377

Berquin, I. M., Min, Y., Wu, R., Wu, J., Perry, D., Cline, J. M., ... Chen, Y. Q. (2007). Modulation of prostate cancer genetic risk by omega-3 and omega-6 fatty acids. *The Journal of Clinical Investigation, 117*(7), 1866–1875. doi:10.1172/JCI31494 PMID:17607361

Bharti, A. C., Donato, N., & Aggarwal, B. B. (2003). Curcumin (diferuloylmethane) inhibits constitutive and IL-6-inducible STAT3 phosphorylation in human multiple myeloma cells. *Journal of Immunology, 171*(7), 3863–71.

Bhui, K., Prasad, S., George, J., & Shukla, Y. (2009). Bromelain inhibits COX-2 expression by blocking the activation of MAPK regulated NF-kappa B against skin tumor-initiation triggering mitochondrial death pathway. *Cancer Letters, 282*(2), 167–176. doi:10.1016/j.canlet.2009.03.003 PMID:19339108

Bonnesen, C., Eggleston, I. M., & Hayes, J. D. (2001). Dietary indoles and isothiocyanates that are generated from cruciferous vegetables can both stimulate apoptosis and confer protection against DNA damage in human colon cell lines. *Cancer Research, 61*(16), 6120–6130. PMID:11507062

Boon, H., & Wong, J. (2004). Botanical medicine and cancer: A review of the safety and efficacy. *Expert Opinion on Pharmacotherapy, 5*(12), 2485–2501. doi:10.1517/14656566.5.12.2485 PMID:15571467

Borchers, A. T., Keen, C. L., & Gershwin, M. E. (2016). The Basis of Structure/Function Claims of Nutraceuticals. *Clinical Reviews in Allergy & Immunology, 51*(3), 370–382. doi:10.100712016-016-8536-9 PMID:27122022

Buhr, G., & Bales, C. W. (2010). Nutritional Supplements for Older Adults: Review and Recommendations—Part II. *Journal of Nutrition for the Elderly*, *29*(1), 42–71. doi:10.1080/01639360903586464 PMID:20391042

Burgain, J., Gaiani, C., Linder, M., & Scher, J. (2011). Encapsulation of probiotic living cells: From laboratory scale to industrial applications. *Journal of Food Engineering*, *104*(4), 467–483. doi:10.1016/j.jfoodeng.2010.12.031

Buyru, N., Tezol, A., Yosunkaya-Fenerci, E., & Dalay, N. (2003). Vitamin D receptor gene polym orphism s in breast cancer. *Experimental & Molecular Medicine*, *35*(6), 550–555. doi:10.1038/emm.2003.72 PMID:14749534

Cárdenas, C., Quesada, A. R., & Medina, M. A. (2006). Evaluation of the anti-angiogenic effect of aloe-emodin. *Cellular and Molecular Life Sciences*, *63*(24), 3083–3089. doi:10.100700018-006-6399-6 PMID:17131052

Carpenter, K. J. (1988). The history of scurvy and vitamin C. Cambridge University Press.

Casto, B. C., Kresty, L. A., Kraly, C. L., & Pearl, D. K. (2004). Chemoprevention of oral cancer by black raspberries. *Anticancer Research*, *22*(6C), 4005–4015. PMID:12553025

Cavalieri, E., Mariotto, S., Fabrizi, C., de Prati, A. C., Gottardo, R., Leone, S., ... Suzuki, H. (2004). α-Bisabolol, a nontoxic natural compound, strongly induces apoptosis in glioma cells. *Biochemical and Biophysical Research Communications*, *315*(3), 589–594. doi:10.1016/j.bbrc.2004.01.088 PMID:14975741

Charoensiri, R., Kongkachuichai, R., Suknicom, S., & Sungpuag, P. (2009). Beta-carotene, lycopene, and alpha-tocopherol contents of selected Thai fruits. *Food Chemistry*, *113*(1), 202–207. doi:10.1016/j.foodchem.2008.07.074

Chen, A., Davis, B. H., Bissonnette, M., Scaglione-Sewell, B., & Brasitus, T. A. (1999). 1,25-Dihydroxyvitamin D(3) stimulates activator protein-1-dependent Caco-2 cell differentiation. *The Journal of Biological Chemistry*, *274*(50), 35505–35513. doi:10.1074/jbc.274.50.35505 PMID:10585423

Chu, Y.-F., Sun, J., Wu, X., & Liu, R. H. (2002). Antioxidant and antiproliferative activities of common vegetables. *Journal of Agricultural and Food Chemistry*, *50*(23), 6910–6916. doi:10.1021/jf020665f PMID:12405796

Chung, T.-W., Moon, S.-K., Chang, Y.-C., Ko, J.-H., Lee, Y.-C., Cho, G., ... Kim, C.-H. (2004). Novel and therapeutic effect of caffeic acid and caffeic acid phenyl ester on hepatocarcinoma cells: Complete regression of hepatoma growth and metastasis by dual mechanism. *The FASEB Journal*, *18*(14), 1670–1681. doi:10.1096/fj.04-2126com PMID:15522912

De Vasconcelos, M., Bennett, R. N., Quideau, S., Jacquet, R., Rosa, E. A. S., & Ferreira-Cardoso, J. V. (2010). Evaluating the potential of chestnut (Castanea sativa Mill.) fruit pericarp and integument as a source of tocopherols, pigments and polyphenols. *Industrial Crops and Products*, *31*(2), 301–311. doi:10.1016/j.indcrop.2009.11.008

De Vrese, M., & Schrezenmeir, J. (2008). Probiotics, Prebiotics, and Synbiotics. *Advances in Biochemical Engineering/Biotechnology*, *111*, 1–66. doi:10.1007/10_2008_097 PMID:18461293

DeFelice, S. (1995). The nutraceutical revolution : Its impact on food industry R & D. *Trends in Food Science & Technology*, *6*(2), 59–61. doi:10.1016/S0924-2244(00)88944-X

Delzenne, N. M., Neyrinck, A. M., Bäckhed, F., & Cani, P. D. (2011). Targeting gut microbiota in obesity: Effects of prebiotics and probiotics. *Nature Reviews. Endocrinology*, *7*(11), 639–646. doi:10.1038/nrendo.2011.126 PMID:21826100

Deorukhkar, A., Krishnan, S., Sethi, G., & Aggarwal, B. B. (2007). Back to basics: How natural products can provide the basis for new therapeutics. *Expert Opinion on Investigational Drugs*, *16*(11), 1753–1773. doi:10.1517/13543784.16.11.1753 PMID:17970636

Dixon, R. A., & Sumner, L. W. (2003). Legume natural products: Understanding and manipulating complex pathways for human and animal health. *Plant Physiology*, *131*(3), 878–885. doi:10.1104/pp.102.017319 PMID:12644640

Douglas, L. C., & Sanders, M. E. (2008). Probiotics and Prebiotics in Dietetics Practice. *Journal of the American Dietetic Association*, *108*(3), 510–521. doi:10.1016/j.jada.2007.12.009 PMID:18313433

Dragsted, L. O., Strube, M., & Larsen, J. C. (1993). Cancer-protective factors in fruits and vegetables: Biochemical and biological background. *Pharmacology & Toxicology*, *72*(Suppl 1), 116–135. doi:10.1111/j.1600-0773.1993.tb01679.x PMID:8474974

Espín, J. C., García-Conesa, M. T., & Tomás-Barberán, F. A. (2007). Nutraceuticals: Facts and fiction. *Phytochemistry*, *68*(22–24), 2986–3008. doi:10.1016/j.phytochem.2007.09.014 PMID:17976666

Facompre, N., & El-Bayoumy, K. (2009). Potential stages for prostate cancer prevention with selenium: Implications for cancer survivors. *Cancer Research*, *69*(7), 2699–2703. doi:10.1158/0008-5472.CAN-08-4359 PMID:19318549

Fazel, M., Sahari, M. A., & Barzegar, M. (2008). Determination of main tea seed oil antioxidants and their effects on common kilka oil. *International Food Research Journal*, *15*(2), 209–217.

Ferguson, L. R., & Philpott, M. (2007). Cancer prevention by dietary bioactive components that target the immune response. *Current Cancer Drug Targets*, *7*(5), 459–464. doi:10.2174/156800907781386605 PMID:17691905

Finley, J. W. (2016). The nutraceutical revolution: Emerging vision or broken dream? Understanding scientific and regulatory concerns. *Clinical Research and Regulatory Affairs*, *33*(1), 1–3. doi:10.3109/10601333.2016.1117096

Finley, J. W., Finley, J. W., Ellwood, K., & Hoadley, J. (2014). Launching a New Food Product or Dietary Supplement in the United States: Industrial, Regulatory, and Nutritional Considerations. *Annual Review of Nutrition*, *34*(1), 421–447. doi:10.1146/annurev-nutr-071813-105817 PMID:24850389

Frost & Sullivan. (2011). *Global Nutraceutical Industry: Investing in healthy living*. Academic Press.

Galli, F., Piroddi, M., Annetti, C., Aisa, C., Floridi, E., & Floridi, A. (2005). Oxidative Stress and Reactive Oxygen Species. In *Cardiovascular Disorders in Hemodialysis* (Vol. 149, pp. 240–260). Basel: KARGER. doi:10.1159/000085686

Garland, C. F., Garland, F. C., Gorham, E. D., Lipkin, M., Newmark, H., Mohr, S. B., & Holick, M. F. (2006). The role of vitamin D in cancer prevention. *American Journal of Public Health*, *96*(2), 252–261. doi:10.2105/AJPH.2004.045260 PMID:16380576

Ghasemzadeh, A., & Jaafar, H. Z. (2013). Profiling of phenolic compounds and their antioxidant and anticancer activities in pandan (Pandanus amaryllifolius Roxb.) extracts from different locations of Malaysia. *BMC Complementary and Alternative Medicine*, *13*(1), 341. doi:10.1186/1472-6882-13-341 PMID:24289290

Gibson, G. R., & Roberfroid, M. B. (1995). Dietary modulation of the human colonic microbiota: Introducing the concept of prebiotics. *The Journal of Nutrition*, *125*(6), 1401–1412. PMID:7782892

Golmakani, M.-T., & Rezaei, K. (2008). Comparison of microwave-assisted hydrodistillation withthe traditional hydrodistillation method in the extractionof essential oils from Thymus vulgaris L. *Food Chemistry*, *109*(4), 925–930. doi:10.1016/j.foodchem.2007.12.084 PMID:26050009

Gosslau, A., & Chen, K. Y. (2004). Nutraceuticals, apoptosis, and disease prevention. *Nutrition (Burbank, Los Angeles County, Calif.)*, *20*(1), 95–102. doi:10.1016/j.nut.2003.09.017 PMID:14698022

Green, D. R. (2000). Apoptotic pathways: Paper wraps stone blunts scissors. *Cell*, *102*(1), 1–4. doi:10.1016/S0092-8674(00)00003-9 PMID:10929706

Guo, Z., Liu, X. M., Zhang, Q. X., Shen, Z., Tian, F. W., Zhang, H., ... Chen, W. (2011). Influence of consumption of probiotics on the plasma lipid profile: A meta-analysis of randomised controlled trials. *Nutrition, Metabolism, and Cardiovascular Diseases*, *21*(11), 844–850. doi:10.1016/j.numecd.2011.04.008 PMID:21930366

Ha, T.-Y., Ko, S.-N., Lee, S.-M., Kim, H.-R., Chung, S.-H., Kim, S.-R., ... Kim, I.-H. (2006). Changes in nutraceutical lipid components of rice at different degrees of milling. *European Journal of Lipid Science and Technology*, *108*(3), 175–181. doi:10.1002/ejlt.200500250

Halliwell, B., & Gutteridge, J. M. C. (1985). *Free radicals in biology and medicine*. Clarendon Press.

Han, S.-S., Chung, S.-T., Robertson, D. A., Ranjan, D., & Bondada, S. (1999). Curcumin Causes the Growth Arrest and Apoptosis of B Cell Lymphoma by Downregulation of egr-1, C-myc, Bcl-XL, NF-κB, and p53. *Clinical Immunology (Orlando, Fla.)*, *93*(2), 152–161. doi:10.1006/clim.1999.4769 PMID:10527691

Hanahan, D., & Weinberg, R. A. (2000). The hallmarks of cancer. *Cell*, *100*(1), 57–70. doi:10.1016/S0092-8674(00)81683-9 PMID:10647931

Hardy, G. (n.d.). Nutraceuticals and functional foods: introduction and meaning. *Nutrition*, *16*(7–8), 688–9.

Hillman, G. G., Singh-Gupta, V., Hoogstra, D. J., Abernathy, L., Rakowski, J., Yunker, C. K., ... Joiner, M. C. (2013). Differential effect of soy isoflavones in enhancing high intensity radiotherapy and protecting lung tissue in a pre-clinical model of lung carcinoma. *Radiotherapy and Oncology: Journal of the European Society for Therapeutic Radiology and Oncology*, *109*(1), 117–125. doi:10.1016/j.radonc.2013.08.015 PMID:24021346

Hirpara, K. V., Aggarwal, P., Mukherjee, A. J., Joshi, N., & Burman, A. C. (2009). Quercetin and its derivatives: Synthesis, pharmacological uses with special emphasis on anti-tumor properties and prodrug with enhanced bio-availability. *Anti-cancer Agents in Medicinal Chemistry*, *9*(2), 138–161. doi:10.2174/187152009787313855 PMID:19199862

(n.d.). Histories of Product Regulation - The 1938 Food. *Drug, and Cosmetic Act.*

Huang, C., Huang, Y., Li, J., & Hu, W. (2002). Inhibition of Benzo(a)pyrene Diol-Epoxide-induced Transactivation of Activated Protein 1 and Nuclear Factor κB by Black Raspberry Extracts. *Cancer Research*, *62*(23). PMID:12460899

Huang, M. T., Ho, C. T., Wang, Z., & Conney, A. H. (1994). Inhibition of skin tumorigenesis by rosemary and its constituents carnosol and ursolic acid. *Cancer Research*, *54*(3), 701–708. PMID:8306331

Ito, K., Nakazato, T., Yamato, K., Miyakawa, Y., Yamada, T., Hozumi, N., ... Kizaki, M. (2004). Induction of apoptosis in leukemic cells by homovanillic acid derivative, capsaicin, through oxidative stress: Implication of phosphorylation of p53 at Ser-15 residue by reactive oxygen species. *Cancer Research*, *64*(3), 1071–1078. doi:10.1158/0008-5472.CAN-03-1670 PMID:14871840

Johnson, J. J. (2011). Carnosol: A promising anti-cancer and anti-inflammatory agent. *Cancer Letters*, *305*(1), 1–7. doi:10.1016/j.canlet.2011.02.005 PMID:21382660

Kaji, I., Tatsuta, M., Iishi, H., Baba, M., Inoue, A., & Kasugai, H. (2001). Inhibition by d-limonene of experimental hepatocarcinogenesis in Sprague-Dawley rats does not involve p21(ras) plasma membrane association. *International Journal of Cancer*, *93*(3), 441–444. doi:10.1002/ijc.1353 PMID:11433412

Kamsteeg, M., Rutherford, T., Sapi, E., Hanczaruk, B., Shahabi, S., Flick, M., ... Mor, G. (2003). Phenoxodiol – an isoflavone analog – induces apoptosis in chemoresistant ovarian cancer cells. *Oncogene*, *22*(17), 2611–2620. doi:10.1038j.onc.1206422 PMID:12730675

Karin, M. (2009). NF- B as a Critical Link Between Inflammation and Cancer. *Cold Spring Harbor Perspectives in Biology*, *1*(5), a000141–a000141. doi:10.1101/cshperspect.a000141 PMID:20066113

Karin, M., & Greten, F. R. (2005). NF-κB: Linking inflammation and immunity to cancer development and progression. *Nature Reviews. Immunology*, *5*(10), 749–759. doi:10.1038/nri1703 PMID:16175180

Kasala, E. R., Bodduluru, L. N., Barua, C. C., & Gogoi, R. (2016). Antioxidant and antitumor efficacy of Luteolin, a dietary flavone on benzo(a)pyrene-induced experimental lung carcinogenesis. *Biomedicine & Pharmacotherapy, 82*, 568–77.

Khan, N., Afaq, F., Saleem, M., Ahmad, N., & Mukhtar, H. (2006). Targeting Multiple Signaling Pathways by Green Tea Polyphenol (−)-Epigallocatechin-3-Gallate. *Cancer Research*, *66*(5), 2500–2505. doi:10.1158/0008-5472.CAN-05-3636 PMID:16510563

Kim, S. O., Chun, K.-S., Kundu, J. K., & Surh, Y.-J. (2004). Inhibitory effects of [6]-gingerol on PMA-induced COX-2 expression and activation of NF-kappaB and p38 MAPK in mouse skin. *BioFactors (Oxford, England)*, *21*(1–4), 27–31. doi:10.1002/biof.552210107 PMID:15630166

Klein, E., Thompson, I., Lippman, S., Goodman, P., Albanes, D., Taylor, P., & Coltman, C. (2000). SELECT: the Selenium and Vitamin E Cancer Prevention Trial: rationale and design. *Prostate Cancer and Prostatic Diseases*, *3*(3), 145–151. doi:10.1038j.pcan.4500412 PMID:12497090

Korutla, L., & Kumar, R. (1994). Inhibitory effect of curcumin on epidermal growth factor receptor kinase activity in A431 cells. *Biochimica et Biophysica Acta*, *1224*(3), 597–600. doi:10.1016/0167-4889(94)90299-2 PMID:7803521

Kotilainen, L., Rajalahti, R., Ragasa, C., & Pehu, E. (2006, June 1). *Health enhancing foods : opportunities for strengthening developing countries*. Academic Press.

Kotzampassi, K., & Giamarellos-Bourboulis, E. J. (2012). Probiotics for infectious diseases: More drugs, less dietary supplementation. *International Journal of Antimicrobial Agents*, *40*(4), 288–296. doi:10.1016/j.ijantimicag.2012.06.006 PMID:22858373

Kresty, L. A., Morse, M. A., Morgan, C., Carlton, P. S., Lu, J., Gupta, A., ... Stoner, G. D. (2001). Chemoprevention of Esophageal Tumorigenesis by Dietary Administration of Lyophilized Black Raspberries. *Cancer Research*, *61*, 6112–6119. PMID:11507061

Kuo, M. L., Huang, T. S., & Lin, J. K. (1996). Curcumin, an antioxidant and anti-tumor promoter, induces apoptosis in human leukemia cells. *Biochimica et Biophysica Acta*, *1317*(2), 95–100. doi:10.1016/S0925-4439(96)00032-4 PMID:8950193

Kwak, N.-S., & Jukes, D. J. (2001). Functional foods. Part 1: The development of a regulatory concept. *Food Control*, *12*(2), 99–107. doi:10.1016/S0956-7135(00)00028-1

Lattimer, J. M., & Haub, M. D. (2010). Effects of Dietary Fiber and Its Components on Metabolic Health. *Nutrients*, *2*(12), 1266–1289. doi:10.3390/nu2121266 PMID:22254008

Lau, B. H. S., Tadi, P. P., & Tosk, J. M. (1990). Allium sativum (Garlic) and cancer prevention. *Nutrition Research (New York, N.Y.)*, *10*(8), 937–948. doi:10.1016/S0271-5317(05)80057-0

Li, Q., Withoff, S., & Verma, I. M. (2005). Inflammation-associated cancer: NF-κB is the lynchpin. *Trends in Immunology*, *26*(6), 318–325. doi:10.1016/j.it.2005.04.003 PMID:15922948

Malaguarnera, G., Leggio, F., Vacante, M., Motta, M., Giordano, M., Bondi, A., ... Salmeri, M. (2012). Probiotics in the gastrointestinal diseases of the elderly. *The Journal of Nutrition, Health & Aging*, *16*(4), 402–410. doi:10.100712603-011-0357-1 PMID:22499466

Mandel, S. A., Avramovich-Tirosh, Y., Reznichenko, L., Zheng, H., Weinreb, O., Amit, T., & Youdim, M. B. H. (2005). Multifunctional Activities of Green Tea Catechins in Neuroprotection. *Neuro-Signals*, *14*(1–2), 46–60. doi:10.1159/000085385 PMID:15956814

Mark-Herbert, C. (2004). Innovation of a new product category - Functional foods. *Technovation*, *24*(9), 713–719. doi:10.1016/S0166-4972(02)00131-1

Marx, J. (2004). CANCER RESEARCH: Inflammation and Cancer: The Link Grows Stronger. *Science*, *306*(5698), 966–968. doi:10.1126cience.306.5698.966 PMID:15528423

Mehta, K., Pantazis, P., McQueen, T., & Aggarwal, B. B. (1997). Antiproliferative effect of curcumin (diferuloylmethane) against human breast tumor cell lines. *Anti-Cancer Drugs*, *8*(5), 470–481. doi:10.1097/00001813-199706000-00010 PMID:9215611

Meier, P., Finch, A., & Evan, G. (2000). Apoptosis in development. *Nature*, *407*(6805), 796–801. doi:10.1038/35037734 PMID:11048731

Melnick, S. J. (2006). Developmental Therapeutics: Review of Biologically Based CAM therapies for Potential Application in Children With Cancer: Part I. *Journal of Pediatric Hematology/Oncology*, *28*(4), 221–230. doi:10.1097/01.mph.0000212922.16427.04 PMID:16679919

Menrad, K. (2003). Market and marketing of functional food in Europe. *Journal of Food Engineering*, *56*(2–3), 181–188. doi:10.1016/S0260-8774(02)00247-9

Murakami, A., Ashida, H., & Terao, J. (2008). Multitargeted cancer prevention by quercetin. *Cancer Letters*, *269*(2), 315–325. doi:10.1016/j.canlet.2008.03.046 PMID:18467024

Nair, H. B., Sung, B., Yadav, V. R., Kannappan, R., Chaturvedi, M. M., & Aggarwal, B. B. (2010). Delivery of antiinflammatory nutraceuticals by nanoparticles for the prevention and treatment of cancer. *Biochemical Pharmacology*, *80*(12), 1833–1843. doi:10.1016/j.bcp.2010.07.021 PMID:20654584

Omenn, G. S., Goodman, G. E., Thornquist, M. D., Balmes, J., Cullen, M. R., Glass, A., ... Hammar, S. (1996). Effects of a Combination of Beta Carotene and Vitamin A on Lung Cancer and Cardiovascular Disease. *The New England Journal of Medicine*, *334*(18), 1150–1155. doi:10.1056/NEJM199605023341802 PMID:8602180

Oyagbemi, A., Saba, A., & Azeez, O. (2010). Capsaicin: A novel chemopreventive molecule and its underlying molecular mechanisms of action. *Indian Journal of Cancer*, *47*(1), 53. doi:10.4103/0019-509X.58860 PMID:20071791

Pala, V., Krogh, V., Muti, P., Chajès, V., Riboli, E., Micheli, A., ... Berrino, F. (2001). Erythrocyte membrane fatty acids and subsequent breast cancer: A prospective Italian study. *Journal of the National Cancer Institute*, *93*(14), 1088–1095. doi:10.1093/jnci/93.14.1088 PMID:11459870

Paliwal, S., Sundaram, J., & Mitragotri, S. (2005). Induction of cancer-specific cytotoxicity towards human prostate and skin cells using quercetin and ultrasound. *British Journal of Cancer*, *92*(3), 499–502. doi:10.1038j.bjc.6602364 PMID:15685239

Pan, M.-H., Lin, C.-C., Lin, J.-K., & Chen, W.-J. (2007). Tea Polyphenol (−)-Epigallocatechin 3-Gallate Suppresses Heregulin-β1-Induced Fatty Acid Synthase Expression in Human Breast Cancer Cells by Inhibiting Phosphatidylinositol 3-Kinase/Akt and Mitogen-Activated Protein Kinase Cascade Signaling. *Journal of Agricultural and Food Chemistry*, *55*(13), 5030–5037. doi:10.1021/jf070316r PMID:17539658

Panossian, A., Wikman, G., & Wagner, H. (1999). Plant adaptogens III. Earlier and more recent aspects and concepts on their mode of action. *Phytomedicine*, *6*(4), 287–300. doi:10.1016/S0944-7113(99)80023-3 PMID:10589450

Pathak, A. K., Bhutani, M., Nair, A. S., Ahn, K. S., Chakraborty, A., Kadara, H., ... Aggarwal, B. B. (2007). Ursolic Acid Inhibits STAT3 Activation Pathway Leading to Suppression of Proliferation and Chemosensitization of Human Multiple Myeloma Cells. *Molecular Cancer Research*, *5*(9), 943–955. doi:10.1158/1541-7786.MCR-06-0348 PMID:17855663

Pecere, T., Gazzola, M. V., Mucignat, C., Parolin, C., Vecchia, F. D., Cavaggioni, A., ... Palù, G. (2000). Aloe-emodin Is a New Type of Anticancer Agent with Selective Activity against Neuroectodermal Tumors. *Cancer Research*, *60*(11). PMID:10850417

Pecorino, L. (2008). *Molecular biology of cancer : mechanisms, targets, and therapeutics*. Oxford University Press.

Pérez-Fons, L., Aranda, F. J., Guillén, J., Villalaín, J., & Micol, V. (2006). Rosemary (Rosmarinus officinalis) diterpenes affect lipid polymorphism and fluidity in phospholipid membranes. *Archives of Biochemistry and Biophysics*, *453*(2), 224–236. doi:10.1016/j.abb.2006.07.004 PMID:16949545

Pérez-Herrero, E., & Fernández-Medarde, A. (2015). Advanced targeted therapies in cancer: Drug nanocarriers, the future of chemotherapy. *European Journal of Pharmaceutics and Biopharmaceutics*, *93*, 52–79. doi:10.1016/j.ejpb.2015.03.018 PMID:25813885

Pericleous, M., Mandair, D., & Caplin, M. E. (2013). Diet and supplements and their impact on colorectal cancer. *Journal of Gastrointestinal Oncology*, *4*(4), 409–423. PMID:24294513

Philip, M., Rowley, D. A., & Schreiber, H. (2004). Inflammation as a tumor promoter in cancer induction. *Seminars in Cancer Biology*, *14*(6), 433–439. doi:10.1016/j.semcancer.2004.06.006 PMID:15489136

Piwocka, K., Zabłocki, K., Wieckowski, M. R., Skierski, J., Feiga, I., Szopa, J., ... Sikora, E. (1999). A novel apoptosis-like pathway, independent of mitochondria and caspases, induced by curcumin in human lymphoblastoid T (Jurkat) cells. *Experimental Cell Research*, *249*(2), 299–307. doi:10.1006/excr.1999.4480 PMID:10366429

Powolny, A. A., & Singh, S. V. (2008). Multitargeted prevention and therapy of cancer by diallyl trisulfide and related Allium vegetable-derived organosulfur compounds. *Cancer Letters*, *269*(2), 305–314. doi:10.1016/j.canlet.2008.05.027 PMID:18579286

Prieto, J. M., Iacopini, P., Cioni, P., & Chericoni, S. (2007). In vitro activity of the essential oils of Origanum vulgare, Satureja montana and their main constituents in peroxynitrite-induced oxidative processes. *Food Chemistry*, *104*(3), 889–895. doi:10.1016/j.foodchem.2006.10.064

Quideau, S. (2006). Flavonoids. Chemistry, Biochemistry and Applications. Edited by Øyvind M. Andersen and Kenneth R. Markham. *Angewandte Chemie*, *45*(41), 6786–6787. doi:10.1002/anie.200685399

Ramachandran, C., & You, W. (1999). Differential sensitivity of human mammary epithelial and breast carcinoma cell lines to curcumin. *Breast Cancer Research and Treatment*, *54*(3), 269–278. doi:10.1023/A:1006170224414 PMID:10445426

Ramawat, K. G., & Merillon, J. M. (2007). *Biotechnology: Secondary metabolites : plants and microbes*. Science Publishers.

Ranjan, D., Johnston, T. D., Reddy, K. S., Wu, G., Bondada, S., & Chen, C. (1999). Enhanced Apoptosis Mediates Inhibition of EBV-Transformed Lymphoblastoid Cell Line Proliferation by Curcumin. *The Journal of Surgical Research*, *87*(1), 1–5. doi:10.1006/jsre.1999.5719 PMID:10527697

Ray, A., Joshi, J., & Gulati, K. (2016). Regulatory Aspects of Nutraceuticals. In Nutraceuticals (pp. 941–946). Elsevier. doi:10.1016/B978-0-12-802147-7.00066-8

Rice-Evans, C. A., & Miller, N. J. (1996). Antioxidant activities of flavonoids as bioactive components of food. *Biochemical Society Transactions*, *24*(3), 790–795. doi:10.1042/bst0240790 PMID:8878849

Ritchie, M. L., & Romanuk, T. N. (2012). A Meta-Analysis of Probiotic Efficacy for Gastrointestinal Diseases. *PLoS One*, *7*(4), e34938. doi:10.1371/journal.pone.0034938 PMID:22529959

de la Rosa, L. A., Alvarez-Parrilla, E., & González-Aguilar, G. A. (2010). Fruit and vegetable phytochemicals: Chemistry, nutritional value, and stability. Wiley-Blackwell.

Roy, P., Madan, E., Kalra, N., Nigam, N., George, J., Ray, R. S., ... Shukla, Y. (2009). Resveratrol enhances ultraviolet B-induced cell death through nuclear factor-kappaB pathway in human epidermoid carcinoma A431 cells. *Biochemical and Biophysical Research Communications*, *384*(2), 215–220. doi:10.1016/j.bbrc.2009.04.100 PMID:19397895

Russell, R. M., & Mayer, J. (2002). Beta-carotene and lung cancer. *Pure and Applied Chemistry*, *74*(8), 1461–1467. doi:10.1351/pac200274081461

Sarkar, F. H., & Li, Y. (2003). Soy isoflavones and cancer prevention. *Cancer Investigation*, *21*(5), 744–757. doi:10.1081/CNV-120023773 PMID:14628433

Schloss, P. D. (2014). Microbiology: An integrated view of the skin microbiome. *Nature*, *514*(7520), 44–45. doi:10.1038/514044a PMID:25279916

Schroeter, H., Boyd, C., Spencer, J. P. E., Williams, R. J., Cadenas, E., & Rice-Evans, C. (n.d.). MAPK signaling in neurodegeneration: influences of flavonoids and of nitric oxide. *Neurobiology of Aging, 23*(5), 861–80.

Sesso, H. D., Buring, J. E., Christen, W. G., Kurth, T., Belanger, C., MacFadyen, J., ... Gaziano, J. M. (2008). Vitamins E and C in the prevention of cardiovascular disease in men: The Physicians' Health Study II randomized controlled trial. *Journal of the American Medical Association*, *300*(18), 2123–2133. doi:10.1001/jama.2008.600 PMID:18997197

Shishodia, S., & Aggarwal, B. B. (2004). Guggulsterone Inhibits NF-κB and IκBα Kinase Activation, Suppresses Expression of Anti-apoptotic Gene Products, and Enhances Apoptosis. *The Journal of Biological Chemistry*, *279*(45), 47148–47158. doi:10.1074/jbc.M408093200 PMID:15322087

Shishodia, S., Potdar, P., Gairola, C. G., & Aggarwal, B. B. (2003). Curcumin (diferuloylmethane) down-regulates cigarette smoke-induced NF- B activation through inhibition of I B kinase in human lung epithelial cells: Correlation with suppression of COX-2, MMP-9 and cyclin D1. *Carcinogenesis*, *24*(7), 1269–1279. doi:10.1093/carcin/bgg078 PMID:12807725

Shukla, S., & Gupta, S. (2005). Dietary Agents in the Chemoprevention of Prostate Cancer. *Nutrition and Cancer*, *53*(1), 18–32. doi:10.120715327914nc5301_3 PMID:16351503

Shukla, Y., & Singh, M. (2007). Cancer preventive properties of ginger: A brief review. *Food and Chemical Toxicology*, *45*(5), 683–690. doi:10.1016/j.fct.2006.11.002 PMID:17175086

Siddiqui, I. A., Shukla, Y., Adhami, V. M., Sarfaraz, S., Asim, M., Hafeez, B., & Mukhtar, H. (2008). Suppression of NFκB and its Regulated Gene Products by Oral Administration of Green Tea Polyphenols in an Autochthonous Mouse Prostate Cancer Model. *Pharmaceutical Research*, *25*(9), 2135–2142. doi:10.100711095-008-9553-z PMID:18317887

Simon, A., Allais, D. P., Duroux, J. L., Basly, J. P., Durand-Fontanier, S., & Delage, C. (1998). Inhibitory effect of curcuminoids on MCF-7 cell proliferation and structure-activity relationships. *Cancer Letters*, *129*(1), 111–116.

Singh, S. V., Mohan, R. R., Agarwal, R., Benson, P. J., Hu, X., Rudy, M., ... Zaren, H. A. (1996). Novel anti-carcinogenic activity of an organosulfide from garlic: Inhibition of H-RAS oncogene transformed tumor growth in vivo by diallyl disulfide is associated with inhibition of p21H-ras processing. *Biochemical and Biophysical Research Communications*, *225*(2), 660–665.

Smith-Warner, S. A., Elmer, P. J., Tharp, T. M., Fosdick, L., Randall, B., Gross, M., ... Potter, J. D. (2000). Increasing vegetable and fruit intake: Randomized intervention and monitoring in an at-risk population. *Cancer Epidemiology, Biomarkers & Prevention*, *9*(3), 307–317. PMID:10750670

Soobrattee, M. A., Bahorun, T., & Aruoma, O. I. (2006). Chemopreventive actions of polyphenolic compounds in cancer. *BioFactors (Oxford, England)*, *27*(1–4), 19–35. doi:10.1002/biof.5520270103 PMID:17012761

Sotiroudis, T. G., & Kyrtopoulos, S. A. (2008). Anticarcinogenic compounds of olive oil and related biomarkers. *European Journal of Nutrition*, *47*(S2), 69–72. doi:10.100700394-008-2008-9 PMID:18458836

Spence, J. T. (2006). Challenges related to the composition of functional foods. *Journal of Food Composition and Analysis*, *19*(SUPPL.), 2005–2007. doi:10.1016/j.jfca.2005.11.007

Sporn, M. B., & Suh, N. (2000). Chemoprevention of cancer. *Carcinogenesis*, *21*(3), 525–530. doi:10.1093/carcin/21.3.525 PMID:10688873

Srinivasan, M., Sudheer, A. R., & Menon, V. P. (2007). Recent Advances in Indian Herbal Drug Research Guest Editor: Thomas Paul Asir Devasagayam Ferulic Acid: Therapeutic Potential Through Its Antioxidant Property. Journal of Clinical Biochemistry and Nutrition, 40(2), 92–100.

Sun, H.-X., Xie, Y., & Ye, Y.-P. (2009). Advances in saponin-based adjuvants. *Vaccine*, *27*(12), 1787–1796. doi:10.1016/j.vaccine.2009.01.091 PMID:19208455

Surh, Y.-J. (2002). Anti-tumor promoting potential of selected spice ingredients with antioxidative and anti-inflammatory activities: A short review. *Food and Chemical Toxicology : An International Journal Published for the British Industrial Biological Research Association*, *40*(8), 1091–1097. doi:10.1016/S0278-6915(02)00037-6 PMID:12067569

Switzer, C. H., Ridnour, L., Cheng, R. Y. S., Sparatore, A., Del Soldato, P., Moody, T. W., ... Wink, D. A. (2009). Dithiolethione compounds inhibit Akt signaling in human breast and lung cancer cells by increasing PP2A activity. *Oncogene*, *28*(43), 3837–3846. doi:10.1038/onc.2009.244 PMID:19701246

Thannickal, V. J., & Fanburg, B. L. (2000). Reactive oxygen species in cell signaling. *American Journal of Physiology. Lung Cellular and Molecular Physiology*, *279*(6), L1005–L1028. doi:10.1152/ajplung.2000.279.6.L1005 PMID:11076791

Trachootham, D., Alexandre, J., & Huang, P. (2009). Targeting cancer cells by ROS-mediated mechanisms: A radical therapeutic approach? *Nature Reviews. Drug Discovery*, *8*(7), 579–591. doi:10.1038/nrd2803 PMID:19478820

Tsao, A. S., Kim, E. S., & Hong, W. K. (2004). Chemoprevention of Cancer. *CA: a Cancer Journal for Clinicians, 54*(3), 150–180. doi:10.3322/canjclin.54.3.150 PMID:15195789

Uedo, N., Tatsuta, M., Iishi, H., Baba, M., Sakai, N., Yano, H., & Otani, T. (1999). Inhibition by D-limonene of gastric carcinogenesis induced by N-methyl-N'-nitro-N-nitrosoguanidine in Wistar rats. *Cancer Letters, 137*(2), 131–136.

Venkatachalam, H., Nayak, Y., & Jayashree, B. S. (2012). Synthesis, Characterization and Antioxidant Activities of Synthetic Chalcones and Flavones. *APCBEE Procedia, 3*, 209–213.

Wang, L.-S., & Stoner, G. D. (2008). Anthocyanins and their role in cancer prevention. *Cancer Letters, 269*(2), 281–290. doi:10.1016/j.canlet.2008.05.020 PMID:18571839

Wang, S., Yang, D., & Lippman, M. E. (2003). Targeting Bcl-2 and Bcl-XL with nonpeptidic small-molecule antagonists. *Seminars in Oncology, 30*(5Suppl 16), 133–142. doi:10.1053/j.seminoncol.2003.08.015 PMID:14613034

Yang, S.-F., Yang, W.-E., Kuo, W.-H., Chang, H.-R., Chu, S.-C., & Hsieh, Y.-S. (2008). Antimetastatic potentials of flavones on oral cancer cell via an inhibition of matrix-degrading proteases. *Archives of Oral Biology, 53*(3), 287–294. doi:10.1016/j.archoralbio.2007.09.001 PMID:17936716

Huang. (2010). Polymethoxy flavones are responsible for the anti-inflammatory activity of citrus fruit peel. *Food Chemistry, 119*(3), 868–873.

Zhao, C., Giusti, M. M., Malik, M., Moyer, M. P., & Magnuson, B. A. (2004). Effects of Commercial Anthocyanin-Rich Extracts on Colonic Cancer and Nontumorigenic Colonic Cell Growth. *Journal of Agricultural and Food Chemistry, 52*(20), 6122–6128. doi:10.1021/jf049517a PMID:15453676

Zhou, C., Lin, H., Ge, X., Niu, J., Wang, J., Wang, Y., ... Tan, X. (2015). The Effects of dietary soybean isoflavones on growth, innate immune responses, hepatic antioxidant abilities and disease resistance of juvenile golden pompano Trachinotus ovatus. *Fish & Shellfish Immunology, 43*(1), 158–166. doi:10.1016/j.fsi.2014.12.014 PMID:25541076

Section 8
Antioxidant

Chapter 13
Clinical Role of Antioxidants in the Treatment of Diseases

Kirti Rani
Amity University, India

ABSTRACT

Antioxidants are our first line of defense against free radical damage and are critical for maintaining optimum healthcare. Although most of the present day research is focused on the potential benefits of antioxidant nutrients or supplements, it has become clear that the best protection against oxidative stress involves a wide assortment of interrelated antioxidants and antioxidant cofactors. Additionally, the combination of several suboptimal concentrations of these kinds of detoxifying supplements may have an additive or even synergistic role to decrease the risk of some of diseases which are caused by aging. Adequate intake of fruit and vegetables have essential antioxidants like B-carotene and vitamin C, which are reported for decreasing the risk of cancer and coronary heart disease (CHD).

INTRODUCTION

Oxygen is a highly reactive atom that is capable of becoming part of potentially damaging molecules commonly called free radicals that are responsible to oxidative stress. Free radicals are capable of causing pathogenesis of healthy cells to lose their structures and functions causing degenerative diseases of aging such as cancer, cardiovascular disease, cataracts, immune system decline, and brain dysfunction. Antioxidants are capable of stabilizing, or deactivating these free radicals before they attack the healthy cells to maintain optimal cellular and systemic health and human well-being. The need for antioxidants becomes more important with increased

DOI: 10.4018/978-1-5225-3267-5.ch013

exposure to free radicals due to pollution, cigarette smoke, drugs, illness, stress, and even exercise can increase free radical exposure that contribute to oxidative stress of every individual. So, many experts believe that the Recommended Dietary Allowance (RDA) for specific antioxidants may be required to live healthy lifestyle and a well-balanced, wholesome diet and adequate antioxidant supplementation to improving free radical protection. Many diseases become more prevalent with the increase of age such as inflammatory diseases, neurodegenerative diseases, diabetes, cancer, and cardiovascular diseases. Reactive oxygen species are believed to be involved in the etiology of these kinds of diseases and conversely, antioxidants are believed to be protective. A balanced diet (including plenty of fruit, vegetables, grains, oils and nuts) should provide most individuals with a complement of antioxidants that is sufficient to protect their body against many diseases. In the treatment of these diseases, antioxidants have a potential role being safe, the toxicity of three selected antioxidants such as vitamin E, beta-carotene, vitamin C and lipoic acid. It is believed that antioxidants have their protective effect by decreasing oxidative damage to DNA and by decreasing abnormal increases in cell division. Cigarette smoking and chronic inflammation have been reported to be two of the major causes of cancer that have strong free radical components in their mechanisms of action as compared to non-smokers are at an increased risk of having cancer and cardiovascular diseases. It can therefore be seen that although antioxidants are generally regarded as safe compounds, even at high concentrations, or after metabolism, reactive species may be generated, which can have a pro-oxidant effect. As well as, it is also important factor to consider in determining the safety of antioxidant supplements on our general health to understand the mechanism of action of antioxidants and their metabolites (both beneficial and toxic activities) which could contribute to a better knowledge of the optimum dose that could have a beneficial effect upon our health, without having a detrimental effect.

Poor diet, stress, lack of exercise, and genetic factors, all of these factors contribute many disease due to aging and tissue or cell degeneration that led to an interest in the potential role of antioxidants to slow down disease progression or prevent its manifestation. Free radicals are electrically charged molecules that have an unpaired electron, which causes them to seek out and capture electrons from other substances in order to neutralize themselves. Although the initial attack causes the free radical to become neutralized, another free radical is formed in the process, causing occurrence of chain reaction. And until subsequent free radicals are deactivated, thousands of free radical reactions can occur within seconds of the initial reactions. Antioxidants are capable of stabilizing, or deactivating, free radicals before they attack cells (Langseth, 1993). Reactive oxygen species (ROS) encompasses all highly reactive, oxygen-containing molecules, including free radicals like hydroxyl radical, the superoxide anion radical, hydrogen peroxide, singlet oxygen, nitric oxide radical, hypochlorite radical, and various lipid peroxides. All are capable of reacting with membrane lipids, nucleic acids, proteins and enzymes, and other small molecules lead to progressive cellular damage (Halliwell, 1994; Jacob, 1995).

Most of the oxidants produced by cells occur as consequence of normal aerobic metabolism and approximately 90% of the oxygen utilized by the cell is consumed by the mitochondrial electron transport system. Oxidative burst from phagocytes (white blood cells) was led to killing of bacteria and viruses due to denaturation of their foreign proteins (antigens) and process is called, detoxification of toxic substances (Sies & Stahl, 1995). Antioxidant enzymes also have an important role in the detoxification of free radicals, and include superoxide dismutase, catalase, and glutathione peroxidase which scavenge free radicals. Decrease in the functioning of antioxidant defense system or an overproduction of free radicals results in oxidative stress which contributes many neurodegenerative diseases and also to ageing. Hence, therapies based on both antioxidants and antioxidant factors have been suggested for many preventing skin aging related diseases and neurodegenerative diseases (Mates, Pérez-Gómez, Núñez, & De Castro, 1999).

ROLE OF ANTIOXIDANTS IN VARIOUS DISEASES PREVENTION

In Inflammatory Diseases

In rheumatoid arthritis, toxic substances are released from the synovium that cause inflammation of the joint tissues, which may lead to the destruction of cartilage. Treatments based on antioxidants may be proved a new therapeutic approach to protect the damage of cartilages in this disease. Antioxidants therefore need to detoxify these species, to minimize the respective adverse effects. The French diet contains a high level of antioxidants, from fruit, vegetables, and red wine that have potency to treat arthritis (Alammanos, Voulgari, & Drosos, 2005). An important polyphenolic antioxidant found in red wine, berries, peanuts and grapes are resveratrol which are potent antioxidant that scavenges free radicals, and up-regulates the activity of various antioxidant enzymes (De La Lastra & Villegas, 2005). Vitamin E-alpha tocopherol scavenges free radicals to react with lipids and proteins which considered a mild anti-inflammatory effect. Vitamin A also has antioxidant properties which has anti-inflammatory effects. Beta-carotene, a precursor of vitamin A may quench singlet oxygen which was reported for decreasing the concentration free radicals and consequently protecting lipids in cell membranes from peroxidation (McAlindon & Felson, 1997).

Pycnogenol (Procyanidine B3) has a role in preventing many inflammatory diseases that increases the intracellular synthesis of antioxidant enzymes, scavenges free radicals, and decreases the production of peroxides by macrophages, thereby protecting cells and tissues from oxidative stress (Rohdewald, 2002). This compound also helps to ensures that cells have a constant supply of vitamins C and E especially in case of in cigarette smoker who have double serum levels of epinephrine that lead to vasoconstriction and increasing platelet aggregation. Pycnogenol also decreases the high level of thromboxanes in smokers, to a normal level, preventing the vasoconstriction (Rohdewald, 2002).

Green tea, *Camellia sinensis*, contains polyphenolic compounds have been shown to reduce the inflammation associated with arthritis in mice and this compounds is called catechins that contain a epigallocatechin gallate (EGCG) which inhibit the breakdown of proteoglycan and collagen (Adcocks, Collin, & Buttle, 2002).

Lipoic acid is a naturally occurring antioxidant, which has been used clinically for the treatment of oxidant-induced diseases that scavenges free radicals and has metal chelating activity, recycles antioxidants, accelerates glutathione synthesis and modulates the activity of transportation factors such as nuclear factor-kB (NF-kB) (Packer, 1998).

In Neurodegenerative Disorders

An increased production of reactive oxygen and nitrogen species have been shown to contribute to several neurodegenerative disorders which could be prevented by using antioxidants. Improved memory is reported with the higher levels of carotenoid and tocopherol in individuals, whereas low levels of antioxidants are associated with a greater risk of brain vascular disease, memory loss, and dementia (Ferrari & Torres, 2003). D, L-alpha-tocopherol was also reported to be administered to patients with moderately severe impairment from this disease, their rate of cognitive decline appeared to be reduced. Resveratrol found in grapes and red wine which may have a neuroprotective effect against Alzheimer's disease (Marambaud Zhao, & Davies, 2005). Some of catechins found in green tea are found to be protective to joint tissues inflammation. Consuming green tea may therefore help to prevent arthritis and benefit patients with arthritis, by reducing inflammation, and slowing down the breakdown of cartilage. So, consumption of green may have a chondroprotective effect. Ascorbate can scavenge reactive species, including the superoxide anion, peroxyl, hydroxyl and peroxynitrite radicals, and lipid hydroperoxides that make catecholamines more stable, preventing them from producing reactive oxygen species (Rice, 2000).

In Obesity and Diabetes Mellitus

Diabetes mellitus is a metabolic disorder, in which the beta cells in the pancreas do not release enough insulin which lead to hyperglycaemia (Westcottet & Muir, 2003; Bhathena & Velasquez, 2002). The isoflavones like genistein and daidzein, are mainly found in soybean and its derived products named, biochanin A and formononetin, respectively have been reported for antioxidant properties. Dietary phytoestrogens, including isoflavones and lignans have a beneficial role in both obesity and diabetes due to their positive regulatory actions on glucose and lipid metabolism as antioxidants. These are found in many plants that are eaten by humans including legumes, seeds and whole grains which have positive effects against menopausal symptoms, cardiovascular disease, cancer, osteoporosis, and renal diseases (Stephen, Wang, Chen, Joseph, & Hu, 2008).

Soy polysaccharides also decrease the steep rise in blood glucose that follows a meal, and decrease triacylglycerol concentration, whereas soy proteins may increase insulin sensitivity, improve glucose control, reduce body weight and reduce high levels of plasma lipids and cholesterol. Flaxseed has the highest concentration of lignans, although they are also found in seeds, whole grains, legumes and vegetables (Bhathena & Velasquez, 2002).

In Cancer Prevention

Carcinogenesis takes place when a normal cell is transformed into cancerous cells due to uncontrolled cell divisions lead to the development of a tumor/ benign /cancer. A number of phytochemicals that are present in edible plants, have anticarcinogenic and antimutagenic effects and can interfere with a particular stage in the development of cancer for achieving lower risk of developing some cancers (particularly of the digestive and respiratory tracts (Surh, 2003). Genistein, the soy isoflavone, can protect individuals against breast and prostate cancers and can inhibit the activity of both AP1 and NF-kappa B (Surh, 2003).

Tea polyphenols may induced apoptosis, cell growth inhibition due to having antioxidant activity through increasing levels of p53, which regulates cell cycle arrest or apoptosis which therefore has a fundamental role in protecting cells from tumorogenesis. So, these antioxidants lead to increase the levels of p53 and altering the redox potential especially, Lutein (a derivative of alpha-carotene) and zeaxanthin (a derivative of beta-carotene) which have been shown to prevent the formation of tumors within the lung, and live in mice (Nishino, Murakoshi, Ii, Takemura, Kuchide, Kanazawa, & Jinno, 2002).

Lycopene is found mainly in tomatoes and has potent antioxidant activity and found to report in preventing the development of tumors (Nishino, Murakoshi, Ii, Takemura, Kuchide, Kanazawa, & Jinno, 2002). The ability of lycopene to scavenge free radicals is also reported for preventing oxidative damage of DNA and also has anticarcinogenic activity (Ferrari & Torres, 2003). Grape seed proanthocyanidin extract (GSPE) may have a antioxidant affect against free radicals, oxidative stress and tissue injury which has been observed in both *in vitro* and *in vivo* models due to the presence of phenolic hydrogens, which allow to quench singlet oxygen for scavenging free radicals (Bagchi, Bagchi, Stohs, Das, Ray, Kuszynski, Joshi, & Pruess, 2000).

In Cardiovascular Diseases Prevention

Polyphenols found in tea include catechins, flavanols, theaflavins, and thearubigins are potent antioxidants which may have a protect effect on the heart, by preventing LDL from being oxidized and decreasing platelet aggregation. The phenolic compounds in wine, including resveratrol, may decrease thrombosis and inflammation by regulating coagulation cascade to reduce the activity of tissue adhesion factor that caused formation of thrombus and also control the production of nitric oxide that lead to the dilation of blood vessels. (Sagara, Kanda, Jelekera, Teramoto, Armitage, Birt, Birt, & Yamori., 2004). Supplements of Omega-3 fatty acids can be able to reduce inflammatory mediators, leukotrienes, and the production of superoxide anions which are also present in good concentration in olive oil, castor oil, flaxseeds oil, jojoba oil and cod liver oil (Westcott & Muir, 2003).

ANTIOXIDANTS TOXICITY

Antioxidants are generally regarded as being healthy and safe. But, toxicity of vitamin E, beta-carotene and lipoic acid have been widely studied previously when their concentration might be increased beyond normal limit in affected individuals. At high concentrations, tocopherol (the most active form of vitamin E) can have an undesirable pro-oxidant effect (Bast & Haenen, 2002; Halliwell, 2000). A similar pro-oxidant effect is seen with high concentrations of vitamin C and vitamin E supplements as well as its interaction with the metal ions result the plaque causing a pro-oxidant effect that lead to increased chance of increase in fatal myocardial infarctions (Halliwell 2000). Vitamin E can be metabolized to form quinone derivatives which are toxic to cells, as they can produce oxygen radicals, which can oxidize lipids and proteins. Beta-carotene is the precursor of vitamin A and supplementation with beta-carotene increased cancer incidence in smokers (Penniston & Tanumihardjo, 2006). Lipoic acid is made from fatty acids and the its R-enantiomer have antioxidant activity, both in its oxidized and reduced forms, although the reduced form, dihydrolipoic acid, can also found to demonstrate a pro-oxidant effect (Bast & Haenen, 2002).

CONCLUSION

So, the chapter provided useful awareness that can be very helpful for depicting oxidative stress and free radicals that responsible for occurrence of many diseases. The antioxidants have a strong potential to be used as current conventional treatments of diseases such as inflammatory disease, neurodegenerative diseases, cancer, diabetes etc. These natural agents may reduce the risk of disease or slow down its progression by acting on the underlying cause of these diseases. So, a balanced diet (including plenty of fruit, vegetables, grains, oils and nuts) have adequate supplements of essential antioxidant such as vitamin A, E, C etc. that are sufficient to protect the body against many diseases despite of genetic and environmental factors, may make disease imminent mostly at any stage or in any specific genetic pool.

ACKNOWLEDGMENT

The author would like also to express cordial appreciation to Amity University Uttar Pradesh, Noida (INDIA).

REFERENCES

Adcocks, C., Collin, P., & Buttle, D. J. (2002). Catechins from Green tea (*Camellia sinensis*) inhibit bovine and human cartilage proteoglycan and Type II collagen degradation *in vitro. The Journal of Nutrition*, *132*(3), 341–346. doi:10.1093/jn/132.3.341 PMID:11880552

Alamanos, Y., Voulgari, P. V., & Drosos, A. A. (2005). Rheumatoid Arthritis in Southern Europe: Epidemiological, Clinical, Radiological and Genetic Considerations. *Current Rheumatology Reviews*, *1*(1), 33–36. doi:10.2174/1573397052954217

Bagchi, D., Bagchi, M., Stohs, S. J., Das, D. K., Ray, S. D., Kuszynski, C. A., ... Pruess, H. G. (2000). Free radicals and grape seed proanthocyanidin extract: Importance in human health and disease prevention. *Toxicol*, *148*(2-3), 187–197. doi:10.1016/S0300-483X(00)00210-9 PMID:10962138

Bast, A., & Haenen, R. M. M. (1998). Interplay between lipoic acid and glutathione in the protection against microsomal lipid peroxidation. *Biochimica et Biophysica Acta*, *963*(3), 558–561. doi:10.1016/0005-2760(88)90326-8 PMID:3143421

Bhathena, S. J., & Velasquez, M. T. (2002). Beneficial role of dietary phytoestrogens in obesity and diabetes. *The American Journal of Clinical Nutrition*, *76*(6), 1191–1201. doi:10.1093/ajcn/76.6.1191 PMID:12450882

De la Lastra, C. A., & Villegas, I. (2005). Resveratrol as an anti-inflammatory and anti-ageing agent: Mechanisms and clinical implications. *Molecular Nutrition & Food Research*, *49*(5), 405–430. doi:10.1002/mnfr.200500022 PMID:15832402

Esposito, E., Rotilio, D., Dimatteo, V., Digiulio, C., Cacchio, M., & Algeri, S. (2002). Di Matteo. V.; Di Giulio, C.; Cacchio, M.; Algeri, S. A. review of specific dietary antioxidants and the effects on biochemical mechanisms related to neurodegenerative processes. *Neurobiology of Aging*, *23*(5), 719–735. doi:10.1016/S0197-4580(02)00078-7 PMID:12392777

Ferrari, C. K. B., & Torres, E. A. F. S. (2003). Biochemical pharmacology of functional foods and prevention of chronic diseases of ageing. *Biomedicine and Pharmacotherapy*, *57*(5-6), 251–260. doi:10.1016/S0753-3322(03)00032-5 PMID:12888262

Halliwell, B. (1994). Free Radicals, Antioxidants, and Human Disease: Curiosity, Cause, or Consequence? *Lancet*, *344*(8924), 721–724. doi:10.1016/S0140-6736(94)92211-X PMID:7915779

Jacob, R. A. (1995). The Integrated Antioxidant System. *Nutrition Research (New York, N.Y.)*, *15*(5), 755–766. doi:10.1016/0271-5317(95)00041-G

Langseth, L. (1993). From the Editor: Antioxidants and Diseases of the Brain. Antioxidant Vitamins Newsletter, 4, 3-5.

Marambaud, P., Zhao, H., & Davies, P. (2005). Resveratrol promotes clearance of Alzheimer's disease Amyloid-β peptides. *The Journal of Biological Chemistry*, *280*(45), 37377–37382. doi:10.1074/jbc.M508246200 PMID:16162502

Matés, J. M., Pérez-Gómez, C., Núñez, I., & De Castro, I. N. (1999). Antioxidant enzymes and human diseases. *Clinical Biochemistry*, *32*(8), 595–603. doi:10.1016/S0009-9120(99)00075-2 PMID:10638941

McAlindon, T., & Felson, D. T. (1997). Nutrition risk factors for Osteoarthritis. *Annals of the Rheumatic Diseases*, *56*(7), 397–402. doi:10.1136/ard.56.7.397 PMID:9485998

Nishino, H., Murakoshi, M., Ii, T., Takemura, M., Kuchide, M., Kanazawa, M., ... Jinno, K. (2002). Carotenoids in cancer chemoprevention. *Cancer and Metastasis Reviews*, *21*(3/4), 257–264. doi:10.1023/A:1021206826750 PMID:12549764

Packer, L. (1998). Alpha-Lipoic acid: A metabolic antioxidant which regulates NF-kappa B signal transduction and protects against oxidative injury. *Drug Metabolism Reviews*, *30*(2), 245–275. doi:10.3109/03602539808996311 PMID:9606603

Penniston, K. L., & Tanumihardjo, S. A. (2006). The acute and chronic toxic effects of vitamin A. *The American Journal of Clinical Nutrition*, *83*(2), 191–201. doi:10.1093/ajcn/83.2.191 PMID:16469975

Rice, M. E. (2000). Ascorbate regulation and its neuroprotective role in the rat brain. *Trends in Neurosciences*, *23*(5), 209–216. doi:10.1016/S0166-2236(99)01543-X PMID:10782126

Rohdewald, P. (2002). A review of the French maritime pine bark extract (Pycnogenol®), a herbal medication with a diverse clinical pharmacology. *International Journal of Clinical Pharmacology and Therapeutics*, *40*(04), 158–168. doi:10.5414/CPP40158 PMID:11996210

Sagara, M., Kanda, T., Jelekera, M. N., Teramoto, T., Armitage, L., Birt, N., ... Yamori, Y. (2004). Effects of Dietary Intake of Soy Protein and Isoflavones on Cardiovascular Disease Risk Factors in High Risk, Middle-Aged Men in Scotland. *Journal of the American College of Nutrition*, *23*(1), 85–91. doi:10.1080/07315724.2004.10719347 PMID:14963058

Sies, H., & Stahl, W. (1995). Vitamins E and C, beta carotene, and other carotenoids as antioxidants. *The American Journal of Clinical Nutrition*, *62*(6suppl), 1315S–1321S. doi:10.1093/ajcn/62.6.1315S PMID:7495226

Stephen, W. J. (2008). Variable Isoflavone Contents of Red Clover Products Affect Intestinal Disposition of Biochanin A, Formononetin, Genistein and Daidzein. *Journal of Alternative and Complementary Medicine (New York, N.Y.)*, *14*(3), 287–297. doi:10.1089/acm.2007.0617 PMID:18370585

Surh, Y.-J. (2003). Cancer Chemoprevention with Dietary Phytochemicals. *National Review*, *3*(10), 768–780. doi:10.1038/nrc1189 PMID:14570043

Westcott, N. R., & Muir, A. D. (2003). Flax seed lignan in disease prevention and health promotion. *Phytochemistry Reviews*, *2*(3), 401–407. doi:10.1023/B:PHYT.0000046174.97809.b6

Section 9
Biochemic and Lactoserum

Chapter 14
Biochemic System of Medicine:
Oldest Form of Nutraceutical Therapy

Srijan Goswami
Indian School of Complementary Therapy and Allied Sciences, India

Sagarika Mitra
Indian School of Complementary Therapy and Allied Sciences, India

Piyasee Paul
Institute of Genetic Engineering, India

Dipjyoti Dey
Indian School of Complementary Therapy and Allied Sciences, India

Sankalan Das
Institute of Genetic Engineering, India

ABSTRACT

The biochemic system of medicine, also known as the inorganic cell salt therapy, pioneered by Dr. Wilhelm Heinrich Schuessler, following the footsteps of Dr. Samuel Hahnemann, is the oldest form of nutraceutical therapy approved and recognized by the World Health Organization as one of the complementary therapies. The chapter presents the fundamental ideology and concepts that underlies the promising system of biochemic medicine as concisely, simply, and to-the-point as possible. The chapter begins with a brief introduction to biochemic system, nutrition science, and concepts of nutraceuticals, followed by a brief history and literature review. It covers biochemic system of medicine and its relevant concepts before closing the chapter with a conclusion.

DOI: 10.4018/978-1-5225-3267-5.ch014

INTRODUCTION

If we could give every individual the right amount of nourishment, not too little and not too much, we would have found the safest way to health. (Hippocrates, n.d.)

The author begins the chapter with the quote, said numerous times by the great Father of Medicine, Hippocrates himself in his scholarly works are appropriate and points out to one of the fundamental aspect that makes the foundation of Biochemic System of Medicine.

The system of medicine using simple inorganic cell salts as medicinal substances for preventing, treating, curing and managing diverse range of both acute and chronic health conditions are completely based on natural laws of biochemistry. Biochemistry is the study of chemical reactions and pathways essential for maintaining healthy life. The system of treatment with inorganic cell salts is approved by World Health Organization and are recognized by several Medical Councils worldwide. According to this system of treatment there are only 12 major natural inorganic components that can prevent and heal almost all types of diseases totally based on the natural laws of cure. Human body is composed several types of inorganic salts and each of them performs specific functions that are crucial for maintaining life and health. Among all the types of inorganic salts, the 12 most abundant and fundamental inorganic salts are mainly used as medicines in this system. There are no side effects of these medicines because the twelve inorganic salts are actually the natural chemical components that makes up the body and are available in nature. Diseases can be cured completely by administering a very small amount of inorganic cell salts in adequate concentration and potency, for a limited period of time. This medicines are suitable for newborns to old age persons. The Biochemic System of Medicine was proved and introduced by Dr. Wilhelm Heinrich Schuessler in the year 1973. According to Dr. Schuessler, when a cell gets all the nutrients and salts that are necessary for performing their regular biochemical activities, the cell stays healthy and no disease can take over the cell, but if somehow there occurs deficiency of the required amount of nutrients or inorganic salts, the cells fails to perform their normal biochemical processes and functions, thus becomes weak and the disease takes over. So somehow if one can maintain or restore the nutrient and salt requirements of the cell, no diseases can take over. Dr. Schuessler explained in his research and the authors quote;

The relationship between the blood and the body is same as that of soil and plant. It is common phenomena that poor exhausted soil will produce only weak, sickly plants. In the same way poor blood lacking its essential constituents will produce disease prone and weak sickly bodies. By enriching the soil, the sick plants can be made to recover and flourish. The recovery of ailing human body can be achieved by a similar process that is by restoring to the blood the constituent in which it is lacking. (Schuessler, n.d.)

The term Nutraceutical also known as Functional Foods, may be new to the world but the underlying concept of treatment using natural products as medicines are very old practice in the history of medical sciences. The term Nutraceutical is composed of two fundamental words,

1. The first one being Nutrition
2. The second one being Pharmaceutical.

The term can be generalized as the use and implementation of nutritional substances found in nature, that are generally acquired though food, as a pharmaceutical substances. As reported by Dr. Tomislav Mestrovic in the year 2015, the term Nutraceuticals was given by Dr. Stephen L De Felice, The founder and chairman of Foundation for Innovation in Medicine, New Jersey, USA. According to Dr. Stephen L De Felice, a Nutraceutical is any substance that is a food or a part of food and provides medical or health benefits, including the prevention and treatment of diseases. Dr. Tomislav Mestrovic in his same article also reported that Nutraceutical is a broad term that connects basic nutritional sciences with core medical practices. These are the food substances containing extra-medicinal value along with their normal nutritional values. Application of Nutraceuticals can be classified as a complementary therapy that can be implemented for maintaining proper health, prevent susceptibility to a disease and cure ailments by filling up the deficiency of the required nutrient by administering it in the perfect size, amount and duration.

This chapter is intended to make medical researchers, students, healthcare practitioners, educators and scientific community aware of the fact that the idea of implementation of Inorganic Salts as medicinal substance using the umbrella term of Nutraceuticals is not new, but a very old medical practice that were kept suppressed for obvious reasons which the authors presented in the chapter. The chapter contains a brief historical review of how pharmaceutical industries suppresses and regulates the medical science research and evidences and completely tries to keep people unaware about the reality of promising simple curative practices. The authors also tried to present the vast field of Biochemic System of Medicine in a concise manner, for easy understanding of the reader. It is not possible to put forth everything about a system of medicine in just one chapter, this chapter provides only the fundamental idea about Biochemic System of Medicine, but the authors tried to keep the concepts simple and to the point as possible.

HISTORICAL BACKGROUND AND REVIEW OF LITERATURE

The greatest medicine of all is teaching people how not to need it. (Hippocrates, n.d.)

At this point the reader must be wondering about the relevance of the above quote with the present chapter. The authors are involved in studying the effectivity of Biochemic System of Medicine in treating diverse array of both chronic and acute disorders since about past five years. But according to the authors writing the literature review section and searching for the latest references of the research work on this promising system of medicine was much more difficult task than curing a patient.

Medical education system and modern healthcare sector are being run under the illusion that they are made for treatment of patients and eradication of serious diseases, but in reality it is designed to operate in a completely biased manner promoting only those medical systems that will generate more and more money at the end of the day. Modern healthcare system are not at all concerned about curing the sick but instead committed on generating permanent customers (Angell, 2005).

It is shocking to see that Biochemic System of Medicine, even after being approved by the World Health Organization for education, treatment and research, there are no such mainstream medical colleges or institutions that teaches Biochemic Medicine System as they teach Conventional Medicine, nor do they encourage students to take the subject as a career and most of the students of biochemistry have no idea that a medicine system like Biochemic Medicine exists, the organizations and institutions do not fund for research to be done on this system of medicine because the funding comes from the pharmaceutical companies themselves. The positive findings and evidences on the effectivity of the Biochemic cell salts and allied complementary therapies like Homoeopathy, Ayurveda, Pranayama, Acupressure etc. are not allowed to be published in the mainstream medical journals or literatures, and are discarded during the review processes because almost all the reputed medical journals are funded, controlled and regulated by pharmaceutical industries directly or indirectly, so they are not allowed to publish anything that might demolish their castle of lies. In one hand the conventional researchers are telling the researchers of complementary therapies to put forth latest research evidences, reviews and citations and on the other hand they kept all the doors closed for the researchers of complementary therapies to perform their research effectively, on purpose (Null, 2010).

History is always written by the winners. When two cultures clash, the loser is obliterated, and the winner writes the history books – books which glorify their own cause and disparage the conquered foe. As Napoleon once said, What is History but a Fable Agreed up on? (Dan Brown. n.d.)

During the five years of their study the authors observed many interesting incidences and one of them is a girl of about 25 years of age gets Measles. As everybody knows that measles is a viral disease and the only way of treating them as per conventional system of medicines are combination of several costly blood tests for detection, followed by prescription of antipyretic drugs, antibiotics, antivirals, side effect suppressing drugs and vitamin supplements and the list goes on. Fortunately the patient in this case was one of the student researching about the effectivity of the Biochemic medicine, took a combination of cell salts namely Ferrum Phosphate 6X, Kalium Muraticum 6X and Kalium Sulphuricum 6X, three tablets three times daily with mild warm water and took complete bed rest to see for herself that does Biochemic Cell salts really works or not, and surprisingly she got cured within 15 days and there were no side effects. If the disease really needed antibiotics and all, then the condition of the patient should have gone worse without the conventional treatment. This is an evidence that Biochemic system of medicine works and much better and faster than conventional treatment.

Another incidence is one of the author had conjunctivitis, and to see for himself whether the cell salts are actually effective against the condition or not, he took Ferrum Phosphoricum 6X, 3 tablets after every 30 minutes with mild warm water. The conjunctivitis got cured within 3 to 4 hours of taking the cell salt and with no side effects. This is where their faith strengthened.

The third incidence was when one of the author got Influenza, which according to conventional medical science is a viral disease and for curing, antipyretic drugs, antivirals and antibiotics are needed. But the condition got cured in about 3 days and without any side effects and without post influenza debility. The author took combination of Ferrum Phosphoricum 6X, Kalium Muraticum 6X, Kalium Sulphuricum 6X, Natrum Muraticum 6X and Natrum Sulphuricum 6X, commercially available as Biocombination 11, 4 tablets, 4 times daily for 2 days with warm water. The fever got aggravated at first few hours followed by slow, steady and complete decline of fever. This is also an evidence that the medicine system is effective and there is no doubt about that.

The authors started studying and observing the effectivity of Biochemic system of medicine seriously after reading several articles about how unscientific and baseless the complementary therapies are and specially going through the statement made by C. E. Cook, Commissioner of Public Health, in Western Australia's Government Gazette of April 12, 1946 and the authors quote;

The following report is issued under section 210 of the Health Act, 1911-1944. It is claimed that the Dr. Schuessler's Cell Salts, Kali Phos. 3X is, indicated in loss of mental power, brain fog, paralysis of any part, nervous headaches, neuralgic pains, general disability and exhaustion and sleeplessness from nervous disorders. The "remedy" has been analyzed and been found to contain potassium dihydrogen phosphate and lactose. The actual quantity of potassium dihydrogen phosphate in the "adult dose" is so minute that over 9,000 tablets would be necessary to give the minimum medicinal dose of this drug. Lactose is a sugar which is of no value in the treatment of any of the above-mentioned maladies. Dr. Schuessler's Cell Salts can therefore have no curative value. They will bring about no improvement in any of the illnesses for which they are said to be indicated. Any expenditure on the purchase of these salts will be money wasted. (Cook, 1946)

But in the above scenarios the authors used 6X potencies, which is considered higher dose as compared to 3X. But still the cell salts worked. It is evident that the statements made by C. E. Cook was totally biased and was based on reductionist idealism.

Biochemic System of Medicine functions on the two distinct principles:

- First, filling up the deficiency of the cell salts.
- Second, Principle of Hormesis.

Hormesis is a phenomena of drug action, it states that when the physiological concentration of a drug decreases, its disease curative properties increases consequently there stays no possibility of adverse drug reactions and above all does not cause dependency of the drug, if required to be administered multiple times. This is very old concept, it is the fundamental mode of action of homoeopathic and biochemic cell salts, banned or omitted from the syllabus of conventional medical and pharmaceutical sciences. A great scientist and Professor B. M. Hegde, wrote in his book titled What Doctors Don't Get to Study in Medical School about the science of Hormesis and the author quotes;

Hormesis is a very important concept in science, but had been killed in its bud by powerful people controlling scientific research. (Hegde, 2014)

Biochemic medicine or treatment system based strictly on the principles of biochemistry was a great breakthrough for mankind. A simple, easily available, inexpensive yet extremely effective form of treatment that actually possess the ability to cure diseases from their root. The ideology of treatment of disease with inorganic cell salts was so simple and in accordance with well-known principles and laws of nature. In year 1832 Dr. George Carey, MD found the following written in Stapf's Archiv:

All essential component parts of human body are great remedies. (Carey, 1832)

And in the same journal, in the year 1846 they found a writing that states:

All constituents of human body act on such organs principally where they have function.

Dr. W. H. Schuessler, of Oldenburg, Germany, developed these suggestions and made the idea anticipated in the above writings the basis of the new system for treatment. In March 1873, in an article entitled: A Shortened Homoeopathic Therapeutics, published in Leipzig Homoeopathic Gazette, Dr. Schuessler narrated his thoughts as follows and authors quotes:

About a year ago I intended to find out by experiments on the sick if it were not possible to heal them, provided their diseases were curable at all, with substances that are natural, i.e., physiological function remedies. (Schuessler, 1873)

As published in one of the writings of Dr. George Carey, the original conversation between Dr. Schuessler and the German journal was translated into English by H. C. G. Luyties, and first published in the Homoeopathic news and later appeared in a small edition by Dr. Constantine Hering, on the Twelve Tissue Remedies, "recommended for investigation". Dr. Boericke and Dewey published a book titled "Twelve Tissue Remedies."

Nutraceuticals is the modern terminology given to the use of nutrient substances as a medical drug. But this is a very old medical practice. As The Father of Medicine, The Great Greek Physician Hippocrates once quoted Let Food Be Your Medicine. And several years later a German Medical Doctor, Dr. Wilhelm Heinrich Schuessler published his work on natural remedies. According to Dr. Schuessler regular nutritional substances available in nature and in the body can be used for maintaining proper health, prevent susceptibility to a disease and cure ailments by filling up the deficiency of the required nutrient by administering it in the perfect size, amount and duration. These great personalities gave the foundation and evidences of the effectivity of Nutritional Therapy or using nutritional substances as medicine for curing diseases. Today medical sciences have evolved a lot and have wide range of sophisticated technologies available for implementing those ideas in a standard and effective manner.

BIOCHEMIC SYSTEM OF MEDICINE AND ITS RELEVENT CONCEPTS

Blood: A Fluid Crucial in Maintaining Health

Blood is a connective tissue. It is one of the means of communication between the cells of different parts of the body and the external environment. The major functions of blood are:

- **Exchange of Gases**: It carries Oxygen from the lungs to the different tissues and carbon dioxide from different tissues to the lungs.
- **Transportation of Nutrients**: It carries nutrients from the alimentary tract to the tissues and cell wastes from the tissues to the excretory organs.
- **Transportation of Hormones**: The hormones secreted by endocrine glands to their target tissues.
- **Thermoregulation**: It regulates temperature by transporting heat generated in the active tissues to other less active tissues.
- **Immune Response:** Transporting protective substances to the area of infection.
- **Protection from Injury**: Accumulation of clotting factors that coagulate blood, minimizing its loss from ruptured blood vessels.

Blood is crucial for maintaining homeostasis, thus contributing in maintaining healthy state of the body. The blood regulates and controls homeostasis by maintaining a sound equilibrium between the following parameters namely Fluid Balance, Temperature Balance, Glucose Balance, Amino acid Balance, Fatty acid Balance, Vitamin and Mineral Balance, Enzyme Balance, pH Balance, Electrolyte Balance and Oxygen-Carbon dioxide Balance. Blood covers about 7% of the body weight. Blood in blood vessels are always in motion. This continuous flow maintains a constant environment for the body cells thus contributing to overall homeostasis.

The Concept of Nutrition and Disease Prevention, Cure and Management: An Overview

Each of the substances of a man's diet acts upon his body and changes it in some way and upon these changes his whole life depends. (Hippocrates, n.d.)

Human body absorbs its nutrients from food materials found in nature. Food substances after being digested, the nutritional substances present in the digested food material, those are essential for the body gets absorbed through the lining of the digestive tract into the blood, and the blood transports the nutrient substances to various parts of the body. The nutrient substances present in blood are taken up by the cells in the amount and form required and excess nutrients and waste substances are excreted from the system. The nutrients or nutritional substances enters each and every cells through pores present in the outer membrane of the cells. In healthy person these pores are of normal size and nutrient substances can enter the cell easily through the pores. But in case of disease or illness or stress the cells becomes weak and their pore size gets altered drastically. As a result the cells becomes unable to take up the nutrient substances directly from digested food materials, as the size of nutritional substance is much larger as compared to the pores of the cells under stress. So even after the presence of nutrients in the circulating blood, the cells of the body could not take up the nutrient derived from food and gradually becomes weaker and weaker. Resulting in deterioration of cellular structure and functionality. This is one of the major cause of nutritional deficiency even after having a balanced diet.

In these cases just providing the patient with nutritional food substances available in the nature directly will not solve the issue. One have to first restore the functionality and structural stability of the cells to its normal form, and when the cells are healthy, they will be able to take up the nutritional substances of their own.

So for restoration of the cellular stability, one need to potentize the nutritional substances found in food. Potentization will amplify the penetration or migration capability of the nutrient substance. Smaller the size of the substance, more it possess the ability for deep action. As soon as the diseased cells finds the smaller nutrient particles in the cell cytoplasm, the internal normal signal transduction pathways gets triggered. Which in turn gradually restores the cells to health. At this point the cells have fully functional metabolic reactions occurring inside it and have the normal healthy pores, and can readily take up the nutrient components from the digested food materials. But it should be kept in mind that long term use of potentized nutritional products may lead to dependency of that substance. So proper expertise and experience is required while administering the nutritional substances in potentized form. It should be determined according to the level of consciousness, constitution and physical status of the patient. The doses should be started with the suitable smallest nutrient particle and gradually increasing the size of the nutritional particle as the cells or tissue recovers and ultimately stop the use of the medicine when the tissues or cells acquires the ability to take up nutrients naturally.

MODE OF ACTION OF BIOCHEMIC MEDICINE

Biochemic System of Medicine and Homoeopathy are two totally separate ideologies but the convergence of the two system gave promising results. Homoeopathy follows the philosophy of *Similia Similibus Curentur* while the Biochemic Medicine is totally based on the underlying principles of biochemistry and follows the philosophy of treating the disease by the *filling up the deficiency* of the inorganic salts. But Hormesis is the fundamental principle behind the mode of action of both the systems.

Since a long time, researchers knew the chemical composition of every body fluid, but these knowledge were not practically implemented for the treatment of the sick until the introduction and development of the science of biochemistry. Before biochemistry became the mainstream science none of the doctors at that time knew with any degree of certainty, the course of action of the drugs they used to administer. Biochemic principles are not a philosophy or hypothesis, it is a well-established science. The food and drink consumed, reaches the stomach, and the air breathed into the lungs furnish all the materials of which the body is made of. The food is dissolved with the help of chemicals released by stomach, liver and pancreas and the essential nutrient particles gets absorbed and gets mixed with the blood. The blood supplies the materials necessary for forming every tissue and fluid in the body and for carrying forward every process (Carey, 1893).

Blood contains organic and inorganic substances. The organic substances are carbohydrates, lipids, proteins, nucleic acids etc. The inorganic substances are water, inorganic salts, vitamins etc. Although inorganic salts are present in small amount but they are the crucial components of the body. Inorganic salts can be viewed as the workers of the body, and uses water and organic substances for building and maintaining the normal structure and function of cells. Inorganic salts controls and regulates each and every biochemical pathways occurring in the body that plays a critical role in maintaining homeostasis. When a deficiency occurs in one or more of these inorganic cell salts, the homeostasis of the body gets disturbed dynamically. This dynamic disturbance in homeostasis are termed as disease, and they are named and classified according to the body parts or organs they manifest. For example diseases that manifests heart are called cardiac diseases, those that manifests lungs are known as pulmonary diseases and so on. But these names of the diseases are up to no good when it comes to treating and curing diseases and restoring the health, because the organs are not isolated or discrete systems because human body works in a nonlinear fashion in any situation. Linear systems do not work in the human body. Every disease that affects one's body is due to the deficiency of one or more of these tissue salts in one's blood (Carey, 1893).

According to Dr. George Carey, the health and strength can be maintained only so long as the system is properly supplied with these inorganic salts. Dr. Carey in his research findings also stated that,

Disease is not a thing, animate or inanimate, but a condition due to lack of some inorganic constituent of blood. Thus the justifiable method of curing the disease

completely based on the natural laws of cure is to provide the inorganic salt that are deficient in the blood. For treating a disease and restoring the health, administering some chemical component that is not a natural component of one's body and that are not a substance that occurs in nature but are synthesized industrially are unnecessary and irrelevant.

The Biochemic system of medicine investigates what is lacking in the body that are disturbing the equilibrium of the homeostasis and administering it just in the form and amount needed. According to Dr. Carey as published in his research findings that, any disturbance in the molecular motion of these cell salts in living tissues constituting disease can be rectified and the requisite equilibrium is reestablished by administering the same mineral salts in small quantities. The idea of system of medicine based on the principles of biochemistry, was established by Dr. Schuessler, and proved that the treatment procedure is purely scientific and is based on natural laws and facts of physiological chemistry and allied sciences.

It is the blood that contains the material essential for every tissue, and supplies nutrient to every organs of the body, helping it to perform their normal functions. The constituent of the blood gets absorbed into the surrounding tissue through the capillary walls, and the required material gets transported to the desired location in the body guided by the signalling mechanism of brain. For building a cell two kinds of components are required, that should be present in blood, namely the organic and inorganic components. The major organic components are carbohydrates, lipids, amino acids, nucleic acids etc. while the inorganic parts are water, calcium, sodium, potassium, magnesium, iron, phosphorous, silica etc. So whenever new cells needs to be formed these organic and inorganic components must be present in blood in sufficient quantity and form. The signalling pathways that governs the developmental and maintenance processes of an organism are strictly regulated by the inorganic salts present in blood. So any disturbance in their quality and quantity during development will lead to developmental and functional derangements of the body, and thus causing disease condition.

Cells are not fed, they feed themselves. Each and every cells possesses their own consciousness, which is derived through evolution. Each and every cells can think and act on their own. As published in the Lecture 14, of the research article, Virchow stated that:

The absorption of matter into the interior of the cells is unquestionably an act of the cells themselves, for we are as yet acquainted with no method enabling us to produce this kind of proliferation in the body, by any mode of experimentation, through the medium of an agency, primarily affecting either the nerves or the vessels.

Virchow also stated in his Lecture 13 that:

Every special function possesses its special elementary cellular organs; every mode of conduction finds paths distinctly traced out for it.

Drugs administered based on the Biochemic system of treatment stimulates the natural self-healing powers of the body and thus enable the system to defeat disease in a natural manner. After the selection and administration of the appropriate remedy in proper potency and dose, it is the duty of the physician to observe the patient carefully in order that one may correctly note and intelligently and reasonably interpret the changes that occurs, for upon these changes in the patient's condition, as revealed by the symptoms, depend the subsequent action in the further treatment of the case under consideration.

The ideal cure or ideal curative procedures are those that restores health rapidly, gently, permanently, possess ability to remove and destroy whole disease in shortest, surest, least harmful way, without causing any drug dependency and are clearly based on natural laws of healing. (Hahnemann, Para 2, Organon)

The first thing to be determined is whether the remedy has acted at all or not. In deciding the question whether the remedy has acted or not, the physician must be careful not to be misled by the opinions or prejudices of the patients or his attendants. Dr. James Tyler Kent and Dr. Constantine Hering, postulated certain interpretations for the situations arising after the first prescription commonly known as Kent's 12 observations and Hering's Law of Direction of Cure, respectively. These postulates are the proven standards for the second prescription as well as planning the management strategy. After administration of a remedy, there could be one of the following reactions which are elaborated in a simple manner in the Table 1.

Hering's Law of Direction of Cure

We must turn to nature itself, to the observations of the body in health and in disease to learn the truth. (Hippocrates, n.d.)

The Natural Laws of Cure was postulated by a Great German Doctor, Constantine Hering, known to the world as the Father of American Homoeopathy in 1830s. The laws are termed as Hering's Laws of the Direction of Cure, which are actually the systematic and logical explanation of how a body responds and tries to eliminate the disease causing agent from the system. Based on his lifelong research and practice

Table 1. Dr. James Tyler Kent's Observations for studying drug action

S. No	Dr. J. T. Kent's Observation	Interpretation	Comment	Intervention
Pattern 1	A prolonged aggravation and final decline of the patient.	The case is incurable. The condition had reached advanced irreversible pathology.	Advanced and irreversible pathologic changes acting as an obstruction to recovery.	Usage of very low or moderately low potency is indicated for providing symptomatic relief.
Pattern 2	Long aggravation but final and slow improvement.	Early stage of the disease having minor tissue change in some organs.	Pathological changes are in early reversible stage.	It is advised to observe the improvement. Do not repeat the medicine.
Pattern 3	Aggravation is quick, short, and strong with rapid improvement of the patient.	The remedy and potency selection are correct.	No irreversible or any structural changes in vital organs.	It is advised to stop the medication. And observe till the improvement takes place.
Pattern 4	No aggravation but steady improvement.	Assessment and potency selection is very good.	No tissue change or tendency of tissue changes.	This is the sign of an ideal cure. At this point it is advised to follow Hering's Law of Cure.
Pattern 5	A brief amelioration first, followed by aggravation.	The medicine acted as palliative.	The case may be incurable.	The case needs a fresh review. In eventuality of incurability, it is advised to use low potencies.
Pattern 6	A short aggravation followed by a very short lasting amelioration	Precarious state, some vital organs having advanced structural changes.	Advanced pathology interfering with the drug action.	Lower potency of the medicine is suggested and patient should be treated with caution.
Pattern 7	Rapid amelioration of the symptoms yet no special relief of the patient.	Excellent palliative action.	If the drug administered completely matched with total symptoms, then the case may be incurable, having latent, advanced or organic changes. Or If the drug administered partially matched the collective symptoms, it acted as palliative.	It is advised to observe the changes in signs and symptoms, it is better to use low potencies at this stage.
Pattern 8	Appearance of new symptoms with every remedy	Idiosyncratic, oversensitive patient, proves every remedy given.	These oversensitive patients often have a low vitality and are incurable.	In this case it is advised to use medication with caution.
Pattern 9	New symptoms appear without appearance of old symptoms	Action of medicine on healthy provers	If the symptom belongs to drug pathogenesis, then the remedy needs to be corrected. Or New symptoms do not belong to drug pathogenesis, the drug symptoms may be missed while proving.	No medication should be administered. The subject is sensitive to drugs and can be a good provers.
Pattern 10	New symptoms appearing after remedy.	Once a new symptom pass away, patient settles down to original state without any improvement.	The prescription is unfavorable	The cased needs fresh review for finding the correct remedy.
Pattern 11	Old symptoms reappear	Patient is on the path of recovery, when symptoms are disappearing in the reverse order of their appearance.	Case is showing a classical recovery.	When old symptoms comes back and disappears, the medication should be stopped immediately. The progress in healing should be observed carefully. If the old symptoms come back to stay, repetition of the dose is necessary.
Pattern 12	Symptoms takes wrong direction	Disease is transferred from circumference to center.	Medicine administered is wrong.	Immediate antidote of the remedy is advised.

of medicine he observed and documented certain specific patterns followed by the body's defense mechanism for curing and healing certain disease.

In a patient who have received the appropriate remedy for certain chronic case, during the period of healing the old symptoms that have been suppressed as a result of faulty medications reappears, though in an attenuated form and shows a tendency to disappear of their own accord. According to Dr. Hering, as he observed based on his studies, no true cure ever took place which does not followed the laws of cure. Dr. Hering published all this research findings on his scholarity works. According to the studies performed by Dr. Hering, the cure takes place only if the symptoms disappear from the directions, above to downwards, inside to outwards, center to periphery, from more vital organs to organs of less priority and in the reverse order of their appearance (Chauhan & Gupta, 2015).

Human body possess its own healing mechanisms and knows how to heal itself, sometimes all it needs an extra push to function efficiently. Whatever may be the system of medicine, be it modern medicine or alternative, if the remedy is appropriate then the curative process will be considered ideal if and only if it strictly follows the Natural Laws of Direction of Cure (Hering, 1845). In 1845, Dr. Constantine Hering published in the preface of the first American edition of Hahnemann's *Chronic Diseases* an extract of an essay *which was never published elsewhere*, called "Guide to the Progressive Development of Homoeopathy" (Saine, 1988). In this essay, Dr. Hering describes that, it was observed and documented by several physicians that ideal curative processes in diseases always takes place from *above downward* and from *within outward* directions. This is the reason why chronic diseases, if they are thoroughly cured, *always* terminates in some cutaneous eruption, which differs according to the different constitutions of the patients. The thorough cure of a widely ramified chronic disease in the organism is indicated by the most important organs being relieved first; *the affection passes off in the order in which the organs had been affected*, the more important being relieved first, the less important next, and the skin last (Saine, 1988). That means body's natural healing mechanism always tends to transfer the disease from organs of high priority to the organs of less priority. This law of order which Dr. Hering have pointed out, accounts for numerous cutaneous eruptions consequent upon homeopathic treatment, even where they never had been seen before (Hering, 1845).

According to the observations documented by Dr. Hahnemann, Dr. Kent, Dr. Hering and Dr. Schuessler and others no true cure ever took place which does not follow this law of cure. The cure takes place only if the symptoms disappear from above-downwards, inside-outwards, Centre to periphery, from more important to less important organs and in the reverse order of their appearance.

THE FUNDAMENTAL TWELVE INORGANIC CELL SALTS

In order to obtain most satisfactory results from Biochemic system of Medicine one should first become familiar with each of the tissue salts individually. A knowledge of the properties and the area and mode of action will be found invaluable when the symptom of any given case are considered. The following section contains a brief idea about the importance of the twelve tissue salts, and for detailed knowledge about the cell salts it is advised to consult Biochemic Materia Medica and Biochemic Practice of Medicine:

1. **Calcarea Fluorica or Calcium Fluoride (Calc Flour):** It gives tissues the quality of elasticity. It combines with the organic substances such as albumin to form elastic tissue and is found in the walls of blood vessels, in muscular tissues in connective tissues, in the surface of bones and in enamel of teeth. Its deficiency results in a loss of elasticity and consequent relaxed condition. Its main function is preservation of contractile power of elastic tissues. Whenever the symptoms are traceable to relaxed condition, for example, relaxed condition of veins and arteries, sluggish circulation, piles, tendency to cracks on skin, this tissue salt is needed. It is also useful in the treatment of diseases affecting the surface of the bones and joint and when teeth becomes loose in their socket and decay rapidly. The elasticity of muscular tissue and supporting membranes becomes impaired when this tissue salt is deficient, resulting in muscular weakness, bearing down pains etc. The symptoms are generally worse in humid condition and are relieved by massage and warmth (Boericke, 1901).
2. **Calcarea Phosphorica or Calcium Phosphate (Calc Phos):** It is a tissue salt concerned with nutrition. It combines with albumin and is indicated when there are albuminous discharges. Without Calcarea Phosphorica there could be no blood coagulation. It will assist the action of a more directly indicated tissue salts and thus produce more rapid results. It promotes healthy cellular activity and restores tone to weakened organs and tissues. It aids in normal growth and development and should be given in cases of backwardness more particularly where there is bone weakness or recurring tooth troubles. It is the Biochemic remedy for rickets. Calcarea Phosphorica is a constituent of saliva and gastric juices. It assists in digestion and assimilation and favors the building up of a sturdy, robust constitution. The restorative power of this inorganic salts will speed up recovery and replenish the body's reserves of strength. It is the tissue salt for weak blood and condition associated with weak and imperfect circulation. It is a great restorative remedy (Boericke, 1901).

3. **Calcarea Sulphurica or Calcium Sulphate (Calc Sulph):** It is the blood purifier and restorer. It is found in the liver where it helps in the removal of waste products from the blood stream and it has a cleansing and purifying influence throughout the system. It cleans out the accumulation of non-functional organic matter in the tissues and causes infiltrated parts to discharge their contents readily, throwing off decaying organic matter, so that it may not lie dormant or slowly decay and thus injure the surrounding tissues. This inorganic salt is indicated in conditions arising from impurities in the blood stream. It supplements the action of Kalium Muraticum in the treatment of catarrh, acne etc. and it should always be given when pimples occur in adolescence. It checks the weakening drain of suppuration too long continued for example, abscess and wounds which will not heal readily and tend to become septic. If taken in early stage, it prevents a sore throat from developing and in the same way it will often cut short a threatening cold. The symptoms are generally worse after getting wet and are better in a warm, dry atmosphere (Boericke, 1901).
4. **Ferrum Phosphorica or Ferrum Phosphate (Ferrum Phos):** It is considered as biochemic first aid. It is the carrier of oxygen and also an important component of haemoglobin. It helps in carrying oxygen from lungs to all the other parts of the body. It provides strength and toughness to the walls of the blood vessels. It is a great remedy for feverish conditions. Bleeding from wounds, cuts and abrasions can be controlled with a little powdered Ferrum Phosphate applied directly to the injured parts. It should also be thought of as a first aid in cases of muscular strains and sprains etc. (Boericke, 1901).
5. **Kalium Muraticum or Potassium Chloride (Kali Mur):** It is a remedy for phlegmatic conditions. Deficiency of this salt renders fibrin nonfunctional. It complements the action of Calcarea Sulphurica as both are concerned with cleansing and purifying blood. It is suitable for second stages of inflammation. The inorganic salt is concerned with the production of saliva and is therefore important in the early stages of digestion. With Natrum Muraticum it is utilized in the production of hydrochloric acid and is thus an essential link in the process of digestion. This tissue salt is useful as a first aid for treatment of burns (Boericke, 1901).
6. **Kalium Phosphoricum or Potassium Phosphate (Kali Phos):** It is a constituent of nerves and nervous system. Deficiency of this salt causes disruption in the nerve signaling processes thus resulting in neurodegenerative conditions. There may be fretfulness, ill humor, bashfulness, laziness and similar indications. It is the remedy for nervous headaches, nervous dyspepsia, sleeplessness, depression, weariness, low vitality, and several other conditions. It covers all those ailments caused by nervous issues (Boericke, 1901).

7. **Kalium Sulphurica or Potassium Sulphate (Kali Sulph):** It works with Ferrum Phosphate as oxygen carrier. It assists in exchange of oxygen from the blood stream to the tissue cells thereby completing the respiratory processes initiated by Ferrum Phosphate. Internal breathing of tissues depends upon Kalium Sulphurica, external breathing is the function of Ferrum Phosphate, if the exchange of gases in the lungs is designated in this manner. It is beneficial on respiration and is indicated in those cases where there is a feeling of stuffiness or desire for cool air. It is also considered as an anti-friction salt, ensuring the smooth working of all organs thus acting as a lubricant. This inorganic salt is indicated where there is a sticky yellowish discharge from skin and mucous membrane. Eruptions on the skin and scalp, with scaling, calls for this remedy. Chilliness, shifting or moving pain are some other striking indications. It is very useful in cases of stomach derangements and in inflammatory condition for promoting perspiration. (Boericke, 1901)
8. **Magnesia Phosphorica or Magnesium Phosphate (Mag Phos):** It is known as anti-spasmodic remedy. Its main function is in nervous system where it supplements the action of Kalium Phosphorica. When a deficiency of Magnesium Phosphate occurs the white nerve fibers contract causing spasms and cramps. This tissue salt is vital to muscular tissues. It quickly relieves pain especially of cramping, shooting, and spasmodic nature. It is indicated for nerve pains such as neuralgia, neuritis, sciatica headaches etc. this inorganic salt is indicated in cases of muscular twitching, cramps, hiccups, convulsive fits, menstrual pains etc. It acts on every kind of pain. The doses are to be taken in frequent intervals with warm water (Boericke, 1901).
9. **Natrum Muraticum or Sodium Chloride (Natrum Mur):** It is the tissue salt that regulates water balance. It enters into the composition of every fluid and solid of the body. Because of its strong affinity for water it controls and regulates the electrolyte balance and flow of the body fluids. Its prime function is to maintain the moisture equilibrium in the body. In absence of this tissue salt cell division and normal growth could not proceed. It is closely associated with nutrition, glandular functioning and bodily secretions which play such an important part of the physiological processes. Excessive moisture or excessive dryness in any part of the system is a clear indication of the deficiency of the mineral salt. An important function of this cell salt is production of hydrochloric acid, so imbalance in the cell salt concentration will result in faulty secretion of the acid and thus causing illness (Boericke, 1901).
10. **Natrum Phosphorica or Sodium Phosphate (Natrum Phos):** It is an acid neutralizer. It is the basic remedy for wide group of diseases arising from an

acid condition of the blood. This tissue salt is also of importance for its action on digestive organs. The assimilation of fats and other nutrient is dependent on the action of this remedy. A deficiency of this mineral in blood allows uric acid to form salts which becomes deposited around the joints and tissues and giving rise to stiffness and swelling and other painful symptoms like that of rheumatism. This salt is indicated whenever symptoms of acidity are present, highly colored urine, golden yellow or creamy coating at the root of the tongue, intestinal worms etc. (Boericke, 1901).

11. **Natrum Sulphurica or Sodium Sulphate (Natrum Sulph):** It regulates the density of the intercellular fluids by eliminating excess water. This tissue salt largely controls the healthy functioning of the liver, it ensures an adequate supply of free flowing, healthy bile essential for several stages of digestion. The removal of toxic metabolic products which are the normal result of the chemical exchange constantly taking place in the tissue cells, is brought about by the action of this particular inorganic salts. If conditions arise which allow this toxic fluids to accumulate in the blood stream and tissues, may lead to self-poisoning. This inorganic salt ensures the disposal of these toxic fluids and its importance in the healing of rheumatic complaints is self-evident. This salt is indicated in the healing of diseases affecting the liver, presence of sandy substance in urine, greenish brown coating on tongue and marked bitter taste of mouth are few of the guiding symptoms. It is the principal remedy in the treatment of influenza. It treats complaints aggravated by humidity (Boericke, 1901).
12. **Silecea or Silica Oxide (Sil):** This salt is categorized as cleanser and eliminator. It is a deep acting remedy and is also known as Surgeon's Knife. It helps the body to eliminate nonfunctional organic matter from the body system. It initiates the healing process by promoting suppurations and breaking up pathological accumulations. This inorganic salt is a constituent of hair, skins, nails and surfaces of the bones. It also acts as in the manner of insulator for the nerves. In conditions of checked perspiration, this inorganic salt restores the activity of the skin, thereby aiding this important cleansing process. It is the Biochemic remedy for offensive perspiration of the feet and armpits. Silecea is indicated in cases of pus formation or threatened suppuration. It is promising in the cases of tonsillitis associated with pus formation, brittle nails etc. This particular mineral salt should be used with caution. This salt should not be given to people having medical implants in their body. For example people with implanted pacemaker or steel plates on bones etc. Since this salt is an eliminator it may try to eliminate the foreign object present in the body (Boericke, 1901).

THE 28 TYPES OF BIOCOMBINATIONS

Based on the tissue affinity and symptoms these twelve cell salts have been combined in 28 different combinations. Each combination works on specific set of symptoms or a specific conditions these are termed as Bio combination. But it is advised that the physician must prepare the biocombinations themselves based on the constitution of the patient. Table 2 describes some of the readily and commercially available biocombinations.

SELECTING THE APPROPRIATE CELL SALTS

Just as the food causes chronic disease, it can be the most powerful cure. (Hippocrates, n.d.)

People often thinks that symptomatic relief means cure. All the medications and treatment procedures implemented by the modern medicine stated that they provides symptomatic relief. One need to understand the fact that symptoms are not disease. It's the modern medicine system that presents symptoms as diseases, which is scientifically not true. And just keeping the symptoms palliated can never cure the underlying problem. Symptoms are actually the body's response to certain stress. They are normal physiological responses that the body naturally meant to exert to evade the agent causing the stress and also provide protection to the body from further damage. Sometimes there comes a situation where those normal physiological responses need to be regulated so that it does not cause any harm to the patient. The best way to deal with the situation is to investigate and point out the reason(s) which triggered the symptom. If the physician can identify the body's need, deficiency of which resulted in the stress and if that particular component is administered to the patient in adequate potency, will restore the normal functioning of the components of the body. As soon as the deficiency of the component is replenished the body starts recovering and symptoms are cured. And when it is seen that body started recovering all the medications should be stopped and the natural healing systems of the body should be allowed to take over. But instead what conventional or modern medicine does is prescribe drugs that acts by suppressing the symptoms or body's response to stress and thus providing instant but short lasting palliation to the patient. They points out the symptoms and charges medicines that by all means will block the signal transduction pathways that is triggering the stress response instead of identifying and filling up the deficiency that lead the body to trigger the stress call. As long as the drug substance is active in the patient's blood stream, that particular

Table 2. List of 28 commercially available Biocombinations, their ingredients and indications

Combination Name	Disease	Cell Salt Composition	Indication
Biocombination 1	Anemia	Calcarea Phosphorica Ferrum Phosphorica Natrum Muraticum Kalium Phosphoricum	Lack of blood, unhealthy conditions, general wasting of tissues, waxy appearance of skin, neurasthenia, mental depression, worry, physical exhaustion, weakness, poor digestion.
Biocombination 2	Asthma	Kalium Phosphoricum Magnesia Phosphoricum Natrum Muraticum Natrum Sulphuricum	Bronchial asthma, humid asthma, dyspnea on exertion, dry tickling cough, spasmodic cough, whooping cough, gasping, irregular pulse.
Biocombination 3	Colic	Kalium Phosphoricum Magnesia Phosphoricum Calcarea Phosphoricum Natrum Sulphuricum Ferrum Phosphoricum	Flatulent colic, colic due to inflammatory conditions, colic in children during teething or due to flatulence or constipation, spasmodic pains.
Biocombination 4	Constipation	Calcarea Phosphoricum Calcarea Flouricum Kalium Muraticum Natrum Muraticum Silecea	Bowels constipated, dry, hard, stool, dull headache, foul breath, coated-tongue.
Biocombination 5	Coryza	Ferrum Phosphoricum Kalium Muraticum Natrum Muraticum Kalium Sulphuricum	Inflammatory, febrile catarrhal condition, Coryza with dull headache, sneezing, watery discharge. Continuous thick white discharge from the nose.
Biocombination 6	Cough, Cold & Catarrh	Ferrum Phosphoricum Kalium Muraticum Magnesia Phosphoricum Natrum Muraticum Natrum Sulphuricum	Indicated in acute inflammatory febrile catarrhal conditions of cough, cold, headache.
Biocombination 7	Diabetes	Calcarea Phosphoricum Ferrum Phosphoricum Kalium Phosphoricum Natrum Phosphoricum Natrum Sulphuricum	It is indicated to relieve many conditions associated with diabetes. It helps better assimilation of glucose. Impaired kidney liver functions are improved.
Biocombination 8	Diarrhoea	Natrum Phosphoricum Calcarea Phosphoricum Ferrum Phosphoricum Kalium Phosphoricum Kalium Sulphuricum Natrum Sulphuricum	Diarrhea during dentition thin watery, greenish stool, foul with undigested food. Stool with blood or yellow, loose morning stools which at times is involuntary while passing flatus.
Biocombination 9	Dysentery	Ferrum Phosphoricum Kalium Muraticum Kalium Phosphoricum Magnesia Phosphoricum	Dysentery with mucus and blood.
Biocombination 10	Enlarged Tonsils	Calcarea Phosphoricum Ferrum Phosphoricum Kalium Muraticum	Inflamed tonsils, follicular tonsillitis painful with white coating or greyish white patches on tongue or tonsils, bad breath with loss or lowered appetite.
Biocombination 11	Pyrexia	Ferrum Phosphoricum Kalium Muraticum Kalium Sulphuricum Natrum Muraticum Natrum Sulphuricum	Inflammatory conditions, chill generally covers all mild febrile conditions.
Biocombination 12	Headache	Ferrum Phosphoricum Kalium Phosphoricum Magnesia Phosphoricum Natrum Muraticum	Headache due to sun-heat, over-exertion, headache of students, vertigo, throbbing headache, nervous headache as a consequence to worries, sleeplessness and sluggish liver functions.
Biocombination 13	Leucorrhoea	Calcarea Sulphuricum Calcarea Phosphoricum Kalium Phosphoricum Kalium Sulphuricum Natrum Muraticum	Discharge like white of eggs, acrid and watery. Indicated for general weakness of young girls with or without functional neuroses.

continued on following page

Table 2. Continued

Combination Name	Disease	Cell Salt Composition	Indication
Biocombination 14	Measles	Ferrum Phosphoricum Kalium Muraticum Kalium Sulphuricum	Sneezing and thin discharge from nose, eyes watery, throbbing headache, cough and fever.
Biocombination 15	Menstrual Troubles	Calcarea Phosphoricum Ferrum Phosphoricum Kalium Phosphoricum Kalium Sulphuricum Magnesia Phosphoricum	Irregular menses, bright red if early, dark red if late, scanty in young girls, excessive in elder women, painful menstruation.
Biocombination 16	Nervous Exhaustion	Calcarea Phosphoricum Ferrum Phosphoricum Kalium Phosphoricum Magnesia Phosphoricum Natrum Muraticum	Lassitude, depression, nervousness, irritability, hysteric behavior, loss of or impaired memory, confusion, sleeplessness, psychosomatic illnesses.
Biocombination 17	Hemorrhoids	Calcarea Flouricum Ferrum Phosphoricum Kalium Muraticum Calcarea Phosphoricum	Bleeding hemorrhoids, fissures, backache, it helps in all kinds of piles.
Biocombination 18	Pyorrhea	Calcarea Flouricum Calcarea Sulphuricum Silecea	Gum boil, unnatural looseness of the teeth, with or without pain, toothache, gums sensitive to cold, abscess at root of teeth, spongy bleeding gums, pus in gums and foul breath.
Biocombination 19	Rheumatism	Calcarea Phosphoricum Ferrum Phosphoricum Kalium Sulphuricum Magnesia Phosphoricum Natrum Sulphuricum	Articular and muscular rheumatism inflammatory and febrile complaints, stiff neck, rheumatic pain in shoulders, shifting, wandering pains, twitching, cramps, writers and players cramps, cracking of joints, lumbago and sciatica.
Biocombination 20	Skin Diseases	Calcarea Fluorica Calcarea Sulphurica Kalium Sulphurica Natrum Muraticum Natrum Sulphurica	Acne, cracks, whitlow, eczema, eruptions on the scalp, seborrhea, psoriasis, herpes.
Biocombination 21	Teething Troubles	Calcarea Phosphorica Ferrum Phosphorica	Tardy dentition and troubles; cuts teeth easy, appetite and digestion are improved; builds the body.
Biocombination 22	Scrofula	Calcarea Phosphorica Ferrum Phosphorica Kalium Muraticum Silecea	It almost covers all symptoms of both dry and suppurating scrupulous glandular abscesses.
Biocombination 23	Toothache	Calcarea Fluorica Ferrum Phosphorica Kalium Muraticum Kalium Phosphorica Silecea	Neuralgic pain or toothache due to unnatural loosing of teeth. Gums bleeding, swelling. Strengthening teeth in their sockets.
Biocombination 24	5 Phos Tonic	Calcarea Phosphorica Ferrum Phosphorica Kalium Phosphorica Magnesia Phosphorica Natrum Phosphorica	The combined phosphates promote tissue building and provides the necessary nutrition to nerves, brain and bones. A general tonic for all chronically wasting diseases, anemia, general debility and exhaustion with lack of vitality.
Biocombination 25	Acidity, Flatulence, Indigestion.	Natrum Phosphorica Natrum Sulphurica Silecea	Gastric disturbances, hyperacidity. Sour eructation, flatulence, flatulent colic dyspepsia, bilious vomiting, heart burn and jaundice.
Biocombination 26	Easy Parturition	Calcarea Fluorica Calcarea Phosphorica Kalium Phosphorica Magnesia Phosphorica	Relieves labor pain and easy delivery. Covers non-specific lower abdomen pain during pregnancy and anxiety states.
Biocombination 27	Lack of vitality	Calcarea Phosphorica Kalium Phosphorica Natrum Sulphurica	Symptoms suggestive of impotence, depression of sexual instinct, lassitude, general debility, quick emission followed by trembling weakness and nervousness.
Biocombination 28	General Tonic	All 12 Biochemic Salts	Helpful in consumption, debilitating diseases, for convalescents. It builds up entire system by providing necessary tissue nutrition, improves resistance to diseases, and helps better utilization of food.

stress response system stays inactivated, and during that point of time if a disease causing agent enters the patient's body, then there will be no active stress response system to protect the body.

The Biochemic cell salts are always selected on the basis of totality of symptoms. Since this is a personalized form of treatment, the idea of conventional reductionism does not apply here. The method and guidelines for selecting the cell salts deficient in the body are given by Dr. Hahnemann, Dr. Schuessler, Dr. Kent, and Dr. Hering in their books and research articles but fundamental principle underlying them remained the same. According to them, symptoms are the body's warning signals. They are the indicators which if carefully observed will tell the remedy required. Symptoms occurs in a variety of forms such as pain, inflammation etc. and their nature and location determines the particular cell salt that are deficient. After the case taking is complete, the next step in selecting the remedy is to compare them with the guiding symptoms and characteristic indications of each of these tissue remedies. It will become evident from the diagnosis that there is one remedy which corresponds most closely to the case for which treatment is required, that tissue salt is known as the Principal remedy.

Other remedies may also be indicated known as supplementary remedy. Each cell salt has its own characteristic symptoms. For example the characteristic symptom of Ferrum phosphate is inflammation while that of Magnesium phosphate is spasms and both contains pain etc. these key symptoms are readily recognized and give a sure led to the treatment called for any given case. Dr. Gold in one of his article mentioned that the key to success in Biochemic system of treatment lies in the accurate linking of the symptom with its appropriate tissue salts. Thorough knowledge and understanding of the metabolic or signal transduction pathways and importance of the inorganic salts in control and regulation of homeostasis is extremely essential for a Biochemic physician.

THE CONCEPT OF POTENCY SCALE

Dr. Samuel Hahnemann, in his attempt to reduce the adverse drug reaction, reduced the dose of the remedy by serially diluting it to a certain range. This is how he discovered the technique of potentization which in today's date known as Hormesis. The crude drugs were documented to act on the living organism in three ways:

1. Mechanical
2. Chemical
3. Dynamic

The process of potentization removes the mechanical and chemical aspect but restores the dynamic properties of the drug. Potentization is a process which reduces the crude drug substances but increases the qualitative, medicinal or therapeutic property of the drug. Potency is the unit of drug strength. In the preparation of potencies generally following three scales are used, but the first one is mainly used in case of Biochemic Medicines. They are as follows:

1. The Decimal Scale, introduced by Dr. C. Hering
2. The Centesimal scale, introduced by Dr. Hahnemann
3. The Fifty Millesimal Scale, introduced by Dr. Hahnemann

Biochemic tissue salts are potentized based on the Decimal Scale. It has a 1:10 ratio and it is prepared in the following manner.

One part of pure inorganic salt is added to 9 parts of sugar of milk and it should be thoroughly mixed in a mortar pestle for uniform distribution. This is the first decimal potency of the cell salt. It is described as for example Ferrum Phos 1X.

The alphabet X denotes the potency scale being used, in this case it denotes Decimal scale, and for denoting Centesimal scale the alphabet C is used.

Similarly if one part of 1X Ferrum Phos is mixed with 9 parts of sugar of milk, the potency thus produced is 2X and so on.

In cases inorganic cell salts are prepared in liquid form in such cases;

One drop of crude extract or mother tincture of the inorganic salt is added to nine parts of water and alcohol mixture. This liquid is then successed ten times in its bottle by firmly hitting the bottle's base against the firm surface. This dilution is called 1X potency.

Here 1 refers to first dilution and Roman numeral X represents the potency scale used.

One part of this 1X potency is again diluted and successed in 9 parts of a water and alcohol mixture to produce a 2X remedy.

It is to be noted that there is no difference between Biochemic 1X potency and Homoeopathic 1X potency. For example, Ferrum Phos 1X in the form of Biochemic tablets and Ferrum Phos 1X of Homoeopathic dilution are same in the mode of action and functionality.

CONSEQUENCES OF LONG TERM USE OF BIOCHEMIC SALTS

Everything in excess is opposed to nature. (Hippocrates, n.d.)

Biochemic cell salts are itself not harmful agents but long term use of any substance leads to its dependency. And the same is also true for Biochemic Cell salts. Cells of our body is supposed to acquire nutrients or mineral salts directly from the food source found in nature. These nutrients enters our cells through pores present in the outer membranes of the cells. These pores have a definite size and shape under healthy condition and thus allows the nutrient particle of appropriate size to enter. And cell requires to provide certain amount of energy to keep the pores open in that way. In cases when the cell is weak and infested with disease its function and structure deteriorates and thus resulting in reduced pore size. Now in this situations the nutrients are provided in the form that could readily enter through the weakened pores of the cell so that the cells could restore its normal structure and function. So when the cell becomes completely healthy and their pore size is restored to normal then the medication should be stopped immediately because the cells of the body may get used to and adapt or modify itself based the availability, size and concentration. At this point the cells have fully functional metabolic reactions occurring inside it and have the normal healthy pores, and can readily take up the nutrient components from the digested food materials. Long term use of potentized nutritional products may lead to dependency of that substance. So proper expertise and experience is required while administering the nutritional substances in potentized form. It should be determined according to the level of consciousness and physical status of the patient. The doses should be started with the suitable smallest nutrient particle and gradually increasing the size of the nutritional particle as the cells or tissue recovers and stop the use of the medicine when the tissues or cells acquires the ability to take up nutrients naturally.

FUTURE PROSPECTS AND CHALLENGES

The first major problem of Biochemic therapy is that the lack of professionally trained Biochemic practitioners who can take on the education, research and treatment based on biochemistry further. The students and researchers studying biochemistry are not aware that such medical system exists other than modern medicine and are approved by WHO. Homoeopaths sometimes use Biochemic tissue salts but in most cases they are not aware the promising capabilities of these simple tissue salts. So proper education and systematic training and research is required in the field of Biochemic System of Medicine.

There are wide diversity of ideologies for treating diseases in this world but they are grouped under two separate categories. The first one being the term modern medicine commonly known to the world as Allopathic Medicine, and the all other medicine system that differed with the ideology of Allopathic form of treatment was given the name of Alternative or Complementary system of medicine. Now comes the question who and on what basis the Allopathic or Systemic form of treatment got classified as modern and mainstream medicine and rest of the treatment ideologies that contradicted with allopathic point of view got classified as Alternative Therapies? Mother Nature did not made this distinction but was forcefully made by practitioners of allopathic medicine with the support of higher authorities many years earlier, especially during the time when Dr. Samuel Hahnemann introduced Homoeopathy. They were aware of the fact that allopathic form of treatment does not cures any disease because that system of medicine was designed to work against the natural laws of healing. Thus it only palliates and suppresses the body's normal physiologic reaction to certain stress and creates an illusion to the patient that his or her disease has been cured, but in reality all it does is suppress the physiological response by the mechanical action of drug. Sadly this distinction was not at all made on the basis of effectivity and disease curing capability of medicine system but it was completely based on which medicine system will generate more money every year. If modern medicine really cured diseases then for example Diabetics would not have to stay dependent on more and more medicines till the rest of their life.

Leave your drugs in chemist's pot if you can heal the patient with food. (Hippocrates, n.d.)

Physicians of Modern Medicine worldwide takes the Hippocratic Oath before receiving their title but very few of them actually keeps that promise they made to themselves and to the patients in the field of service. Patients comes to the doctors in their deepest darkest times, when they are helpless and desperate. They comes to the doctors believing that the doctor will cure his disease and will save his life. The patient considers the doctors equivalent to God. But what they are actually doing is making the patient dependent on more and more drugs till the rest of their life in the illusion of curing the disease. The practitioners of modern medicine ridicules the vital force theory proposed by Dr. Hahnemann saying that it is a pseudoscience. But in reality what Dr. Samuel Hahnemann designated as The Vital Force, in today's date after development of biochemistry it can be related to Homeostasis of the body or collective interdependency and coordination of numerous biochemical reactions working together in our body for maintaining what we call life and health. Allopathic practitioners knew this concept very well and this is why they ridicule this theory in defense so that people does not become aware of the potential that the natural system of medicines possesses over allopathic practices in curing both acute and chronic conditions permanently. Same kind of situation happened when Gregor Mendel discovered the principles of heredity and named the components involved as Factors, the scientific community at that time ridiculed his findings but several years later after evolution of the science of microscopy it was accepted that the findings of Mendel was true and the Factors in reality are Genes or Chromosomes. The theory got accepted because it did not interfere with the image of mainstream medicine. But the case of Vital Force theory and Homeostasis is different, it will lead to the rise of the Alternative therapies over so called mainstream therapies.

The mainstream medicine is acknowledging that their ideology of treatment has drawbacks. And with the completion of Human Genome Project and several Genomics and Proteomics research it was proved what modern medicine was trying to hide all these time. These discoveries proved that One Drug Fits All approach followed by mainstream medicine does not cures disease at all, instead it suppresses and palliates the complaints and converts the disease from superficial to much deeper state. The idea of personalized treatment and treatment with natural product is not the ideology they invented, they just coined and defined the terminologies like Personalized Medicine or Nutraceuticals etc. These ideologies existed since long time and all these time these forms of treatment were ridiculed and was tagged as non-scientific or as a pseudoscience until in modern days they found the ways to implement those practices under their own terms. Trying to overcome the drawbacks faced by modern medicine with the integration of ideas from alternative therapies is a good thing. But the major concern are the natural therapies that already are very cheap, easily available and easily affordable and does not possesses any side effects, when these will be manufactured under large industries and will be sold and controlled like pharmaceutical product, will result in exponential rise in its cost and lots of people will not be able to afford it. The best solution is to educate people and make them aware about the alternative natural therapies approved by World Health Organization for treatment purposes and make the systematic and harmonic use of several medical practices. Mainstream medicine should be implemented once the natural system of treatments have failed. This will protect the patient of unnecessary toxic effects of the drug materials of synthetic medicine because the great Hippocrates himself told that *natural forces within us are the true healers of the diseases.* Last but not the least, it is evident that the biochemic system of medicine strictly follows and satisfies the postulates and treatise of great Hippocrates in relation to art of medicine and curing of diseases much more than conventional system of medicine does. So Biochemic system of medicine and the practitioners of biochemic system should be given the position and honour they deserve for the service to the mankind and for following the path shown by the great Father of Medicine himself in serving those who are sick.

Wherever the art of medicine is loved, there is also a love for humanity. (Hippocrates, n.d.)

REFERENCES

Abramson, J. (2008). *Overdosed America: The Broken Promise of American Medicine (P.S)*. Harper Perennial.

Angell, M. (2005). *The Truth about The Drug Companies: How they Deceive Us and What To Do About It*. Random House Publisher.

Boericke, W. (1901). *Pocket Manual of Homeopathic Materia Medica*. Retrieved from http://www.materiamedica.info/en/materia-medica/william-boericke/index

Boericke, W. (1927). Pocket manual of homoeopathic materia medica: comprising the characteristic and guiding symptoms of all remedies (clinical and pathogenetic). Santa Rosa, CA: Academic Press.

Carey, G. W. (1894). *Biochemic System of Medicine*. The Theory, Pathological Action, Therapeutical Application, MateriaMedica, and Repertory of Schuessler's Twelve Tissue Remedies.

Cassels, A., & Moyninan, R. (2005). *Selling Sickness: How Drug Companies Are Turning Us All into Patients*. Orion Publishing Group.

Glidden, P. (2010). The MD Emperor has No Clothes. Academic Press.

Goswami, S. (2017). *Proteomics in Personalized Medicine: An Evolution Not a Revolution. In Applying big Data Analytics in Bioinformatics & Medicine*. IGI Global.

Gyorgyi, A. S. (1960). Introduction to a Submolecular Biology. Academic Press.

Hegde, B. M. (2014). What Doctors Don't Get to Study. In *Medical School* (4th ed.). Paras Medical Publisher.

Hering, C. (1836). Preface to the first American edition. In the Organon of Homeopathic Medicine. New York: William Radde.

Hering, C. (1879). *The Guiding Symptoms of our MateriaMedica, V(1).* Philadelphia: The American Publishing Society.

Kent, J. T. (1929). *Lectures on Homeopathic Philosophy* (2nd ed.). Chicago: Ehrhart & Karl.

Ludwig, E. (1943). *The Hippocratic Oath: Test, Translation and Interpretation.* Baltimore, MD: John Hopkins Press.

New York Health Department. (1932). *Practical Homeopathic Therapeutics.* New York: Oxford University Press.

Schuessler, W. H. (2013). *The Biochemic Handbook. An introduction to the cellular therapy and practical application of the twelve tissue cell salts in accordance with the Biochemic system of Medicine.* Retrieved from http://www.campbellmgold.com

ADDITIONAL READING

Abramson, J. (2008). *Overdosed America: The Broken Promise of American Medicine (P.S).* Harper Perennial.

Angell, M. (2005). *The Truth about The Drug Companies: How they Deceive Us and What To Do About It.* Random House Publisher.

Bollinger, (2016). *The Truth About Cancer: What you need to know about cancer's History, Treatment and Prevention.* Hey House Inc.

Geriatric Medicine. (2017).An Evidence-Based Approach (4th Ed.), Available from: https://www.researchgate.net/publication/245662227_Geriatric_Medicine_An_Evidence-Based_Approach_4th_Ed [accessed Oct 08 2017].

Guyton, A., & Hall, J. (2009). *Biochemistry. Human Metabolism in Health and Disease. Textbook of Medical Physiology. Elsevier Saunders* (11th ed.). Wiley.

Hahnemann, S. (1982). *Organon of Medicine.* Germany: The Hahnemann Foundation.

Molony, E., (2014), Ageing and Cancer: A Complex Relationship. *4th Year Cancer Council Australia.*

Null, G. (2010). *Death by Medicine*. Axios Press. DVD Ed.

Owen, D. (2007). *Principles and Practice of Homoeopathy. The therapeutic and Healing Process*. London: Elsevier.

Roberts, H. A. (1942). *The Principles and Art of Cure by Homeopathy* (2nd Rev Ed.). Rustington: Health Science Press.

Ruesch, H. (1986). *Naked Empress or The Great Medical Fraud*. Civis Publications.

Chapter 15
Lactoserum:
As a Complete Nutraceutical

Charu Gupta
Amity University, India

Consuelo Pacheco
Universidad Nacional del Sur, Argentina

Dhan Prakash
Amity University, India

ABSTRACT

Lactoserum, a byproduct of cheese industry, is rich in nutrients, but it is discharged directly into the environment. It has many human applications that promise to be a complete nutraceutical for the future generations. It is of high nutritive value and its products can be used as functional ingredients in food and pharmaceutical applications and as nutrients in dietary and health foods. They contain full spectrum of amino acids including essential and branched-chain amino acids which are important in tissue growth and repair. The other biological activities of lactoserum are antibiotic, anti-cancer, anti-toxin, immune-enhancer, and prebiotic (growth enhancement of gut microflora such as bifidobacteria). Lactoserum can thus be used as nutraceutical in various products like infant formulas, food supplements, cheese spreads, sports bars, and beverages to meet a variety of health goals for people of all ages, including animal feed.

INTRODUCTION

Lactoserum is a by-product of cheese or casein in the dairy industry and contains usually high levels of lactose, low levels of nitrogenous compounds, protein, salts, lactic acid and small amounts of vitamins and minerals. It is obtained by following

DOI: 10.4018/978-1-5225-3267-5.ch015

acid, heat or rennet driven coagulation (Kargi, & Ozmihci., 2006). Lactoserum, also known as cheese whey, is an opaque liquid, greenish yellow in colour with total solid content ranging in 6-6.5% w/v and biochemical oxygen demand (BOD) of at least 30,000.

Cheese whey is usually produced all over the world according to the traditional protocols and in small scale through denaturation of whey proteins but it is chiefly generated from ovine whey in the Mediterranean basin. About 9 kgs of whey are usually produced from 1 kg of cheese production (Zafar & Owais, 2005). It is well known that cheese whey is rich in nutrients but it is discharged directly into the environment that constitutes significant loss of protein and energy source. The BOD of whey varies from 30,000 to 50,000 mg/g depending upon the wastage of milk in the whey (Mukhopadhyay, Talukdar, Chatterjee, & Guha, 2003). There are mainly two types of cheese whey (lactoserum): Sweet whey and Acid whey.

Sweet whey is produced by precipitation of casein by proteolytic enzymes such as chymosine and pepsin or microbial enzymes produced from *Mucor miehei* and *M. pusillus*. It comes from the production of cheddar, Swiss and Italian varieties of cheese. It contains approximately 93% water and 6.35% solids, with about 76% of the solids being lactose (Delfour Jolles, Alais, & Jolles, 1965).

Acid whey is produced by precipitation of caseins during cheese making. It comes from soft cheese with cottage cheese as a predominant product. Precipitation is achieved by acidification not above pH 5.1. Acid whey is rich in minerals due to solubilization of colloidal calcium phosphate of casein micelles that occurs concomitantly with acidification. Its composition is similar to sweet whey except that it has higher lactic acid and ash contents (Delfour Jolles, Alais, & Jolles, 1965).

The composition of cheese whey depends on various factors like source of cheese (bovine, caprine or ovine), composition of cheese (i.e. breed, stage of lactation, feeding regime and type of cheese), ratio of whey to milk (if milk or cream is added to whey prior to manufacturing cheese) and technological practices or the manufacturing procedure followed (i.e. heat temperature, ripening temperature, time, batch vs. continuous processes and possible use of ultrafiltration) (Ong & Shah, 2009).

MICROBIOLOGY OF LACTOSERUM

The predominating microflora in cheese whey are *Lactococcus lactis subsp. cremoris, L. lactis* subsp. *lactis, Lactobacillus helveticus, Streptococcus thermophilus, Enterococcus faecium, Leuconostoc mesenteroides, Leuconostoc pseudomesenteroides, Lactobacillus plantarum, Lactobacillus pentosus, Lactobacillus paracasei, Lactobacillus plantarum, Enterococcus faecalis,*

Pediococcus pentosaceus, Buttiauxella agrestis, Hafnia alvei, Escherichia coli (Rossetti, Carminati, Zago, & Giraffa., 2009).

Factors Influencing or Controlling the Microbial Community

The diversity of cheese-manufacturing protocols, ripening regimens, and composition makes Lactoserum (cheese whey) a complex subject microbiologically. Each individual cheese has its own unique microflora regardless of the starter or any deliberately added secondary ripening microorganisms (e.g., molds or yeasts). There are varieties of microorganism that can grow in or on cheese whey, but their presence is governed by chance. These nonstarters, non-deliberately added microbes are contaminants to milk, cheese or cheese whey. Thus, the contaminants that are found in any cheese whey results because the specific microbes happen to be in milk or on equipment, in air, or on humans that had direct contact with the milk or cheese. It is extremely difficult to interpret data on microbial content of cheese whey because of chance contamination (Rossetti, 2008).

In addition, the cheese environment plays a critical role in growth of microorganisms. Microorganisms that grow in cheese whey follow the same set of criteria (pH, moisture, salt, acidity/type of acid, redox potential, nutrient availability, competition, temperature, anaerobic/aerobic conditions) as in any food product. Two factors determine the microflora of cheese whey (Lactoserum): presence and survival of the microorganism and ability of the microorganism to grow (Rossetti, 2008). During cheese maturation, environmental conditions can change sufficiently to allow growth of initially inhibited contaminants, or conditions may become even more inhospitable. Thus cheese whey environment is dynamic (Jessup & Forde, 2008).

Methods Used to Quantify or Identify the Microbial Community in Lactoserum

Molecular techniques are used to determine the presence of individual species and strains of bacteria in cheese whey. The polymerase chain reaction (PCR) is a rapid procedure for *in vitro* enzymatic amplification of a defined segment of DNA. A unique oligo-nucleotide sequence (probe) is used specifically to identify the presence of DNA from particular bacteria in cheese whey. These tools are generally based on 16S ribosomal DNA sequences and exploit either hybridization or PCR techniques (Duthoit, Godon, & Montel, 2003).

Recently complete or partial genomes of various LAB and bifidobacteria have been determined that offer omics-based approaches to analyze the activity of the bacteria provided that the mechanisms of their action are known. Finally, fluorescent probes coupled to flow cytometry are used to monitor the physiological capacity of bacterial cells *in situ*. All these approaches can be used for the screening and selection of LAB, assessing their role in fermentation and flavor development in fermented products.

PCR-based approaches other than RAPD and AFLP have been used for molecular typing, such as amplified ribosomal DNA restriction analysis (ARDRA) (Delley & Germond., 2002), repetitive extragenic palindromic PCR (Rep-PCR) (Ventura, Meylan, & Zink, 2003), and triplicate arbitrary primed PCR (TAP-PCR), and have been shown to offer a high discriminatory power for the identification and differentiation of LAB.

For analyzing the viability of lactic acid bacteria, fluorescent techniques in combination with flow cytometry (FCM) offers a powerful tool to analyze a cell population at the single-cell level. Fluorescent probes including carboxy fluorescein diacetate, oxonol and propidium iodide are used to monitor the esterase activity, membrane potential, and membrane permeability of bile salt–stressed bifidobacteria (Ben Amor, Breeuwer, Verbaarschot, Rombouts, Akkermans, De Vos, & Abee, 2002). These physiological parameters serve as good indicators to assess viable, injured and dead cells.

LACTOSERUM AS NUTRACEUTICAL

Antibiotic Property

Lactoserum contains several unique components that possess some important antimicrobial and antiviral properties. They are immunoglobulins (Igs), lactoferrin (Lf), lactoperoxidase (Lp), glycomacropeptide GMP) and sphingolipids. All these compounds survive passage through the stomach and small intestine and exert their biological effects in the large intestine. The best-known whey components that provide antimicrobial action in the intestinal tract are the immunoglobulins. They fall into several subclasses like IgG, IgM and IgA. IgGs predominate in milk-derived sources such as whey. It comprises up to 1% of the total wt. of whey proteins. IgG binds the toxin produced by *Clostridium difficile* thereby reducing the deleterious effects of infection like diarrhea, dehydration and muscle aches. It is therefore being suggested that in the absence of antibiotics, fermented cheese whey can be used to treat diarrhea especially in rural areas where there may not be quick access to convectional antibiotics (Adetuyi, Olorunfemi, & Adebolu, 2009). GMP inhibits cholera toxin binding to receptors in the intestinal tract.

Lactoferrin, an iron binding protein, is a whey derived compound that possesses antibacterial properties. It sequesters iron from bacteria (Lonnerdal, 2009). Since pathogens in particular have high iron requirements for metabolism and growth, this property of lactoferrin makes it broadly antimicrobial in nature. Lactobacilli can utilize lactoferrin bound iron, thus allowig lactoferrin to both inhibit pathogenic bacteria and support the growth of lactobacilli (Baker & Baker, 2009).

Additionally, lactoferrin has been shown to possess important antiviral properties. It directly interacts with selected viral pathogens, inhibits virus replication and their ability to attach to colonic epithelial cells. Viral inhibition also results through immune modulation benefits of lactoferrin (Yen, Lin, Chong, Tsai, Shen, Lin, Su, Chen, & Chen, 2009).

Another whey derived protein with potent antimicrobial properties is lactoperoxidase (Lp). Lp catalyzes the oxidation of thiocyanate into hypothiocynate ion, which is a strong oxidizing agent. Hypothiocynate ions cause damage to bacterial cell membranes. This "Lp system" is also used as a milk-preservative system (Defaie, Sharieat, & Divsalar, 2010).

Whey derived phospholipids such as sphingolipids are metabolized in the GI tract and produce sphingosine and lysosphingomyelin. These compounds possess powerful bactericidal agents in vitro (Duan, 2005).

Anti-Cancer Property

Some whey components possess anticancer properties. The first are the sulphur containing amino-acids (cysteine and methionine) that are found in high levels in whey protein. Cysteine and methionine are utilized in glutathione synthesis. Glutathione is a substrate for two classes of enzymes that catalyze detoxification compounds and bind mutagens and carcinogens, facilitating their elimination from the body. Lactoferrin's ability to bind iron is another benefit in the area of colon cancer. They induce apoptosis in tumour cells and so are useful adjunct in colon cancer therapy (Commane, Hughes, Shortt, & Rowland, 2005).

Sphingomyelin, one of the most abundant whey derived sphingolipids, have potential to inhibit colon cancer. Sphingomyelins also regulate growth factor receptors, such as transforming growth factor beta family (TGF-β) (Huang, Chen, Lin, & Lin, 2011).

TGF-βs are a multifunctional family of growth factors that regulate cell growth in a variety of normal and tumour cells by suppressing proliferation, inducing differentiation and apoptosis. TGF-β passes out unaffected through the stomach and maintains bioactivity in colon by withstanding enzymatic proteolysis (Le, Yu, Ruan, Wang, Qi, Zhu… Wang, 2005).

Immune-Enhancer

IgGs, Lp and Lf concentrated from whey participates in host immunity. IgGs binds with bacterial toxins and lowers the bacterial load in the large bowel. Dietary Lp and Lf also play an important role in host immunity through their antibacterial action on pathogenic microorganisms. Thus using whey derived adjuncts shifts the balance of intestinal microflora and aids in immune enhancement. Calcium by virtue of its probiotic activity and influence on macrophages–neutrophils and other WBC subtypes are also classified as immune-modifying minerals (Mehra, Marnila, & Korhonen, 2006).

Lf provides immune modulation as it is a natural component of the human immune system. It is found in body's mucous substances including saliva (Puddu, Valenti, & Gessani, 2009).

TGFs are abundant in milk (1-2mg/L) and colostrum (20-40mg/L) and serves major role in GI integrity of new born animals. TGF-b2 resides locally near the tops of the intestinal villi, inhibits proliferation and signals neutrophils as a part of innate host immunity (Le, Yu, Ruan, Wang, Qi, Zhu… Wang, 2005).

Prebiotic Properties

There are some whey-derived carbohydrate components that possess prebiotic activity. Lactose support LAB (such as *Bifidobacteria* and *Lactobacilli*). Stallic acids (type of oligosaccharides that are commonly found in whey), are typically attached to proteins and have been shown to possess prebiotic properties. Besides, three other non-carbohydrate prebiotics from whey has also been found. The first is a protein called glycol-macropeptide (GMP). It is derived from the partial enzymatic breakdown of kappa-casein during cheese production. GMP supports the growth of bifidobacteria (Bruck, Redgrave, Tuohy, Lonnerdal, Graverholt, Hernell, & Gibson, 2006).

The second whey derived probiotic is lactoferrin (Lf) which supports the growth of bifidobacteria and lactobacilli. The third component with prebiotic potential is mineral, calcium in form of calcium phosphate. It selectively stimulates the growth of intestinal lactobacilli and decreases the severity of *Salmonella* infections in rats (Yen, Lin, Chong, Tsai, Shen, Lin…Chen, 2009).

NUTRITIONAL VALUE OF LACTOSERUM PROTEINS

The proteins present in lactoserum are considered to have the highest nutritional values of all food proteins. They contain all the amino acids required by humans, in the right proportions. Whey proteins are rich in branched chain amino acids, components that provide energy for people undergoing intense or prolonged periods of exercise and help prevent loss of body mass and muscle. They are also readily digestible and completely bio-available. Whey proteins supply additional nutritional benefits, for example, α-lactalbumin, the second most abundant whey protein, has a high content of the amino acid tryptophan, a precursor of the vitamin niacin (Somaye, Marzieh, & Lale, 2008).

The health and nutritional value of the components of lactoserum include high quality nutritional source of amino acids, supply additional nutritional benefits like α-lactalbumin, has a high content of the amino acid tryptophan (precursor of the vitamin niacin); leucine (branched-chain amino acid) that plays a critical role in insulin and glucose metabolism. The other components of lactoserum are immunoglobulins (Igs), lactoferrin (Lf), lactoperoxidase (Lp), glycomacropeptide GMP) and sphingolipids. The main advantage of all these compounds is that they can survive passage through the stomach and small intestine and exert their biological effects in the large intestine.

BIOLOGICAL PROPERTIES OF WHEY PROTEINS

Whey proteins have been reported to have one or more biological functions in food. The health and nutritional value of the components of whey include high quality nutritional source of amino acids; anti-microbial action; growth enhancement of beneficial gut microflora, such as bifidobacteria; immuno-enhancing properties; control of specific diseases, including cancer and antitoxin activity (Thomä-Worringer, Sørensen, & López-Fandiño, 2006). Lactoserum proteins are unique in their ability to optimize a number of aspects of the immune system, primarily by boosting glutathione (GSH) levels in various tissues. GSH, the centerpiece of the body's antioxidant defense system, protects cells against free radical damage, pollution, toxins, infection and UV exposure.

FUNCTIONAL PROPERTIES OF LACTOSERUM PROTEINS

Lactoserum (whey) proteins bring a wide range of valuable functional properties as food ingredients. They can modify some or all of the organoleptic, visual, hydration, surfactant, structural, textural and rheological properties of food, resulting in improved consumer acceptance of the food product. Lactoserum proteins in their native state are highly soluble in food and beverage systems and are used for applications such as whipping/foaming. They act at oil/water interfaces to form and stabilize emulsions. In their under-natured form, whey proteins have the ability to form rigid, heat-induced irreversible gels that hold water, fat and provide structural support. In addition, they play an important role in controlling the texture of many food products and are used to modify the rheological properties of foods (Alfaifi & Stathopoulos, 2010). There are numerous applications of whey protein:

Body Composition

Due to its high concentration of essential amino-acids (EAAs) and branched chain amino acids (BCAAs), lactoserum protein helps individuals to maintain muscle tissue. This can be particularly important for seniors, active individuals and those trying to maintain or lose weight.

Weight Management

Lactoserum protein can play an important role in weight management. Specific factors in whey protein are being investigated for their ability to promote weight loss by increasing satiety, influencing glucose homeostasis and maintaining lean body mass (Volpi, 2003).

Immunity

Lactoserum proteins are unique in their ability to optimize a number of aspects of the immune system, primarily by boosting glutathione (GSH) levels in various tissues. GSH, the centerpiece of the body's antioxidant defense system, protects cells against free radical damage, pollution, toxins, infection and UV exposure. GSH levels are typically depressed in individuals with cancer, HIV, chronic fatigue syndrome and other immune-compromising conditions. GSH also decreases with age and may be partially responsible for diseases such as Alzheimer's disease, cataracts, Parkinson's disease and arteriosclerosis, e.g. the concentration of immunoglobulins in bovine milk is 0.6-1.0 g/kg (Mehra, Marnila, & Korhonen, 2006). Thus, incorporating whey proteins into the diet may protect the health of not just those with a compromised immune system but those of all ages.

The specific components in lactoserum that are believed to play a role in enhancing the immune system are *Cysteine* – an amino acid found in high levels in whey proteins, is involved in the intracellular production of GSH (Liang, Du, & Chen, 2008).

Lactoferrin – has been shown to exhibit immune-modulating activity through both antimicrobial and antitoxin activity; it may also provide protection against viruses such as hepatitis, cytomegalovirus and influenza (Puddu, Valenti, & Gessani, 2009).

Immunoglobulins – may confer disease protection to infants through passive immunity and to adults by promoting the activity level of the immune system (Mehra, Marnila, & Korhonen, 2006).

Branched chain amino acids (BCAAs) – are metabolized in the muscle to manufacture glutamine, a precursor to GSH and another important component of the immune system (Calder, 2006).

Lactoserum Induces Cell Senescence

Peptides from water buffalo cheese whey induce senescence cell death in human colon adeno-carcinoma cell line through ceramide secretion. Milk proteins are a source of bioactive peptides. Recent studies have indicated that protein-derived peptides released in buffalo cheese acid whey exert a cyto-modulatory effect in human epithelial colon cancer ($CaCo_2$) cells (De Simone, Ferranti, Picariello, Scognamiglio, Dicitore, Addeo, Chianese, & Stiuso, 2010).

USE OF LACTOSERUM IN VALUE ADDED PRODUCTS

Lactoserum/Cheese whey is usually treated as a waste and discharged in nature without any treatment which creates pollution problems. However they can be used to obtain value added products as discussed below.

Ethanol

Cheese whey or whey-permeate has a relative cost advantage as a substrate for ethanol production. There have been some researches concerning the use of cheese whey fermentation to produce ethanol (Zafar & Owais, 2005). Whey proteins can be recovered by ultra- filtration leaving behind the milk lactose in permeates. This lactose can be converted into ethanol that can be used as a valuable fuel resource. The traditional *Saccharomyces cerevisiae* cannot be used to produce ethanol from cheese whey because the yeast lacks assimilatory mechanisms for lactose. New yeast strain *Kluyveromyces marxianus* (formerly *K. fragilis*) named as UFV-3 is used because of its high β-galactosidase activity. Its high β-galactosidase activity is also accompanied with high lactose permeate activity because the two genes LAC 4 and LAC 12, encoding β-galactosidase and lactose permease respectively, are contiguously placed on the chromosome and controlled by a common bi-directional promoter that responds to a same activator protein (Kargi & Ozmihci, 2006). Some other examples of lactose-fermenting yeasts are *Torula cremoris*, *Candida psudotropicalis* and *Candida kefir* (Agustriyanto & Fatmawati, 2009).

Cheddar cheese whey is ultra-filtered, with the retentate destined for whey protein concentrate (WPC) powders and permeate is used as a feedstock for the ethanol fermenters. Although food-grade ethanol can be converted into other products such as acetic acid, but most important use for ethanol is in gasoline blends.

Vinegar

Ethanol produced from whey can be used as a substrate for production of vinegar. *Acetobacter* and *Gluconobacter* species are used to convert alcohol to acetic acid. The pre-requirement for the process is that there must be a plentiful supply of oxygen (Parrondo, Garcia, & Diaz, 2009).

Wine

The production of wine from whey is a good way for its utilization. Straight whey wine, flavored whey wine, and whey wine blended with fruit or berry show promise for commercial development (Koutinas, Athanasiadis, Bekatorou, Psarianos, Kanellaki, Agouridis, & Blekas, 2007).

Whey Wines

Whey wines can be made from whey or it's permeates with a final alcohol content of about 2.25–14.0%. The alcohol content of wine derived from cheese whey is approximately 2.4%, assuming there is an efficiency of approximately 90% conversion of the lactose to ethanol (Koutinas, Athanasiadis, Bekatorou, Psarianos, Kanellaki, Agouridis, & Blekas, 2007).

Whey Champagne

Serwovit, whey champagne, is produced in Poland. The starting material is de-proteinated acid whey, sucrose and caramelized sugar, a dry yeast, fruit flavors and water. Caramelization of the lactose develops a flavor suggestive of dried malt. Yeast and fruit flavorings are added to the pasteurized base of whey, water and sugars. The mixture is bottled and the fermentation occurs in the bottle at 18°C in 8–12 h (Koutinas, Athanasiadis, Bekatorou, Psarianos, Kanellaki, Agouridis, & Blekas, 2007).

Whey Beers

A malted whey beer contains a maximum of 30% whey and is brewed with hops. Bottom-fermenting yeasts are used with this product. A whey malt beer is a sweeter beverage that contains a maximum of 50% whey and additional fermentable carbohydrates such as starch and glucose syrup. A whey-nutrient beer is weakly alcoholic. It is brewed from de-proteinated whey and hops and has a mineral mix added to it before fermentation. The product is pasteurized before bottling (Koutinas, Athanasiadis, Bekatorou, Psarianos, Kanellaki, Agouridis, & Blekas, 2007).

Other Fermented Beverages

Rivella has been a popular sparkling fermented whey beverage with an alpine herb flavor (Tranjan, Cruz, Walter, Faria, Bolini, Moura, & Carvalho, 2009). It is fermented de-proteinized whey that is condensed to a 7:1 concentration. It was first introduced in Switzerland in 1952. Flavors and sugar are added to the concentrate, and it is re-filtered, diluted to beverage strength, and carbonated before bottling.

Gefilus, available in Europe, is an apricot-peach flavored drink prepared by fermenting lactose hydrolyzed cheese whey with a patented strain of *Lactobacillus casei* subsp. *rhamnosum* (*Lactobacillus* GG or Gefilac). The whey drink contains 10^8 colony-forming units per milliliter of the strain GG. The drink is accepted by consumers who do not like traditional fermented dairy products (Tranjan, Cruz, Walter, Faria, Bolini, Moura, & Carvalho, 2009).

Single Cell Protein

Several categories of whey protein ingredients are commonly used in food and nutrition products, including whey powder, whey protein concentrate and whey protein isolate (Somaye, Marzieh, & Lale, 2008). The variation in composition is due to the difference in extent and method of processing.

Whey powder is produced by taking the whey directly from cheese production. It is then clarified, pasteurized and dried to provide a fine white powder known as whey powder.

Whey concentrate typically uses ultra-filtration membrane technology to filter or concentrate whey components based on the membrane pore size and/ or molecular wt. The fluid whey is allowed to pass through a semi-permeable membrane thereby removing lactose and ash and concentrating the protein content (Somaye, Marzieh, & Lale, 2008).

Whey protein isolate have a protein content of 90% or greater and is produced through a variety of processes like microfiltration and ion exchange. Microfiltration removes additional lactose and fat to increase protein concentration to up to 90% or higher. This process maintains the naturally occurring bioactive components in whey. Advanced chromatography technology can be used to further separate the individual protein components such as Lf and Lp from the main whey proteins (alpha-lactalbumin, beta-lactglobulin and bovine serum albumin). Advanced membrane technology is used for the enrichment of whey concentrate with whey bioactive components such as sphingolipids, Lf, Igs, GMP and TGF-betas (Le, Yu, Ruan, Wang, Qi, Zhu…Wang, 2005). The whey solids are used as concentrated whey for human and animal food, as rich source of proteins (Somaye, Marzieh, & Lale, 2008).

Whey proteins can be separated from the cheese milk permeate (native whey) prior to cheese manufacture by microfiltration (MF) that allows whey proteins to be further processed into value-added whey products such as a native whey protein concentrate as a liquid (Marcelo & Rizvi, 2008).

Whey is used in various products like infant formulas, food supplements, sport bars and beverages, to meet a variety of health goals for people of all ages (Anon, 2006). Whey proteins refer to a group of individual proteins or fractions that separate out from the casein during cheese-making. These fractions are purified to different concentrations, depending on the end composition desired, and can vary in their content of protein, lactose, carbohydrates, immunoglobulins, minerals and fat. Whey protein is a complete, high quality protein with a rich amino acid (AA) profile. It contains the full spectrum of amino acids (AAs) including essential AAs (EAAs) and branched-chain AAs (BCAAs) which are important in tissue growth and repair. Leucine is a key BCAA in protein synthesis and has recently been identified as playing a critical role in insulin and glucose metabolism. The EAAs and BCAAs in whey protein are not only present in higher concentrations than in other protein sources such as soy, corn and wheat; they are also efficiently absorbed and utilized (Thomä-Worringer, Sørensen, & López-Fandiño, 2006).

Culture Media

A low-cost alternative to nonfat dry milk or commercial bacteriophage-inhibitory media was developed for propagation of lactic starter cultures for cheese makers from fresh Cheddar or Swiss cheese whey by Richardson *et al.,* (1977). Cheese whey served as a source of a phosphate that provided protection for the lactic starter culture organisms against bacteriophage action and provided minerals and vitamins needed for acceptable activity. Recently, a culture medium for LAB was developed based on de-proteinated whey supplemented with yeast autolysate and de-lipidated egg yolk. Few selective media were formulated and their potential for LAB selection and enumeration was examined. A pH indicator and some inhibitory compounds were also added to select the LAB flora of various dairy products including milk, disinfected or not, fermented milk and yoghurt (Baida, Messaouda, & Abdeltif, 2010). Cheese whey was used as an inexpensive medium to produce bacteriocin by *Bacillus sp.* P11 (Leães, Natália, Voltaire, & Adriano, 2010).

Animal Feed

Dried whey has been widely used as a feed for cattle although its nutritional value is low, because of its low organic nitrogen content. Liquid whey can be used as a carrier of non-protein nitrogen components such as urea or ammonium salts to make crude protein supplements. Whey has a good supply of minerals especially calcium and phosphorus.

The advantages of using cheese whey in farms are numerous. Lactoserum easily replaces 100% of water intake at the farm; provides a low cost alternative to liquid feeds; improves feed palatability, texture and dust control of feed lot rations; provides a balanced nutrition of energy, protein, minerals and a safety factor to compensate for poor or variable quality diets; being a pumpable supplement, whey can save on feeding overheads as it requires less labour and feeding and mixing equipment. It can provide an economic and convenient method to feed urea supplements, vitamins, minerals and feed additives (Costa, Filho, Medeiros, Vilarroel, Cruz, & Santos, 2009).

INDUSTRIAL PRODUCTS

Lactic Acid

Lactic acid from cheese whey is produced commercially in Slovakia, Italy, and the United States. Although the synthetic production from acetaldehyde or lactonitrile is cheaper, the low cost of whey makes a large-scale production facility competitive (Altiok, Tokatli, & Harsa, 2006). The starting materials for lactic acid production include rennet and acid whey and their respective permeates. Lactic acid bacteria such as *Lactococcus lactis, Lactobacillus delbrueckii* subsp. *bulgaricus, Lb. acidophilus, Lb. helveticus, Lb. casei*, and mixed cultures of these organisms have been successfully used to convert lactose to lactic acid. Recently it has been discovered that fermentation of lactose into lactic acid can be enhanced in cheese whey by using recombinants between *Lactobacillus* and *Tetragenococcus* (Zaied, Kawther, Kash, Essawy & Aliaa, 2009).

Propionic Acid

Propionic acid is widely used in chemical, food and pharmaceutical industries as an important intermediate. Propionic acid is produced by fermentation with *Propionibacterium freundenrichii* from lactose and lactate (Feng, Chen, Xu, Wu, Yao, Ying, & Ouyang, 2010). Whey was fortified with pulverized limestone, which led to formation of calcium salts of propionic and acetic acids and then the salts are recovered. A preferred use of calcium and sodium propionates is in bakery products. They have relatively no effect on yeast growth, but inhibit growth of spoilage molds and *Bacillus* species, which causes ropiness in bakery products. Recently, research has been done to increase propionic acid production by using enzyme inhibitors, such as calcium-EGTA and o-iodosobenzoate. These enzyme inhibitors divert the metabolic flux to the propionic acid pathway. Addition of 0.3 mM of o-iodosobenzoate results in an increase of cell growth and a 2.4-fold increase in the propionic acid (Morales, Choi, & Kim, 2006).

Butanol and Butyric Acid

Cheese whey can be fermented to produce butanol and butyric acid by using immobilized *Clostridium acetobutylicum* in a continuous packed bed reactor. The medium contains a solution of lactose (15–30g/L) and yeast extracts (3g/L) to emulate the cheese whey, an abundant lactose-rich wastewater (Napoli, Olivieri, Russo, Marzocchella, & Salatino, 2010).

Calcium Magnesium Acetate

An innovative product proposed at Ohio State University was the production of calcium magnesium acetate (CMA) for use as a road deicer. A sequential conversion of lactose to lactate and then to acetate with a yield of greater than 90% was developed. Improvement of acetate production was observed from lactose by growing *Clostridium thermolacticum* in mixed batch culture. The use of this thermophilic anaerobic consortium opens new opportunities for the efficient valorization of lactose, the main waste from the cheese industry and production of calcium–magnesium acetate, an environmentally friendly road deicer (Collet, Schwitzguébel, & Péringer, 2003).

Biogas

The lactose content of whey (lactoserum) is readily degraded by acidogenic bacteria. An up-flow anaerobic sludge-fixed film (UASFF) reactor is a granular sludge bioreactor that is used for the rapid biological conversion of organic matter to biogas with the help of aggregated microbial consortium. The up-flow anaerobic fixed film section caused the flocculated biomass to be trapped in the sludge blanket and the delivery of biogas was easily performed. The gaseous biofuels (hydrogen and methane) and electricity can be produced from cheese whey. Hydrogen and methane production from cheese whey is a two-stage process. At a lab scale it is carried in a continuous stirred tank reactor (CSTR) of 3 L and a periodic anaerobic baffled reactor of 15 L (Stamatelatou, Georgia, Tremouli, & Lyberatos, 2011).

Encapsulation of Bioactives

The encapsulation process, which permits to entrap active agents into particles, pursues diverse objectives, namely protection of active compounds against ambient conditions such as temperature, oxygen, and light; minimization of degradative interactions during processing and storage; functionalization of the active compound; and improvement of its organoleptic properties (Zuidam & Shimoni, 2010; Gunasekaran & Ko, 2014).

Because of their high nutrition value and unique functional properties, including their ability to form gels and emulsions, food proteins can serve as excellent matrixes for the encapsulation of bioactive compounds (Chen, Remondetto, & Subirade, 2006). They are widely available, inexpensive, natural and they possess good sensorial properties (Gunasekaran, Xiao, & Eleya, 2006; Gunasekaran, Ko, & Xiao, 2007).

Different encapsulation techniques have made use of whey proteins as wall material. Coacervation exploits their ability to denature, dissociate, and aggregate under different conditions of pH, ionic strength, and temperature to form particles entrapping the active ingredient (Chen, Remondetto, & Subirade, 2006). Several works have been published on the topic (Lee, Ahn, Lee, & Kwak, 2004; Friedmann, Lumsdon, & Green, 2009; Bortlik, Saucy, Duruz, Richelle, Lambelet, Baur, & Pfeifer, 2005; Eratte, Wang, Dowling, Barrow, & Adhikari, 2014). Spray-drying, a one-step process which converts a liquid feed into solid particles by the evaporation of the solvent also includes whey protein among its encapsulating agents (Pillai, Prabhasankar, Jena, & Anandharamakrishnan, 2012). Whey proteins have also been used to encapsulate bioactive ingredients by freeze-drying (Premarajah, 2014).

Numerous active ingredients have been encapsulated in whey protein based matrixes namely, probiotics (Bosnea, Moschakis, & Biliaderis, 2014); oils and essential fatty acids (Bae & Lee, 2008); antioxidants (Koga, Andrade, Ferruzzi, & Lee, 2015; Al-Ismail, El-Dijani, Al-Khatib, & Saleh, 2016); extracts (Esfanjani, Jafari, Assadpoor, & Mohammadi, 2015; Saponjac, Cetkovic, Canadanovic-Brunet, Pajin, Djilas, Petrovic… Vulic, 2016) and flavors (Baranauskiene, Venskutonis, Dewettinck, & Verhé, 2006).

OTHER APPLICATIONS OF LACTOSERUM

In Land Reclamation

Lactoserum can improve the physical condition of sodic soils or those susceptible to erosion by increasing their aggregate stability. Lactoserum has significant potential as an amendment for land reclamation, particularly in those areas where soils can be affected by relatively large amounts of sodium and/or lime. The low pH of the whey decreases soil solution pH and thus increases calcium solubility. As microorganisms decompose the lactose and proteins in the whey, they produce CO_2 and organic acids that also increase calcium solubility.

All of these processes will speed the leaching of exchangeable sodium from a sodic soil profile when sufficient water is passed through the soil (Watkinsa & Nash, 2010).

Food and Dairy Industry

Whey protein precipitates are used for the manufacture of cheese spreads. Cheese whey (called Myzithra) is also used for the preparation of certain foods and cheese pies in Greece. Dry Myzithra is used in food seasoning after grating (Cruz, Sant'Ana, Macchione, Teixeira, & Schmidt, 2009).

As Lactoserum Intimate Liquid Soap for External Hygiene

Lactic acid plus lactoserum intimate liquid soap for external hygiene has also been studied in the prevention of bacterial vaginosis (BV) recurrence after metronidazole oral treatment. A total of 123 women with diagnosis of BV with the following criteria: homogeneous vaginal discharge without inflammation of the vagina or vulva; vaginal pH ≥ 4.5; 3) positive Whiff test; and "clue cells" in more than 20% of the epithelial cells in the vagina were studied. A Nugent score ≥ 4 in the vaginal bacterioscopy was also used. After BV diagnosis, metronidazole 500 mg was administered orally bid during 7 days. Patients cured of BV were then instructed to use 7.5 to 10 mL of a lactic acid plus lactoserum liquid soap once-a-day for hygiene of the external genital region. A questionnaire was applied in the form of visual analogue scale (VAS) in all the visits regarding:

1. Level of comfort at the genital region;
2. Malodorous external genitalia;
3. Comfort in sexual intercourse;

4. Satisfaction with intimate hygiene; and
5. Self-esteem.

Quality of life was evaluated in the 42 women who completed the four visits schedule and there were significant improvement in the five domains assessed. It was finally concluded that a lactic acid plus lactoserum liquid soap for external intimate hygiene may be an option for the prevention of BV recurrence after treatment and cure with oral metronidazole (Bahamondes, Portugal, Brolazo, Simões, & Bahamondes, 2011).

CONCLUSION

Although previously lactoserum was considered as a potent pollutant with high BOD but nowadays it is evolving into a most sought-after product because of the lactose, minerals, and proteins as well as the functional properties that it imparts to food. Whey derived ingredients such as lactose, lactoferrin, lactoperoxidase, immunoglobulins, glycomacropeptide, transforming growth factors, sphingolipids and calcium can be used as concentrated bioactive whey ingredients for the promotion of intestinal health through the action on the intestinal microflora. These compounds also have broad spectrum anti-microbial, anticancer and immune-potentiating properties, which provide added benefits over traditional fiber-based probiotics.

To conclude, as exciting intestinal health benefits of lactoserum-derived bioactives continue to emerge, companies are stepping up to provide innovative, evidence based nutritional products to the wellness and medical consumer markets. Thus lactoserum can serve as an attractive ecofriendly, cost effective alternate to other nutraceuticals.

ACKNOWLEDGMENT

The authors are grateful to Dr. Ashok K. Chauhan, Founder President and Mr. Atul Chauhan, Chancellor, Amity University UP, Noida, India for the encouragement, research facilities and financial support.

REFERENCES

Adetuyi, F. C., Olorunfemi, O. B., & Adebolu, T. T. (2009). Antibacterial activities of *Micrococcus lactis* strain isolated from Nigerian fermented cheese whey against diarrhea-causing organisms. *Research Journal of Biological Sciences*, *1*, 24–27.

Agustriyanto, R., & Fatmawati, A. (2009). Model of Continuous Cheese Whey Fermentation by *Candida pseudotropicalis*. *World Academy of Science, Engineering and Technology*, *57*, 213–217.

Al-Ismail, K., El-Dijani, L., Al-Khatib, H., & Saleh, M. (2016). Effect of Microencapsulation of Vitamin C with Gum Arabic, Whey Protein. *Journal of Scientific and Industrial Research*, *75*, 176–180.

Alfaifi, M. S., & Stathopoulos, C. E. (2010). Effect of egg yolk substitution by sweet whey protein isolate on texture, stability and colour of Gelato-style vanilla ice cream. *International Journal of Dairy Technology*, *63*(4), 593–598. doi:10.1111/j.1471-0307.2010.00609.x

Altiok, D., Tokatli, F., & Harsa, S. (2006). Kinetic modeling of lactic acid production from whey by *Lactobacillus casei* (NRRL B-441). *Journal of Chemical Technology and Biotechnology (Oxford, Oxfordshire)*, *81*(7), 1190–1197. doi:10.1002/jctb.1512

Amor, K. B., Vaughan, E. E., & de Vos, W. M. (2007). Advanced Molecular Tools for the identification of lactic acid bacteria. *The Journal of Nutrition*, *137*(3), 741S–747S. doi:10.1093/jn/137.3.741S PMID:17311970

Anon. (2006). *Comprehensive review of scientific literature pertaining to nitrogen protein conversion factors, IDF Bulletin 405*. Brussels: International Dairy Federation.

Bae, E. K., & Lee, S. J. (2008). Microencapsulation of avocado oil by spray drying using whey protein and maltodextrin. *Journal of Microencapsulation*, *25*(8), 549–560. doi:10.1080/02652040802075682 PMID:18465295

Bahamondes, M. V., Portugal, P. M., Brolazo, E. M., Simões, J. A., & Bahamondes, L. (2011). Use of a lactic acid plus lactoserum intimate liquid soap for external hygiene in the prevention of bacterial vaginosis recurrence after metronidazole oral treatment. *Revista da Associação Médica Brasileira*, *57*(4), 415–420. doi:10.1590/S0104-42302011000400015 PMID:21876923

Baida, D.-H., Messaouda, B., & Abdeltif, A. (2010). Formulation and evaluation of a selective medium for lactic acid bacteria-validation on some dairy products. *American Journal of Agricultural and Biological Sciences*, *5*(2), 148–153. doi:10.3844/ajabssp.2010.148.153

Baker, E. N., & Baker, H. M. (2009). A structural framework for understanding the multifunctional character of lactoferrin. *Biochimie*, *91*(1), 3–10. doi:10.1016/j.biochi.2008.05.006 PMID:18541155

Baranauskiene, R., Venskutonis, P. R., Dewettinck, K., & Verhé, R. (2006). Properties of oregano (*Origanum vulgare L.*), citronella (*Cymbopogon nardus G.*) and marjoram (*Majorana hortensis L.*) flavors encapsulated into milk protein-based matrices. *Food Research International*, *39*(4), 413–425. doi:10.1016/j.foodres.2005.09.005

Ben Amor, K., Breeuwer, P., Verbaarschot, P., Rombouts, F. M., Akkermans, A. D. L., De Vos, W. M., & Abee, T. (2002). Multi-parametric flow cytometry and cell sorting for the assessment of viable, injured, and dead *Bifidobacterium* cells during bile salt stress. *Applied and Environmental Microbiology*, *68*(11), 5209–5216. doi:10.1128/AEM.68.11.5209-5216.2002 PMID:12406706

Bortlik, K., Saucy, F., Duruz, E., Richelle, M., Lambelet, P., Baur, M., & Pfeifer, A.M.A. (2005). *Primary composition comprising a lipophilic bioactive compound*. US 2005/0106219 A1.

Bosnea, L. A., Moschakis, T., & Biliaderis, C. G. (2014). Complex Coacervation as a Novel Microencapsulation Technique to Improve Viability of Probiotics under Different Stresses. *Food and Bioprocess Technology*, *7*(10), 2767–2781. doi:10.100711947-014-1317-7

Bruck, W. M., Redgrave, M., Tuohy, K. M., Lonnerdal, B., Graverholt, G., Hernell, O., & Gibson, G. R. (2006). Effects of bovine alpha-lactalbumin and casein glycomacropeptide-enriched infant formulae on faecal microbiota in healthy term infants. *Journal of Pediatric Gastroenterology and Nutrition*, *43*(5), 673–679. doi:10.1097/01.mpg.0000232019.79025.8f PMID:17130747

Calder, P. C. (2006). Branched-chain amino acids and immunity. *The Journal of Nutrition*, *136*(1), 288S–293S. doi:10.1093/jn/136.1.288S PMID:16365100

Chen, L., Remondetto, G. E., & Subirade, M. (2006). Food protein-based materials as nutraceutical delivery systems. *Trends in Food Science & Technology*, *17*(5), 272–283. doi:10.1016/j.tifs.2005.12.011

Collet, C., Schwitzguébel, J.-P., & Péringer, P. (2003). Improvement of acetate production from lactose by growing *Clostridium thermolacticum* in mixed batch culture. *Journal of Applied Microbiology*, *95*(4), 824–831. doi:10.1046/j.1365-2672.2003.02060.x PMID:12969297

Commane, D., Hughes, R., Shortt, C., & Rowland, I. (2005). The potential mechanisms involved in the anti-carcinogenic action of probiotics. *Mutation Research*, *591*(1-2), 276–289. doi:10.1016/j.mrfmmm.2005.02.027 PMID:16095630

Costa, R. G., Filho, E. M. B., Medeiros, G. R., Vilarroel, A. S., Cruz, S. E. S. B. S., & Santos, E. M. (2009). Replacement of goat milk by cheese whey in the feed of Alpine kids. *Tropical and Subtropical Agroecosystems*, *11*, 87–90.

Cruz, A. G., Sant'Ana, A. S., Macchione, M. M., Teixeira, A. M., & Schmidt, F. L. (2009). Milk drink using whey butter cheese (Queijo manteiga) and Acerola juice as a potential source of vitamin C. *Food and Bioprocess Technology*, *2*(4), 368–373. doi:10.100711947-008-0059-9

De Simone, C., Ferranti, P., Picariello, G., Scognamiglio, I., Dicitore, A., Addeo, F., ... Stiuso, P. (2010). Peptides from water buffalo cheese whey induced senescence cell death via ceramide secretion in human colon adenocarcinoma cell line. *Molecular Nutrition & Food Research*, *55*(2), 229–238. doi:10.1002/mnfr.201000074 PMID:20725925

de Wit, J. N. (1998). Nutritional and functional characteristics of whey proteins in food systems. *Journal of Dairy Science*, *81*(3), 597–608. doi:10.3168/jds.S0022-0302(98)75613-9 PMID:9565865

Defaie, S. Z., Sharieat, S., & Divsalar, A. (2010). Kinetic Investigation on Lactoperoxidase upon Interaction with Lead ion M. *International Journal of Environmental Sciences and Development*, *1*(1), 97–100. doi:10.7763/IJESD.2010.V1.19

Delfour, A., Jolles, J., Alais, C., & Jolles, P. (1965). Caseino-glycopeptides: Characterization of a methionine residue and of the N-terminal sequence. *Biochemical and Biophysical Research Communications*, *19*(4), 452–455. doi:10.1016/0006-291X(65)90145-2 PMID:14338991

Delley, M., & Germond, J. E. (2002). Differentiation of *Lactobacillus helveticus, Lactobacillus delbrueckii subsp bulgaricus, subsp lactis, and subsp delbrueckii* using physiological and genetic tools and reclassification of some strains from the ATCC collection. *Systematic and Applied Microbiology*, *25*(2), 228–231. doi:10.1078/0723-2020-00106 PMID:12353877

Duan, R. D. (2005). Anticancer compounds and sphingolipid metabolism in the colon. *In Vivo (Athens, Greece)*, *19*, 293–300. PMID:15796189

Duthoit, F., Godon, J. J., & Montel, M. C. (2003). Bacterial community dynamics during production of registered designation of origin salers cheese as evaluated by 16SrRNA gene single-strand conformation polymorphism analysis. *Applied and Environmental Microbiology*, *69*(7), 3840–3848. doi:10.1128/AEM.69.7.3840-3848.2003 PMID:12839752

Eratte, D., Wang, B., Dowling, K., Barrow, C. J., & Adhikari, B. P. (2014). Complex coacervation with whey protein isolate and gum arabic for the microencapsulation of omega-3 rich tuna oil. *Food & Function*, *5*(11), 2743–2750. doi:10.1039/C4FO00296B PMID:25008146

Esfanjani, A. F., Jafari, S. M., Assadpoor, E., & Mohammadi, E. (2015). Nano-encapsulation of saffron extract through double-layered multiple emulsions of pectin and whey protein concentrate. *Journal of Food Engineering*, *165*, 149–155. doi:10.1016/j.jfoodeng.2015.06.022

Feng, X. H., Chen, F., Xu, H., Wu, B., Yao, J., Ying, H. J., & Ouyang, P. K. (2010). Propionic acid fermentation by *Propionibacterium freudenreichii* CCTCC M207015 in a multi-point fibrous-bed bioreactor. *Bioprocess and Biosystems Engineering*, *33*(9), 1077–1085. doi:10.100700449-010-0433-7 PMID:20589397

Friedmann, T.E., Lumsdon, S.O., & Green, J.H. (2009). *Encapsulation of oils by coacervation*. US 2009/0189304 A1.

Gunasekaran, S., & Ko, S. (2014). Rationales of Nano- and Microencapsulation for Food Ingredients. In H. S. Kwak (Ed.), *Nano- and Microencapsulation for Foods*. John Wiley & Sons, Ltd. doi:10.1002/9781118292327.ch3

Gunasekaran, S., Ko, S., & Xiao, L. (2007). Use of whey proteins for encapsulation and controlled delivery applications. *Journal of Food Engineering*, *83*(1), 31–40. doi:10.1016/j.jfoodeng.2006.11.001

Gunasekaran, S., Xiao, L., & Eleya, M. M. (2006). Whey protein concentrates hydrogels as bioactive carriers. *Journal of Applied Polymer Science*, *99*(5), 2470–2476. doi:10.1002/app.22838

Huang, W.-C., Chen, C.-L., Lin, Y.-S., & Lin, C.-F. (2011). Apoptotic Sphingolipid Ceramide in Cancer Therapy. Journal of Lipids.

Jessup, C. M., & Forde, S. E. (2008). Ecology and evolution in microbial systems: The generation and maintenance of diversity in phage-host interactions. *Research in Microbiology*, *159*(5), 382–389. doi:10.1016/j.resmic.2008.05.006 PMID:18582563

Kargi, F., & Ozmihci, S. (2006). Utilization of cheese whey powder (CWP) for ethanol fermentations: Effect of operating parameters. *Enzyme and Microbial Technology*, *38*(5), 711–718. doi:10.1016/j.enzmictec.2005.11.006

Koga, C. C., Andrade, J. E., Ferruzzi, M. G., & Lee, Y. (2015). Stability of Trans-Resveratrol Encapsulated in a Protein Matrix Produced Using Spray Drying to UV Light Stress and Simulated Gastro-Intestinal Digestion. *Journal of Food Science*, *81*(2), 292–300. doi:10.1111/1750-3841.13176 PMID:26677808

Koutinas, A. A., Athanasiadis, I., Bekatorou, A., Psarianos, C., Kanellaki, M., Agouridis, N., & Blekas, G. (2007). Kefir-yeast technology: Industrial scale- up of alcoholic fermentation of whey, promoted by raisin extracts, using kefir-yeast granular biomass. *Enzyme and Microbial Technology*, *41*(5), 576–582. doi:10.1016/j.enzmictec.2007.05.013

Le, Y., Yu, X., Ruan, L., Wang, O., Qi, D., Zhu, J., ... Wang, J. M. (2005). The immuno-pharmacological properties of transforming growth factor beta. *International Immunopharmacology*, *5*(13-14), 1771–1782. doi:10.1016/j.intimp.2005.07.006 PMID:16275614

Leães, F.L., Natália G.V., Voltaire, S.A., & Adriano, B. (2010). Use of Byproducts of Food Industry for Production of Antimicrobial Activity by *Bacillus sp.* P11 (Communication). *Food and Bioprocess Technology,* 133-140.

Lee, J. B., Ahn, J. B., Lee, J., & Kwak, H. S. (2004). L-Ascorbic Acid Microencapsulated with Polyacylglycerol Monostearate for Milk Fortification. *Bioscience, Biotechnology, and Biochemistry*, *68*(3), 495–500. doi:10.1271/bbb.68.495 PMID:15056878

Liang, G. B., Du, G. C., & Chen, J. (2008). A novel strategy of enhanced glutathione production in high cell density cultivation of *Candida utilis*-Cysteine addition combined with dissolved oxygen controlling. *Enzyme and Microbial Technology*, *42*(3), 284–289. doi:10.1016/j.enzmictec.2007.10.008

Lonnerdal, B. (2009). Nutritional roles of lactoferrin. *Current Opinion in Clinical Nutrition and Metabolic Care*, *12*(3), 293–297. doi:10.1097/MCO.0b013e328328d13e PMID:19318940

Marcelo, P. A., & Ritzvi, S. S. H. (2008). Physicochemical properties of liquid virgin whey protein isolate. *International Dairy Journal*, *18*(3), 236–246. doi:10.1016/j.idairyj.2007.08.011

Mehra, R., Marnila, P., & Korhonen, H. (2006). Milk immunoglobulins for health promotion. *International Dairy Journal*, *16*(11), 1262–1271. doi:10.1016/j.idairyj.2006.06.003

Morales, J., Choi, J.-S., & Kim, D.-S. (2006). Production rate of propionic acid in fermentation of cheese whey with enzyme inhibitors. *Environment and Progress*, *25*(3), 228–234. doi:10.1002/ep.10153

Mukhopadhyay, R., Talukdar, D., Chatterjee, B. P., & Guha, A. K. (2003). Whey processing with chitosan and isolation of lactose. *Process Biochemistry*, *39*(3), 381–385. doi:10.1016/S0032-9592(03)00126-2

Napoli, F., Olivieri, G., Russo, M. E., Marzocchella, A., & Salatino, P. (2010). Butanol production by *Clostridium acetobutylicum* in a continuous packed bed reactor. *Journal of Industrial Microbiology & Biotechnology*, *37*(6), 603–608. doi:10.100710295-010-0707-8 PMID:20349108

Ong, L., & Shah, N. P. (2009). Probiotic Cheddar cheese: Influence of ripening temperatures on survival of probiotic microorganisms, cheese composition and organic acid profiles. *Food Science and Technology (Campinas)*, *42*, 1260–1268.

Parrondo, J., Garcia, L. A., & Diaz, M. (2009). Whey Vinegars. In Vinegars of the World. Springer.

Pillai, D. S., Prabhasankar, P., Jena, B. S., & Anandharamakrishnan, C. (2012). Microencapsulation of *Garcinia cowa* Fruit Extract and Effect of its use on Pasta Process and Quality. *International Journal of Food Properties*, *15*(3), 590–604. do i:10.1080/10942912.2010.494756

Premarajah, R. (2014). *The effects of drying conditions and carrier selection on the production of an antioxidant rich powder* (MPhil thesis). The University of Sydney.

Puddu, P., Valenti, P., & Gessani, S. (2009). Immunomodulatory effects of lactoferrin on antigen presenting cells. *Biochimie*, *91*(1), 11–18. doi:10.1016/j.biochi.2008.05.005 PMID:18539153

Richardson, G. H., Cheng, C. T., & Young, R. (1977). Lactic bulk culture system utilizing a whey-based bacteriophage inhibitory medium and pH control: Applicability to American style cheese. *Journal of Dairy Science*, *60*(3), 378–386. doi:10.3168/jds.S0022-0302(77)83876-9

Rossetti, L., Carminati, D., Zago, M., & Giraffa, G. (2009). A qualified presumption of safety approach for the safety assessment of Grana Padano whey starters. *International Journal of Food Microbiology*, *130*(1), 70–73. doi:10.1016/j.ijfoodmicro.2009.01.003 PMID:19187995

Rossetti, L., Fornasari, M., Gatti, M., Lazzi, C., Neviani, E., & Giraffa, G. (2008). Grana Padano cheese whey starters: Microbial composition and strain distribution. *International Journal of Food Microbiology*, *127*(1-2), 168–171. doi:10.1016/j.ijfoodmicro.2008.06.005 PMID:18620769

Šaponjac, V. T., Cetkovic, G., Canadanovic-Brunet, J., Pajin, B., Djilas, S., Petrovic, J., ... Vulic, J. (2016). Sour cherry pomace extract encapsulated in whey and soy proteins: Incorporation in cookies. *Food Chemistry*, *207*, 27–33. doi:10.1016/j.foodchem.2016.03.082 PMID:27080876

Somaye, F., Marzieh, M. N., & Lale, N. (2008). Single cell protein (SCP) production from UF cheese whey by *Kluyveromyces marxianus*. *18th National Congress on Food Technology*.

Stamatelatou, K., Georgia, A., Tremouli, A., & Lyberatos, G. (2011). Production of gaseous biofuels and electricity from cheese whey. *Industrial & Engineering Chemistry Research*, *50*(2), 639–644. doi:10.1021/ie1002262

Thomä-Worringer, C., Sørensen, J., & López-Fandiño, R. (2006). Health effects and technological features of caseinomacropeptide. *International Dairy Journal*, *16*(11), 1324–1333. doi:10.1016/j.idairyj.2006.06.012

Tranjan, B. C., Cruz, A. G., Walter, E. H. M., Faria, J. A. F., Bolini, H. M. A., Moura, M. R. L., & Carvalho, L. M. J. (2009). Development of goat cheese whey-flavoured beverages. *International Journal of Dairy Technology*, *62*(3), 438–443. doi:10.1111/j.1471-0307.2009.00491.x

Ventura, M., Meylan, V., & Zink, R. (2003). Identification and tracing of *Bifidobacterium* species by use of enterobacterial repetitive intergenic consensus sequences. *Journal of Applied and Environmental Microbiology*, *69*(7), 4296–4301. doi:10.1128/AEM.69.7.4296-4301.2003 PMID:12839818

Volpi, E., Kobayashi, H., Sheffield-Moore, M., Mittendorfer, B., & Wolfe, R. R. (2003). Essential amino acids are primarily responsible for the amino acid stimulation of muscle protein anabolism in healthy elderly adults. *The American Journal of Clinical Nutrition*, *78*(5), 250–258. doi:10.1093/ajcn/78.2.250 PMID:12885705

Watkinsa, M., & Nash, D. (2010). Dairy factory wastewaters, their use on land and possible environmental impacts – A mini review. *The Open Agriculture Journal*, *4*(1), 1–9. doi:10.2174/1874331501004010001

Yen, C. C., Lin, C. Y., Chong, K. Y., Tsai, T. C., Shen, C. J., Lin, M. F., ... Chen, C. M. (2009). Lactoferrin as a natural regimen for selective decontamination of the digestive tract: Recombinant porcine lactoferrin expressed in the milk of transgenic mice protects neonates from pathogenic challenge in the gastrointestinal tract. *The Journal of Infectious Diseases*, *199*(4), 590–598. doi:10.1086/596212 PMID:19125673

Zafar, S., & Owais, M. (2005). Ethanol production from crude whey by *Kluyveromyces marxianus*. *Biochemical Engineering Journal*, *27*(3), 295–298. doi:10.1016/j.bej.2005.05.009

Zaied, K.A., Kawther, S., & Kash, E.A., & Aliaa, A.D. (2009). Enhancement the Fermentation of Lactose–Whey Using Recombinants between *Lactobacillus* and *Tetragenococcus*. *Australian Journal of Basic and Applied Sciences*, *3*(2), 761–775.

Zuidam, N., & Shimoni, E. (Eds.). (2010). Encapsulation Technologies for Active Food Ingredients and Food Processing. Springer Science Plus Business Media.

Compilation of References

(n.d.). Histories of Product Regulation - The 1938 Food. *Drug, and Cosmetic Act.*

Aasheim, E. T., Hofso, D., Hjelmesaeth, J., Birkeland, K. I., & Bohmer, T. (2008). Vitamin status in morbidly obese patients: A cross-sectional study. *The American Journal of Clinical Nutrition*, *87*(2), 362–369. doi:10.1093/ajcn/87.2.362 PMID:18258626

Abramson, J. (2008). *Overdosed America: The Broken Promise of American Medicine (P.S).* Harper Perennial.

Abumrad, N. A., & Davidson, N. O. (2012). Role of the gut in lipid homeostasis. *Physiological Reviews*, *92*(3), 1061–1085. doi:10.1152/physrev.00019.2011 PMID:22811425

Adams, J. B., Audhya, T., McDonough-Means, S., Rubin, R. A., Quig, D., Geis, E., & Lee, W. (2011). Effect of a vitamin/mineral supplement on children and adults with autism. *BMC Pediatrics*, *11*(1), 111. doi:10.1186/1471-2431-11-111 PMID:22151477

Adcocks, C., Collin, P., & Buttle, D. J. (2002). Catechins from Green tea (*Camellia sinensis*) inhibit bovine and human cartilage proteoglycan and Type II collagen degradation *in vitro*. *The Journal of Nutrition*, *132*(3), 341–346. doi:10.1093/jn/132.3.341 PMID:11880552

Addeo, F., Chianese, L., Salzano, A., Sacchi, R., Cappuccio, U., Ferranti, P., & Malorni, A. (1992). Characterization of the 12% trichloroacetic acid-insoluble oligopeptides of Parmigiano-Reggiano cheese. *The Journal of Dairy Research*, *59*(03), 401–411. doi:10.1017/S0022029900030673

Adetuyi, F. C., Olorunfemi, O. B., & Adebolu, T. T. (2009). Antibacterial activities of *Micrococcus lactis* strain isolated from Nigerian fermented cheese whey against diarrhea-causing organisms. *Research Journal of Biological Sciences*, *1*, 24–27.

Afroz, R., Tanvir, E., & Little, P. J. (2016). Honey-derived flavonoids: Natural products for the prevention of atherosclerosis and cardiovascular diseases. *Clinical & Experimental Pharmacology*, *6*(3).

Agarwal, K. N. (2001). Iron and the brain: Neurotransmitter receptors and magnetic resonance spectroscopy. *British Journal of Nutrition*, *85*(S2), S147. doi:10.1079/BJN2000307 PMID:11509103

Aggarwal, B. B. (2010). Targeting inflammation-induced obesity and metabolic diseases by curcumin and other nutraceuticals. *Annual Review of Nutrition*, *21*(30), 173–199. doi:10.1146/annurev.nutr.012809.104755 PMID:20420526

Aggarwal, B. B., & Shishodia, S. (2006a). Molecular targets of dietary agents for prevention and therapy of cancer. *Biochemical Pharmacology*, *71*(10), 1397–1421. doi:10.1016/j.bcp.2006.02.009 PMID:16563357

Aggarwal, B. B., & Shishodia, S. (2006b). *Resveratrol in health and disease*. CRC Taylor & Francis.

Aggarwal, B. B., Surh, Y.-J., & Shishodia, S. (Eds.). (2007). *The Molecular Targets and Therapeutic Uses of Curcumin in Health and Disease* (Vol. 595). Boston, MA: Springer US. doi:10.1007/978-0-387-46401-5_1

Aggarwal, S., Takada, Y., Singh, S., Myers, J. N., & Aggarwal, B. B. (2004). Inhibition of growth and survival of human head and neck squamous cell carcinoma cells by curcumin via modulation of nuclear factor B signaling. *International Journal of Cancer*, *111*(5), 679–692. doi:10.1002/ijc.20333 PMID:15252836

Agricultural Research Service USDA (2010). *What we eat in America.* NHANES 2007-2008.

Agustriyanto, R., & Fatmawati, A. (2009). Model of Continuous Cheese Whey Fermentation by *Candida pseudotropicalis. World Academy of Science, Engineering and Technology*, *57*, 213–217.

Ahmad, A., Husain, A., Mujeeb, M., Khan, S. A., Najmi, A. K., Siddique, N. A., ... Anwar, F. (2013). A review on therapeutic potential of Nigella sativa: A miracle herb. *Asian Pacific Journal of Tropical Biomedicine*, *3*(5), 337–352. doi:10.1016/S2221-1691(13)60075-1 PMID:23646296

Ajala, O., English, P., & Pinkney, J. (2013). Systematic review and meta-analysis of different dietary approaches to the management of type 2 diabetes. *The American Journal of Clinical Nutrition*, *97*(3), 505–516. doi:10.3945/ajcn.112.042457 PMID:23364002

Ajjawi, I., & Shintani, D. (2004). Engineered plants with elevated vitamin E: A nutraceutical success story. *Trends in Biotechnology*, *22*(3), 104–107. doi:10.1016/j.tibtech.2004.01.008 PMID:15043044

Akihisa, T., Kokke, W., & Tamura, T. (1991). Naturally occurring sterols and related compounds from plants. In G. W. Peterson & W. D. Nes (Eds.), *Physiology and Biochemistry of Sterols* (pp. 172–178). Champaign, IL: AOCS.

Akinsulie, A. O., Temiye, E. O., Akanmu, A. S., Lesi, F. E. A., & Whyte, C. O. (2005). Clinical evaluation of extract of Cajanuscajan (Ciklavit®) in sickle cell anemia. *Journal of Tropical Pediatrics*, *51*(4), 200–205. doi:10.1093/tropej/fmh097 PMID:15917266

Aksoy, N., Dogan, Y., Iriadam, M., Bitiren, M., Uzer, E., Ozgonul, A., & Aksoy, S. (2012). Protective and therapeutic effects of licorice in rats with acute tubular necrosis. *Journal of Renal Nutrition: The Official Journal of the Council on Renal Nutrition of the National Kidney Foundation*, *22*(3), 336–343. doi:10.1053/j.jrn.2011.07.002 PMID:22047711

Alamanos, Y., Voulgari, P. V., & Drosos, A. A. (2005). Rheumatoid Arthritis in Southern Europe: Epidemiological, Clinical, Radiological and Genetic Considerations. *Current Rheumatology Reviews*, *1*(1), 33–36. doi:10.2174/1573397052954217

Alam, M. A., Kauter, K., & Brown, L. (2013). Naringin improves diet-induced cardiovascular dysfunction and obesity in high carbohydrate, high fat diet-fed rats. *Nutrients*, *5*(3), 637–650. doi:10.3390/nu5030637 PMID:23446977

Alam, S., Subhan, N., Rahman, M. M., Uddin, S. J., Reza, H. M., & Sarker, S. D. (2014). Effect of citrus flavonoids, naringin and naringenin, on metabolic syndrome and their mechanisms of action. *Advances in Nutrition*, *5*(4), 404–417. doi:10.3945/an.113.005603 PMID:25022990

Albert, C. M., Gaziano, J. M., Willett, W. C., & Manson, J. E. (2002). Nut Consumption and Decreased Risk of Sudden Cardiac Death in the Physicians' Health Study. *Archives of Internal Medicine*, *162*(12), 1382–1387. doi:10.1001/archinte.162.12.1382 PMID:12076237

Alberti, K. G. M. M., Eckel, R. H., Grundy, S. M., Zimmet, P. Z., Cleeman, J. I., & Donato, K. A. (2009). Harmonizing the metabolic syndrome: a joint interim statement of the International Diabetes Federation Task Force on Epidemiology and Prevention; National Heart, Lung, and Blood Institute; American Heart Association; World Heart Federation; International Atherosclerosis Society; and International Association for the Study of Obesity. *Circulation*, *120*(16), 1640–1645. .19264410.1161/CIRCULATIONAHA.109

Aldana, S. G., Greenlaw, R., Salberg, A., Merrill, R. M., Hager, R., & Jorgensen, R. B. (2007). The effects of an intensive lifestyle modification program on carotid artery intima-media thickness: A randomized trial. *American Journal of Health Promotion: AJHP*, *21*(6), 510–516. doi:10.4278/0890-1171-21.6.510 PMID:17674638

Alfaifi, M. S., & Stathopoulos, C. E. (2010). Effect of egg yolk substitution by sweet whey protein isolate on texture, stability and colour of Gelato-style vanilla ice cream. *International Journal of Dairy Technology*, *63*(4), 593–598. doi:10.1111/j.1471-0307.2010.00609.x

Al-Ismail, K., El-Dijani, L., Al-Khatib, H., & Saleh, M. (2016). Effect of Microencapsulation of Vitamin C with Gum Arabic, Whey Protein. *Journal of Scientific and Industrial Research*, *75*, 176–180.

Aljuraiban, G. S., Griep, L. M. O., Chan, Q., Daviglus, M. L., Stamler, J., Horn, L. V., ... Frost, G. S. (2015). Total, insoluble and soluble dietary fibre intake in relation to blood pressure: The INTERMAP Study - CORRIGENDUM. *British Journal of Nutrition*, *114*(9), 1534–1534. doi:10.1017/S0007114515003876 PMID:26388506

Al-Lahham, S. H., Roelofsen, H., Priebe, M., Weening, D., Dijkstra, M., Hoek, A., ... Vonk, R. J. (2010). Regulation of adipokine production in human adipose tissueby propionic acid. *European Journal of Clinical Investigation*, *40*(5), 401–407. doi:10.1111/j.1365-2362.2010.02278.x PMID:20353437

Allen, L. H., De Benoist, B., Dary, O., & Hurrell, R. (2006). *Guidelines on food fortification with micronutrients*. WHO.

Al-Naqeep, Al-Zubairi, Ismail, Amom, & Esa. (2011). Antiatherogenic Potential of Nigella sativa Seeds and Oil in Diet-Induced Hypercholesterolemia in Rabbits. *Evidence-based Complementary and Alternative Medicine: eCAM, 2011*. doi: 10.1093/ecam/neq071

Al-Solaiman, Y., Jesri, A., Mountford, W. K., Lackland, D. T., Zhao, Y., & Egan, B. M. (2010). DASH Lowers Blood Pressure in Obese Hypertensives Beyond Potassium, Magnesium and Fiber. *Journal of Human Hypertension*, *24*(4), 237–246. doi:10.1038/jhh.2009.58 PMID:19626043

Altiok, D., Tokatli, F., & Harsa, S. (2006). Kinetic modeling of lactic acid production from whey by *Lactobacillus casei* (NRRL B-441). *Journal of Chemical Technology and Biotechnology (Oxford, Oxfordshire)*, *81*(7), 1190–1197. doi:10.1002/jctb.1512

Aluko, R. E. (2012). *Functional foods and nutraceuticals*. New York: Springer. doi:10.1007/978-1-4614-3480-1

Alves-Silva, J. M., Monica, Z., Carla, M., Ligia, S., & Henrique, G. (2016). Protective effects of terpenes on the cardiovascular system: Current advances and future perspectives. *Current Medicinal Chemistry*. PMID:27604093

Amagase, H., & Nance, D. M. (2008). A randomized, double-blind, placebo-controlled, clinical study of the general effects of a standardized Lycium barbarum (goji) juice, GoChi™. *Journal of Alternative and Complementary Medicine (New York, N.Y.)*, *14*(4), 403–412. doi:10.1089/acm.2008.0004 PMID:18447631

Amagase, H., Sun, B., & Borek, C. (2009). Lycium barbarum (goji) juice improves in vivo antioxidant biomarkers in serum of healthy adults. *Nutrition Research (New York, N.Y.)*, *29*(1), 19–25. doi:10.1016/j.nutres.2008.11.005 PMID:19185773

Amara, A. A., & Shibl, A. (2015). Role of Probiotics in health improvement, infection control and disease treatment and management. *Saudi Pharmaceutical Journal*, *23*(2), 107–114. doi:10.1016/j.jsps.2013.07.001 PMID:25972729

Ameh, S. J., Tarfa, F. D., & Ebeshi, B. U. (2012). Traditional herbal management of sickle cell anemia: Lessons from Nigeria. *Anemia*. PMID:23198140

Amer, M. S., Elawam, A. E., Khater, M. S., Omar, O. H., Mabrouk, R. A., & Taha, H. M. (2011). Association of high-sensitivity C-reactive protein with carotid artery intima-media thickness in hypertensive older adults. *Journal of the American Society of Hypertension: JASH*, *5*(5), 395–400. doi:10.1016/j.jash.2011.03.004 PMID:21524639

Ames, B. N., Shigenaga, M. K., & Gold, L. S. (1993). DNA lesions, inducible DNA repair, and cell division: three key factors in mutagenesis and carcinogenesis. *Environmental Health Perspectives, 101*(Suppl 5), 35–44.

Amor, K. B., Vaughan, E. E., & de Vos, W. M. (2007). Advanced Molecular Tools for the identification of lactic acid bacteria. *The Journal of Nutrition*, *137*(3), 741S–747S. doi:10.1093/jn/137.3.741S PMID:17311970

Amri, A., Chaumeil, J. C., Sfar, S., & Charrueau, C. (2012). Administration of resveratrol: What formulation solutions to bioavailability limitations? *Journal of Controlled Release, 158*(2), 182–193. doi:10.1016/j.jconrel.2011.09.083 PMID:21978644

Anadón, A., Martínez-Larrañaga, M. R., Arés, I., & Martínez, M. A. (2016). Prebiotics and Probiotics: An Assessment of Their Safety and Health Benefits. In Probiotics, Prebiotics, and Synbiotic. Elsevier Inc. doi:10.1016/B978-0-12-802189-7.00001-0

Anderson, K. M., Wilson, P. W., Odell, P. M., & Kannel, W. B. (1991). An updated coronary risk profile. A statement for health professionals. *Circulation, 83*(1), 356–362. doi:10.1161/01.CIR.83.1.356 PMID:1984895

Anderson, R. C., Cookson, A. L., McNabb, W. C., Park, Z., McCann, M. J., Kelly, W. J., & Roy, N. C. (2010). Lactobacillus plantarum MB452 enhances the function of the intestinal barrier by increasing the expression levels of genes involved in tight junction formation. *BMC Microbiology, 10*(1), 316. doi:10.1186/1471-2180-10-316 PMID:21143932

Andersson, A. F., Lindberg, M., Jakobsson, H., Backhed, F., Nyren, P., & Engstrand, L. (2008). Comparative analysis of human gut microbiota by barcoded pyrosequencing. *PLoS One, 3*(7), e2836. doi:10.1371/journal.pone.0002836 PMID:18665274

Ando, C., Takahashi, N., Hirai, S., Nishimura, K., Lin, S., Uemura, T., ... Kawada, T. (2009). Luteolin, a food derived flavonoid, suppresses adipocyte-dependent activation of macrophages by inhibiting JNK activation. *FEBS Letters, 583*(22), 3649–3654. doi:10.1016/j.febslet.2009.10.045 PMID:19854181

Angell, M. (2005). *The Truth about The Drug Companies: How they Deceive Us and What To Do About It*. Random House Publisher.

Ankolekar, C., Terry, T., Johnson, K., Johnson, D., Barbosa, A. C. L., & Shetty, K. (2011). Anti-hyperglycemia properties of Tea (Camellia sinensis) bioactives using in vitro assay models and influence of extraction time. *Journal of Medicinal Food, 14*(10), 1190–1197. doi:10.1089/jmf.2010.0291 PMID:21859352

Annweiler, C., Llewellyn, D. J., & Beauchet, O. (2013). Low serum vitamin D concentrations in Alzheimer's disease: A systematic review and meta-analysis. *Journal of Alzheimer's Disease, 33*(3), 659–674. PMID:23042216

Annweiler, C., Rolland, Y., Schott, A. M., Blain, H., Vellas, B., Herrmann, F. R., & Beauchet, O. (2012). Higher vitamin D dietary intake is associated with lower risk of alzheimer's disease: A 7-year follow-up. *The Journals of Gerontology. Series A, Biological Sciences and Medical Sciences, 67*(11), 1205–1211. doi:10.1093/gerona/gls107 PMID:22503994

Anon. (1989). Analysis of steryl glycosides. In W. D. Nes & E. J. Parish (Eds.), *Analysis of sterols and other biologically significant steroids*. San Diego, CA: Academic Press Inc.

Anon. (2003). *Functional foods fact sheet: Plant stenols and sterols*. Available: http://ific.org/

Anon. (2005). *Phytosterol esters (Plant sterols and stenols esters).* Available: http://www.ifst.org/hottop29.htm

Anon. (2006). *Comprehensive review of scientific literature pertaining to nitrogen protein conversion factors, IDF Bulletin 405*. Brussels: International Dairy Federation.

Appel, L. J. (2003). The effects of protein intake on blood pressure and cardiovascular disease. *Current Opinion in Lipidology*, *14*(1), 55–59. doi:10.1097/00041433-200302000-00010 PMID:12544662

Appel, L. J., Moore, T. J., Obarzanek, E., Vollmer, W. M., Svetkey, L. P., Sacks, F. M., & Karanja, N. (1997). A clinical trial of the effects of dietary patterns on blood pressure. DASH Collaborative Research Group. *The New England Journal of Medicine*, *336*(16), 1117–1124. doi:10.1056/NEJM199704173361601 PMID:9099655

Appel, L. J., Sacks, F. M., Carey, V. J., Obarzanek, E., Swain, J. F., Miller, E. R., ... OmniHeart Collaborative Research Group. (2005). Effects of protein, monounsaturated fat, and carbohydrate intake on blood pressure and serum lipids: Results of the OmniHeart randomized trial. *Journal of the American Medical Association*, *294*(19), 2455–2464. doi:10.1001/jama.294.19.2455 PMID:16287956

Appendino, G., Belcaro, G., Cornelli, U., Luzzi, R., Togni, S., Dugall, M., ... Pellegrini, L. (2011). Potential role of curcumin phytosome (Meriva) in controlling the evolution of diabetic microangiopathy.A pilot study. *Panminerva Medica*, *53*(3Suppl 1), 43–49. PMID:22108476

Appleby, P. N., Thorogood, M., Mann, J. I., & Key, T. J. (1999). The Oxford Vegetarian Study: An overview. *The American Journal of Clinical Nutrition*, *70*(3Suppl), 525S–531S. doi:10.1093/ajcn/70.3.525s PMID:10479226

Aprikian, O., Duclos, V., Guyot, S., Besson, C., Manach, C., Bernalier, A., ... Demigne, C. (2003). Apple Pectin and a Polyphenol-Rich Apple Concentrate Are More Effective Together than Separately on Cecal Fermentations and Plasma Lipids in Rats. *The Journal of Nutrition*, *133*(6), 1860–1865. doi:10.1093/jn/133.6.1860 PMID:12771330

Aragon, G., Graham, D. B., Borum, M., & Doman, D. B. (2010). Probiotic therapy for irritable bowel syndrome. *Gastroenterology & Hepatology*, *6*(1), 39–44. PMID:20567539

Arai, S. (1996). Studies on functional foods in Japan--state of the art. *Bioscience, Biotechnology, and Biochemistry*, *60*(1), 9–15. doi:10.1271/bbb.60.9 PMID:8824819

Aranda, F. J., & Villala, J. (1997). The interaction of abietic acid with phospholipid membranes. *Biochimica et Biophysica Acta*, *1327*(2), 171–180. doi:10.1016/S0005-2736(97)00054-0 PMID:9271259

Arnold, J. W., Roach, J., & Azcarate-Peril, M. A. (2016). Emerging Technologies for Gut Microbiome Research. *Trends in Microbiology*, *24*(11), 887–901. doi:10.1016/j.tim.2016.06.008 PMID:27426971

Arora, T., Anastasovska, J., Gibson, G., Tuohy, K., Sharma, R. K., Bell, J., & Frost, G. (2012). Effect of Lactobacillus acidophilus NCDC 13 supplementation on the progression of obesity in diet-induced obese mice. *British Journal of Nutrition, 108*(08), 1382–1389. doi:10.1017/S0007114511006957 PMID:22289627

Arora, T., Sharma, R., & Frost, G. (2011). Propionate. Anti-obesity and satiety enhancing factor. *Appetite, 56*(2), 511–515. doi:10.1016/j.appet.2011.01.016 PMID:21255628

Ashari, A., Omar, J., Hashim, A., & Hamid, S. (2016). Apolipoprotein E Gene Polymorphism and Its Association with Cardiovascular Heart Disease Risk Factors in Type 2 Diabetes Mellitus. *World Academy of Science, Engineering and Technology, International Journal of Medical, Health, Biomedical. Bioengineering and Pharmaceutical Engineering, 10*(9), 471–476.

Ashor, A. W., Siervo, M., Lara, J., Oggioni, C., Afshar, S., & Mathers, J. C. (2015). Effect of vitamin C and vitamin E supplementation on endothelial function: A systematic review and meta-analysis of randomised controlled trials. *British Journal of Nutrition, 113*(08), 1182–1194. doi:10.1017/S0007114515000227 PMID:25919436

Assini, J. M., Mulvihill, E. E., & Huff, M. W. (2013). Citrus flavonoids and lipid metabolism. *Current Opinion in Lipidology, 24*(1), 34–40. doi:10.1097/MOL.0b013e32835c07fd PMID:23254473

Astrup, A., Bulow, J., Christensen, N. J., Madsen, J., & Quaade, F. (1986). Facultative thermogenesis induced by carbohydrate: A skeletal muscle component mediated by epinephrine. *The American Journal of Physiology, 250*, E226–E229. PMID:3513610

Augustin, M. A. (2001). Functional foods : An adventure in food formulation. *Food Australia, 53*(10), 428–432.

Avila, M. A., Velasco, J. A., Cansado, J., & Notario, V. (1994). Quercetin mediates the down-regulation of mutant p53 in the human breast cancer cell line MDA-MB468. *Cancer Research, 54*(9), 2424–2428. PMID:8162591

Awad, A. B., Chen, Y. C., Fink, C. S., & Hennessey, T. (n.d.). beta-Sitosterol inhibits HT-29 human colon cancer cell growth and alters membrane lipids. *Anticancer Research, 16*(5A), 2797–804.

Awad, A. B., & Fink, C. S. (2000). Phytosterols as anticancer dietary components: Evidence and mechanism of action. *The Journal of Nutrition, 130*(9), 2127–2130. doi:10.1093/jn/130.9.2127 PMID:10958802

Awad, A. B., Karen, C. C., Downie, A. C., & Fink, C. S. (2000). Peanuts as a source of B-sitosterol, a Sterol with anticancer properties. *Nutrition and Cancer, 36*(2), 238–241. doi:10.1207/S15327914NC3602_14 PMID:10890036

Awad, E. M., & Binder, B. R. (2005). In vitro induction of endothelial cell fibrinolytic alterations by Nigella sativa. *Phytomedicine, 12*(3), 194–202. doi:10.1016/j.phymed.2003.09.008 PMID:15830841

Axona. (2017, March 13). In *Wikipedia*. Retrieved from https://en.wikipedia.org/w/index.php?title=Axona&oldid=770058091

Ayabe, T., Satchell, D. P., Wilson, C. L., Parks, W. C., Selsted, M. E., & Ouellette, A. J. (2000). Secretion of microbicidal alpha defensins by intestinal Paneth cells in response to bacteria. *Nature Immunology*, *1*(2), 113–118. doi:10.1038/77783 PMID:11248802

Baba, S., Natsume, M., Yasuda, A., Nakamura, Y., Tamura, T., Osakabe, N., ... Kondo, K. (2007). Plasma LDL and HDL cholesterol and oxidized LDL concentrations are altered in normo- and hypercholesterolemic humans after intake of different levels of cocoa powder. *The Journal of Nutrition*, *137*(6), 1436–1441. doi:10.1093/jn/137.6.1436 PMID:17513403

Bacigalupo, A. (2007). Aplastic anemia: Pathogenesis and treatment. *Hematology*, *2007*(1), 23–28. doi:10.1182/asheducation-2007.1.23 PMID:18024605

Badimon, L., Vilahur, G., & Padro, T. (2010). Nutraceuticals and atherosclerosis: Human trials. *Cardiovascular Therapeutics*, *28*(4), 202–215. doi:10.1111/j.1755-5922.2010.00189.x PMID:20633023

Bae, E. K., & Lee, S. J. (2008). Microencapsulation of avocado oil by spray drying using whey protein and maltodextrin. *Journal of Microencapsulation*, *25*(8), 549–560. doi:10.1080/02652040802075682 PMID:18465295

Bagchi, D., Bagchi, M., Stohs, S. J., Das, D. K., Ray, S. D., Kuszynski, C. A., ... Pruess, H. G. (2000). Free radicals and grape seed proanthocyanidin extract: Importance in human health and disease prevention. *Toxicology*, *148*(2), 187–197. doi:10.1016/S0300-483X(00)00210-9 PMID:10962138

Bagger, M., Andersen, O., Nielsen, J. B., & Ryttig, K. R. (1996). Dietary fibres reduce blood pressure, serum total cholesterol and platelet aggregation in rats. *British Journal of Nutrition*, *75*(3), 483–493. doi:10.1079/BJN19960149 PMID:8785220

Bahamondes, M. V., Portugal, P. M., Brolazo, E. M., Simões, J. A., & Bahamondes, L. (2011). Use of a lactic acid plus lactoserum intimate liquid soap for external hygiene in the prevention of bacterial vaginosis recurrence after metronidazole oral treatment. *Revista da Associação Médica Brasileira*, *57*(4), 415–420. doi:10.1590/S0104-42302011000400015 PMID:21876923

Baida, D.-H., Messaouda, B., & Abdeltif, A. (2010). Formulation and evaluation of a selective medium for lactic acid bacteria-validation on some dairy products. *American Journal of Agricultural and Biological Sciences*, *5*(2), 148–153. doi:10.3844/ajabssp.2010.148.153

Baker, E. N., & Baker, H. M. (2009). A structural framework for understanding the multifunctional character of lactoferrin. *Biochimie*, *91*(1), 3–10. doi:10.1016/j.biochi.2008.05.006 PMID:18541155

Bakken, J. S. (2009). Fecal bacteriotherapy for recurrent Clostridium difficile infection. *Anaerobe*, *15*(6), 285–289. doi:10.1016/j.anaerobe.2009.09.007 PMID:19778623

Ballard, C., Margallo-Lana, M., Juszczak, E., Douglas, S., Swann, A., Thomas, A., ... Lee, L. (2005). Quetiapine and rivastigmine and cognitive decline in Alzheimer9s disease: Randomised double blind placebo controlled trial. *BMJ (Clinical Research Ed.)*, *330*(7496), 874. doi:10.1136/bmj.38369.459988.8F PMID:15722369

Ballard, H. S. (1997). The hematological complications of alcoholism. *Alcohol Health and Research World*, *21*, 42–52. PMID:15706762

Balunas, M. J., & Kinghorn, A. D. (2005). Drug discovery from medicinal plants. *Life Sciences*, *78*(5), 431–441. doi:10.1016/j.lfs.2005.09.012 PMID:16198377

Bandmann, O., Weiss, K. H., & Kaler, S. G. (2015). Wilson's disease and other neurological copper disorders. *Lancet Neurology*, *14*(1), 103–113. doi:10.1016/S1474-4422(14)70190-5 PMID:25496901

Banerjee, S. K., & Maulik, S. K. (2002). Effect of garlic on cardiovascular disorders: A review. *Nutrition Journal*, *1*(1), 4. doi:10.1186/1475-2891-1-4 PMID:12537594

Bansal, S., Mangal, M., Sharma, S. K., & Gupta, R. K. (2016). Non-Dairy based probiotics: A healthy treat for intestine. *Critical Reviews in Food Science and Nutrition*, *56*(11), 1856–1867. doi:10.1080/10408398.2013.790780 PMID:25747894

Baranauskiene, R., Venskutonis, P. R., Dewettinck, K., & Verhé, R. (2006). Properties of oregano (*Origanum vulgare L.*), citronella (*Cymbopogon nardus G.*) and marjoram (*Majorana hortensis L.*) flavors encapsulated into milk protein-based matrices. *Food Research International*, *39*(4), 413–425. doi:10.1016/j.foodres.2005.09.005

Barb, D., Williams, C. J., Neuwirth, A. K., & Mantzoros, C. S. (2007). Adiponectin in relation to malignancies: A review of existing basic research and clinical evidence. *The American Journal of Clinical Nutrition*, *86*(3), s858–s866. doi:10.1093/ajcn/86.3.858S PMID:18265479

Barrow, C., & Shahidi, F. (Eds.). (2007). *Marine nutraceuticals and functional foods*. CRC Press.

Bartlett, J. G. (2002). Antibiotic-associated diarrhoea. *The New England Journal of Medicine*, *346*(5), 334–339. doi:10.1056/NEJMcp011603 PMID:11821511

Basch, E., Ulbricht, C., Kuo, G., Szapary, P., & Smith, M. (2003). Therapeutic applications of fenugreek. *Alternative Medicine Review*, *8*(1), 20–27. PMID:12611558

Bast, A., & Haenen, R. M. M. (1998). Interplay between lipoic acid and glutathione in the protection against microsomal lipid peroxidation. *Biochimica et Biophysica Acta*, *963*(3), 558–561. doi:10.1016/0005-2760(88)90326-8 PMID:3143421

Basu, A., Betts, N. M., Nguyen, A., Newman, E. D., Fu, D., & Lyons, T. J. (2014). Freeze-dried strawberries lower serum cholesterol and lipid peroxidation in adults with abdominal adiposity and elevated serum lipids. *The Journal of Nutrition*, *144*(6), 830–837. doi:10.3945/jn.113.188169 PMID:24670970

Basu, A., Rhone, M., & Lyons, T. J. (2010). Berries: Emerging impact on cardiovascular health. *Nutrition Reviews*, *68*(3), 168–177. doi:10.1111/j.1753-4887.2010.00273.x PMID:20384847

Batetta, B., Griinari, M., Carta, G., Murru, E., Ligresti, A., Cordeddu, L., ... Banni, S. (2009). Endo-cannabinoids may mediate the ability of (n-3) fatty acids to reduce ectopic fat and inflammatory mediators in obese Zucker rats. *The Journal of Nutrition*, *139*(8), 1495–1501. doi:10.3945/jn.109.104844 PMID:19549757

Batterham, R. L., Cowley, M. A., Small, C. J., Herzog, H., Cohen, M. A., & Deakin, C. L. (2002). Gut hormone PYY(3-36) physiologically inhibits food intake. *Nature*, *418*(6898), 415–421. doi:10.1038/nature00887 PMID:12167864

Bazinet, R. P., & Layé, S. (2014). Polyunsaturated fatty acids and their metabolites in brain function and disease. *Nature Reviews. Neuroscience*, *15*(12), 771–785. doi:10.1038/nrn3820 PMID:25387473

Beilin, L. J., & Burke, V. (1995). Vegetarian diet components, protein and blood pressure: Which nutrients are important? *Clinical and Experimental Pharmacology & Physiology*, *22*(3), 195–198. doi:10.1111/j.1440-1681.1995.tb01979.x PMID:7554413

Ben Amor, K., Breeuwer, P., Verbaarschot, P., Rombouts, F. M., Akkermans, A. D. L., De Vos, W. M., & Abee, T. (2002). Multi-parametric flow cytometry and cell sorting for the assessment of viable, injured, and dead *Bifidobacterium* cells during bile salt stress. *Applied and Environmental Microbiology*, *68*(11), 5209–5216. doi:10.1128/AEM.68.11.5209-5216.2002 PMID:12406706

Berdanier, C. D. (1994). Nutrient-gene interactions: Today and tomorrow. *The FASEB Journal*, *8*(1), 1. doi:10.1096/fasebj.8.1.8299881 PMID:8299881

Berer, K., Mues, M., Koutrolos, M., Rasbi, Z. A., Boziki, M., Johner, C., ... Krishnamoorthy, G. (2011). Commensal microbiota and myelin autoantigen cooperate to trigger autoimmune demyelination. *Nature*, *479*(7374), 538–541. doi:10.1038/nature10554 PMID:22031325

Berger, A., & Jones, P. J. H. (2004). Plant sterols: Factors affecting their efficacy and safety as functional food ingredients. *Lipids in Health and Disease*, *3*(1), 1–54. doi:10.1186/1476-511X-3-1 PMID:15070410

Bermudez-Brito, M., Plaza-Díaz, J., Muñoz-Quezada, S., Gómez-Llorente, C., & Gil, A. (2012). Probiotic Mechanisms of Action. *Annals of Nutrition & Metabolism*, *61*(2), 160–174. doi:10.1159/000342079 PMID:23037511

Bernstein, A. M., Sun, Q., Hu, F. B., Stampfer, M. J., Manson, J. E., & Willett, W. C. (2010). Major dietary protein sources and risk of coronary heart disease in women. *Circulation*, *122*(9), 876–883. doi:10.1161/CIRCULATIONAHA.109.915165 PMID:20713902

Berquin, I. M., Min, Y., Wu, R., Wu, J., Perry, D., Cline, J. M., ... Chen, Y. Q. (2007). Modulation of prostate cancer genetic risk by omega-3 and omega-6 fatty acids. *The Journal of Clinical Investigation*, *117*(7), 1866–1875. doi:10.1172/JCI31494 PMID:17607361

Berry, C. E., & Hare, J. M. (2004). Xanthine oxidoreductase and cardiovascular disease: Molecular mechanisms and pathophysiological implications. *The Journal of Physiology*, *555*(Pt 3), 589–606. doi:10.1113/jphysiol.2003.055913 PMID:14694147

Berthoud, H. R., Lenard, N. R., & Shin, A. C. (2011). Food reward, hyperphagia, and obesity. *American Journal of Physiology. Regulatory, Integrative and Comparative Physiology*, *300*(6), R1266–R1277. doi:10.1152/ajpregu.00028.2011 PMID:21411768

Bertomeu, V., & Castillo-Castillo, J. (2008). Situación de la enfermedad cardiovascular en España. Del riesgo a la enfermedad. *Revista Espanola de Cardiologia*, *8*(Supl.E), 2–9.

Bhagwat, Haytowitz, & Holden. (2014). USDA Database for the Flavonoid Content of Selected Foods Release 3.1. U.S. Department of Agriculture Agricultural Research Service.

Bhagwat, R. R. (2015). Novel drug delivery systems: an overview. *International Journal of Pharmaceutical Sciences and Research*. Retrieved April 12, 2017, from http://ijpsr.com/bft-article/novel-drug-delivery-systems-an-overview/?view=fulltext

Bhandari, P. R., & Kamdod, M. A. (2012). *Emblica officicalis* (Amla): A review on potential therapeutic applications. *International Journal of Green Pharmacy*, *6*(4), 257–269. doi:10.4103/0973-8258.108204

Bhardwaj, S., Passi, S. J., & Misra, A. (2011). Overview of trans fatty acids: Biochemistry and health effects. *Diabetes & Metabolic Syndrome*, *5*(3), 161–164. doi:10.1016/j.dsx.2012.03.002 PMID:22813572

Bharti, A. C., Donato, N., & Aggarwal, B. B. (2003). Curcumin (diferuloylmethane) inhibits constitutive and IL-6-inducible STAT3 phosphorylation in human multiple myeloma cells. *Journal of Immunology, 171*(7), 3863–71.

Bhathena, S. J., & Velasquez, M. T. (2002). Beneficial role of dietary phytoestrogens in obesity and diabetes. *The American Journal of Clinical Nutrition*, *76*(6), 1191–1201. doi:10.1093/ajcn/76.6.1191 PMID:12450882

Bhatnagar, S., & Taneja, S. (2001). Zinc and cognitive development. *British Journal of Nutrition*, *85*(S2Suppl 2), S139–S145. doi:10.1079/BJN2000306 PMID:11509102

Bhui, K., Prasad, S., George, J., & Shukla, Y. (2009). Bromelain inhibits COX-2 expression by blocking the activation of MAPK regulated NF-kappa B against skin tumor-initiation triggering mitochondrial death pathway. *Cancer Letters*, *282*(2), 167–176. doi:10.1016/j.canlet.2009.03.003 PMID:19339108

Bibiloni, R., Fedorak, R. N., Tannock, G. W., Madsen, K. L., Gionchetti, P., Campieri, M., ... Sartor, R. B. (2005). VSL#3 probiotic-mixture induces remission in patients with active ulcerative colitis. *The American Journal of Gastroenterology*, *100*(7), 1539–1546. doi:10.1111/j.1572-0241.2005.41794.x PMID:15984978

Bierbaum, G., & Sahl, H. G. (2009). Lantibiotics: Mode of action, biosynthesis and bioengineering. *Current Pharmaceutical Biotechnology*, *10*(1), 2–18. doi:10.2174/138920109787048616 PMID:19149587

Bischoff, S., & Crowe, S. E. (2004). Food allergy and the gastrointestinal tract. *Current Opinion in Gastroenterology*, *20*(2), 156–161. doi:10.1097/00001574-200403000-00018 PMID:15703638

Bitanihirwe, B. K. Y., & Cunningham, M. G. (2009). Zinc: The brain's dark horse. *Synapse (New York, N.Y.)*, *63*(11), 1029–1049. doi:10.1002yn.20683 PMID:19623531

Blaser, M. (2011). Antibiotic overuse: Stop the killing of beneficial bacteria. *Nature*, *476*(7361), 393–394. doi:10.1038/476393a PMID:21866137

Blasina, F., Vaamonde, L., Silvera, F., Tedesco, A. C., & Dajas, F. (2015). Intravenous nanosomes of quercetin improve brain function and hemodynamic instability after severe hypoxia in newborn piglets. *Neurochemistry International*, *89*, 149–156. doi:10.1016/j.neuint.2015.08.007 PMID:26297982

Block, G., Mangels, A. R., Norkus, E. P., Patterson, B. H., Levander, O. A., & Taylor, P. R. (2001). Ascorbic acid status and subsequent diastolic and systolic blood pressure. *Hypertension (Dallas, Tex.: 1979)*, *37*(2), 261–267.

Boericke, W. (1901). *Pocket Manual of Homeopathic Materia Medica*. Retrieved from http://www.materiamedica.info/en/materia-medica/william-boericke/index

Boericke, W. (1927). Pocket manual of homoeopathic materia medica: comprising the characteristic and guiding symptoms of all remedies (clinical and pathogenetic). Santa Rosa, CA: Academic Press.

Bogani, P., Galli, C., Villa, M., & Visioli, F. (2007). Postprandial anti-inflammatory and antioxidant effects of extra virgin olive oil. *Atherosclerosis*, *190*(1), 181–186. doi:10.1016/j.atherosclerosis.2006.01.011 PMID:16488419

Bohnen, N. I., Kaufer, D. I., Hendrickson, R., Ivanco, L. S., Lopresti, B., Davis, J. G., & DeKosky, S. T. (2005). Cognitive correlates of alterations in acetylcholinesterase in Alzheimer's disease. *Neuroscience Letters*, *380*(1–2), 127–132. doi:10.1016/j.neulet.2005.01.031 PMID:15854764

Boltin, D. (in press). Probiotics in Helicobacter *pylori*-induced peptic ulcer disease. *Best Practice & Research. Clinical Gastroenterology*. doi:10.1016/j.bpg.2015.12.003 PMID:27048901

Bonnesen, C., Eggleston, I. M., & Hayes, J. D. (2001). Dietary indoles and isothiocyanates that are generated from cruciferous vegetables can both stimulate apoptosis and confer protection against DNA damage in human colon cell lines. *Cancer Research*, *61*(16), 6120–6130. PMID:11507062

Boon, H., & Wong, J. (2004). Botanical medicine and cancer: A review of the safety and efficacy. *Expert Opinion on Pharmacotherapy*, *5*(12), 2485–2501. doi:10.1517/14656566.5.12.2485 PMID:15571467

Boothby, L. A., & Doering, P. L. (2005). Vitamin C and vitamin E for Alzheimer's disase. *The Annals of Pharmacotherapy*, *39*(12), 2073–2080. doi:10.1345/aph.1E495 PMID:16227450

Boque, N., Iglesia, R., Garza, A. L., Milagro, F. I., Olivares, M., Bañuelos, O., ... Campión, J. (2013). Prevention of Diet-Induced Obesity by Apple Polyphenols in Wistar Rats through Regulation of Adipocyte Gene Expression and DNA Methylation Patterns. *Molecular Nutrition & Food Research*, *57*(8), 1473–1478. doi:10.1002/mnfr.201200686 PMID:23529981

Borchers, A. T., Keen, C. L., & Gershwin, M. E. (2016). The Basis of Structure/Function Claims of Nutraceuticals. *Clinical Reviews in Allergy & Immunology*, *51*(3), 370–382. doi:10.100712016-016-8536-9 PMID:27122022

Bortlik, K., Saucy, F., Duruz, E., Richelle, M., Lambelet, P., Baur, M., & Pfeifer, A.M.A. (2005). *Primary composition comprising a lipophilic bioactive compound.* US 2005/0106219 A1.

Bose, K. S., & Sarma, R. H. (1975). Delineation of the intimate details of the backbone conformation of pyridine nucleotide coenzymes in aqueous solution. *Biochemical and Biophysical Research Communications*, *66*(4), 1173–1179. doi:10.1016/0006-291X(75)90482-9 PMID:2

Bose, M., Lambert, J. D., Ju, J., Reuhl, K. R., Shapses, S. A., & Yang, C. S. (2008). The major green tea polyphenol, (-)-epigallocatechin-3-gallate, inhibits obesity, metabolic syndrome, and fatty liver disease in high-fat-fed mice. *The Journal of Nutrition*, *138*(9), 1677–1683. doi:10.1093/jn/138.9.1677 PMID:18716169

Bosnea, L. A., Moschakis, T., & Biliaderis, C. G. (2014). Complex Coacervation as a Novel Microencapsulation Technique to Improve Viability of Probiotics under Different Stresses. *Food and Bioprocess Technology*, *7*(10), 2767–2781. doi:10.100711947-014-1317-7

Bothwell, T. H., & Charlton, R. W. (1981). *Iron deficiency in women: a report of the International Nutritional Anemia Consultative Group (INACG).* New York: The Nutrition Foundation.

Bouhallab, S., & Bouglé, D. (2004). Biopeptides of milk: Caseinophosphopeptides and mineral bioavailability. *Reproduction, Nutrition, Development*, *44*(5), 493–498. doi:10.1051/rnd:2004053 PMID:15636166

Bousvaros, A., Guandalini, S., Baldassano, R. N., Botelho, C., Evans, J., Ferry, G. D., ... Hibberd, P. L. (2005). A randomized, double-blind trial of *Lactobacillus GG* versus placebo in addition to standard maintenance therapy for children with Crohn's disease. *Inflammatory Bowel Diseases*, *11*(9), 833–839. doi:10.1097/01.MIB.0000175905.00212.2c PMID:16116318

Bovell-Benjamin, A. C., Allen, L. H., Frankel, E. N., & Guinard, J. X. (1999). Sensory quality and lipid oxidation of maize porridge as affected by iron amino acid chelates and EDTA. *Journal of Food Science*, *64*(2), 371–376. doi:10.1111/j.1365-2621.1999.tb15903.x

Bovell-Benjamin, A. C., Allen, L. H., & Guinard, J. X. (1999). Toddlers' acceptance of whole maize meal porridge fortified with ferrous bisglycinate. *Food Quality and Preference*, *10*(2), 123–128. doi:10.1016/S0950-3293(98)00058-5

Bovell-Benjamin, A. C., Viteri, F. E., & Allen, L. H. (2000). Iron absorption from ferrous bisglycinate and ferric trisglycinate in whole maize is regulated by iron status. *The American Journal of Clinical Nutrition*, *71*(6), 1563–1569. doi:10.1093/ajcn/71.6.1563 PMID:10837299

Boyle, R. J., Robins-Browne, R. M., & Tang, M. L. K. (2006). Probiotic use in clinical practice: What are the risks? *The American Journal of Clinical Nutrition*, *83*(6), 1256–1264. doi:10.1093/ajcn/83.6.1256 PMID:16762934

Brand-Miller, J. C., Holt, S. H., Pawlak, D. B., & McMillan, J. (2002). Glycemic index and obesity. *The American Journal of Clinical Nutrition*, *76*(1), 281S–285S. doi:10.1093/ajcn/76.1.281S PMID:12081852

Brimson, J. M., Brimson, S. J., Brimson, C. A., Rakkhitawatthana, V., & Tencomnao, T. (2012). Rhinacanthus nasutus Extracts Prevent Glutamate and Amyloid-β Neurotoxicity in HT-22 Mouse Hippocampal Cells: Possible Active Compounds Include Lupeol, Stigmasterol and β-Sitosterol. *International Journal of Molecular Sciences*, *13*(4), 5074–5097. doi:10.3390/ijms13045074 PMID:22606031

Broadhurst, C. L. (1997). Balanced intakes of natural triglycerides for optimum nutrition: An evolutionary and phytochemical perspective. *Medical Hypotheses*, *49*(3), 247–261. doi:10.1016/S0306-9877(97)90210-3 PMID:9293470

Broekaert, W. F., Courtin, C. M., Verbeke, K., Vandewiele, T., Verstraete, W., & Delcour, J. A. (2011). Prebiotic and other health-related effects of cereal-derived arabinoxylans, arabinoxylan-oligosaccharides, and xylooligosaccharides. *Critical Reviews in Food Science and Nutrition*, *51*(2), 178–194. doi:10.1080/10408390903044768 PMID:21328111

Broekmans, W. M., Klöpping-Ketelaars, I. A., Schuurman, C. R., Verhagen, H., van den Berg, H., Kok, F. J., & van Poppel, G. (2000). Fruits and vegetables increase plasma carotenoids and vitamins and decrease homocysteine in humans. *The Journal of Nutrition*, *130*(6), 1578–1583. doi:10.1093/jn/130.6.1578 PMID:10827213

Bron, P. A., Baarlen, P. V., & Kleerebezem, M. (2012). Emerging molecular insights into the interaction between probiotics and the host intestinal mucosa. *Nature*, *10*(1), 66–78. PMID:22101918

Bruck, W. M., Redgrave, M., Tuohy, K. M., Lonnerdal, B., Graverholt, G., Hernell, O., & Gibson, G. R. (2006). Effects of bovine alpha-lactalbumin and casein glycomacropeptide-enriched infant formulae on faecal microbiota in healthy term infants. *Journal of Pediatric Gastroenterology and Nutrition*, *43*(5), 673–679. doi:10.1097/01.mpg.0000232019.79025.8f PMID:17130747

Brüll, F., Mensink, R. P., van den Hurk, K., Duijvestijn, A., & Plat, J. (2010). TLR2 activation is essential to induce a Th1 shift in human peripheral blood mononuclear cells by plant stanols and plant sterols. *The Journal of Biological Chemistry*, *285*(5), 2951–2958. doi:10.1074/jbc.M109.036343 PMID:19948716

Brumfield, K. M., Moroney, J. V., Moore, T. S., Simms, T. A., & Donze, D. (2010). Functional characterization of the *Chlamydomonas reinhardtii ERG3* Ortholog, a gene involved in the biosynthesis of ergosterol. *PLoS One*, *5*(1), e8659. doi:10.1371/journal.pone.0008659 PMID:20084111

Bruun, J. M., Lihn, A. S., Pedersen, S. B., & Richelsen, B. (2005). Monocyte chemoattractant protein-1 release is higher in visceral than subcutaneous human adipose tissue (AT): Implication of macrophages resident in the AT. *The Journal of Clinical Endocrinology and Metabolism*, *90*(4), 2282–2289. doi:10.1210/jc.2004-1696 PMID:15671098

Buck, B. L., Altermann, E., Svingerud, T., & Klaenhammer, T. R. (2005). Functional analysis of putative adhesion factors in *Lactobacillus acidophilus* NCNCFM. *Applied and Environmental Microbiology*, *71*(12), 8344–8351. doi:10.1128/AEM.71.12.8344-8351.2005 PMID:16332821

Buckland, G., & Gonzalez, C. A. (2015). The role of olive oil in disease prevention: A focus on the recent epidemiological evidence from cohort studies and dietary intervention trials. *British Journal of Nutrition*, *113*(S2Suppl 2), S94–S101. doi:10.1017/S0007114514003936 PMID:26148926

Buhr, G., & Bales, C. W. (2010). Nutritional Supplements for Older Adults: Review and Recommendations—Part II. *Journal of Nutrition for the Elderly*, *29*(1), 42–71. doi:10.1080/01639360903586464 PMID:20391042

Bullock, N. R., Booth, J. C., & Gibson, G. R. (2004). Comparative composition of bacteria in the human intestinal microflora during remission and active ulcerative colitis. *Current Issues in Intestinal Microbiology*, *5*, 59–64. PMID:15460067

Burgain, J., Gaiani, C., Linder, M., & Scher, J. (2011). Encapsulation of probiotic living cells: From laboratory scale to industrial applications. *Journal of Food Engineering*, *104*(4), 467–483. doi:10.1016/j.jfoodeng.2010.12.031

Burr, M. L., & Butland, B. K. (1988). Heart disease in British vegetarians. *The American Journal of Clinical Nutrition*, *48*(3Suppl), 830–832. doi:10.1093/ajcn/48.3.830 PMID:3414590

Burr, M. L., Fehily, A. M., Gilbert, J. F., Rogers, S., Holliday, R. M., Sweetnam, P. M., ... Deadman, N. M. (1989). Effects of changes in fat, fish, and fibre intakes on death and myocardial reinfarction: Diet and reinfarction trial (DART). *Lancet (London, England)*, *2*(8666), 757–761. doi:10.1016/S0140-6736(89)90828-3 PMID:2571009

Buyru, N., Tezol, A., Yosunkaya-Fenerci, E., & Dalay, N. (2003). Vitamin D receptor gene polym orphism s in breast cancer. *Experimental & Molecular Medicine*, *35*(6), 550–555. doi:10.1038/emm.2003.72 PMID:14749534

Caballero, B., Finglas, P., & Toldrá, F. (2015). *Encyclopedia of food and health*. Oxford, UK: Academic Press.

Calder, P. C. (2006). Branched-chain amino acids and immunity. *The Journal of Nutrition*, *136*(1), 288S–293S. doi:10.1093/jn/136.1.288S PMID:16365100

Campos-Esparza, M. R., Sánchez-Gómez, M. V., & Matute, C. (2009). Molecular mechanisms of neuroprotection by two natural antioxidant polyphenols. *Cell Calcium*, *45*(4), 358–368. doi:10.1016/j.ceca.2008.12.007 PMID:19201465

Canani, R. B., Cirillo, P., Terrin, G., Cesarano, L., Spagnuolo, M. I., De Vicenzo, A., ... Guarino, A. (2007). Probiotics for treatment of acute diarrhoea in children: Randomised clinical trial of five different preparations. *British Medical Journal*, *335*(7615), 340. doi:10.1136/bmj.39272.581736.55 PMID:17690340

Canini, A., Alesiani, D., D'Arcangelo, G., & Tagliatesta, P. (2007). Gas chromatography–mass spectrometry analysis of phenolic compounds from Carica papaya L. leaf. *Journal of Food Composition and Analysis*, *20*(7), 584–590. doi:10.1016/j.jfca.2007.03.009

Cani, P. D., Possemiers, S., Van de Wiele, T., Guiot, Y., Everard, A., Rottier, O., ... Delzenne, N. M. (2009). Changes in gut microbiota control inflammation in obese mice through a mechanism involving GLP-2-driven improvement of gut permeability. *Gut*, *58*(8), 1091–1103. doi:10.1136/gut.2008.165886 PMID:19240062

Cantrill, R., & Kawamura, Y. (2008). Phytosterols, phytostanols and their esters Chemical and technical assessment. *Proceedings of 69th JECFA*, 1-13.

Capozzi, V., Russo, P., Duenas, M. T., Lopez, P., & Spano, G. (2012). Lactic acid bacteria producing B-group vitamins: A great potential for functional cereals products. *Applied Microbiology and Biotechnology*, *96*(6), 1383–1394. doi:10.100700253-012-4440-2 PMID:23093174

Cappellini, M. D., & Fiorelli, G. (2008). Glucose-6-phosphate dehydrogenase deficiency. *Lancet*, *371*(9606), 64–74. doi:10.1016/S0140-6736(08)60073-2 PMID:18177777

Cárdenas, C., Quesada, A. R., & Medina, M. A. (2006). Evaluation of the anti-angiogenic effect of aloe-emodin. *Cellular and Molecular Life Sciences*, *63*(24), 3083–3089. doi:10.100700018-006-6399-6 PMID:17131052

Cardoso, B. R., Roberts, B. R., Bush, A. I., & Hare, D. J. (2015). Selenium, selenoproteins and neurodegenerative diseases. *Metallomics*, *7*(8), 1213–1228. doi:10.1039/C5MT00075K PMID:25996565

Carey, G. W. (1894). *Biochemic System of Medicine*. The Theory, Pathological Action, Therapeutical Application, MateriaMedica, and Repertory of Schuessler's Twelve Tissue Remedies.

Carmena, R., Duriez, P., & Fruchart, J.-C. (2004). Atherogenic Lipoprotein Particles in Atherosclerosis. *Circulation*, *109*(23suppl 1), III-2–III-7. doi:10.1161/01.cir.0000131511.50734.44 PMID:15198959

Carpenter, K. J. (1988). The history of scurvy and vitamin C. Cambridge University Press.

Carroll, D. N., & Roth, M. T. (2002). Evidence for the cardioprotective effects of omega-3 Fatty acids. *The Annals of Pharmacotherapy*, *36*(12), 1950–1956. doi:10.1345/aph.1A314 PMID:12452760

Cassels, A., & Moyninan, R. (2005). *Selling Sickness: How Drug Companies Are Turning Us All into Patients*. Orion Publishing Group.

Castelli, W.P. (1988). Cholesterol and lipids in the risk of coronary artery disease--the Framingham Heart Study. *Canadian Journal of Cardiology, 4*(A), 5A-10A.

Casto, B. C., Kresty, L. A., Kraly, C. L., & Pearl, D. K. (2004). Chemoprevention of oral cancer by black raspberries. *Anticancer Research*, *22*(6C), 4005–4015. PMID:12553025

Cater, N. B. (2000). Plant stanol ester: Review of cholesterol-lowering efficacy and implications for coronary heart disease risk reduction. *Preventive Cardiology*, *3*(3), 121–130. doi:10.1111/j.1520-037X.2000.80370.x PMID:11834929

Cavalieri, E., Mariotto, S., Fabrizi, C., de Prati, A. C., Gottardo, R., Leone, S., ... Suzuki, H. (2004). α-Bisabolol, a nontoxic natural compound, strongly induces apoptosis in glioma cells. *Biochemical and Biophysical Research Communications*, *315*(3), 589–594. doi:10.1016/j.bbrc.2004.01.088 PMID:14975741

Cencic, A., & Chingwaru, W. (2010). The role of functional foods, nutraceuticals, and food supplements in intestinal health. *Nutrients*, *2*(6), 611–625. doi:10.3390/nu2060611 PMID:22254045

Cesar, T. B., Aptekmann, N. P., Araujo, M. P., Vinagre, C. C., & Maranhão, R. C. (2010). Orange juice decreases low-density lipoprotein cholesterol in hypercholesterolemic subjects and improves lipid transfer to high-density lipoprotein in normal and hypercholesterolemic subjects. *Nutrition Research (New York, N.Y.)*, *30*(10), 689–694. doi:10.1016/j.nutres.2010.09.006 PMID:21056284

Chadha, R., Bhalla, Y., Vashisht, M. K., & Chadha, K. (2015). Cocrystallization in Nutraceuticals. In *Recrystallization in Materials Processing*. InTech. doi:10.5772/59365

Chang, C. K., & Ulrich, C. M. (2003). Hyperinsulinaemia and hyperglycaemia: Possible risk factors of colorectal cancer among diabetic patients. *Diabetologia*, *46*(5), 595–607. doi:10.100700125-003-1109-5 PMID:12764580

Chang-Claude, J., Hermann, S., Eilber, U., & Steindorf, K. (2005). Lifestyle determinants and mortality in German vegetarians and health-conscious persons: Results of a 21-year follow-up. *Cancer Epidemiology, Biomarkers & Prevention*, *14*(4), 963–968. doi:10.1158/1055-9965.EPI-04-0696 PMID:15824171

Chang, M.-H., Hahn, R., Teutsch, S. M., & Hutwagner, L. C. (2001). Multiple risk factors and and population attributable risk for ischemic heart disease mortality in the United States, 1971-1992. *Journal of Clinical Epidemiology*, *54*(6), 634–644. doi:10.1016/S0895-4356(00)00343-7 PMID:11377125

Chang-Mu, C., Jen-Kun, L., Shing-Hwa, L., & Shoei-Yn, L.-S. (2010). Characterization of neurotoxic effects of NMDA and the novel neuroprotection by phytopolyphenols in mice. *Behavioral Neuroscience*, *124*(4), 541–553. doi:10.1037/a0020050 PMID:20695653

Chan, L.-N. (2002). Drug-nutrient interaction in clinical nutrition. *Current Opinion in Clinical Nutrition and Metabolic Care*, *5*(3), 327–332. doi:10.1097/00075197-200205000-00014 PMID:11953660

Chan, Y. M., Demonty, I., Pelled, D., & Jones, P. J. H. (2006). Olive oil containing olive oil fatty acid esters of plant sterols and dietary diacylglycerol reduces low-density lipoprotein cholesterol and decreases the tendency for peroxidation in hypercholesterolaemic subjects. *British Journal of Nutrition*, *98*(03), 563–570. doi:10.1017/S0007114507730775 PMID:17559697

Charoensiri, R., Kongkachuichai, R., Suknicom, S., & Sungpuag, P. (2009). Beta-carotene, lycopene, and alpha-tocopherol contents of selected Thai fruits. *Food Chemistry*, *113*(1), 202–207. doi:10.1016/j.foodchem.2008.07.074

Chasapis, C. T., Loutsidou, A. C., Spiliopoulou, C. A., & Stefanidou, M. E. (2012). Zinc and human health: An update. *Archives of Toxicology*, *86*(4), 521–534. doi:10.100700204-011-0775-1 PMID:22071549

Chaturvedi, S., Sharma, P. K., Garg, V. K., & Bansal, M. (2011). Role of nutraceuticals in health promotion. *Health*, *4*, 5.

Chauhan, N. B., & Mehla, J. (2014). Ameliorative Effects of Nutraceuticals in Neurological Disorders. Elsevier Inc.

Chauhan, B., Kumar, G., Kalam, N., & Ansari, S. H. (2013). Current concepts and prospects of herbal nutraceutical: A review. *Journal of Advanced Pharmaceutical Technology & Research*, *4*(1), 4. doi:10.4103/2231-4040.107494 PMID:23662276

Cha, Y. S. (2008). Effects of l-carnitine on obesity, diabetes, and as an ergogenic aid. *Asia Pacific Journal of Clinical Nutrition*, *17*(1), 306–308. PMID:18296364

Chen, A., Davis, B. H., Bissonnette, M., Scaglione-Sewell, B., & Brasitus, T. A. (1999). 1,25-Dihydroxyvitamin D(3) stimulates activator protein-1-dependent Caco-2 cell differentiation. *The Journal of Biological Chemistry*, *274*(50), 35505–35513. doi:10.1074/jbc.274.50.35505 PMID:10585423

Chen, C.-W., Lin, Y.-L., Lin, T.-K., Lin, C.-T., Chen, B.-C., & Lin, C.-L. (2008). Total cardiovascular risk profile of Taiwanese vegetarians. *European Journal of Clinical Nutrition*, *62*(1), 138–144. doi:10.1038j.ejcn.1602689 PMID:17356561

Chen, G., Shaw, M. H., Kim, Y. G., & Nuñez, G. (2009). NOD-like receptors: Role in innate immunity and inflammatory disease. *Annual Review of Pathology*, *4*(1), 365–398. doi:10.1146/annurev.pathol.4.110807.092239 PMID:18928408

Chen, G., Wang, H., Zhang, X., & Yang, S.-T. (2014). Nutraceuticals and functional foods in the management of hyperlipidemia. *Critical Reviews in Food Science and Nutrition*, *54*(9), 1180–1201. doi:10.1080/10408398.2011.629354 PMID:24499150

Chen, H.-Y., & Yen, G.-C. (2007). Antioxidant activity and free radical-scavenging capacity of extracts from guava (Psidium guajava L.) leaves. *Food Chemistry*, *101*(2), 686–694. doi:10.1016/j.foodchem.2006.02.047

Chen, L., Remondetto, G. E., & Subirade, M. (2006). Food protein-based materials as nutraceutical delivery systems. *Trends in Food Science & Technology*, *17*(5), 272–283. doi:10.1016/j.tifs.2005.12.011

Chen, Q., Gruber, H., Swist, E., Coville, K., Pakenham, C., Ratnayake, W. M. N., & Scoggan, K. A. (2010). Dietary phytosterols and phytostanols decrease cholesterol levels but increase blood pressure in WKY inbred rats in the absence of salt-loading. *Nutrition and Metabolism*, *7*(1), 11–20. doi:10.1186/1743-7075-7-11 PMID:20637058

Chin, SP, Jeyaindran, S, Azhari, R, Wan Azman, WA, Omar, I, Robaayah, Z, & Sim, KH. (2008). Acute Coronary Syndrome (ACS) Registry - Leading the charge for National Cardiovascular Disease (NCVD) Database. *Med J Malaysia, 63 Supplemen C*, 29-36.

Chirovsky, D. R., Fedirko, V., Cui, Y., Sazonov, V., & Barter, P. (2009). Prospective studies on the relationship between high-density lipoprotein cholesterol and cardiovascular risk: A systematic review. *European Journal of Cardiovascular Prevention and Rehabilitation*, *16*(4), 404–423. doi:10.1097/HJR.0b013e32832c8891 PMID:19465856

Chobanian, A. V., Bakris, G. L., Black, H. R., Cushman, W. C., Green, L. A., & Izzo, J. L. (2003). Seventh report of the Joint National Committee on Prevention, Detection, Evaluation, and Treatment of High Blood Pressure. *Hypertension (Dallas, Tex.: 1979)*, *42*(6), 1206–1252. 10.1161/01.HYP.0000107251.49515.c2

Choi, D. W., Monyer, H., Giffard, R. G., Goldberg, M. P., & Christine, C. W. (1990). Acute brain injury, NMDA receptors, and hydrogen ions: Observations in cortical cell cultures. *Advances in Experimental Medicine and Biology*, *268*, 501–504. doi:10.1007/978-1-4684-5769-8_55 PMID:2150160

Chopra, M., O'Neill, M. E., Keogh, N., Wortley, G., Southon, S., & Thurnham, D. I. (2000). Influence of increased fruit and vegetable intake on plasma and lipoprotein carotenoids and LDL oxidation in smokers and nonsmokers. *Clinical Chemistry*, *46*(11), 1818–1829. PMID:11067818

Choumenkovitch, S. F., McKeown, N. M., Tovar, A., Hyatt, R. R., Kraak, V. I., Hastings, A. V., et al. (2013). Whole grain consumption is inversely associated with BMI Z-score in rural school-aged children. *Public Health and Nutrition*, *16*(2), 212-218.

Christiansen, L. I., Lahteenmaki, P. L. A., Mannelin, M. R., Seppänen-Laakso, T. E., Hiltunen, R. V., & Yliruusi, J. K. (2001). Cholesterol-lowering effect of spreads enriched with microcrystalline plant sterols in hypercholesterolemic subjects. *European Journal of Nutrition*, *40*(2), 66–73. doi:10.1007003940170017 PMID:11518201

Chrysohoou, C., Panagiotakos, D. B., Pitsavos, C., Skoumas, I., Papademetriou, L., Economou, M., & Stefanadis, C. (2007). The implication of obesity on total antioxidant capacity in apparently healthy men and women: The ATTICA study. *Nutrition, Metabolism, and Cardiovascular Diseases*, *17*(8), 590–597. doi:10.1016/j.numecd.2006.05.007 PMID:16901682

Chung, T.-W., Moon, S.-K., Chang, Y.-C., Ko, J.-H., Lee, Y.-C., Cho, G., ... Kim, C.-H. (2004). Novel and therapeutic effect of caffeic acid and caffeic acid phenyl ester on hepatocarcinoma cells: Complete regression of hepatoma growth and metastasis by dual mechanism. *The FASEB Journal*, *18*(14), 1670–1681. doi:10.1096/fj.04-2126com PMID:15522912

Chu, Y.-F., & Liu, R. H. (2005). Cranberries inhibit LDL oxidation and induce LDL receptor expression in hepatocytes. *Life Sciences*, *77*(15), 1892–1901. doi:10.1016/j.lfs.2005.04.002 PMID:15982671

Chu, Y.-F., Sun, J., Wu, X., & Liu, R. H. (2002). Antioxidant and antiproliferative activities of common vegetables. *Journal of Agricultural and Food Chemistry*, *50*(23), 6910–6916. doi:10.1021/jf020665f PMID:12405796

Cilla, A., Alegría, A., Attanzio, A., Garcia-Llatas, G., Tesoriere, L., & Livrea, M. A. (2017). Dietary phytochemicals in the protection against oxysterol-induced damage. *Chemistry and Physics of Lipids*, *207*, 192–205. doi:10.1016/j.chemphyslip.2017.03.001 PMID:28267434

Cinq-Mars, C. D., Hu, C., Kitts, D. D., & Li-Chan, E. C. Y. (2008). Investigations into inhibitor type and mode, simulated gastrointestinal digestion, and cell transport of the angiotensin I-converting enzyme-inhibitory peptides in Pacific hake (Merluccius productus) fillet hydrolysate. *Journal of Agricultural and Food Chemistry*, *56*(2), 410–419. doi:10.1021/jf072277p PMID:18163568

Clausen, M. R., Bonnen, H., Tvede, M., & Mortensen, P. B. (1991). Colonic fermentation to short-chain fatty acids is decreased in antibiotic-associated diarrhea. *Gastroenterology*, *101*(6), 1497–1504. doi:10.1016/0016-5085(91)90384-W PMID:1955116

Clayton, P. E., Banerjee, I., Murray, P. G., & Renehan, A. G. (2011). Growth hormone, the insulin-like growth factor axis, insulin and cancer risk. *Nature Reviews. Endocrinology*, *7*(1), 11–24. doi:10.1038/nrendo.2010.171 PMID:20956999

Clifton, P. (2012). Effects of a high protein diet on body weight and comorbidities associated with obesity. *British Journal of Nutrition*, *108*(2), S122-S129.

Clifton, P. (2002). Plant sterol and stanols-comparison and contrasts. Sterol versus stanols in cholesterol lowering: Is there a difference? *Atherosclerosis*, *3*(3), 5–9. doi:10.1016/S1567-5688(02)00020-X PMID:12429167

Clifton, P. (2009). Lowering cholesterol: A review on the role of plant sterols. *Reprint from Australian Family Physician*, *38*(4), 218–221. PMID:19350071

Collet, C., Schwitzguébel, J.-P., & Péringer, P. (2003). Improvement of acetate production from lactose by growing *Clostridium thermolacticum* in mixed batch culture. *Journal of Applied Microbiology*, *95*(4), 824–831. doi:10.1046/j.1365-2672.2003.02060.x PMID:12969297

Comin, L. M., Temelli, F., & Saldaña, M. A. (2011). Supercritical CO2 extraction of flax lignans. *Journal of the American Oil Chemists' Society*, *88*(5), 707–715. doi:10.100711746-010-1704-9

Commane, D., Hughes, R., Shortt, C., & Rowland, I. (2005). The potential mechanisms involved in the anti-carcinogenic action of probiotics. *Mutation Research*, *591*(1-2), 276–289. doi:10.1016/j.mrfmmm.2005.02.027 PMID:16095630

Cook, N. C., & Samman, S. (1996). Flavonoids - Chemistry, metabolism, cardioprotective effects, and dietary sources. *The Journal of Nutritional Biochemistry*, *7*(2), 66–76. doi:10.1016/0955-2863(95)00168-9

Coppen, A., & Bolander-Gouaille, C. (2005). Treatment of depression: Time to consider folic acid and vitamin B12. *Journal of Psychopharmacology (Oxford, England), 19*(1), 59–65. doi:10.1177/0269881105048899 PMID:15671130

Corradini, C., Galanti, R., & Nicoletti, I. (2002). Characterization of nutraceuticals and functional foods by innovative HPLC methods. *Annali di Chimica, 92*(4), 387–396. PMID:12073884

Costa, L. G., Garrick, J., Roque, P. J., & Pellacani, C. (2016). Nutraceuticals in CNS Diseases: Potential Mechanisms of Neuroprotection. In R. C. Gupta (Ed.), *Nutraceuticals* (pp. 3–13). Boston: Academic Press. doi:10.1016/B978-0-12-802147-7.00001-2

Costa, R. G., Filho, E. M. B., Medeiros, G. R., Vilarroel, A. S., Cruz, S. E. S. B. S., & Santos, E. M. (2009). Replacement of goat milk by cheese whey in the feed of Alpine kids. *Tropical and Subtropical Agroecosystems, 11*, 87–90.

Council for Responsible Nutrition. (2003). Retrieved April 15, 2017, from http://www.crnusa.org/

Covian, D. R., Madiedo, P. R., Margolles, A., Gueimonde, M., Gavilan, C. G. D. L. R., & Salazar, N. (2016). Intestinal short chain fatty acids and their link with diet and human health. *Frontiers in Microbiology, 7*(185), 1–9. PMID:26834723

Crowther, M. A. (2005). Pathogenesis of Atherosclerosis. *Hematology, 2005*(1), 436–441. doi:10.1182/asheducation-2005.1.436 PMID:16304416

Crozier, A., Yokota, T., Jaganath, I. B., Marks, S., Saltmarsh, M., & Clifford, M. N. (2007). *Secondary Metabolites in Fruits, Vegetables, Beverages and Other Plant-based Dietary Components. In Plant Secondary Metabolites* (pp. 208–302). Blackwell Publishing Ltd.

Cruchet, S., Obregon, M. C., Salazar, G., Diaz, E., & Gottenland, M. (2003). Effect of the ingestion of a dietary product containing *Lactobacillus johnsonii* La1 on *Helicobacter pylori* colonization in children. *Nutrition (Burbank, Los Angeles County, Calif.), 19*(9), 716–721. doi:10.1016/S0899-9007(03)00109-6 PMID:12921879

Crujeiras, A. B., Parra, M. D., Rodríguez, M. C., Martínez de Morentin, B. E., & Martínez, J. A. (2006). A Role for Fruit Content in Energy-Restricted Diets in Improving Antioxidant Status in Obese Women during Weight Loss. *Nutrition (Burbank, Los Angeles County, Calif.), 22*(6), 593–599. doi:10.1016/j.nut.2006.03.008 PMID:16704952

Cruz, A. G., Sant'Ana, A. S., Macchione, M. M., Teixeira, A. M., & Schmidt, F. L. (2009). Milk drink using whey butter cheese (Queijo manteiga) and Acerola juice as a potential source of vitamin C. *Food and Bioprocess Technology, 2*(4), 368–373. doi:10.100711947-008-0059-9

Cryan, J. J., & Dinan, T. G. (2012). Mind-altering microorganisms: The impact of the gut microbiota on brain and behaviour. *Nature Reviews. Neuroscience, 13*(10), 701–712. doi:10.1038/nrn3346 PMID:22968153

Csiszar, A., Ungvari, Z., Edwards, J. G., Kaminski, P., Wolin, M. S., Koller, A., & .... (2002). Aging-induced phenotypic changes and oxidative stress impair coronary arteriolar function. *Circulation Research, 90*(11), 1159–1166. doi:10.1161/01.RES.0000020401.61826.EA PMID:12065318

Csont, T., Sárközy, M., Szűcs, G., Szűcs, C., Bárkányi, J., Bencsik, P., ... Ferdinandy, P. (2013). Effect of a multivitamin preparation supplemented with phytosterol on serum lipids and infarct size in rats fed with normal and high cholesterol diet. *Lipids in Health and Disease*, *12*(1), 138. doi:10.1186/1476-511X-12-138 PMID:24063587

Culligan, E. P., Hill, C., Sleator, R. D., (2009). Probiotics and gastrointestinal disease: successes, problems and future prospects. *Gut Pathogens, 1*(19), 1-12.

Da Costa, J. P. (2017). A current look at nutraceuticals – Key concepts and future prospects. *Trends in Food Science & Technology*, *62*, 68–78. doi:10.1016/j.tifs.2017.02.010

Dai, F. J., Hsu, W. H., Huang, J. J., & Wu, S. C. (2013). Effect of pigeon pea (Cajanus cajan L.) on high-fat diet-induced hypercholesterolemia in hamsters. *Food Chemistry and Toxicology*, *53*, 384-391.

Dai, J., & Mumper, R. J. (2010). Plant phenolics: Extraction, analysis and their antioxidant and anticancer properties. *Molecules (Basel, Switzerland)*, *15*(10), 7313–7352. doi:10.3390/molecules15107313 PMID:20966876

Daliri, E.B.M., Lee, B. H. (in press). New perspectives on probiotics in health and disease. *Food Science and Human Wellness*. .10.1016/j.fshw.2015.06.002

Dallman, P. R. (1992). Changing iron needs from birth through adolescence. Nestle nutrition workshop series (USA).

Damaskos, D., & Kolios, G. (2008). Probiotics and prebiotics in inflammatory bowel disease: Microflora 'on the scope'. *British Journal of Clinical Pharmacology*, *65*(4), 453–467. doi:10.1111/j.1365-2125.2008.03096.x PMID:18279467

Dandona, P., Ghanim, H., Chaudhuri, A., Dhindsa, S., & Kim, S. S. (2010). Macronutrient intake induces oxidative and inflammatory stress: Potential relevance to atherosclerosis and insulin resistance. *Experimental & Molecular Medicine*, *42*(4), 245–253. doi:10.3858/emm.2010.42.4.033 PMID:20200475

Dao, H. H., Frelut, M. L., Oberlin, F., Peres, G., Bourgeois, P., & Navarro, J. (2004). Effects of a multidisciplinary weight loss intervention on body composition in obese adolescents. *International Journal of Obesity and Related Metabolic Disorders*, *28*(2), 290–299. doi:10.1038j.ijo.0802542 PMID:14970838

Darmadi-Blackberry, I., Wahlqvist, M. L., Kouris-Blazos, A., Steen, B., Lukito, W., Horie, Y., & Horie, K. (2004). Legumes: The most important dietary predictor of survival in older people of different ethnicities. *Asia Pacific Journal of Clinical Nutrition*, *13*(2), 217–220. PMID:15228991

Dash, S. K. (2014). Probiotics - an overview the value of chitosan healthful ingredients that address the major health concerns of aging consumers. *Nutraceuticals Now.* Retrieved from http://superbakrill.com/wp-content/uploads/2013/08/NN-pages-1.pdf

Das, L., Bhaumik, E., Raychaudhuri, U., & Chakraborty, R. (2012). Role of nutraceuticals in human health. *Journal of Food Science and Technology*, *49*(2), 173–183. doi:10.100713197-011-0269-4 PMID:23572839

Das, U. N. (2003). Folic acid says NO to vascular diseases. *Nutrition (Burbank, Los Angeles County, Calif.)*, *19*(7-8), 686–692. doi:10.1016/S0899-9007(02)01044-4 PMID:12831960

Dauchy, R. T., Blask, D. E., Sauer, L. A., Davidson, L. K., Krause, J. A., Smith, L. C., & Dauchy, E. M. (2003). Physiologic melatonin concentration, omega-3-fatty acids, and conjugated linoleic acid inhibit fatty acid transport in rodent hind limb skeletal muscle in vivo. *Comparative Medicine*, *53*(2), 186–190. PMID:12784853

Davidson, L. E., Fiorino, A. M., Snydman, D. R., & Hibberd, P. L. (2011). *Lactobacillus GG* as an immune adjuvant for live-attenuated influenza vaccine in healthy adults: A randomized double-blind placebo-controlled trial. *European Journal of Clinical Nutrition*, *65*(4), 501–507. doi:10.1038/ejcn.2010.289 PMID:21285968

De Biase, S. G., Fernandes, S. F. C., Gianini, R. J., & Duarte, J. L. G. (2007). Vegetarian diet and cholesterol and triglycerides levels. *Arquivos Brasileiros de Cardiologia*, *88*(1), 35–39. doi:10.1590/S0066-782X2007000100006 PMID:17364116

De Jong, A., Plat, J., Bast, A., Godschalk, R. W., Basu, S., & Mensink, R. P. (2008). Effects of plant sterol and stanol ester consumption on lipid metabolism, antioxidant status and markers of oxidative stress, endothelial function and low-grade inflammation in patients on current statin treatment. *European Journal of Clinical Nutrition*, *62*(2), 263–273. doi:10.1038j.ejcn.1602733 PMID:17487211

De la Lastra, C. A., & Villegas, I. (2005). Resveratrol as an anti-inflammatory and anti-ageing agent: Mechanisms and clinical implications. *Molecular Nutrition & Food Research*, *49*(5), 405–430. doi:10.1002/mnfr.200500022 PMID:15832402

de la Rosa, L. A., Alvarez-Parrilla, E., & González-Aguilar, G. A. (2010). Fruit and vegetable phytochemicals: Chemistry, nutritional value, and stability. Wiley-Blackwell.

de Lucia, C., Komici, K., Borghetti, G., Femminella, G. D., Bencivenga, L., Cannavo, A., ... Rengo, G. (2017). microRNA in Cardiovascular Aging and Age-Related Cardiovascular Diseases. *Frontiers in Medicine*, *4*, 74. doi:10.3389/fmed.2017.00074 PMID:28660188

De Simone, C., Ferranti, P., Picariello, G., Scognamiglio, I., Dicitore, A., Addeo, F., ... Stiuso, P. (2010). Peptides from water buffalo cheese whey induced senescence cell death via ceramide secretion in human colon adenocarcinoma cell line. *Molecular Nutrition & Food Research*, *55*(2), 229–238. doi:10.1002/mnfr.201000074 PMID:20725925

De Vasconcelos, M., Bennett, R. N., Quideau, S., Jacquet, R., Rosa, E. A. S., & Ferreira-Cardoso, J. V. (2010). Evaluating the potential of chestnut (Castanea sativa Mill.) fruit pericarp and integument as a source of tocopherols, pigments and polyphenols. *Industrial Crops and Products*, *31*(2), 301–311. doi:10.1016/j.indcrop.2009.11.008

De vrese, M., & Schrezenmeir, J. (2008). Probiotics, prebiotics, and synbiotics. In *Advances in Biochemical Engineering and Biotechnology: Food Biotechnology* (pp. 1-66). Springer Publishing.

De Vrese, M., & Schrezenmeir, J. (2008). Probiotics, Prebiotics, and Synbiotics. *Advances in Biochemical Engineering/Biotechnology*, *111*, 1–66. doi:10.1007/10_2008_097 PMID:18461293

de Wit, J. N. (1998). Nutritional and functional characteristics of whey proteins in food systems. *Journal of Dairy Science*, *81*(3), 597–608. doi:10.3168/jds.S0022-0302(98)75613-9 PMID:9565865

DeAngelis, C. D., & Fontanarosa, P. B. (2003). Drugs Alias Dietary Supplements. *Journal of the American Medical Association*, *290*(11), 1519–1520. doi:10.1001/jama.290.11.1519 PMID:13129996

Defaie, S. Z., Sharieat, S., & Divsalar, A. (2010). Kinetic Investigation on Lactoperoxidase upon Interaction with Lead ion M. *International Journal of Environmental Sciences and Development*, *1*(1), 97–100. doi:10.7763/IJESD.2010.V1.19

DeFelice, S. L. (1995). The nutraceutical revolution: Its impact on food industry R&D. *Trends in Food Science & Technology*, *6*(2), 59–61. doi:10.1016/S0924-2244(00)88944-X

Defronzo, R. A. (1992). Insulin resistance, hyperinsulimemia and coronary artery disease a complex metabolic. *Journal of Cardiovascular Pharmacology*. PMID:1284137

Delfour, A., Jolles, J., Alais, C., & Jolles, P. (1965). Caseino-glycopeptides: Characterization of a methionine residue and of the N-terminal sequence. *Biochemical and Biophysical Research Communications*, *19*(4), 452–455. doi:10.1016/0006-291X(65)90145-2 PMID:14338991

Delley, M., & Germond, J. E. (2002). Differentiation of *Lactobacillus helveticus, Lactobacillus delbrueckii subsp bulgaricus, subsp lactis, and subsp delbrueckii* using physiological and genetic tools and reclassification of some strains from the ATCC collection. *Systematic and Applied Microbiology*, *25*(2), 228–231. doi:10.1078/0723-2020-00106 PMID:12353877

Delzenne, N. M., Neyrinck, A. M., Bäckhed, F., & Cani, P. D. (2011). Targeting gut microbiota in obesity: Effects of prebiotics and probiotics. *Nature Reviews. Endocrinology*, *7*(11), 639–646. doi:10.1038/nrendo.2011.126 PMID:21826100

Demonty, I., Chan, Y. M., Pelled, D., & Jones, P. J. H. (2006). Fish-oil esters of plant sterols improve the lipid profile of dyslipidemic subjects more than do fish-oil or sunflower oil esters of plant sterols. *The American Journal of Clinical Nutrition*, *84*(6), 1534–1542. doi:10.1093/ajcn/84.6.1534 PMID:17158440

Demonty, I., Ras, R. T., van der Knaap, H. C. M., Duchateau, G. S. M. J. E., Meijer, L., Zock, P. L., ... Trautwein, E. A. (2009). Continuous dose-response relationship of the LDL-cholesterol-lowering effect of phytosterol intake. *The Journal of Nutrition*, *139*(2), 271–284. doi:10.3945/jn.108.095125 PMID:19091798

Demrow, H. S., Slane, P. R., & Folts, J. D. (1995). Administration of wine and grape juice inhibits in vivo platelet activity and thrombosis in stenosed canine coronary arteries. *Circulation*, *91*(4), 1182–1188. doi:10.1161/01.CIR.91.4.1182 PMID:7850957

Deorukhkar, A., Krishnan, S., Sethi, G., & Aggarwal, B. B. (2007). Back to basics: How natural products can provide the basis for new therapeutics. *Expert Opinion on Investigational Drugs*, *16*(11), 1753–1773. doi:10.1517/13543784.16.11.1753 PMID:17970636

Depeint, F., Bruce, W. R., Shangari, N., Mehta, R., & O'Brien, P. J. (2006). Mitochondrial function and toxicity: Role of the B vitamin family on mitochondrial energy metabolism. *Chemico-Biological Interactions*, *163*(1), 94–112. doi:10.1016/j.cbi.2006.04.014 PMID:16765926

Desai, V., & Kaler, S. G. (2008). Role of copper in human neurological disorders. *The American Journal of Clinical Nutrition*, *88*(3), 855S–858S. doi:10.1093/ajcn/88.3.855S PMID:18779308

Dhingra, D., Michael, M., Rajput, H., & Patil, R. T. (2012). Dietary fibre in foods: A review. *Journal of Food Science and Technology*, *49*(3), 255–266. doi:10.100713197-011-0365-5 PMID:23729846

Dietary fibre and blood pressure. (2004). Dietary fibre and blood pressure. *Journal of Hypertension*. Retrieved April 13, 2017, from http://journals.lww.com /jhypertension/Fulltext/2004/01000/Dietaryfibreandbloodpressure.5.aspx

Dietary Reference Intakes. (2011). *Dietary Reference Intakes: Proposed Definition of Dietary Fiber*. The National Academies Press. Retrieved April 13, 2017, from https://www.nap.edu/catalog/10161/dietary-reference-intakes-proposed-definition-of-dietary-fiber

Dietary Supplem, C. for F. S. and A. (2015). U S Food and Drug Administration. Retrieved from https://www.fda.gov/Food/DietarySupplements/

Dietary Supplement Regulation in the United States. (n.d.). Retrieved from http://www.springer.com/in/book/9783319015019

Dillard, C. J., & German, J. B. (2000). Phytochemicals: Nutraceuticals and human health. *Journal of the Science of Food and Agriculture*, *80*(12), 1744–1756. doi:10.1002/1097-0010(20000915)80:12<1744::AID-JSFA7253.0.CO;2-W

Dixon, R. A., & Sumner, L. W. (2003). Legume natural products: Understanding and manipulating complex pathways for human and animal health. *Plant Physiology*, *131*(3), 878–885. doi:10.1104/pp.102.017319 PMID:12644640

Dolpady, J., Sorini, C., Pietro, C. D., Cosorich, I., Ferrarese, R., Saita, D., Clementi, M., Canducci, F., Falcone, M. (2016). Oral probiotic *VSL#3* prevents autoimmune diabetes by modulating microbiota and promoting indoleamine 2,3-dioxygenase-enriched tolerogenic intestinal environment. *Journal of Diabetes Research*. .10.1155/2016/7569431

Douglas, L. C., & Sanders, M. E. (2008). Probiotics and Prebiotics in Dietetics Practice. *Journal of the American Dietetic Association*, *108*(3), 510–521. doi:10.1016/j.jada.2007.12.009 PMID:18313433

Dragsted, L. O., Strube, M., & Larsen, J. C. (1993). Cancer-protective factors in fruits and vegetables: Biochemical and biological background. *Pharmacology & Toxicology*, *72*(Suppl 1), 116–135. doi:10.1111/j.1600-0773.1993.tb01679.x PMID:8474974

Duan, R. D. (2005). Anticancer compounds and sphingolipid metabolism in the colon. *In Vivo (Athens, Greece)*, *19*, 293–300. PMID:15796189

Dubey, A. P., Rajeshwari, K., Chakravarty, A., & Famularo, G. (2008). Use of VSL#3 in the treatment of rotavirus diarrhea in children: Preliminary results. *Journal of Clinical Gastroenterology*, *42*(Suppl. 3 Pt. 1), S126–S129. doi:10.1097/MCG.0b013e31816fc2f6 PMID:18806703

Dugo, P., Presti, M. L., Öhman, M., Fazio, A., Dugo, G., & Mondello, L. (2005). Determination of flavonoids in citrus juices by micro-HPLC-ESI/MS. *Journal of Separation Science*, *28*(11), 1149–1156. doi:10.1002/jssc.200500053 PMID:16116991

Duncan, B. (2013). Prebiotics, Probiotics, and Health Promotion: An Overview. In *Bioactive Food as Dietary Interventions for Liver and Gastrointestinal Disease* (pp. 449–463). Elsevier Inc. doi:10.1016/B978-0-12-397154-8.00005-1

Duranti, M. (2006). Grain legume proteins and nutraceutical properties. *Fitoterapia*, *77*(2), 67–82. doi:10.1016/j.fitote.2005.11.008 PMID:16406359

Dureja, H., Kaushik, D., & Kumar, V. (2003). Developments in nutraceuticals. *Indian Journal of Pharmacology*, *35*(6), 363–372.

Duthoit, F., Godon, J. J., & Montel, M. C. (2003). Bacterial community dynamics during production of registered designation of origin salers cheese as evaluated by 16SrRNA gene single-strand conformation polymorphism analysis. *Applied and Environmental Microbiology*, *69*(7), 3840–3848. doi:10.1128/AEM.69.7.3840-3848.2003 PMID:12839752

Dutta, P. C. (2004). Chemistry, analysis, and occurrence of phytosterol oxidation products in foods. In P. C. Dutta (Ed.), Phytosterols as Functional Food Components and Nutraceuticals (pp. 397–417). Academic Press.

Dyck, D. J. (2000). Dietary fat intake, supplements, and weight loss. *Canadian Journal of Applied Physiology*, *25*(6), 495–523. doi:10.1139/h00-033 PMID:11187927

Dyerberg, J., Eskesen, D. C., Andersen, P. W., Astrup, A., Buemann, B., Christensen, J. H., ... Stender, S. (2004). Effects of trans- and n-3 unsaturated fatty acids on cardiovascular risk markers in healthy males. An 8 weeks' dietary intervention study. *European Journal of Clinical Nutrition*, *58*(7), 1062–1070. doi:10.1038j.ejcn.1601934 PMID:15220949

Eaton, S. B., Eaton, S. B., & Konner, M. J. (1997). Paleolithic nutrition revisited: A twelve-year retrospective on its nature and implications. *European Journal of Clinical Nutrition*, *51*(4), 207–216. doi:10.1038j.ejcn.1600389 PMID:9104571

Ebel, B., Lemetais, G., Beney, L., Cachon, R., Sokol, H., Langella, P., & Gervais, P. (2014). Impact of probiotics on risk factors for cardiovascular diseases: A Review. *Critical Reviews in Food Science and Nutrition*, *54*(2), 175–189. doi:10.1080/10408398.2011.579361 PMID:24188267

Ebrahimi, A., & Schluesener, H. (2012). Natural polyphenols against neurodegenerative disorders: Potentials and pitfalls. *Ageing Research Reviews*, *11*(2), 329–345. doi:10.1016/j.arr.2012.01.006 PMID:22336470

EFSA Panel on Dietetic Products, N. and A. (NDA). (2011). Scientific Opinion on the substantiation of health claims related to polyphenols in olive and protection of LDL particles from oxidative damage (ID 1333, 1638, 1639, 1696, 2865), maintenance of normal blood HDL cholesterol concentrations (ID 1639), maintenance of normal blood pressure (ID 3781), "anti-inflammatory properties" (ID 1882), "contributes to the upper respiratory tract health" (ID 3468), "can help to maintain a normal function of gastrointestinal tract" (3779), and "contributes to body defences against external agents" (ID 3467) pursuant to Article 13(1) of Regulation (EC) No 1924/2006. *EFSA Journal, 9*(4). 10.2903/j.efsa.2011.2033

EFSA Panel on Dietetic Products. (2011). Scientific Opinion on the substantiation of health claims related to oleic acid intended to replace saturated fatty acids (SFAs) in foods or diets and maintenance of normal blood LDL-cholesterol concentrations (ID 673, 728, 729, 1302, 4334) and maintenanc: Health claims related to oleic acid intended to replace saturated fatty acids (SFAs) in foods or diets. *EFSA Journal*, *9*(4), 2043. doi:10.2903/j.efsa.2011.2043

Eftekhari, A., Mathiassen, O. N., Buus, N. H., Gotzsche, O., Mulvany, M. J., & Christensen, K. L. (2011). Disproportionally impaired microvascular structure in essential hypertension. *Journal of Hypertension*, *29*(5), 896–905. doi:10.1097/HJH.0b013e3283447a1c PMID:21330935

Eidelman, R. S., Hollar, D., Hebert, P. R., Lamas, G. A., & Hennekens, C. H. (2004). Randomized trials of vitamin E in the treatment and prevention of cardiovascular disease. *Archives of Internal Medicine*, *164*(14), 1552–1556. doi:10.1001/archinte.164.14.1552 PMID:15277288

El-Bahai, M. N., Al-Hariri, M. T., Yar, T., & Bamosa, A. O. (2009, January 24). Cardiac inotropic and hypertrophic effects of Nigella sativa supplementation in rats. *International Journal of Cardiology*, *131*(3), e115–e117. doi:10.1016/j.ijcard.2007.07.075 PMID:17931720

Elliott, P. (2003). Protein intake and blood pressure in cardiovascular disease. *The Proceedings of the Nutrition Society*, *62*(2), 495–504. doi:10.1079/PNS2003266 PMID:14506897

Engelhard, Y. N., Gazer, B., & Paran, E. (2006). Natural antioxidants from tomato extract reduce blood pressure in patients with grade-1 hypertension: A double-blind, placebo-controlled pilot study. *American Heart Journal*, *151*(1), 100. doi:10.1016/j.ahj.2005.05.008 PMID:16368299

Eratte, D., Wang, B., Dowling, K., Barrow, C. J., & Adhikari, B. P. (2014). Complex coacervation with whey protein isolate and gum arabic for the microencapsulation of omega-3 rich tuna oil. *Food & Function*, *5*(11), 2743–2750. doi:10.1039/C4FO00296B PMID:25008146

Erickson, D., O'Dell, D., Jiang, L., Oncescu, V., Gumus, A., Lee, S., ... Mehta, S. (2014). Smartphone technology can be transformative to the deployment of lab-on-chip diagnostics. *Lab on a Chip*, *14*(17), 3159–3164. doi:10.1039/C4LC00142G PMID:24700127

Erkkilä, A. T., & Lichtenstein, A. H. (2006). Fiber and cardiovascular disease risk: How strong is the evidence? *The Journal of Cardiovascular Nursing*, *21*(1), 3–8. doi:10.1097/00005082-200601000-00003 PMID:16407729

Esfanjani, A. F., Jafari, S. M., Assadpoor, E., & Mohammadi, E. (2015). Nano-encapsulation of saffron extract through double-layered multiple emulsions of pectin and whey protein concentrate. *Journal of Food Engineering*, *165*, 149–155. doi:10.1016/j.jfoodeng.2015.06.022

Espín, J. C., García-Conesa, M. T., & Tomás-Barberán, F. A. (2007). Nutraceuticals: Facts and fiction. *Phytochemistry*, *68*(22–24), 2986–3008. doi:10.1016/j.phytochem.2007.09.014 PMID:17976666

Esposito, E., Iacono, A., Bianco, G., Autore, G., Cuzzocrea, S., Vajro, P., ... Meli, R. (2009). Probiotics reduce the inflammatory response induced by a highfatdiet in the liver of young rats. *The Journal of Nutrition*, *139*(5), 905–911. doi:10.3945/jn.108.101808 PMID:19321579

Esposito, E., Rotilio, D., Dimatteo, V., Digiulio, C., Cacchio, M., & Algeri, S. (2002). Di Matteo. V.; Di Giulio, C.; Cacchio, M.; Algeri, S. A. review of specific dietary antioxidants and the effects on biochemical mechanisms related to neurodegenerative processes. *Neurobiology of Aging*, *23*(5), 719–735. doi:10.1016/S0197-4580(02)00078-7 PMID:12392777

European Cardiovascular Disease Statistics 2017 - EHN - European Heart Network. (n.d.). Retrieved April 13, 2017, from http://www.ehnheart.org/cvd-statistics.html

European Society of Hypertension-European Society of Cardiology guidelines for the management of arterial hypertension. (2003). Retrieved April 13, 2017, from https://www.ncbi.nlm.nih.gov/pubmed/12777938

Evans, W. C. (1996). Trease and Evans' pharmacognosy (14th ed.). London: WB Saunders.

Evenepoel, P., Meijers, B. K. I., Bammens, B. R. M., & Verbeke, K. (2009). Uremic toxins originating from colonic microbial metabolism. *Kidney International. Supplement*, *114*, S12–S19. doi:10.1038/ki.2009.402 PMID:19946322

Expert Panel on Detection, Evaluation, and Treatment of High Blood Cholesterol in Adults. (2001). Executive Summary of the Third Report of The National Cholesterol Education Program (NCEP) Expert Panel on Detection, Evaluation, And Treatment of High Blood Cholesterol In Adults (Adult Treatment Panel III). *Journal of the American Medical Association*, *285*(19), 2486–2497. doi:10.1001/jama.285.19.2486 PMID:11368702

Fa, G., & A, M. (2007). Inflammation in high blood pressure: a clinician perspective. *Journal of the American Society of Hypertension: JASH*, *1*(2), 113–119. 10.1016/ j.jash.2007.01.004

Facompre, N., & El-Bayoumy, K. (2009). Potential stages for prostate cancer prevention with selenium: Implications for cancer survivors. *Cancer Research*, *69*(7), 2699–2703. doi:10.1158/0008-5472.CAN-08-4359 PMID:19318549

Falagas, M. E., Betsi, G. I., & Athanasiou, S. (2007). Probiotics for the treatment of women with bacterial vaginosis. *Clinical Microbiology and Infection*, *13*(7), 657–664. doi:10.1111/j.1469-0691.2007.01688.x PMID:17633390

Fall, A. B., Vanhaelen-Fastré, R., Vanhaelen, M., Lo, I., Toppet, M., Ferster, A., & Fondu, P. (1999). In vitro antisickling activity of a rearranged limonoid isolated from Khayasenegalensis. *Planta Medica*, *65*(03), 209–212. doi:10.1055-1999-14083 PMID:10232063

Fang, C. Y., Lu, J. R., Chen, B. J., Wu, C., Chen, Y. P., & Chen, M. J. (2014). Selection of uremic toxin-reducing probiotics *in vitro* and *in vivo*. *Journal of Functional Foods*, *7*(1), 407–415. doi:10.1016/j.jff.2014.01.018

FAO/WHO. (2002). *Joint FAO/WHO Working Group on Drafting Guidelines for the Evaluation of Probiotics in Food. Guidelines for the evaluation of probiotics in food: report of a Joint FAO/ WHO Working Group on Drafting Guidelines for the Evaluation of Probiotics in Food.* London, ON, Canada: FAO/WHO.

Fatima, M., Kesharwani, R. K., Misra, K., & Rizvi, S. I. (2013). Protective effect of theaflavin on erythrocytes subjected to in vitro oxidative stress. *Biochemistry Research International*. PMID:24455262

Faujdar, S. S., Mehrishi, P., Bishnoi, S., & Sharma, A. (2016). Role of Probiotics in human health and disease: An update. *International Journal of Current Microbiology and Applied Sciences*, *5*(3), 328–344. doi:10.20546/ijcmas.2016.503.040

Fazel, M., Sahari, M. A., & Barzegar, M. (2008). Determination of main tea seed oil antioxidants and their effects on common kilka oil. *International Food Research Journal*, *15*(2), 209–217.

Fedorak, R. N. (2008). Understanding why probiotic therapies can be effective in treating IBD. *Journal of Clinical Gastroenterology*, *42*(Suppl 3 Pt 1), S111–S115. doi:10.1097/MCG.0b013e31816d922c PMID:18806699

Fedorak, R. N., & Madsen, K. L. (2004). Probiotics and the Management of Inflammatory Bowel Disease. *Inflammatory Bowel Diseases*, *10*(3), 286–299. doi:10.1097/00054725-200405000-00018 PMID:15290926

Feldstein, A. E., Werneburg, N. W., Canbay, A., Guicciardi, M. E., Bronk, S. F., Rydzewski, R., ... Gores, G. J. (2004). Free fatty acids promote hepatic lipotoxicity by stimulating TNF-alpha expression via a lysosomal pathway. *Hepatology (Baltimore, Md.)*, *40*(1), 185–194. doi:10.1002/hep.20283 PMID:15239102

Feng, X. H., Chen, F., Xu, H., Wu, B., Yao, J., Ying, H. J., & Ouyang, P. K. (2010). Propionic acid fermentation by *Propionibacteriumfreudenreichii* CCTCC M207015 in a multi-point fibrous-bed bioreactor. *Bioprocess and Biosystems Engineering*, *33*(9), 1077–1085. doi:10.100700449-010-0433-7 PMID:20589397

Fenton, M. (1992). Chromatographic separation of cholesterol in foods. *Journal of Chromatography. A*, *624*(1-2), 369–388. doi:10.1016/0021-9673(92)85689-Q PMID:1494014

Ferguson, L. R., & Philpott, M. (2007). Cancer prevention by dietary bioactive components that target the immune response. *Current Cancer Drug Targets*, *7*(5), 459–464. doi:10.2174/156800907781386605 PMID:17691905

Ferna'ndez-Sa'nchez, A., Madrigal-Santillán, E., Bautista, M., Esquivel-Soto, J., Morales-González, Á., Esquivel-Chirino, C., ... Morales-González, J. A. (2011). Inflammation, oxidative stress, and obesity. *International Journal of Molecular Sciences*, *12*(5), 3117–3132. doi:10.3390/ijms12053117 PMID:21686173

Ferrari, C. K. B., & Torres, E. A. F. S. (2003). Biochemical pharmacology of functional foods and prevention of chronic diseases of aging. *Biomedicine and Pharmacotherapy*, *57*(5–6), 251–260. doi:10.1016/S0753-3322(03)00032-5 PMID:12888262

Fibre in food, D. of H. & H. (2017). *Fibre in food*. Retrieved April 13, 2017, from https://www.betterhealth.vic.gov.au:443/health/healthyliving/fibre-in-food

Fielding, P. E., Ishikawa, Y., & Fielding, C. J. (1989). Apolipoprotein E mediates binding of normal very low density lipoprotein to heparin but is not required for high affinity receptor binding. *The Journal of Biological Chemistry*, *264*(21), 12462–12466. PMID:2745454

Figueiredo, M. S. (2015). The compound state: Hb S/beta-thalassemia. *Revista Brasileira de Hematologia e Hemoterapia*, *37*(3), 150–152. doi:10.1016/j.bjhh.2015.02.008 PMID:26041415

Finkelstein, E. A., Trogdon, J. G., Cohen, J. W., & Dietz, W. (2009). Annual medical spending attributable to obesity: Payer and service-specific estimates. *Health Affairs (Project Hope)*, *28*(5), 822–831. doi:10.1377/hlthaff.28.5.w822 PMID:19635784

Finley, J. W. (2016). The nutraceutical revolution: Emerging vision or broken dream? Understanding scientific and regulatory concerns. *Clinical Research and Regulatory Affairs*, *33*(1), 1–3. doi:10.3109/10601333.2016.1117096

Finley, J. W., Finley, J. W., Ellwood, K., & Hoadley, J. (2014). Launching a New Food Product or Dietary Supplement in the United States: Industrial, Regulatory, and Nutritional Considerations. *Annual Review of Nutrition*, *34*(1), 421–447. doi:10.1146/annurev-nutr-071813-105817 PMID:24850389

Firmansyah, A., Penn, D., & Lebenthal, E. (1989). Isolated colonocyte metabolism of glucose, glutamine, n-butyrate, and beta-hydroxy-butyrate in malnutrition. *Gastroenterology*, *97*(3), 622–629. doi:10.1016/0016-5085(89)90633-1 PMID:2753323

Fischer, H., Gottschlich, R., & Seelig, A. (1998). Blood-Brain Barrier Permeation: Molecular Parameters Governing Passive Diffusion. *The Journal of Membrane Biology*, *165*(3), 201–211. doi:10.1007002329900434 PMID:9767674

Fisher, A. (2008). Cholinergic treatments with emphasis on m1 muscarinic agonists as potential disease-modifying agents for Alzheimer's disease. *Neurotherapeutics; the Journal of the American Society for Experimental NeuroTherapeutics*, *5*(3), 433–442. doi:10.1016/j.nurt.2008.05.002 PMID:18625455

FitzGerald, R. J., Murray, B. A., & Walsh, D. J. (2004). Hypotensive peptides from milk proteins. *The Journal of Nutrition*, *134*(4), 980S–988S. doi:10.1093/jn/134.4.980S PMID:15051858

Fitzmaurice, C., Allen, C., Barber, R. M., Barregard, L., Bhutta, Z. A., ... Naghavi, M. (2017). Global, Regional, and National Cancer Incidence, Mortality, Years of Life Lost, Years Lived With Disability, and Disability-Adjusted Life-years for 32 Cancer Groups, 1990 to 2015: A Systematic Analysis for the Global Burden of Disease Study. *JAMA Oncology*, *3*(4), 524–548. doi:10.1001/jamaoncol.2016.5688 PMID:27918777

Flint, H. J. (2012). The impact of nutrition on the human microbiome. *Nutrition Reviews*, *70*(Suppl. 1), S10–S13. doi:10.1111/j.1753-4887.2012.00499.x PMID:22861801

Flint, H. J., Scott, K. P., Louis, P., & Duncan, S. H. (2012). The role of the gut microbiota in nutrition and health. *Nature Reviews. Gastroenterology & Hepatology*, *9*(10), 577–589. doi:10.1038/nrgastro.2012.156 PMID:22945443

Flores, G., Dastmalchi, K., Wu, S.-B., Whalen, K., Dabo, A. J., Reynertson, K. A., ... Kennelly, E. J. (2013). Phenolic-rich extract from the Costa Rican guava (Psidium friedrichsthalianum) pulp with antioxidant and anti-inflammatory activity. Potential for COPD therapy. *Food Chemistry*, *141*(2), 889–895. doi:10.1016/j.foodchem.2013.03.025 PMID:23790863

Folsom, A. R., Parker, E. D., & Harnack, L. J. (2007). Degree of concordance with DASH diet guidelines and incidence of hypertension and fatal cardiovascular disease. *American Journal of Hypertension*, *20*(3), 225–232. doi:10.1016/j.amjhyper.2006.09.003 PMID:17324731

Food and Agriculture Organization of the United Nations. (2007). *Report on functional foods, food quality and standards service (AGNS)*. Retrieved November 25, 2007, from http://www.fao.org/ag/agn/agns/files/Functional_Foods_Report_Nov 2007.pdf

Foods That Lower Cholesterol. (2007, April 17). Retrieved April 13, 2017, http://health.howstuffworks.com/diseases-conditions/cardiovascular/cholesterol/foods-that-lower-cholesterol.htm

Forman. (2015). *Part D. Ch 2: Dietary Patterns - 2015 Advisory Report - health.gov*. Retrieved April 13, 2017, from https://health.gov/dietaryguidelines/2015-scientific-report/07-chapter-2

Foroughi, M., Akhavanzanjani, M., Maghsoudi, Z., Ghiasvand, R., Khorvash, F., & Askari, G. (2013). Stroke and Nutrition: A Review of Studies. *International Journal of Preventive Medicine*, *4*(Suppl 2), S165–S179. PMID:23776719

Franz, C. M., Huch, M., Abriouel, H., Holzapfel, W. H., & Gálvez, A. (2011). *Enterococci* as probiotics and their implications in food safety. *International Journal of Food Microbiology*, *151*(2), 125–140. doi:10.1016/j.ijfoodmicro.2011.08.014 PMID:21962867

Fraser, G. E. (1999). Associations between diet and cancer, ischemic heart disease, and all-cause mortality in non-Hispanic white California Seventh-day Adventists. *The American Journal of Clinical Nutrition*, *70*(3Suppl), 532S–538S. doi:10.1093/ajcn/70.3.532s PMID:10479227

Friedmann, T.E., Lumsdon, S.O., & Green, J.H. (2009). *Encapsulation of oils by coacervation*. US 2009/0189304 A1.

Friesen, J. A., & Rodwell, V. W. (2004). The 3-hydroxy-3-methylglutaryl coenzyme-A (HMG-CoA) reductases. *Genome Biology*, *5*(11), 1. doi:10.1186/gb-2004-5-11-248 PMID:15535874

Frost & Sullivan. (2011). *Global Nutraceutical Industry: Investing in healthy living*. Academic Press.

Fuhrman, B., Elis, A., & Aviram, M. (1997). Hypocholesterolemic effect of lycopene and β-carotene is related to suppression of cholesterol synthesis and augmentation of LDL receptor activity in macrophages. [Article]. *Biochemical and Biophysical Research Communications*, *233*(3), 658–662. doi:10.1006/bbrc.1997.6520 PMID:9168909

Furrie, E., Macfarlane, S., Kennedy, A., Cummings, J. H., Walsh, S. V., O'neil, D. A., & Macfarlane, G. T. (2005). Synbiotic therapy *(Bifidobacteriumlongum*/Synergy 1) initiates resolution of inflammation in patients with active ulcerative colitis: A randomised controlled pilot trial. *Gut*, *54*(2), 242–249. doi:10.1136/gut.2004.044834 PMID:15647189

Galli, F., Piroddi, M., Annetti, C., Aisa, C., Floridi, E., & Floridi, A. (2005). Oxidative Stress and Reactive Oxygen Species. In *Cardiovascular Disorders in Hemodialysis* (Vol. 149, pp. 240–260). Basel: KARGER. doi:10.1159/000085686

Gallo, R. L., & Hooper, L. V. (2012). Epithelial antimicrobial defence of the skin and intestine. *Nature Reviews. Immunology*, *12*(7), 503–516. doi:10.1038/nri3228 PMID:22728527

Ganz, T. (2003). Defensins: Antimicrobial peptides of innate immunity. *Nature Reviews. Immunology*, *3*(9), 710–720. doi:10.1038/nri1180 PMID:12949495

Gareau, M. G., Sherman, P. M., & Walker, W. A. (2010). Probiotics and the gut microbiota in intestinal health and disease. *Nature Reviews. Gastroenterology & Hepatology*, *7*(9), 503–514. doi:10.1038/nrgastro.2010.117 PMID:20664519

Garland, C. F., Garland, F. C., Gorham, E. D., Lipkin, M., Newmark, H., Mohr, S. B., & Holick, M. F. (2006). The role of vitamin D in cancer prevention. *American Journal of Public Health*, *96*(2), 252–261. doi:10.2105/AJPH.2004.045260 PMID:16380576

Gault, P. M., Allen, K. R., & Newton, K. E. (2005). Plasma aluminium: A redundant test for patients on dialysis? *Annals of Clinical Biochemistry*, *42*(1), 51–54. doi:10.1258/0004563053026862 PMID:15802033

Gawkowski, D., & Chikindas, M. L. (2013). Non-dairy probiotic beverages: The next step into human health. *Beneficial Microbes*, *4*(2), 127–142. doi:10.3920/BM2012.0030 PMID:23271064

Gaziano, T. A. (2005). Cardiovascular disease in the developing world and its cost-effective management. *Circulation*, *112*(23), 3547–3553. doi:10.1161/CIRCULATIONAHA.105.591792 PMID:16330695

Gaziano, T., Reddy, K. S., Paccaud, F., Horton, S., & Chaturvedi, V. (2010). *Cardiovascular Disease Control Priorities in Developing Countries* (2nd ed.). Washington, DC: National Academies Press (US).

Geier, M. S., Butler, R. N., & Howarth, G. S. (2006). Probiotics, prebiotics and synbiotics: A role in chemoprevention for colorectal cancer? *Cancer Biology & Therapy*, *5*(10), 1265–1269. doi:10.4161/cbt.5.10.3296 PMID:16969130

Geier, M. S., Butler, R. N., & Howarth, G. S. (2007). Inflammatory bowel disease: Current insights into pathogenesis and new therapeutic options; probiotics, prebiotics and synbiotics. *International Journal of Food Microbiology*, *115*(1), 1–11. doi:10.1016/j.ijfoodmicro.2006.10.006 PMID:17137666

Gellman, J., Hare, J. M., Lowenstein, C. J., Gerstenblith, G., Coombs, V., Langenberg, P., ... Resar, J. R. (2004). L-arginine ameliorates the abnormal sympathetic response of the dysfunctional human coronary microvasculature. *Angiology*, *55*(1), 1–8. doi:10.1177/000331970405500101 PMID:14759083

GEN. (2005). *GEN, 25*(9). Retrieved from http://www.genengnews.com/gen-articles/opportunities-and-challenges-for-developing-functional-foods/361

Genser, D. (2008). Food and drug interaction: Consequences for the nutrition/health status. *Annals of Nutrition & Metabolism*, *52*(Suppl 1), 29–32. doi:10.1159/000115345 PMID:18382075

Georgiev, V., Ananga, A., & Tsolova, V. (2014). Recent advances and uses of grape flavonoids as nutraceuticals. *Nutrients*, *6*(1), 391–415. doi:10.3390/nu6010391 PMID:24451310

Ghasemzadeh, A., & Jaafar, H. Z. (2013). Profiling of phenolic compounds and their antioxidant and anticancer activities in pandan (Pandanus amaryllifolius Roxb.) extracts from different locations of Malaysia. *BMC Complementary and Alternative Medicine*, *13*(1), 341. doi:10.1186/1472-6882-13-341 PMID:24289290

Gibson, G. R., Probert, H. M., van Loo, J. A. E., Rastall, R. A., & Roberfroid, M. B. (2004). Dietary modulation of the human colonic microbiota: Updating the concept of prebiotics. *Nutrition Research Reviews*, *17*(2), 259–275. doi:10.1079/NRR200479 PMID:19079930

Gibson, G. R., & Roberfroid, M. B. (1995). Dietary modulation of the human colonic microbiota: Introducing the concept of prebiotics. *The Journal of Nutrition*, *125*(6), 1401–1412. PMID:7782892

Gilbert, R., Thompson, M. D., & Grundy, S. M. (2005). History and development of plant sterol and stanol esters for cholesterol-lowering purposes. *The American Journal of Cardiology*, *96*(1suppl.), 3D–9D. doi:10.1016/j.amjcard.2005.03.013 PMID:15992509

Glidden, P. (2010). The MD Emperor has No Clothes. Academic Press.

Glik, Sharif, Tucker, Tejada, Prelip, Ammerman, & ... Jilcott Pitts. (2016). Community-engagement to support cardiovascular disease prevention in disparities populations: Three case studies. *Journal of Health Disparities Research and Practice*, *9*(1), 6.

Gliozzi, M., Walker, R., Muscoli, S., Vitale, C., Gratteri, S., Carresi, C., ... Mollace, V. (2013). Bergamot polyphenolic fraction enhances rosuvastatin-induced effect on LDL-cholesterol, LOX-1 expression and protein kinase B phosphorylation in patients with hyperlipidemia. *International Journal of Cardiology*, *170*(2), 140–145. doi:10.1016/j.ijcard.2013.08.125 PMID:24239156

Golbitz, P. (1995). Traditional soyfoods: Processing and products. *The Journal of Nutrition*, *125*(3Suppl), 570S–572S. PMID:7884535

Goldman, C. G., Barrado, D. A., Balcarce, N., Rua, E. C., Oshiro, M., Calcagno, M. L., ... Boccio, J. R. (2006). Effect of a probiotic food as an adjuvant to triple therapy for eradication of *Helicobacter pylori* infection in children. *Nutrition (Burbank, Los Angeles County, Calif.)*, *22*(10), 984–988. doi:10.1016/j.nut.2006.06.008 PMID:16978844

Goldstein, J. L., & Brown, M. S. (2009). The LDL Receptor. *Arteriosclerosis, Thrombosis, and Vascular Biology*, *29*(4), 431–438. doi:10.1161/ATVBAHA.108.179564 PMID:19299327

Golmakani, M.-T., & Rezaei, K. (2008). Comparison of microwave-assisted hydrodistillation withthe traditional hydrodistillation method in the extractionof essential oils from Thymus vulgaris L. *Food Chemistry*, *109*(4), 925–930. doi:10.1016/j.foodchem.2007.12.084 PMID:26050009

Gomes, A. C., Bueno, A. A., Souza, R. G. M. D., & Mota, J. F. (2014). Gut microbiota, probiotics and diabetes. *Nutrition Journal*, *13*(60), 1–13. PMID:24939063

Gómez-Llorente, C., Muñoz, S., & Gil, A. (2010). Role of Toll-like receptors in the development of immune tolerance mediated by probiotics. *The Proceedings of the Nutrition Society*, *69*(03), 381–389. doi:10.1017/S0029665110001527 PMID:20416121

Gooch, C. L., Pracht, E., & Borenstein, A. R. (2017). The burden of neurological disease in the United States: A summary report and call to action: Burden of Neurological Disease. *Annals of Neurology*, *81*(4), 479–484. doi:10.1002/ana.24897 PMID:28198092

Gooda, S. N., Abdul-Hamid, A., Saari, N., Abas, F., Pak Dek, M. S., & Rahim, M. (2012). Anti-pancreatic lipase and antioxidant activity of selected tropical herbs. *International Journal of Food Properties*, *15*(3), 569-578.

Goodman, B. E. (2010). Insights into digestion and absorption of major nutrients in humans. *Advances in Physiology Education*, *34*(2), 44–53. doi:10.1152/advan.00094.2009 PMID:20522896

Gosslau, A., & Chen, K. Y. (2004). Nutraceuticals, apoptosis, and disease prevention. *Nutrition (Burbank, Los Angeles County, Calif.)*, *20*(1), 95–102. doi:10.1016/j.nut.2003.09.017 PMID:14698022

Goswami, S. (2017). *Proteomics in Personalized Medicine: An Evolution Not a Revolution. In Applying big Data Analytics in Bioinformatics & Medicine*. IGI Global.

Gotteland, M., Andrews, M., Toledo, M., Muñoz, L., Caceres, P., Anziani, A., ... Salazar, G. (2008). Modulation of *Helicobacter pylori* colonization with cranberry juice and *Lactobacillus johnsonii*La1 in children. *Nutrition (Burbank, Los Angeles County, Calif.)*, *24*(5), 421–426. doi:10.1016/j.nut.2008.01.007 PMID:18343637

Gotteland, M., Poliak, L., Cruchet, S., & Brunser, O. (2005). Effect of regular ingestion of *Saccharomyces boulardii*plus inulin or *Lactobacillus acidophilus* LB in children colonized by *Helicobacter pylori. Acta Paediatrica (Oslo, Norway)*, *94*(12), 1747–1751. doi:10.1111/j.1651-2227.2005.tb01848.x PMID:16421034

Granato, D., Branco, G. F., Cruz, A. G., Faria, J. A. F., & Shah, N. P. (2010). Probiotic dairy products as functional foods. *Comprehensive Reviews in Food Science and Food Safety*, *9*(5), 455–470. doi:10.1111/j.1541-4337.2010.00120.x

Grand View Research. (2016, November 17). *Functional Foods Market Is Expected To Reach $255.10 Billion By 2024*. Grand View Research, Inc. Retrieved April 14, 2017, from http://www.prnewswire.com/news-releases/functional-foods-market-is-expected-to-reach-25510-billion-by-2024-grand-view-research-inc-601642985.html

Grassi, D., Lippi, C., Necozione, S., Desideri, G., & Ferri, C. (2005). Short-term administration of dark chocolate is followed by a significant increase in insulin sensitivity and a decrease in blood pressure in healthy persons. *The American Journal of Clinical Nutrition*, *81*(3), 611–614. doi:10.1093/ajcn/81.3.611 PMID:15755830

Greenburg, A. G. (1996). Pathophysiology of anemia. *The American Journal of Medicine*, *101*(2), 7S–11S. doi:10.1016/S0002-9343(96)00161-1 PMID:8831424

Green, D. R. (2000). Apoptotic pathways: Paper wraps stone blunts scissors. *Cell*, *102*(1), 1–4. doi:10.1016/S0092-8674(00)00003-9 PMID:10929706

Griffiths, M., Payne, P. R. A. J., Rivers, J. P. W., Cox, M., & Stunkard, A. J. (1990). Metabolic rate and physical development in children at risk of obesity. *Lancet*, *336*(8707), 76–78. doi:10.1016/0140-6736(90)91592-X PMID:1975323

Grönlund, M. M., Arvilommi, H., Kero, P., Lehtonen, O. P., & Isolauri, E. (2000). Importance of intestinal colonisation in the maturation of humoral immunity in early infancy: A prospective follow up study of healthy infants aged 0-6 months. *Archives of Disease in Childhood. Fetal and Neonatal Edition*, *83*(3), F186–F192. doi:10.1136/fn.83.3.F186 PMID:11040166

Grundy, M., Pasternak, R., Greenland, P., Smith, S., & Fuster, V. (1999). Assessment of Cardiovascular Risk by Use of Multiple-Risk Factor Assessment Equations: A statement for Healthcare Professionals From The American Heart Association and The American College of Cardiology. *100*, 1481-1492.

Guandalini, S., Pensabene, L., Zikri, M. A., Dias, J. A., Casali, L. G., Hoekstra, H., ... Weizman, Z. (2000). *Lactobacillus* GG administered in oral rehydration solution to children with acute diarrhea: A multicenter European study. *Journal of Pediatric Gastroenterology and Nutrition*, *30*(1), 54–60. doi:10.1097/00005176-200001000-00018 PMID:10630440

Guglielmetti, S., Mora, D., Gschwender, M., & Popp, K. (2011). Randomised clinical trial: *Bifidobacterium bifidum* MIMBb75 significantly alleviates irritable bowel syndrome and improves quality of life a double-blind, placebo-controlled study. *Alimentary Pharmacology & Therapeutics*, *33*(10), 1123–1132. doi:10.1111/j.1365-2036.2011.04633.x PMID:21418261

Gunasekaran, S., & Ko, S. (2014). Rationales of Nano- and Microencapsulation for Food Ingredients. In H. S. Kwak (Ed.), *Nano- and Microencapsulation for Foods*. John Wiley & Sons, Ltd. doi:10.1002/9781118292327.ch3

Gunasekaran, S., Ko, S., & Xiao, L. (2007). Use of whey proteins for encapsulation and controlled delivery applications. *Journal of Food Engineering*, *83*(1), 31–40. doi:10.1016/j.jfoodeng.2006.11.001

Gunasekaran, S., Xiao, L., & Eleya, M. M. (2006). Whey protein concentrates hydrogels as bioactive carriers. *Journal of Applied Polymer Science*, *99*(5), 2470–2476. doi:10.1002/app.22838

Guo, J., Gan, X. T., Haist, J. V., Rajapurohitam, V., Zeidan, A., Faruq, N. S., & Karmazyn, M. (2011). Ginseng inhibits cardiomyocyte hypertrophy and heart failure via NHE-1 inhibition and attenuation of calcineurin activation. *Circulation: Heart Failure*, *4*(1), 79–88. doi:10.1161/CIRCHEARTFAILURE.110.957969 PMID:20971938

Guo, Z., Liu, X. M., Zhang, Q. X., Shen, Z., Tian, F. W., Zhang, H., ... Chen, W. (2011). Influence of consumption of probiotics on the plasma lipid profile: A meta-analysis of randomised controlled trials. *Nutrition, Metabolism, and Cardiovascular Diseases*, *21*(11), 844–850. doi:10.1016/j.numecd.2011.04.008 PMID:21930366

Gupta, S. C., Patchva, S., & Aggarwal, B. B. (2013). Therapeutic roles of curcumin: Lessons learned from clinical trials. *The AAPS Journal*, *15*(1), 195–218. doi:10.120812248-012-9432-8 PMID:23143785

Gupta, S., & Abu-Ghannam, N. (2012). Probiotic fermentation of plant based products: Possibilities and opportunities. *Critical Reviews in Food Science and Nutrition*, *52*(2), 183–199. doi:10.1080/10408398.2010.499779 PMID:22059963

Gylling, H., & Miettinen, T. A. (1999). Cholesterol reduction by different plant sterol and stanol esters for cholesterol lowering purposes. *The American Journal of Cardiology*, *96*(suppl.), 3D–9D.

Gyorgyi, A. S. (1960). Introduction to a Submolecular Biology. Academic Press.

H, K., Fc, L., & Dn, M. (2009). Role of the immune system in hypertensive target organ damage. *Trends in Cardiovascular Medicine, 19*(7), 242–246. 10.1016/j.tcm.2010.02.004

Hager, K., Marahrens, A., Kenklies, M., Riederer, P., & Münch, G. (2001). Alpha-lipoic acid as a new treatment option for Azheimer type dementia. *Archives of Gerontology and Geriatrics*, *32*(3), 275–282. doi:10.1016/S0167-4943(01)00104-2 PMID:11395173

Hakansson, A., & Molin, G. (2011). Gut microbiota and inflammation. *Nutrients*, *3*(6), 637–682. doi:10.3390/nu3060637 PMID:22254115

Hallberg, L., Hôgdahl, A. M., Nilsson, L., & Rybo, G. (1966). Menstrual blood loss–a population study. *Acta Obstetricia et Gynecologica Scandinavica*, *45*(3), 320–351. doi:10.3109/00016346609158455 PMID:5922481

Halliwell, B. (1994). Free Radicals, Antioxidants, and Human Disease: Curiosity, Cause, or Consequence? *Lancet*, *344*(8924), 721–724. doi:10.1016/S0140-6736(94)92211-X PMID:7915779

Halliwell, B., & Gutteridge, J. M. C. (1985). *Free radicals in biology and medicine*. Clarendon Press.

Halsted, C. H., Villanueva, J. A., Devlin, A. M., & Chandler, C. J. (2002). Metabolic interactions of alcohol and folate. *The Journal of Nutrition*, *132*(8), 2367S–2372S. doi:10.1093/jn/132.8.2367S PMID:12163694

Hamilton, J. A. (2004). Fatty acid interactions with proteins: What X-ray crystal and NMR solution structures tell us. *Progress in Lipid Research*, *43*(3), 177–199. doi:10.1016/j.plipres.2003.09.002 PMID:15003394

Hanafy, M. S., & Hatem, M. E. (1991). Studies on the antimicrobial activity of Nigella sativa seed (black cumin). *Journal of Ethnopharmacology*, *34*(2-3), 275–278. doi:10.1016/0378-8741(91)90047-H PMID:1795532

Hanahan, D., & Weinberg, R. A. (2000). The hallmarks of cancer. *Cell*, *100*(1), 57–70. doi:10.1016/S0092-8674(00)81683-9 PMID:10647931

Han, S.-S., Chung, S.-T., Robertson, D. A., Ranjan, D., & Bondada, S. (1999). Curcumin Causes the Growth Arrest and Apoptosis of B Cell Lymphoma by Downregulation of egr-1, C-myc, Bcl-XL, NF-κB, and p53. *Clinical Immunology (Orlando, Fla.)*, *93*(2), 152–161. doi:10.1006/clim.1999.4769 PMID:10527691

Hansen, T. H., Gobel, R. J., Hansen, T., & Pedersen, O. (2015). The gut microbiome in cardio-metabolic health. *Genome Medicine*, *7*(1), 1–16. doi:10.118613073-015-0157-z PMID:25825594

Harats, D., Chevion, S., Nahir, M., Norman, Y., Sagee, O., & Berry, E. M. (1998). Citrus fruit supplementation reduces lipoprotein oxidation in young men ingesting a diet high in saturated fat: Presumptive evidence for an interaction between vitamins C and E in vivo. *The American Journal of Clinical Nutrition*, *67*(2), 240–245. doi:10.1093/ajcn/67.2.240 PMID:9459371

Hardy, G. (n.d.). Nutraceuticals and functional foods: introduction and meaning. *Nutrition*, *16*(7–8), 688–9.

Hardy, G. (2000). Nutraceuticals and functional foods: Introduction and meaning. *Nutrition (Burbank, Los Angeles County, Calif.)*, *16*(7), 688–689. doi:10.1016/S0899-9007(00)00332-4 PMID:10906598

Harisa, G. I., & Alanazi, F. K. (2013). Low density lipoprotein bionanoparticles: From cholesterol transport to delivery of anti-cancer drugs. *Saudi Pharmaceutical Journal*. PMID:25561862

Harper, S., Lynch, J., & Smith, G. D. (2011). Social determinants and the decline of cardiovascular diseases: Understanding the links. *Annual Review of Public Health*, *32*(1), 39–69. doi:10.1146/annurev-publhealth-031210-101234 PMID:21219168

Haslam, D. W., & James, W. P. (2005). Obesity. *Lancet*, *366*(9492), 1197–1209. doi:10.1016/S0140-6736(05)67483-1 PMID:16198769

Hasler, C. M. (2002). The cardiovascular effects of soy products. *The Journal of Cardiovascular Nursing*, *16*(4), 50–63, quiz 75–76. doi:10.1097/00005082-200207000-00006 PMID:12597262

Hassan, M., Kjos, M., Nes, I. F., Diep, D. B., & Lotfipour, F. (2012). Natural antimicrobial peptides from bacteria: Characteristics and potential applications to fight against antibiotic resistance. *Journal of Applied Microbiology*, *113*(4), 723–736. doi:10.1111/j.1365-2672.2012.05338.x PMID:22583565

Hasslof, P., Hedberg, M., Twetman, S., & Stecksén-Blicks, C. (2010). Growth inhibition of oral mutans *streptococci* and candida by commercial probiotic *lactobacilli* an *in vitro* study. *BMC Oral Health*, *10*(18), 1–6. PMID:20598145

Ha, T.-Y., Ko, S.-N., Lee, S.-M., Kim, H.-R., Chung, S.-H., Kim, S.-R., ... Kim, I.-H. (2006). Changes in nutraceutical lipid components of rice at different degrees of milling. *European Journal of Lipid Science and Technology*, *108*(3), 175–181. doi:10.1002/ejlt.200500250

Hatakka, K., Ahola, A. J., Yli-Knuuttila, H., Richardson, M., Poussa, T., Meurman, J. H., & Korpela, R. (2007). Probiotics reduce the prevalence of oral *Candida* in the elderly-A randomized controlled trial. *Journal of Dental Research*, *86*(2), 125–130. doi:10.1177/154405910708600204 PMID:17251510

Hathcock, J. (2001). Dietary supplements: How they are used and regulated. *The Journal of Nutrition*, *131*(33s), 1114S–1117S. doi:10.1093/jn/131.3.1114S PMID:11238828

Health Information. (2017). *Fibre Sources and Fibre Supplements Information*. Retrieved April 13, 2017, from https://patient.info/in/health/fibre-and-fibre-supplements

Heber, D. (1999). Dietary supplement or drug? The case for cholestin. *The American Journal of Clinical Nutrition*, *70*(1), 106–108. doi:10.1093/ajcn/70.1.106 PMID:10393149

He, F., Ouwehand, A. C., Isolauri, E., Hashimoto, H., Benno, Y., & Salminen, S. (2001). Comparison of mucosal adhesion and species identification of bifidobacteria isolated from healthy and allergic infants. *FEMS Immunology and Medical Microbiology*, *30*(1), 43–47. doi:10.1111/j.1574-695X.2001.tb01548.x PMID:11172990

Hegde, B. M. (2014). What Doctors Don't Get to Study. In *Medical School* (4th ed.). Paras Medical Publisher.

He, J., Klag, M. J., Whelton, P. K., Chen, J. Y., Qian, M. C., & Het, G. Q. (1995). Dietary macronutrients and blood pressure in southwestern China. *Journal of Hypertension*, *13*(11), 1267–1274. doi:10.1097/00004872-199511000-00008 PMID:8984124

He, J., Streiffer, R. H., Muntner, P., Krousel-Wood, M. A., & Whelton, P. K. (2004). Effect of dietary fiber intake on blood pressure: A randomized, double-blind, placebo-controlled trial. *Journal of Hypertension*, *22*(1), 73–80. doi:10.1097/00004872-200401000-00015 PMID:15106797

He, K., Merchant, A., Rimm, E. B., Rosner, B. A., Stampfer, M. J., Willett, W. C., & Ascherio, A. (2003). Dietary fat intake and risk of stroke in male US healthcare professionals: 14 year prospective cohort study. *BMJ (Clinical Research Ed.)*, *327*(7418), 777–782. doi:10.1136/bmj.327.7418.777 PMID:14525873

Hekmat, S., & McMahon, D. J. (1997). Manufacture and quality of iron-fortified yogurt. *Journal of Dairy Science*, *80*(12), 3114–3122. doi:10.3168/jds.S0022-0302(97)76282-9 PMID:9436092

Hemaiswarya, S., Raja, R., Ravikumar, R., & Isabel, S. C. (2013). Mechanism of action of probiotics. *Brazilian Archives of Biology and Technology*, *56*(1), 113–119. doi:10.1590/S1516-89132013000100015

Hempel, S., Newberry, S. J., Maher, A. R., Wang, Z., Miles, J. N., Shanman, R., ... Shekelle, P. G. (2012). Probiotics for the prevention and treatment ofantibiotic-associated diarrhea: A systematic review and meta-analysis. *Journal of the American Medical Association*, *307*, 1959–1969. doi:10.1001/jama.2012.3507 PMID:22570464

Hering, C. (1836). Preface to the first American edition. In the Organon of Homeopathic Medicine. New York: William Radde.

Hering, C. (1879). *The Guiding Symptoms of our MateriaMedica, V(1)*. Philadelphia: The American Publishing Society.

Hernández-Díaz, S., Werler, M. M., Walker, A. M., & Mitchell, A. A. (2000). Folic acid antagonists during pregnancy and the risk of birth defects. *The New England Journal of Medicine*, *343*(22), 1608–1614. doi:10.1056/NEJM200011303432204 PMID:11096168

Herrada, A. A., Campino, C., Amador, C. A., Michea, L. F., Fardella, C. E., & Kalergis, A. M. (2011). Aldosterone as a modulator of immunity: Implications in the organ damage. *Journal of Hypertension*, *29*(9), 1684–1692. doi:10.1097/HJH.0b013e32834a4c75 PMID:21826023

High Blood Pressure. (2014). *High Blood Pressure (Hypertension) Information | cdc.gov*. Retrieved April 13, 2017, from https://www.cdc.gov/bloodpressure/index.htm

Hil, J. O., & Peters, J. C. (2002). Biomarkers and functional foods for obesity and diabetes. *British Journal of Nutrition*, *88*(S2), 213–218. doi:10.1079/BJN2002685 PMID:12495462

Hillman, G. G., Singh-Gupta, V., Hoogstra, D. J., Abernathy, L., Rakowski, J., Yunker, C. K., ... Joiner, M. C. (2013). Differential effect of soy isoflavones in enhancing high intensity radiotherapy and protecting lung tissue in a pre-clinical model of lung carcinoma. *Radiotherapy and Oncology: Journal of the European Society for Therapeutic Radiology and Oncology*, *109*(1), 117–125. doi:10.1016/j.radonc.2013.08.015 PMID:24021346

Hilton, E., Kolakowski, P., Singer, C., & Smith, M. (1997). Efficacy of *Lacto-bacillus* GG as a diarrheal preventive in travelers. *Journal of Travel Medicine*, *4*(1), 41–92. doi:10.1111/j.1708-8305.1997.tb00772.x PMID:9815476

Hilty, F. M., Arnold, M., Hilbe, M., Teleki, A., Knijnenburg, J. T., Ehrensperger, F., & Zimmermann, M. B. (2010). Iron from nanocompounds containing iron and zinc is highly bioavailable in rats without tissue accumulation. *Nature Nanotechnology*, *5*(5), 374–380. doi:10.1038/nnano.2010.79 PMID:20418865

Hipsley, E. H. (1953). Dietary "Fibre" and Pregnancy Toxaemia. *British Medical Journal*, *2*(4833), 420–422. doi:10.1136/bmj.2.4833.420 PMID:13066743

Hirai, S., Takahashi, N., Goto, T., Lin, S., Uemura, T., Yu, R., & Kawada, T. (2010). Functional food targeting the regulation of obesity-induced inflammatory responses and pathologies. *Mediators of Inflammation. Article ID, 367838*. doi:10.1155/2010/367838

Hirano, J., Yoshida, T., Sugiyama, T., Koide, N., Mori, I., & Yokochi, T. (2003). The effect of *Lactobacillus rhamnosus*on enterohemorrhagic*Escherichia coli* infection of human intestinal cells in vitro. *Microbiology and Immunology*, *47*(6), 405–409. doi:10.1111/j.1348-0421.2003.tb03377.x PMID:12906100

Hirpara, K. V., Aggarwal, P., Mukherjee, A. J., Joshi, N., & Burman, A. C. (2009). Quercetin and its derivatives: Synthesis, pharmacological uses with special emphasis on anti-tumor properties and prodrug with enhanced bio-availability. *Anti-cancer Agents in Medicinal Chemistry*, *9*(2), 138–161. doi:10.2174/187152009787313855 PMID:19199862

Hoarau, C., Lagaraine, C., Martin, I., Velge-Roussel, F., & Lecranchu, Y. (2006). Supernatant of Bifidobacterium breve induces dendritic cell maturation, activation, and survival through a Toll-like receptor pathway. *The Journal of Allergy and Clinical Immunology*, *117*(3), 696–702. doi:10.1016/j.jaci.2005.10.043 PMID:16522473

Hollman, P. C. H., Hertog, M. G. L., & Katan, M. B. (1996). Analysis and health effects of flavonoids. *Food Chemistry*, *57*(1), 43–46. doi:10.1016/0308-8146(96)00065-9

Homan, M., & Orel, R. (2015). Are probiotics useful in *Helicobacter pylori* eradication? *World Journal of Gastroenterology*, *21*(37), 10644–10653. doi:10.3748/wjg.v21.i37.10644 PMID:26457024

Hong, Y. (2009). Burden of Cardiovascular Disease in Asia: Big Challenges and Ample Opportunities for Action and Making a Difference. *Clinical Chemistry*, *55*(8), 1450–1452. doi:10.1373/clinchem.2009.125369 PMID:19498049

Ho, P., & Ross, D. A. (2017). More than a gut feeling: The implications of the gut microbiota in psychiatry. *Biological Psychiatry*, *81*(5), e35–e37. doi:10.1016/j.biopsych.2016.12.018 PMID:28137375

Hosseinzadeh, H., & Parvardeh, S. (2004). Anticonvulsant effects of thymoquinone, the major constituent of Nigella sativa seeds, in mice. *Phytomedicine*, *11*(1), 56–64. doi:10.1078/0944-7113-00376 PMID:14971722

Hotamisligil, G. S. (2006). Inflammation and metabolic disorders. *Nature*, *444*(7121), 860–867. doi:10.1038/nature05485 PMID:17167474

Hotamisligil, G. S., Peraldi, P., Budavari, A., Ellis, R., White, M. F., & Spiegelman, B. M. (1996). IRS-1-mediated inhibition of insulin receptor tyrosine kinase activity in TNF-alpha- and obesity-induced insulin resistance. *Science*, *271*(5249), 665–668. doi:10.1126cience.271.5249.665 PMID:8571133

Hotamisligil, G. S., Shargill, N. S., & Spiegelman, B. M. (1993). Adipose expression of tumor necrosis factor-α: Direct role I obesity-linked insulin resistance. *Science*, *259*(5091), 87–91. doi:10.1126cience.7678183 PMID:7678183

Houston, M. (2014). The role of nutrition and nutraceutical supplements in the treatment of hypertension. *World Journal of Cardiology*, *6*(2), 38–66. doi:10.4330/wjc.v6.i2.38 PMID:24575172

Houston, M. C. (2005). Nutraceuticals, vitamins, antioxidants, and minerals in the prevention and treatment of hypertension. *Progress in Cardiovascular Diseases*, *47*(6), 396–449. doi:10.1016/j.pcad.2005.01.004 PMID:16115519

Houston, M. C., & Harper, K. J. (2008). Potassium, magnesium, and calcium: Their role in both the cause and treatment of hypertension. *Journal of Clinical Hypertension (Greenwich, Conn.)*, *10*(7Suppl 2), 3–11. doi:10.1111/j.1751-7176.2008.08575.x PMID:18607145

Hsiao, E. Y., McBride, S. W., Hsien, S., Sharon, G., Hyde, E. R., McCue, T., ... Mazmanian, S. K. (2013). Microbiota modulate behavioral and physiological abnormalities associated with neurodevelopmental disorders. *Cell*, *155*(7), 1451–1463. doi:10.1016/j.cell.2013.11.024 PMID:24315484

Hsueh, W. A., & Law, R. E. (1998). Diabetes is a vascular disease. *Journal of Investigative Medicine*, *46*(8), 387–390. PMID:9805424

Huang, W.-C., Chen, C.-L., Lin, Y.-S., & Lin, C.-F. (2011). Apoptotic Sphingolipid Ceramide in Cancer Therapy. Journal of Lipids.

Huang. (2010). Polymethoxy flavones are responsible for the anti-inflammatory activity of citrus fruit peel. *Food Chemistry*, *119*(3), 868–873.

Huang, C. L., & Sumpio, B. E. (2008). Olive oil, the mediterranean diet, and cardiovascular health. *Journal of the American College of Surgeons*, *207*(3), 407–416. doi:10.1016/j.jamcollsurg.2008.02.018 PMID:18722947

Huang, C., Huang, Y., Li, J., & Hu, W. (2002). Inhibition of Benzo(a)pyrene Diol-Epoxide-induced Transactivation of Activated Protein 1 and Nuclear Factor κB by Black Raspberry Extracts. *Cancer Research*, *62*(23). PMID:12460899

Huang, M. T., Ho, C. T., Wang, Z., & Conney, A. H. (1994). Inhibition of skin tumorigenesis by rosemary and its constituents carnosol and ursolic acid. *Cancer Research*, *54*(3), 701–708. PMID:8306331

Hu, B., Kou, L., Li, C., Zhu, L. P., Fan, Y. R., Wu, Z. W., ... Xu, G. X. (2009). *Bifidobacterium longum* as a delivery system of TRAIL and endostatin cooperates with chemotherapeutic drugs to inhibit hypoxic tumor growth. *Cancer Gene Therapy*, *16*(8), 655–663. doi:10.1038/cgt.2009.7 PMID:19229287

Hudson, S. A., Ecroyd, H., Dehle, F. C., Musgrave, I. F., & Carver, J. A. (2009). (-)-epigallocatechin-3-gallate (EGCG) maintains kappa-casein in its pre-fibrillar state without redirecting its aggregation pathway. *Journal of Molecular Biology*, *392*(3), 689–700. doi:10.1016/j.jmb.2009.07.031 PMID:19616561

Hu, F. B., Stampfer, M. J., Manson, J. E., Rimm, E., Colditz, G. A., Speizer, F. E., ... Willett, W. C. (1999). Dietary protein and risk of ischemic heart disease in women. *The American Journal of Clinical Nutrition*, *70*(2), 221–227. doi:10.1093/ajcn.70.2.221 PMID:10426698

Hu, F., Koon, C. M., Chan, J. Y., Lau, K. M., & Fung, K. P. (2012). The cardioprotective effect of danshen and gegen decoction on rat hearts and cardiomyocytes with post-ischemia reperfusion injury. *BMC Complementary and Alternative Medicine*, *12*(1), 249. doi:10.1186/1472-6882-12-249 PMID:23228089

Hulston, C. J., Churnside, A. A., & Venables, M. C. (2015). Probiotic supplementation prevents high-fat, overfeeding-induced insulin resistance in human subjects. *British Journal of Nutrition*, *113*(4), 596–602. doi:10.1017/S0007114514004097 PMID:25630516

Humphrey, B. D., Huang, N., & Klasing, K. C. (2002). Rice expressing lactoferrin and lysozyme has antibiotic-like properties when fed to chicks. *The Journal of Nutrition*, *132*(6), 1214–1218. doi:10.1093/jn/132.6.1214 PMID:12042436

Hutchins, A. M., Slavin, J. L., & Lampe, J. W. (1995). Urinary isoflavonoid phytoestrogen and lignan excretion after consumption of fermented and unfermented soy products. *Journal of the American Dietetic Association*, *95*(5), 545–551. doi:10.1016/S0002-8223(95)00149-2 PMID:7722188

Huurre, A., Laitinen, K., Rautava, S., Korkeamäki, M., & Isolauri, E. (2008). Impact of maternal atopy and probiotic supplementation during pregnancy on infant sensitization. *Clinical and Experimental Allergy*, *38*(8), 1342–1348. doi:10.1111/j.1365-2222.2008.03008.x PMID:18477013

Hwang, E. S., & Bowen, P. E. (2004). Cell cycle arrest and induction of apoptosis by lycopene in LNCaP human prostate cancer cells. *Journal of Medicinal Food*, *7*(3), 284–289. doi:10.1089/jmf.2004.7.284 PMID:15383220

Hyun, Y. J., Kim, O. Y., Kang, J. B., Lee, J. H., Jang, Y., Liponkoski, L., & Salo, P. (2005). Plant stanol esters in low-fat yoghurt reduce total and low density lipoprotein cholesterol and low-density lipoprotein oxidation in normocholesterolemic and mildly hypercholesterolemic subjects. *Nutrition Research (New York, N.Y.)*, *25*(8), 743–753. doi:10.1016/j.nutres.2005.08.004

Ikeda, I., Sugano, M., Yoshida, K., Sasaki, E., Iwamoto, Y., & Hatano, K. (1993). Effects of chitosan hydrolyzates on lipid absorption and on serum and liver lipid concentration in rats. *Journal of Agricultural and Food Chemistry*, *41*(3), 431–435. doi:10.1021/jf00027a016

International Obesity Task Force (IOTF). (2005). *Obesity in Europe*. EU Platform Briefing Paper. Retrieved from http://www.iaso.org/

Irizar, A., Barnett, C. R., Flatt, P. R., & Ioannides, C. (1995). Defective expression of cytochrome P450 proteins in the liver of the genetically obese Zucker rat. *European Journal of Pharmacology*, *293*(4), 385–393. doi:10.1016/0926-6917(95)90059-4 PMID:8748692

Irondi, E. A., Agboola, S. O., Oboh, G., Boligon, A. A., Athayde, M. L., & Shode, F. O. (2016). Guava leaves polyphenolics-rich extract inhibits vital enzymes implicated in gout and hypertension in vitro. *J Intercult Ethnopharmacol*, *5*(2), 122. doi:10.5455/jice.20160321115402 PMID:27104032

Isa, Y., Miyakawa, Y., Yanagisawa, M., Goto, T., Kang, M. S., Kawada, T., ... Tsuda, T. (2008). 6-Shogaol and 6-gingerol, the pungent of ginger, inhibit TNF-α mediated down regulation of adiponectin expression via different mechanisms in 3T3-L1 adipocytes. *Biochemical and Biophysical Research Communications*, *373*(3), 429–434. doi:10.1016/j.bbrc.2008.06.046 PMID:18577375

Ishibashi, N., & Yamazaki, S. (2001). Probiotics and safety. *The American Journal of Clinical Nutrition*, *73*(2Suppl.), 465S–470S. doi:10.1093/ajcn/73.2.465s PMID:11157359

Ishimwe, N., Daliri, E., Lee, B., Fang, F., & Du, G. (2015). The perspective on cholesterol-lowering mechanisms of probiotics. *Molecular Nutrition & Food Research*, *59*(1), 94–105. doi:10.1002/mnfr.201400548 PMID:25403164

Isolauri, E. (2001). Probiotics in human disease. *The American Journal of Clinical Nutrition*, *73*(6), 1142S–1146S. doi:10.1093/ajcn/73.6.1142S PMID:11393192

Ito, K., Nakazato, T., Yamato, K., Miyakawa, Y., Yamada, T., Hozumi, N., ... Kizaki, M. (2004). Induction of apoptosis in leukemic cells by homovanillic acid derivative, capsaicin, through oxidative stress: Implication of phosphorylation of p53 at Ser-15 residue by reactive oxygen species. *Cancer Research*, *64*(3), 1071–1078. doi:10.1158/0008-5472.CAN-03-1670 PMID:14871840

Iyer, A., Panchal, S., Poudyal, H., & Brown, L. (2009). Potential health benefits of Indian spices in the symptoms of the metabolic syndrome: A review. *Indian Journal of Biochemistry & Biophysics*, *46*(6), 467–481. PMID:20361710

J. C., Ursell, L.K., Parfrey, L. W., Knight, R. (2012). The Impact of the Gut Microbiota on Human Health: An Integrative View. *Cell*, *148*(16), 1258–1270. PMID:22424233

Jackson, R., Lawes, C. M. M., Bennett, D. A., Milne, R. J., & Rodgers, A. (2005). Treatment with drugs to lower blood pressure and blood cholesterol based on an individual's absolute cardiovascular risk. *Lancet (London, England)*, *365*(9457), 434–441. doi:10.1016/S0140-6736(05)70240-3 PMID:15680460

Jacob, R. A. (1995). The Integrated Antioxidant System. *Nutrition Research (New York, N.Y.)*, *15*(5), 755–766. doi:10.1016/0271-5317(95)00041-G

Jagerstad, M., & Skog, K. (2005). Genotoxicity of heat-processed foods. *Mutation Research*, *574*(1-2), 156–172. doi:10.1016/j.mrfmmm.2005.01.030 PMID:15914214

Jain, A., Jain, K., Kesharwani, P., & Jain, N. K. (2013). Low density lipoproteins mediated nanoplatforms for cancer targeting. *Journal of Nanoparticle Research*, *15*(9), 1–38. doi:10.100711051-013-1888-7

Jallouli, Y., Paillard, A., Chang, J., Sevin, E., & Betbeder, D. (2007). Influence of surface charge and inner composition of porous nanoparticles to cross blood–brain barrier in vitro. *International Journal of Pharmaceutics*, *344*(1–2), 103–109. doi:10.1016/j.ijpharm.2007.06.023 PMID:17651930

Jamal, P., & Akbar, I. (2016). Process Development for Maximum Lycopene Production from Selected Fruit Waste and its Antioxidant and Antiradical Activity. *Journal of Food Processing & Technology*, *07*(04). doi:10.4172/2157-7110.1000576

James, P. A., Oparil, S., Carter, B. L., Cushman, W. C., Dennison-Himmelfarb, C., Handler, J., ... Ortiz, E. (2014). 2014 Evidence-Based Guideline for the Management of High Blood Pressure in Adults: Report from the Panel Members Appointed to the Eighth Joint National Committee (JNC 8). *Journal of the American Medical Association*, *311*(5), 507–520. doi:10.1001/jama.2013.284427 PMID:24352797

Janca, A., Aarli, J. A., Prilipko, L., Dua, T., Saxena, S., & Saraceno, B. (2006). WHO/WFN Survey of neurological services: A worldwide perspective. *Journal of the Neurological Sciences*, *247*(1), 29–34. doi:10.1016/j.jns.2006.03.003 PMID:16624322

Jeffery, I. B., Toole, P. W. O., Human, L. O., Claesson, M. J., Deane, J., Quigley, E. M. M., & Simren, M. (2012). An irritable bowel syndrome subtype defined by species-specific alterations in faecal microbiota. *Gut*, *61*(7), 997–1006. doi:10.1136/gutjnl-2011-301501 PMID:22180058

Jenkins, D. J. A., Kendall, C. W. C., Marchie, A., Faulkner, D. A., Wong, J. M. W., de Souza, R., ... Connelly, P. W. (2005). Direct comparison of a dietary portfolio of cholesterol-lowering foods with a statin in hypercholesterolemic participants. *The American Journal of Clinical Nutrition*, *81*(2), 380–387. doi:10.1093/ajcn.81.2.380 PMID:15699225

Jeppesen, J., Hein, H. O., Suadicani, P., & Gyntelberg, F. (1998). Triglyceride concentration and ischemic heart disease: An eight-year follow-up in the Copenhagen Male Study. *Circulation*, *97*(11), 1029–1036. doi:10.1161/01.CIR.97.11.1029 PMID:9531248

Jessup, C. M., & Forde, S. E. (2008). Ecology and evolution in microbial systems: The generation and maintenance of diversity in phage-host interactions. *Research in Microbiology*, *159*(5), 382–389. doi:10.1016/j.resmic.2008.05.006 PMID:18582563

Jiang, T., Sun, Q., & Chen, S. (2016). Oxidative stress: A major pathogenesis and potential therapeutic target of antioxidative agents in Parkinson's disease and Alzheimer's disease. *Progress in Neurobiology*, *147*, 1–19. doi:10.1016/j.pneurobio.2016.07.005 PMID:27769868

Johansson, M. L., Sanni, A., Likner, C., & Molin, G. (1995). Phenotypically based taxonomy using API 50CH of lactobacilli from Nigerian ogi, and the occurrence of starch fermenting strains. *International Journal of Food Microbiology*, *25*(2), 159–168. doi:10.1016/0168-1605(94)00096-O PMID:7547147

Johnson, J. J. (2011). Carnosol: A promising anti-cancer and anti-inflammatory agent. *Cancer Letters, 305*(1), 1–7. doi:10.1016/j.canlet.2011.02.005 PMID:21382660

Johnston, B. C., Goldenberg, J. C., Vandvik, P. O., Sun, X., & Guyatt, G. H. (2011). Probiotics for the prevention of pediatric-associated diarrhea. *Cochrane Database of Systematic Reviews*, CD004827. PMID:22071814

Jones, P. J. H. J., & AbuMweis, S. S. (2009). Phytosterols as functional food ingredients: Linkages to cardiovascular disease and cancer. *Current Opinion in Clinical Nutrition and Metabolic Care, 12*(2), 147–151. doi:10.1097/MCO.0b013e328326770f PMID:19209468

Jong, A., Plat, J., & Mensink, R. P. (2003). Metabolic effects of plant sterols and stanols. *The Journal of Nutritional Biochemistry, 14*(7), 362–369. doi:10.1016/S0955-2863(03)00002-0 PMID:12915216

Joseph, T. (2014). *Pharmacotherapy: A Pathophysiologic Approach, Access Pharmacy*. McGraw-Hill Medical. Retrieved April 13, 2017, from http://accesspharmacy.mhmedical.com/book.aspx?bookid=689

Joseph, J. A., Shukitt-Hale, B., Brewer, G. J., Weikel, K. A., Kalt, W., & Fisher, D. R. (2010). Differential protection among fractionated blueberry polyphenolic families against DA-, Aβ42 and LPS-induced decrements in Ca2+ buffering in primary hippocampal cells. *Journal of Agricultural and Food Chemistry, 58*(14), 8196–8204. doi:10.1021/jf100144y PMID:20597478

Jungbauer, A., & Medjakovic, S. (2012). Anti-inflammatory properties of culinary herbs and spices that ameliorate the effects of metabolic syndrome. *Maturitas, 71*(3), 227-239.

Kabanov, A. V., & Gendelman, H. E. (2007). Nanomedicine in the diagnosis and therapy of neurodegenerative disorders. *Progress in Polymer Science, 32*(8–9), 1054–1082. doi:10.1016/j.progpolymsci.2007.05.014 PMID:20234846

Kajantie, E., Fall, C. H., Seppälä, M., Koistinen, R., Dunkel, L., Ylihärsilä, H., ... Eriksson, J. (2003). Serum insulin-like growth factor (IGF)-I and composition, size at birth, and childhood growth. *The Journal of Clinical Endocrinology and Metabolism, 88*(3), 1059–1065. doi:10.1210/jc.2002-021380 PMID:12629086

Kajantie, E., Fall, C. H., Seppala, M., Koistinen, R., Dunkel, L., Yliharsila, H., ... Yu, R. (2007). Capsaicin, a spicy component of hot peppers, modulates adipokine gene expression and protein release from obese mouse adipose tissues and isolated adipocytes, and suppresses the inflammatory responses of adipose tissue macrophages. *FEBS Letters, 581*(23), 4389–4396. doi:10.1016/j.febslet.2007.07.082 PMID:17719033

Kaji, I., Tatsuta, M., Iishi, H., Baba, M., Inoue, A., & Kasugai, H. (2001). Inhibition by d-limonene of experimental hepatocarcinogenesis in Sprague-Dawley rats does not involve p21(ras) plasma membrane association. *International Journal of Cancer, 93*(3), 441–444. doi:10.1002/ijc.1353 PMID:11433412

Kaliora, A. C., Dedoussis, G. V. Z., & Schmidt, H. (2006). Dietary antioxidants in preventing atherogenesis. *Atherosclerosis*, *187*(1), 1–17. doi:10.1016/j.atherosclerosis.2005.11.001 PMID:16313912

Kalix, B., Meynet, M. C., Garin, M. C., & James, R. W. (2001). The apolipoprotein epsilon2 allele and the severity of coronary artery disease in Type 2 diabetic patients. *Diabetic Medicine*, *18*(6), 445–450. doi:10.1046/j.1464-5491.2001.00497.x PMID:11472462

Kalliomaki, M., & Isolauri, E. (2002). Pandemic of atopic diseases—a lack of microbial exposure in early infancy? *Current Drug Targets. Infectious Disorders*, *2*(3), 193–199. doi:10.2174/1568005023342452 PMID:12462124

Kalliomäki, M., Salminen, S., Arvilommi, H., Kero, P., Koskinen, P., & Isolauri, E. (2001). Probiotics in primary prevention of atopic 392 disease: A randomised placebo-controlled trial. *Lancet*, *357*(9262), 1076–1079. doi:10.1016/S0140-6736(00)04259-8 PMID:11297958

Kalliomäki, M., Salminen, S., Poussa, T., & Isolauri, E. (2007). Probiotics during the first 7 years of life: A cumulative risk reduction of 388 eczema in randomized, placebo-controlled trial. *The Journal of Allergy and Clinical Immunology*, *119*(4), 1019–1021. doi:10.1016/j.jaci.2006.12.608 PMID:17289135

Kalra, E. K. (2003). Nutraceutical--definition and introduction. *AAPS PharmSci*, *5*(3), E25. doi:10.1208/ps050325 PMID:14621960

Kampoli, A.-M., Tousoulis, D., Antoniades, C., Siasos, G., & Stefanadis, C. (2009). Biomarkers of premature atherosclerosis. *Trends in Molecular Medicine*, *15*(7), 323–332. doi:10.1016/j.molmed.2009.06.001 PMID:19577961

Kamsteeg, M., Rutherford, T., Sapi, E., Hanczaruk, B., Shahabi, S., Flick, M., ... Mor, G. (2003). Phenoxodiol – an isoflavone analog – induces apoptosis in chemoresistant ovarian cancer cells. *Oncogene*, *22*(17), 2611–2620. doi:10.1038j.onc.1206422 PMID:12730675

Kargi, F., & Ozmihci, S. (2006). Utilization of cheese whey powder (CWP) for ethanol fermentations: Effect of operating parameters. *Enzyme and Microbial Technology*, *38*(5), 711–718. doi:10.1016/j.enzmictec.2005.11.006

Karin, M. (2009). NF- B as a Critical Link Between Inflammation and Cancer. *Cold Spring Harbor Perspectives in Biology*, *1*(5), a000141–a000141. doi:10.1101/cshperspect.a000141 PMID:20066113

Karin, M., & Greten, F. R. (2005). NF-κB: Linking inflammation and immunity to cancer development and progression. *Nature Reviews. Immunology*, *5*(10), 749–759. doi:10.1038/nri1703 PMID:16175180

Kasala, E. R., Bodduluru, L. N., Barua, C. C., & Gogoi, R. (2016). Antioxidant and antitumor efficacy of Luteolin, a dietary flavone on benzo(a)pyrene-induced experimental lung carcinogenesis. *Biomedicine & Pharmacotherapy, 82*, 568–77.

Kasbia, G. S. (2005). Functional foods and nutraceuticals in the management of obesity. *Nutrition & Food Science*, *35*(5), 344–351. doi:10.1108/00346650510625557

Kasili, E. G. (1989). Malnutrition and infections as causes of childhood anemia in tropical Africa. *The American Journal of Pediatric Hematology/Oncology*, *12*(3), 375–377. doi:10.1097/00043426-199023000-00023 PMID:2122763

Kassis, A. N., Vanstone, C. A., AbuMweis, S. S., & Jones, P. J. H. J. (2008). Efficacy of plant sterol is not influenced by dietary cholesterol intake in hypercholesterolemic individuals. *Metabolism: Clinical and Experimental*, *57*(3), 339–346. doi:10.1016/j.metabol.2007.10.008 PMID:18249205

Katan, M. B. (2002). Nutrition in the Prevention and Treatment of Disease. *The New England Journal of Medicine*, *346*(22), 1754–1754. doi:10.1056/NEJM200205303462221

Kataoka, S., Robbins, D. C., Cowan, L. D., Go, O., Yeh, J. L., Devereux, R. B., ... Howard, B. V. (1996). Apolipoprotein E polymorphism in American Indians and its relation to plasma lipoproteins and diabetes. The Strong Heart Study. *Arteriosclerosis, Thrombosis, and Vascular Biology*, *16*(8), 918–925. doi:10.1161/01.ATV.16.8.918 PMID:8696954

Katare, C., Agrawal, S., Jain, M., Rani, S., Saxena, S., Prakash, S. B., & Godavarthi, B. K. S. P. (2011). Lagenaria siceraria: A potential source of anti-hyperlipidemic and other pharmacological agents. *Current Nutrition and Food Science*, *7*(4), 1–7. doi:10.2174/157340111804586501

Katelaris, P. H., Salam, I., & Farthing, M. J. (1995). *Lactobacilli* to preventtraveler's diarrhea? *The New England Journal of Medicine*, *333*(20), 1360–1391. doi:10.1056/NEJM199511163332016 PMID:7566045

Kearney, P. M., Whelton, M., Reynolds, K., Muntner, P., Whelton, P. K., & He, J. (2005). Global burden of hypertension: Analysis of worldwide data. *Lancet*, *365*(9455), 217–223. doi:10.1016/S0140-6736(05)70151-3 PMID:15652604

Keats, S., & Wiggins, S. (2014). *The overseas development institute (ODI). Future diets: Implications for agriculture and food prices*. Retrieved January 20, 2014, from http://www.odi.org.uk/sites/odi.org.uk/files/odi-assets/publications-opinion-files/8776.pdf

Kechagia, M., Basoulis, D., Konstantopoulou, S., Dimitriadi, D., Gyftopoulou, K., Skarmoutsou, N., & Fakiri, E. M. (2012). *Health benefits of probiotics: A Review*. Hindawi Publishing Corporation ISRN Nutrition. .10.5402/2013/481651

Kekkonen, R. A., Sysi-Aho, M., Seppanen-Laakso, T., Julkunen, I., Vapaatalo, H., Oresic, M., & Korpela, R. (2008). Effect of probiotic *Lactobacillus rhamnosus* GG intervention on global serum lipidomic profiles in healthy adults. *World Journal of Gastroenterology*, *14*(20), 3188–3194. doi:10.3748/wjg.14.3188 PMID:18506924

Kelsey, N. A., Wilkins, H. M., & Linseman, D. A. (2010). Nutraceutical antioxidants as novel neuroprotective agents. *Molecules (Basel, Switzerland)*, *15*(11), 7792–7814. doi:10.3390/molecules15117792 PMID:21060289

Kent, J. T. (1929). *Lectures on Homeopathic Philosophy* (2nd ed.). Chicago: Ehrhart & Karl.

Kesaniemi, Y. A., Ehnholm, C., & Miettinen, T. A. (1987). Intestinal cholesterol absorption efficiency in man is related to apoprotein E phenotype. *The Journal of Clinical Investigation*, *80*(2), 578–581. doi:10.1172/JCI113107 PMID:3611358

Keservani, R. K., Kesharwani, R. K., Sharma, A. K., Vyas, N., & Chadoker, A. (2010a). Nutritional supplements: An overview. *Int J Curr Pharm Rev Res*, *1*, 59–75.

Keservani, R. K., Kesharwani, R. K., Vyas, N., Jain, S., Raghuvanshi, R., & Sharma, A. K. (2010b). Nutraceutical and functional food as future food: A review. *Der Pharmacia Lett*, *2*, 106–116.

Keservani, R. K., Sharma, A. K., & Kesharwani, R. K. (2016). Medicinal effect of nutraceutical fruits for the cognition and brain health. *Scientifica*. PMID:26966612

Khan, N., Afaq, F., Saleem, M., Ahmad, N., & Mukhtar, H. (2006). Targeting Multiple Signaling Pathways by Green Tea Polyphenol (−)-Epigallocatechin-3-Gallate. *Cancer Research*, *66*(5), 2500–2505. doi:10.1158/0008-5472.CAN-05-3636 PMID:16510563

Khatib, R., McKee, M., Shannon, H., Chow, C., Rangarajan, S., Teo, K., ... Yusuf, S. (2016). Availability and affordability of cardiovascular disease medicines and their effect on use in high-income, middle-income, and low-income countries: An analysis of the PURE study data. *Lancet*, *387*(10013), 61–69. doi:10.1016/S0140-6736(15)00469-9 PMID:26498706

Khoo, H. E., Azlan, A., Kong, K. W., & Ismail, A. (2016). Phytochemicals and Medicinal Properties of Indigenous Tropical Fruits with Potential for Commercial Development. *Evidence-Based Complementary and Alternative Medicine*, *7591951*. doi:10.1155/2016/7591951 PMID:27340420

Khor, E.-S., & Wong, N.-K. (2014). Potential antioxidant and cytotoxic properties of secondary metabolite extracts from Carica Papaya fruits and seeds. *International Journal of Pharmacy and Pharmaceutical Sciences*, *6*(7), 220–224.

Khoruts, A., Dicksved, J., Jansson, J. K., & Sadowsky, M. J. (2010). Changes in the composition of the human fecal microbiome after bacteriotherapy for recurrent Clostridium difficile-associated diarrhea. *Journal of Clinical Gastroenterology*, *44*, 354–360. PMID:20048681

Kim, Y., Lee, D., Kim, D., Cho, J., Yang, J., Chung, M., Kim, K., & Ha, N. (2008). Inhibition of proliferation in colon cancer cell lines and harmful enzyme activity of colon bacteria by Bifidobacteriumadolescentis SPM0212. *Archives of Pharmcal Research*, 468–473.

Kim, H. J., Vazquez Roque, M. I., Camilleri, M., Stephens, D., Burton, D. D., Baxter, K., ... Zinsmeister, A. R. (2005). A randomized controlled trial of a probiotic combination *VSL#3* and placebo in irritable bowel syndrome with bloating. *Neurogastroenterology and Motility*, *17*(5), 687–696. doi:10.1111/j.1365-2982.2005.00695.x PMID:16185307

Kim, L. S., Axelrod, L. J., Howard, P., Buratovich, N., & Waters, R. F. (2006). Efficacy of methylsulfonylmethane (MSM) in osteoarthritis pain of the knee: A pilot clinical trial. *Osteoarthritis and Cartilage*, *14*(3), 286–294. doi:10.1016/j.joca.2005.10.003 PMID:16309928

Kim, S. H., Park, H. S., Lee, M. S., Cho, Y. J., Kim, Y. S., Hwang, J. T., ... Kwon, D. Y. (2008). Vitisin A inhibits adipocyte differentiation through cell cycle arrest in 3T3-L1 cells. *Biochemical and Biophysical Research Communications*, *372*(1), 108–113. doi:10.1016/j.bbrc.2008.04.188 PMID:18482581

Kim, S. O., Chun, K.-S., Kundu, J. K., & Surh, Y.-J. (2004). Inhibitory effects of [6]-gingerol on PMA-induced COX-2 expression and activation of NF-kappaB and p38 MAPK in mouse skin. *BioFactors (Oxford, England)*, *21*(1–4), 27–31. doi:10.1002/biof.552210107 PMID:15630166

Kim, S., Jin, Y., Choi, Y., & Park, T. (2011). Resveratrol exerts anti-obesity effects via mechanisms involving down-regulation of adipogenic and inflammatory processes in mice. *Biochemical Pharmacology*, *81*(11), 1343–1351. doi:10.1016/j.bcp.2011.03.012 PMID:21439945

Kimura, I., Inoue, D., Hirano, K., & Tsujimoto, G. (2014). The SCFA receptor GPR43 and energy metabolism. *Frontiers in Endocrinology*, *5*(85), 7–14. PMID:24926285

Kizhakekuttu, T. J., & Widlansky, M. E. (2010). Natural antioxidants and hypertension: Promise and challenges. *Cardiovascular Therapeutics*, *28*(4), e20–e32. doi:10.1111/j.1755-5922.2010.00137.x PMID:20370791

Klein, E., Thompson, I., Lippman, S., Goodman, P., Albanes, D., Taylor, P., & Coltman, C. (2000). SELECT: the Selenium and Vitamin E Cancer Prevention Trial: rationale and design. *Prostate Cancer and Prostatic Diseases*, *3*(3), 145–151. doi:10.1038j.pcan.4500412 PMID:12497090

Kobyliak, N., Conte, C., Cammarota, G., Haley, A. P., Styriak, I., Gaspar, L., ... Kruzliak, P. (2016). Probiotics in prevention and treatment of obesity: A critical view. *Nutrition and Metabolism*, *13*(1), 14. doi:10.118612986-016-0067-0 PMID:26900391

Koçyildiz, Z. C., Birman, H., Olgaç, V., Akgün-Dar, K., Melikoğlu, G., & Meriçli, A. H. (2006). Crataegus tanacetifolia leaf extract prevents L-NAME-induced hypertension in rats: A morphological study. *Phytotherapy Research: PTR*, *20*(1), 66–70. doi:10.1002/ptr.1808 PMID:16397846

Koga, C. C., Andrade, J. E., Ferruzzi, M. G., & Lee, Y. (2015). Stability of Trans-Resveratrol Encapsulated in a Protein Matrix Produced Using Spray Drying to UV Light Stress and Simulated Gastro-Intestinal Digestion. *Journal of Food Science*, *81*(2), 292–300. doi:10.1111/1750-3841.13176 PMID:26677808

Kohlmeier, M. (2015). *Nutrient metabolism: structures, functions, and genes*. Retrieved from http://alltitles.ebrary.com/Doc?id=11055728

Kollaritsch, H. (1989). Traveller's diarrhea among Austrian touriststowarm climate countries: II Clinical features. *European Journal of Epidemiology*, *5*(3), 355–362. doi:10.1007/BF00144838 PMID:2792310

Konno, S., Hirooka, Y., Araki, S., Koga, Y., Kishi, T., & Sunagawa, K. (2008). Azelnidipine decreases sympathetic nerve activity via antioxidant effect in the rostral ventrolateral medulla of stroke-prone spontaneously hypertensive rats. *Journal of Cardiovascular Pharmacology*, *52*(6), 555–560. doi:10.1097/FJC.0b013e318192690e PMID:19057394

Koo, M., Kim, S. H., Lee, N., Yoo, M. Y., Ryu, S. Y., Kwon, D. Y., & Kim, Y. S. (2008). 3-Hydroxy-3-methylglutaryl-CoA (HMG-CoA) reductase inhibitory effect of Vitis vinifera. *Fitoterapia*, *79*(3), 204–206. doi:10.1016/j.fitote.2007.11.005 PMID:18191910

Koppe, L., Mafra, D., & Fouque, D. (2015). Probiotics and chronic kidney disease. *Kidney International*, *88*(5), 958–966. doi:10.1038/ki.2015.255 PMID:26376131

Kopp-Hoolihan, L. (2001). Prophylactic and therapeutic uses of probiotics: A review. *Journal of the American Dietetic Association*, *101*(2), 229–238, quiz 239–241. doi:10.1016/S0002-8223(01)00060-8 PMID:11271697

Korutla, L., & Kumar, R. (1994). Inhibitory effect of curcumin on epidermal growth factor receptor kinase activity in A431 cells. *Biochimica et Biophysica Acta*, *1224*(3), 597–600. doi:10.1016/0167-4889(94)90299-2 PMID:7803521

Kotilainen, L., Rajalahti, R., Ragasa, C., & Pehu, E. (2006, June 1). *Health enhancing foods : opportunities for strengthening developing countries*. Academic Press.

Kotzampassia, K., & Giamarellos-Bourboulis, E. J. (2012). Probiotics for infectious diseases: More drugs, less dietary supplementation. *International Journal of Antimicrobial Agents*, *40*(4), 288–296. doi:10.1016/j.ijantimicag.2012.06.006 PMID:22858373

Koutinas, A. A., Athanasiadis, I., Bekatorou, A., Psarianos, C., Kanellaki, M., Agouridis, N., & Blekas, G. (2007). Kefir-yeast technology: Industrial scale- up of alcoholic fermentation of whey, promoted by raisin extracts, using kefir-yeast granular biomass. *Enzyme and Microbial Technology*, *41*(5), 576–582. doi:10.1016/j.enzmictec.2007.05.013

Kresty, L. A., Morse, M. A., Morgan, C., Carlton, P. S., Lu, J., Gupta, A., ... Stoner, G. D. (2001). Chemoprevention of Esophageal Tumorigenesis by Dietary Administration of Lyophilized Black Raspberries. *Cancer Research*, *61*, 6112–6119. PMID:11507061

Kreuter, J. (2007). Nanoparticles-a historical perspective. *International Journal of Pharmaceutics*, *331*(1), 1–10. doi:10.1016/j.ijpharm.2006.10.021 PMID:17110063

Krinsky, N. I., & Johnson, E. J. (2005). Carotenoid actions and their relation to health and disease. *Molecular Aspects of Medicine*, *26*(6), 459–516. doi:10.1016/j.mam.2005.10.001 PMID:16309738

Kristen, A. V., Lehrke, S., Buss, S., Mereles, D., Steen, H., Ehlermann, P., ... Katus, H. A. (2012). Green tea halts progression of cardiac transthyretin amyloidosis: An observational report. *Clinical Research in Cardiology; Official Journal of the German Cardiac Society*, *101*(10), 805–813. doi:10.100700392-012-0463-z PMID:22584381

Kritchevsky, D., & Chen, S. C. (2005). Phytosterols-health benefits and potential concerns: A review. *Nutrition Research (New York, N.Y.)*, *25*(5), 413–428. doi:10.1016/j.nutres.2005.02.003

Kruis, W., Chrubasik, S., Boehm, S., Stange, C., & Schulze, J. (2012). A double-blind placebo-controlled trial to study therapeutic effects of probiotic *Escherichia coli Nissle* 1917 in subgroups of patients with irritable bowel syndrome. *International Journal of Colorectal Disease*, *27*(4), 467–474. doi:10.100700384-011-1363-9 PMID:22130826

Kruis, W., Schutz, E., Fric, P., Fixa, B., Judmaier, G., & Stolte, M. (1997). Double-blind comparison of an oral *E. coli* preparation and mesalazine in maintaining remission of ulcerative colitis. *Aliment Pharmacology & Theraputics*, *11*(5), 853–858. doi:10.1046/j.1365-2036.1997.00225.x PMID:9354192

Kukkonen, K., Savilahti, E., Haahtela, T., Juntunen-Backman, K., Korpela, R., Poussa, T., ... Kuitunen, M. (2008). Long-term safety and impacton infection rates of postnatal probiotic and prebiotic(synbiotic) treatment: Randomized, double-blind, placebo-controlled trial. *Pediatrics*, *122*(1), 8–12. doi:10.1542/peds.2007-1192 PMID:18595980

Kumar, A., & Sharma, S. S. (2010). NF-kB inhibitory action of resveratrol: A probable mechanism of neuro protection in experimental diabetic neuropathy. *Biochemical and Biophysical Research Communications*, *394*(2), 360–365. doi:10.1016/j.bbrc.2010.03.014 PMID:20211601

Kumar, B. V., Vijayendra, S. V. N., & Reddy, O. V. S. (2015). Trends in dairy and non-dairy probiotic products - a review. *Journal of Food Science and Technology*, *5*(10), 6112–6124. doi:10.100713197-015-1795-2 PMID:26396359

Kumari, S., Rakavi, R., & Mangaraj, M. (2016). Effect of Guava in Blood Glucose and Lipid Profile in Healthy Human Subjects: A Randomized Controlled Study. *Journal of Clinical and Diagnostic Research: JCDR*, *10*(9), BC04–BC07. doi:10.7860/JCDR/2016/21291.8425 PMID:27790420

Kumar, K., & Kumar, S. (2015). Role of nutraceuticals in health and disease prevention: A review. *South Asian J Food Technol Environ*, *1*, 116–121.

Kumar, M., Nagpal, R., Kumar, R., Hemalatha, R., Verma, V., Kumar, A., ... Yadav, H. (2012). Cholesterol-lowering probiotics as potential biotherapeutics for metabolic diseases. *Experimental Diabetes Research*, *2012*, 902917. doi:10.1155/2012/902917 PMID:22611376

Kuna, A., & Poshadri, A. (2012). Phytosterol- A functional ingredient for Indian food industry. *Indian Food Industry*, *30*(3), 21–28.

Kuna, A., Raju, P. N., & Poshadri, A. (2011). Phytosterols as functional ingredients for dairy foods. *Indian Journal of Dairy Science*, *64*(5), 359–367.

Kuo, M. L., Huang, T. S., & Lin, J. K. (1996). Curcumin, an antioxidant and anti-tumor promoter, induces apoptosis in human leukemia cells. *Biochimica et Biophysica Acta*, *1317*(2), 95–100. doi:10.1016/S0925-4439(96)00032-4 PMID:8950193

Kuo, Y.-C., & Su, F.-L. (2007). Transport of stavudine, delavirdine, and saquinavir across the blood–brain barrier by polybutylcyanoacrylate, methylmethacrylate-sulfopropylmethacrylate, and solid lipid nanoparticles. *International Journal of Pharmaceutics*, *340*(1–2), 143–152. doi:10.1016/j.ijpharm.2007.03.012 PMID:17418986

Kurmann, J. A., Rasic, J. L. J., & Kroger, M. (1992). *Encyclopedia of fermented fresh milk products: An International inventory of fermented milk, Cream, Buttermilk, Whey, and related products*. New York: Van Nostrand Reinhold, Springer.

Kuroyanagi, K., Kang, M. S., Goto, T., Hirai, S., Ohyama, K., Kusudo, T., ... Kawada, T. (2008). Citrus auraptene acts as an agonist for PPARs and enhances adiponectin production and MCP-1 reduction in 3T3-L1 adipocytes. *Biochemical and Biophysical Research Communications*, *366*(1), 219–225. doi:10.1016/j.bbrc.2007.11.119 PMID:18060855

Kushi, L. H., Folsom, A. R., Prineas, R. J., Mink, P. J., Wu, Y., & Bostick, R. M. (1996). Dietary antioxidant vitamins and death from coronary heart disease in postmenopausal women. *The New England Journal of Medicine*, *334*(18), 1156–1162. doi:10.1056/NEJM199605023341803 PMID:8602181

Kwak, H.-M., Jeon, S.-Y., Sohng, B.-H., Kim, J.-G., Lee, J.-M., Lee, K.-B., & Song, K.-S. (2005). beta-Secretase (BACE1) inhibitors from pomegranate (Punica granatum) husk. *Archives of Pharmacal Research*, *28*(12), 1328–1332. doi:10.1007/BF02977896 PMID:16392663

Kwak, N.-S., & Jukes, D. J. (2001). Functional foods. Part 1: The development of a regulatory concept. *Food Control*, *12*(2), 99–107. doi:10.1016/S0956-7135(00)00028-1

Kwak, N.-S., & Jukes, D. J. (2001). Functional foods. Part 2: The impact on current regulatory terminology. *Food Control*, *12*(2).

Kwon, O., Eck, P., Chen, S., Corpe, C. P., Lee, J. H., Kruhlak, M., & Levine, M. (2007). Inhibition of the intestinal glucose transporter GLUT 2 by flavonoids. *The FASEB Journal*, *21*(2), 366–377. doi:10.1096/fj.06-6620com PMID:17172639

Ladanyia, M., & Ladaniya, M. (2010). *Citrus fruit: biology, technology and evaluation*. Academic press.

Lan, A., Lagadic-Gossmann, D., Lemaire, C., & Jan, G. (2007). Acidic extracellular pH shifts colorectal cancer cell death from apoptosis to necrosis upon exposure to propionate and acetate, major end-products of the human probiotic propionibacteria. *Apoptosis*, *12*(3), 573–591. doi:10.100710495-006-0010-3 PMID:17195096

Lang, K. S., Roll, B., Myssina, S., Schittenhelm, M., Scheel-Walter, H. G., Kanz, L., & Wieder, T. (2002). Enhanced erythrocyte apoptosis in sickle cell anemia, thalassemia and glucose-6-phosphate dehydrogenase deficiency. *Cellular Physiology and Biochemistry*, *12*(5-6), 365–372. doi:10.1159/000067907 PMID:12438773

Langseth, L. (1993). From the Editor: Antioxidants and Diseases of the Brain. Antioxidant Vitamins Newsletter, 4, 3-5.

Lattimer, J. M., & Haub, M. D. (2010). Effects of Dietary Fiber and Its Components on Metabolic Health. *Nutrients*, *2*(12), 1266–1289. doi:10.3390/nu2121266 PMID:22254008

Latvala, J., Parkkila, S., & Niemelä, O. (2004). Excess alcohol consumption is common in patients with cytopenia: Studies in blood and bone marrow cells. *Alcoholism, Clinical and Experimental Research, 28*(4), 619–624. doi:10.1097/01.ALC.0000122766.54544.3B PMID:15100613

Lau, B. H. S., Tadi, P. P., & Tosk, J. M. (1990). Allium sativum (Garlic) and cancer prevention. *Nutrition Research (New York, N.Y.), 10*(8), 937–948. doi:10.1016/S0271-5317(05)80057-0

Law, M. (2000). Plant sterol and stanol margarines and health. *British Medical Journal, 320*(7238), 861–864. doi:10.1136/bmj.320.7238.861 PMID:10731187

Layne, J., Majkova, Z., Smart, E. J., Toborek, M., & Hennig, B. (2011). Caveolae: A regulatory platform for nutritional modulation of inflammatory diseases. *The Journal of Nutritional Biochemistry, 22*(9), 807–811. doi:10.1016/j.jnutbio.2010.09.013 PMID:21292468

Leães, F.L., Natália G.V., Voltaire, S.A., & Adriano, B. (2010). Use of Byproducts of Food Industry for Production of Antimicrobial Activity by *Bacillus sp.* P11 (Communication). *Food and Bioprocess Technology,* 133-140.

Leblond, J. D., Dahmen, A. S., Lebret, K., & Rengefors, K. (2013). Sterols of the green-pigmented, freshwater raphidophyte, *Gonyostomum semen*, from Scandinavian lakes. *The Journal of Eukaryotic Microbiology, 60*(4), 399–405. doi:10.1111/jeu.12050 PMID:23731265

Lee, E. S., Vedanthan, R., Jeemon, P., Kamano, J. H., Kudesia, P., Rajan, V., ... Moran, A. E. (2016). Quality improvement for cardiovascular disease care in low-and middle-income countries: A systematic review. *PLoS One, 11*(6), e0157036. doi:10.1371/journal.pone.0157036 PMID:27299563

Lee, H. Y., Park, J. H., Seok, S. H., Baek, M. W., Kim, D. J., Lee, K. E., ... Park, J. H. (2006). Human originated bacteria, Lactobacillus rhamnosus PL60, produce conjugated linoleic acid and show anti-obesity effects in diet induced obese mice. *Biochimica et Biophysica Acta, 1761*(7), 736–744. doi:10.1016/j.bbalip.2006.05.007 PMID:16807088

Lee, J. B., Ahn, J. B., Lee, J., & Kwak, H. S. (2004). L-Ascorbic Acid Microencapsulated with Polyacylglycerol Monostearate for Milk Fortification. *Bioscience, Biotechnology, and Biochemistry, 68*(3), 495–500. doi:10.1271/bbb.68.495 PMID:15056878

Lee, J., Koo, N., & Min, D. B. (2004). Reactive oxygen species, aging, and antioxidative nutraceuticals. *Comprehensive Reviews in Food Science and Food Safety, 3*(1), 21–33. doi:10.1111/j.1541-4337.2004.tb00058.x

Lee, Y.-B., Lee, H. J., & Sohn, H. S. (2005). Soy isoflavones and cognitive function. *The Journal of Nutritional Biochemistry, 16*(11), 641–649. doi:10.1016/j.jnutbio.2005.06.010 PMID:16169201

Lehto, S., Rönnemaa, T., Pyörälä, K., & Laakso, M. (2000). Cardiovascular risk factors clustering with endogenous hyperinsulinaemia predict death from coronary heart disease in patients with Type II diabetes. *Diabetologia, 43*(2), 148–155. doi:10.1007001250050023 PMID:10753035

Lercker, G., & Rodriguez-Estrada, M. T. (2002). Cholesterol oxidation mechanisms. In F. Guardiola, P. C. Dutta, R. Codony, & G. P. Savage (Eds.), *Cholesterol and Phytosterol Oxidation Products* (pp. 1–25). Champaign, IL: AOCS Press.

Levitan, I., Volkov, S., & Subbaiah, P. V. (2010). Oxidized LDL: Diversity, Patterns of Recognition, and Pathophysiology. *Antioxidants & Redox Signalling*, *13*(1), 39–75. doi:10.1089/ars.2009.2733 PMID:19888833

Lewington, S., Clarke, R., Qizilbash, N., Peto, R., & Collins, R.. (2002). Age-specific relevance of usual blood pressure to vascular mortality: A meta-analysis of individual data for one million adults in 61 prospective studies. *Lancet (London, England)*, *360*(9349), 1903–1913. doi:10.1016/S0140-6736(02)11911-8 PMID:12493255

Le, Y., Yu, X., Ruan, L., Wang, O., Qi, D., Zhu, J., ... Wang, J. M. (2005). The immunopharmacological properties of transforming growth factor beta. *International Immunopharmacology*, *5*(13-14), 1771–1782. doi:10.1016/j.intimp.2005.07.006 PMID:16275614

Ley, R. E., Turnbaugh, P. J., Klein, S., & Gordon, J. I. (2006). Microbial ecology: Human gut microbes associated with obesity. *Nature*, *444*(7122), 1022–1023. doi:10.1038/4441022a PMID:17183309

Liang, G. B., Du, G. C., & Chen, J. (2008). A novel strategy of enhanced glutathione production in high cell density cultivation of *Candida utilis*-Cysteine addition combined with dissolved oxygen controlling. *Enzyme and Microbial Technology*, *42*(3), 284–289. doi:10.1016/j.enzmictec.2007.10.008

Libby, P. (2002). Inflammation in atherosclerosis. *Nature*, *420*(6917), 868–874. doi:10.1038/nature01323 PMID:12490960

Libby, P. (2005). Act local, act global: Inflammation and the multiplicity of "vulnerable" coronary plaques. *Journal of the American College of Cardiology*, *45*, 1600–1602. doi:10.1016/j.jacc.2005.02.058 PMID:15893173

Lichtenstein, A. H. (1998). Soy Protein, Isoflavones and Cardiovascular Disease Risk. *The Journal of Nutrition*, *128*(10), 1589–1592. doi:10.1093/jn/128.10.1589 PMID:9772121

Lichtenstein, A. H., & Deckelbaum, R. J. (2001). AHA Science Advisory. Stanol/sterol ester-containing foods and blood cholesterol levels. A statement for healthcare professionals from the Nutrition Committee of the Council on Nutrition, Physical Activity, and Metabolism of the American Heart Association. *Circulation*, *103*(8), 1177–1179. doi:10.1161/01.CIR.103.8.1177 PMID:11222485

Li, D., Wang, P., Wang, P., Hu, X., & Chen, F. (2016). The gut microbiota: A treasure for human health. *Biotechnology Advances*, *34*(7), 1210–1224. doi:10.1016/j.biotechadv.2016.08.003 PMID:27592384

Lin, D., & Zhao, Y. (2007). Innovations in the development and application of edible coatings for fresh and minimally processed fruits and vegetables. *Comprehensive Reviews in Food Science and Food Safety*, *6*(3), 60–75. doi:10.1111/j.1541-4337.2007.00018.x

Ling, B., Aziz, C., Wojnarowicz, C., Olkowski, A., & Alcorn, J. (2010). Timing and Duration of Drug Exposure Affects Outcomes of a Drug-Nutrient Interaction During Ontogeny. *Pharmaceutics*, *2*(4), 321–338. doi:10.3390/pharmaceutics2040321 PMID:27721360

Ling, W. H., & Jones, P. J. H. (1995). Dietary phytosterols; a review of metabolism, benefits and side effects. *Life Sciences*, *57*(3), 195–206. doi:10.1016/0024-3205(95)00263-6 PMID:7596226

Linnenkamp, U., Guariguata, L., Beagley, J., Whiting, D. R., & Cho, N. H. (2014). The IDF Diabetes Atlas methodology for estimating global prevalence of hyperglycaemia in pregnancy. *Diabetes Research and Clinical Practice*, *103*(2), 186–196. doi:10.1016/j.diabres.2013.11.004 PMID:24300016

Lin, X., Racette, S. B., Lefevre, M., Spearie, C. A., Most, M., Ma, L., & Ostlund, R. E. Jr. (2010). The effects of phytosterols present in natural food matrices on cholesterol metabolism and LDL-cholesterol: A controlled feeding trial. *European Journal of Clinical Nutrition*, *64*(12), 1481–1487. doi:10.1038/ejcn.2010.180 PMID:20808333

Lin, Y. L., Chang, Y. Y., Yang, D. J., Tzang, B. S., & Chen, Y. C. (2013). Beneficial Effects of Noni (*Morinda citrifolia* L.) Juice on Livers of High-Fat Dietary Hamsters. *Food Chemistry*, *140*(1-2), 31–38. doi:10.1016/j.foodchem.2013.02.035 PMID:23578611

Lipid modification: Cardiovascular risk assessment and the modification of blood lipids for the primary and secondary prevention of cardiovascular disease | Guidance and guidelines | NICE. (n.d.). Retrieved April 12, 2017, from https://www.nice.org.uk

Lipton, S. A. (2007). Pathologically-Activated Therapeutics for Neuroprotection: Mechanism of NMDA Receptor Block by Memantine and S-Nitrosylation. *Current Drug Targets*, *8*(5), 621–632. doi:10.2174/138945007780618472 PMID:17504105

Li, Q., Withoff, S., & Verma, I. M. (2005). Inflammation-associated cancer: NF-κB is the lynchpin. *Trends in Immunology*, *26*(6), 318–325. doi:10.1016/j.it.2005.04.003 PMID:15922948

Liu, S., Han, Y., & Zhou, Z. (2011). Lactic acid bacteria in traditional fermented Chinese foods. *Food Research International*, *44*(3), 643–651. doi:10.1016/j.foodres.2010.12.034

Loban, K. M., Polozok, E. S., Efimov, L. S., & Khorin, A. T. (1987). Treatment of imported tropical malaria caused by chloroquine-resistant strains of P. falciparum. *Terapevticheskii Arkhiv*, *59*(1), 69–72. PMID:3551176

Lobo, V., Patil, A., Phatak, A., & Chandra, N. (2010). Free radicals, antioxidants and functional foods: Impact on human health. *Pharmacognosy Reviews*, *4*(8), 118. doi:10.4103/0973-7847.70902 PMID:22228951

Lockwood, B. (2007). *Nutraceuticals: a guide for healthcare professionals*. Pharmaceutical Press.

Loizou, S., Lekakis, I., Chrousos, G. P., & Moutsatsou, P. (2010). Beta-Sitosterol exhibits anti-inflammatory activity in human aortic endothelial cells. *Molecular Nutrition & Food Research*, *54*(4), 551–558. doi:10.1002/mnfr.200900012 PMID:19937850

Lonnerdal, B. (2009). Nutritional roles of lactoferrin. *Current Opinion in Clinical Nutrition and Metabolic Care*, *12*(3), 293–297. doi:10.1097/MCO.0b013e328328d13e PMID:19318940

Lonnermark, E., Friman, V., Lappas, G., Sandberg, T., Berggren, A., & Adlerberth, I. (2010). Intake of *Lactobacillus plantarum* reduces certain gastrointestinal symptoms during treatment with antibiotics. *Journal of Clinical Gastroenterology*, *44*(2), 106–112. doi:10.1097/MCG.0b013e3181b2683f PMID:19727002

Loos, R. J. F., & Bouchard, C. (2003). Obesity – is it a genetic disorder? *Journal of Internal Medicine*, *254*(5), 401–425. doi:10.1046/j.1365-2796.2003.01242.x PMID:14535962

Lopez, A. D., & Murray, C. C. (1998). The global burden of disease, 1990-2020. *Nature Medicine*, *4*(11), 1241–1243. doi:10.1038/3218 PMID:9809543

Lopez-Varela, S., Gonzalez-Gross, M., & Marcos, A. (2002). Functional foods and the immune system: A review. *European Journal of Clinical Nutrition*, *56*(S3), S29–S33. doi:10.1038j.ejcn.1601481 PMID:12142958

Lucas, M. L., Blair, J. A., Cooper, B., & Matty, A. J. (1975). Further investigations with pH microelectrodes into the jejunal microclimate in rat and man. *Gut*, *16*(10), 844. PMID:1331

Ludwig, E. (1943). *The Hippocratic Oath: Test, Translation and Interpretation*. Baltimore, MD: John Hopkins Press.

Luft, F. C. (2012). Neural regulation of the immune system modulates hypertension-induced target-organ damage. *Journal of the American Society of Hypertension: JASH*, *6*(1), 23–26. doi:10.1016/j.jash.2011.09.006 PMID:22047671

Lü, J.-H., Guo, J., & Yang, W.-H. (2006). Effects of green tea polyphenol on the behaviour of Alzheimer' s disease like mice induced by D-galactose and Abeta25-35. *Zhong Yao Cai*, *29*(4), 352–354. PMID:16913491

Lutsey, P. L., Jacobs, D. R., Kori, S., Mayer-Davis, E., Shea, S., Steffen, L. M., ... Tracy, R. (2007). Whole grain intake and its cross-sectional association with obesity, insulin resistance, inflammation, diabetes and subclinical CVD: The MESA Study. *British Journal of Nutrition*, *98*(2), 397–405. doi:10.1017/S0007114507700715 PMID:17391554

Lye, H. S., Rahmat-Ali, G. R., & Liong, M. T. (2010). Mechanisms of cholesterol removal by lactobacilli under conditions that mimic the human gastrointestinal tract. *International Dairy Journal*, *20*(3), 169–175. doi:10.1016/j.idairyj.2009.10.003

Macfarlane, G. T., & Macfarlane, S. (2011). Fermentation in the human large intestine its physiologic consequences and the potential contribution of prebiotics. *Journal of Clinical Gastroenterology*, *45*(Suppl.), S120–S127. doi:10.1097/MCG.0b013e31822fecfe PMID:21992950

Mack, D. R., Ahrne, S., Hyde, L., Wei, S., & Hollingsworth, M. A. (2003). Extracellular MUC3 mucin secretion follows adherence of *Lactobacillus* strains to intestinal epithelial cells in vitro. *Gut*, *52*(6), 827–833. doi:10.1136/gut.52.6.827 PMID:12740338

Madsen, K., Cornish, A., Soper, P., McKaigney, C., Jijon, H., Yachimec, C., ... De Simone, C. (2001). Probiotic bacteria enhance murine and human intestinal epithelial barrier function. *Gastroenterology*, *121*(3), 580–591. doi:10.1053/gast.2001.27224 PMID:11522742

Maeda, G., Takara, K., Wada, K., Oki, T., Masuda, M., Ichiba, T., ... Suda, I. (2006). Evaluation of Antioxidant Activity of Vegetables from Okinawa Prefecture and Determination of Some Antioxidative Compounds. *Food Science and Technology Research*, *12*(1), 8–14. doi:10.3136/fstr.12.8

Maeda, N., Shimomura, I., Kishida, K., Nishizawa, H., Matsuda, M., Nagaretani, H., ... Matsuzawa, Y. (2002). Diet-induced insulin resistance in mice lacking adiponectin/ACRP30. *Nature Medicine*, *8*(7), 731–737. doi:10.1038/nm724 PMID:12068289

Magrone, T., Perez de Heredia, F., Jirillo, E., Morabito, G., Marcos, A., & Serafini, M. (2013). Functional foods and nutraceuticals as therapeutic tools for the treatment of diet-related diseases [1]. *Canadian Journal of Physiology and Pharmacology*, *91*(6), 387–396. doi:10.1139/cjpp-2012-0307 PMID:23745830

Mahley, R. W. (1988). Apolipoprotein E: Cholesterol transport protein with expanding role in cell biology. *Science*, *240*(4852), 622–630. doi:10.1126cience.3283935 PMID:3283935

Malaguarnera, G., Leggio, F., Vacante, M., Motta, M., Giordano, M., Bondi, A., ... Salmeri, M. (2012). Probiotics in the gastrointestinal diseases of the elderly. *The Journal of Nutrition, Health & Aging*, *16*(4), 402–410. doi:10.100712603-011-0357-1 PMID:22499466

Mancia, G., Fagard, R., Narkiewicz, K., Redón, J., Zanchetti, A., & Böhm, M. (2013). ESH/ESC Guidelines for the management of arterial hypertension: The Task Force for the management of arterial hypertension of the European Society of Hypertension (ESH) and of the European Society of Cardiology (ESC). *Journal of Hypertension*, *31*(7), 1281–1357. doi:10.1097/01.hjh.0000431740.32696.cc PMID:23817082

Mandel, S. A., Avramovich-Tirosh, Y., Reznichenko, L., Zheng, H., Weinreb, O., Amit, T., & Youdim, M. B. H. (2005). Multifunctional Activities of Green Tea Catechins in Neuroprotection. *Neuro-Signals*, *14*(1–2), 46–60. doi:10.1159/000085385 PMID:15956814

Mano, R., Ishida, A., Ohya, Y., Todoriki, H., & Takishita, S. (2009). Dietary intervention with Okinawan vegetables increased circulating endothelial progenitor cells in healthy young women. *Atherosclerosis*, *204*(2), 544–548. doi:10.1016/j.atherosclerosis.2008.09.035 PMID:19013573

Mansbach, C. M. II, & Gorelick, F. (2007). Development and Physiological Regulation of Intestinal Lipid Absorption. II. Dietary lipid absorption, complex lipid synthesis, and the intracellular packaging and secretion of chylomicrons. *American Journal of Physiology. Gastrointestinal and Liver Physiology*, *293*(4), G645–G650. doi:10.1152/ajpgi.00299.2007 PMID:17627968

Mansego, M. L., Solar, G. D. M., Alonso, M. P., Martínez, F., Sáez, G. T., Escudero, J. C. M., ... Chaves, F. J. (2011). Polymorphisms of antioxidant enzymes, blood pressure and risk of hypertension. *Journal of Hypertension, 29*(3), 492–500. doi:10.1097/HJH.0b013e328341f1b2 PMID:21178785

Marambaud, P., Zhao, H., & Davies, P. (2005). Resveratrol promotes clearance of Alzheimer's disease Amyloid-β peptides. *The Journal of Biological Chemistry, 280*(45), 37377–37382. doi:10.1074/jbc.M508246200 PMID:16162502

Marcelo, P. A., & Ritzvi, S. S. H. (2008). Physicochemical properties of liquid virgin whey protein isolate. *International Dairy Journal, 18*(3), 236–246. doi:10.1016/j.idairyj.2007.08.011

Marchesi, J. R., Adams, D. H., Fava, F., Hermes, G. D., Hirschfield, G. M., Hold, G., ... Hart, A. (2016). The gut microbiota and host health: A new clinical frontier. *Gut, 65*(2), 330–339. doi:10.1136/gutjnl-2015-309990 PMID:26338727

Market and Standard Market. (2015). Retrieved September 25, 2015, from http://www.marketsandmarkets.com/Market-Reports/ prebiotics-ingredients-market-219677001.html

Marketou, M. E., Kontaraki, J. E., Zacharis, E. A., Kochiadakis, G. E., Giaouzaki, A., Chlouverakis, G., & Vardas, P. E. (2012). TLR2 and TLR4 gene expression in peripheral monocytes in nondiabetic hypertensive patients: The effect of intensive blood pressure-lowering. *Journal of Clinical Hypertension (Greenwich, Conn.), 14*(5), 330–335. doi:10.1111/j.1751-7176.2012.00620.x PMID:22533660

Mark-Herbert, C. (2004). Innovation of a new product category - Functional foods. *Technovation, 24*(9), 713–719. doi:10.1016/S0166-4972(02)00131-1

Marlett, J. A., & Slavin, J. L. (1997). Position of the American Dietetic Association. *Journal of the American Dietetic Association, 97*(10), 1157–1159. doi:10.1016/S0002-8223(97)00279-4 PMID:9336564

Marsanasco, M., Márquez, A. L., Wagner, J. R., Alonso, S. D. V., & Chiaramoni, N. S. (2011). Liposomes as vehicles for vitamins E and C: An alternative to fortify orange juice and offer vitamin C protection after heat treatment. *Food Research International, 44*(9), 3039–3046. doi:10.1016/j.foodres.2011.07.025

Marteau, P., Lemann, M., & Seksik, P. (2005). Ineffectiveness of *Lactobacillus johnsonii*la1 for prophylaxis of postoperative recurrence in Crohn's disease: A randomised, double-blind, placebo-controlled getaid trial. *Gut, 23*, 443–454.

Marteau, P., & Shanahan, F. (2003). Basic aspects and pharmacology of probiotics: An overview of pharmacokinetics, mechanisms of action and side-effects. *Best Practice & Research. Clinical Gastroenterology, 17*(5), 725–740. doi:10.1016/S1521-6918(03)00055-6 PMID:14507584

Martínez-González, M. Á., Corella, D., Salas-Salvadó, J., Ros, E., Covas, M. I., Fiol, M., ... Estruch, R. (2012). Cohort profile: Design and methods of the PREDIMED study. *International Journal of Epidemiology, 41*(2), 377–385. doi:10.1093/ije/dyq250 PMID:21172932

Martínez-González, M. A., García-López, M., Bes-Rastrollo, M., Toledo, E., Martínez-Lapiscina, E. H., Delgado-Rodriguez, M., ... Beunza, J. J. (2011). Mediterranean diet and the incidence of cardiovascular disease: A Spanish cohort. *Nutrition, Metabolism, and Cardiovascular Diseases, 21*(4), 237–244. doi:10.1016/j.numecd.2009.10.005 PMID:20096543

Martınez-Navarrete, N., Camacho, M. M., Martınez-Lahuerta, J., Martınez-Monzó, J., & Fito, P. (2002). Iron deficiency and iron fortified foods—a review. *Food Research International, 35*(2), 225–231. doi:10.1016/S0963-9969(01)00189-2

Martirosyan, D. M., & Singh, J. (2015). A new definition of functional food by FFC: What makes a new definition unique? *Functional Foods in Health and Disease, 5*(6), 209–223.

Martorell, R., Kettel Khan, L., Hughes, M. L., & Grummer-Strawn, L. M. (2000). Overweight and obesity in preschool children from developing countries. *International Journal of Obesity and Related Metabolic Disorders, 24*(8), 959–967. doi:10.1038j.ijo.0801264 PMID:10951533

Marx, J. (2004). CANCER RESEARCH: Inflammation and Cancer: The Link Grows Stronger. *Science, 306*(5698), 966–968. doi:10.1126cience.306.5698.966 PMID:15528423

Masters, R. C., Liese, A. D., Haffner, S. M., Wagenknecht, L. E., & Hanley, A. J. (2010). Whole and Refined Grain Intakes Are Related to Inflammatory Protein Concentrations in Human Plasma. *The Journal of Nutrition, 140*(3), 587–594. doi:10.3945/jn.109.116640 PMID:20089789

Mastretta, E., Longo, P., Laccisaglia, A., & Gianino, P. (2002). Effect of *Lactobacillus* GG and breast-feeding in the prevention of rotavirus nosocomial infection. *Journal of Pediatric Gastroenterology and Nutrition, 35*(4), 527–531. doi:10.1097/00005176-200210000-00013 PMID:12394379

Matés, J. M., Pérez-Gómez, C., Núñez, I., & De Castro, I. N. (1999). Antioxidant enzymes and human diseases. *Clinical Biochemistry, 32*(8), 595–603. doi:10.1016/S0009-9120(99)00075-2 PMID:10638941

Mat, M. C., Mohamed, A. S., & Hamid, S. S. (2011). Primary human monocyte differentiation regulated by Nigella sativa pressed oil. *Lipids in Health and Disease, 10*(1), 216–216. doi:10.1186/1476-511X-10-216 PMID:22104447

Matsunaga, S., Azuma, K., Watanabe, M., Tsuka, T., Imagawa, T., Osaki, T., & Okamoto, Y. (2014). Onion Peel Tea Ameliorates Obesity and Affects Blood Parameters in a Mouse Model of High-Fat-Diet-Induced Obesity. *Experimental and Therapeutic Medicine, 7*(2), 379–382. doi:10.3892/etm.2013.1433 PMID:24396409

Matsuoka, K., & Kanai, T. (2015). The gut microbiota and inflammatory bowel disease. *Seminars in Immunopathology, 37*(1), 47–55. doi:10.100700281-014-0454-4 PMID:25420450

Matsuura, H. (2001). Saponins in garlic as modifiers of the risk of cardiovascular disease. *The Journal of Nutrition, 131*(33s), 1000S–1005S. doi:10.1093/jn/131.3.1000S PMID:11238805

Matsuyama, T., Tanaka, Y., Kamimaki, I., Nagao, T., & Tokimitsu, I. (2008). Catechin Safely Improved Higher Levelsof Fatness, Blood Pressure, and Cholesterol in Children. *Obesity (Silver Spring, Md.)*, *16*(6), 1338–1348. doi:10.1038/oby.2008.60 PMID:18356827

Mattson, F. H., Grundy, S. M., & Crouse, J. R. (1982). Optimizing the effect of plant sterols on cholesterol absorption in man. *The American Journal of Clinical Nutrition*, *35*(4), 697–700. doi:10.1093/ajcn/35.4.697 PMID:7072622

McAlindon, T., & Felson, D. T. (1997). Nutrition risk factors for Osteoarthritis. *Annals of the Rheumatic Diseases*, *56*(7), 397–402. doi:10.1136/ard.56.7.397 PMID:9485998

McCarty, M. F. (2005). A chlorogenic acid-induced increase in GLP-1 production may mediate the impact of heavy coffee consumption on diabetes risk. *Medical Hypotheses*, *64*(4), 848–853. doi:10.1016/j.mehy.2004.03.037 PMID:15694706

McCook-Russell, K. P., Nair, M. G., Facey, P. C., & Bowen-Forbes, C. S. (2012). Nutritional and nutraceutical comparison of Jamaican Psidium cattleianum (strawberry guava) and Psidium guajava (common guava) fruits. *Food Chemistry*, *134*(2), 1069–1073. doi:10.1016/j.foodchem.2012.03.018 PMID:23107729

McDougall, G. J., Austin-Wells, V., & Zimmerman, T. (2005). Utility of Nutraceutical Products Marketed for Cognitive and Memory Enhancement. *Journal of Holistic Nursing : Official Journal of the American Holistic Nurses'. Association*, *23*(4), 415–433.

McFarland, L. V. (2008). Antibiotic-associated diarrhoea: Epidemiology, trends and treatment. *Future Microbiology*, *3*(5), 563–578. doi:10.2217/17460913.3.5.563 PMID:18811240

McFarland, L. V. (2010). Probiotics and diarrhea. *Annals of Nutrition & Metabolism*, *57*(1), 10–11. doi:10.1159/000309016 PMID:20829585

McFarland, L. V. (2010). Systematic review and meta-analysis of *Saccharomyces boulardii*in adult patients. *World Journal of Gastroenterology*, *16*(18), 2202–2222. doi:10.3748/wjg.v16.i18.2202 PMID:20458757

McGill, H. C. Jr. (1979). The relationship of dietary cholesterol to serum cholesterol concentration and to atherosclerosis in man. *The American Journal of Clinical Nutrition*, *32*(12Suppl), 2664–2702. doi:10.1093/ajcn/32.12.2664 PMID:389024

McGroarty, J. A. (1993). Probiotic use of lactobacilli in the human female urogenital tract. *FEMS Immunology and Medical Microbiology*, *6*(4), 251–264. doi:10.1111/j.1574-695X.1993.tb00337.x PMID:8499891

McKie, A. T., Barrow, D., Latunde-Dada, G. O., Rolfs, A., Sager, G., Mudaly, E., & Peters, T. J. (2001). An iron-regulated ferric reductase associated with the absorption of dietary iron. *Science*, *291*(5509), 1755–1759. doi:10.1126cience.1057206 PMID:11230685

McNamara, D. J. (2000). Dietary cholesterol and atherosclerosis. *Biochimica et Biophysica Acta*, *1529*(1-3), 310–320. doi:10.1016/S1388-1981(00)00156-6 PMID:11111098

Medjakovic, S., & Jungbauer, A. (2013). Pomegranate: a fruit that ameliorates metabolic syndrome. *Food Functions*, *4*(1), 19-39.

Medjakovic, S., & Jungbauer, A. (2013). Pomegranate: A Fruit That Ameliorates Metabolic Syndrome. *Food & Function*, *4*(1), 19–39. doi:10.1039/C2FO30034F PMID:23060097

Mehra, R., Marnila, P., & Korhonen, H. (2006). Milk immunoglobulins for health promotion. *International Dairy Journal*, *16*(11), 1262–1271. doi:10.1016/j.idairyj.2006.06.003

Mehta, K., Pantazis, P., McQueen, T., & Aggarwal, B. B. (1997). Antiproliferative effect of curcumin (diferuloylmethane) against human breast tumor cell lines. *Anti-Cancer Drugs*, *8*(5), 470–481. doi:10.1097/00001813-199706000-00010 PMID:9215611

Meier, P., Finch, A., & Evan, G. (2000). Apoptosis in development. *Nature*, *407*(6805), 796–801. doi:10.1038/35037734 PMID:11048731

Mel'nikova, V. M., Gracheva, N. M., Belikov, G. P., Blatun, L. A., & Shcherbakova, E. G. (1993). The chemoprophylaxis and chemotherapy of opportunistic infections. *Antibiotiki I Khimioterapiia*, *38*(10–11), 44–48.

Melnick, S. J. (2006). Developmental Therapeutics: Review of Biologically Based CAM therapies for Potential Application in Children With Cancer: Part I. *Journal of Pediatric Hematology/Oncology*, *28*(4), 221–230. doi:10.1097/01.mph.0000212922.16427.04 PMID:16679919

Mendis, S. (2014). *Global status report on non communicable diseases*. World Health Organization.

Mendis, S., Puska, P., & Norrving, B. (2011). *Global atlas on cardiovascular disease prevention and control*. World Health Organization.

Menrad, K. (2003). Market and marketing of functional food in Europe. *Journal of Food Engineering*, *56*(2–3), 181–188. doi:10.1016/S0260-8774(02)00247-9

Mensink, R. P., Ebbing, S., Lindhout, M., Plat, J., & Heugten, M. M. (2002). Effects of plant-stanol esters supplied in low-fat yoghurt on serum lipids and lipoproteins, non-cholesterol sterols and fat soluble antioxidant concentrations. *Atherosclerosis*, *160*(1), 205–213. doi:10.1016/S0021-9150(01)00562-7 PMID:11755939

Messina, M. J., Persky, V., Setchell, K. D., & Barnes, S. (1994). Soy intake and cancer risk: A review of the in vitro and in vivo data. *Nutrition and Cancer*, *21*(2), 113–131. doi:10.1080/01635589409514310 PMID:8058523

Micallef, M. A., & Garg, M. L. (2008). The lipid-lowering effects of phytosterols and (n-3) polyunsaturated fatty acids are synergistic and complementary in hyperlipidemic men and women. *The Journal of Nutrition*, *138*(6), 1086–1090. doi:10.1093/jn/138.6.1086 PMID:18492838

Michel, M. (2014). Warm autoimmune hemolytic anemia: Advances in pathophysiology and treatment. *La Presse Medicale*, *43*(4), e97–e104. doi:10.1016/j.lpm.2014.02.009 PMID:24680421

Miller, L. E. (2013). Lorcaserin for Weight Loss: Insights into US Food and drug administration approval. *Journal of the Academy of Nutrition and Dietetics*, *113*(1), 25–30. doi:10.1016/j.jand.2012.08.028 PMID:23260720

Minemura, M., & Shimizu, Y. (2015). Gut microbiota and liver diseases. *World Journal of Gastroenterology*, *21*(6), 1691–1702. doi:10.3748/wjg.v21.i6.1691 PMID:25684933

Ministry of health and family, New Delhi, India, (2006). *Home*. Retrieved April 15, 2017, from http://www.fssai.gov.in/home

Mischke, M., & Plosch, T. (2013). More than just a gut instinct—The potential interplay between a baby's nutrition, its gut microbiome and the epigenome. *American Journal of Physiology. Regulatory, Integrative and Comparative Physiology*, *304*(12), R1065–R1069. doi:10.1152/ajpregu.00551.2012 PMID:23594611

Mishra, B., Malhotra, P., Ratho, R. K., Singh, M. P., Varma, S., & Varma, N. (2005). Human parvovirus B19 in patients with aplastic anemia. *American Journal of Hematology*, *79*(2), 166–167. doi:10.1002/ajh.20347 PMID:15929106

Miura, T., Itoh, Y., Iwamoto, N., Kato, M., & Ishida, T. (2004). Suppressive activity of the fruit of Momordica charantia with exercise on blood glucose in type 2 diabetic mice. *Biological & Pharmaceutical Bulletin*, *27*(2), 248–250. doi:10.1248/bpb.27.248 PMID:14758046

Mizrahi, A., Knekt, P., Montonen, J., Laaksonen, M. A., Heliövaara, M., & Järvinen, R. (2009). Plant foods and the risk of cerebrovascular diseases: A potential protection of fruit consumption. *British Journal of Nutrition*, *102*(7), 1075–1083. doi:10.1017/S0007114509359097 PMID:19646291

Mocchegiani, E., Bertoni-Freddari, C., Marcellini, F., & Malavolta, M. (2005). Brain, aging and neurodegeneration: Role of zinc ion availability. *Progress in Neurobiology*, *75*(6), 367–390. doi:10.1016/j.pneurobio.2005.04.005 PMID:15927345

Mohammadi, F., Mohammadi, M., Bagheri, A., & Roozbahani, H. (2013). Probiotics in human health. *European Journal of Experimental Biology*, *3*(2), 116–120.

Mollet, B., & Lacroix, C. (2007). Where biology and technology meet for better nutrition and health. *Current Opinion in Biotechnology*, *18*(2), 154–155. doi:10.1016/j.copbio.2007.03.003

Moncheva, P., Chipeva, V., Kujumzieva, A., Ivanova, I., Dousset, X., & Gocheva, B. (2003). The composition of the microflora of boza, an original Bulgarian beverage. *Biotechnology, Biotechnological Equipment*, *17*(1), 164–168. doi:10.1080/13102818.2003.10819214

Monu, E., Blank, G., Holley, R., & Zawistowski, J. (2008). Phytosterol effects on milk and yoghurt microflora. *Journal of Food Science*, *00*, M1–M6. PMID:18387114

Monzon Ballarin, S., Lopez-Matas, M. A., Saenz Abad, D., Perez-Cinto, N., & Carnes, J. (2011). Anaphylaxis associated with the ingestion of Goji berries (Lycium barbarum). *Journal of Investigational Allergology & Clinical Immunology*, *21*(7), 567–570. PMID:22312943

Moo-Huchin, V. M., Moo-Huchin, M. I., Estrada-Leon, R. J., Cuevas-Glory, L., Estrada-Mota, I. A., Ortiz-Vazquez, E., ... Sauri-Duch, E. (2015). Antioxidant compounds, antioxidant activity and phenolic content in peel from three tropical fruits from Yucatan, Mexico. *Food Chemistry*, *166*, 17–22. doi:10.1016/j.foodchem.2014.05.127 PMID:25053022

Morales, J., Choi, J.-S., & Kim, D.-S. (2006). Production rate of propionic acid in fermentation of cheese whey with enzyme inhibitors. *Environment and Progress*, *25*(3), 228–234. doi:10.1002/ep.10153

Moreno, D. A., Carvajal, M., López-Berenguer, C., & García-Viguera, C. (2006). Chemical and biological characterisation of nutraceutical compounds of broccoli. *Journal of Pharmaceutical and Biomedical Analysis*, *41*(5), 1508–1522. doi:10.1016/j.jpba.2006.04.003 PMID:16713696

Morotomi, M. (1996). Properties of *Lactobacillus casei*Shirota strain as probiotics. *Asia Pacific Journal of Clinical Nutrition*, *5*, 29–30. PMID:24394462

Morreau, R. A., Whitaker, B. D., & Hicks, K. B. (2002). Phytosterols, phytostanols, and their conjugates in foods: Structural diversity, quantitative analysis, and health-promoting uses. *Progress in Lipid Research*, *41*(6), 457–500. doi:10.1016/S0163-7827(02)00006-1 PMID:12169300

Mozaffarian, D. (2008). Fish and n-3 fatty acids for the prevention of fatal coronary heart disease and sudden cardiac death. *The American Journal of Clinical Nutrition*, *87*(6), 1991S–1996S. doi:10.1093/ajcn/87.6.1991S PMID:18541600

Mozaffarian, D., Benjamin, E. J., Go, A. S., Arnett, D. K., Blaha, M. J., Cushman, M., ... Turner, M. B. (2016). Heart Disease and Stroke Statistics—2016 Update: A Report From the American Heart Association. *Circulation*, *133*(4), e38–e360. doi:10.1161/CIR.0000000000000350 PMID:26673558

Mukherjee, A. K. (1995). India's health - today and tomorrow. *Journal of the Indian Medical Association*, *93*(8), 312–315. PMID:8713248

Mukhopadhyay, R., Talukdar, D., Chatterjee, B. P., & Guha, A. K. (2003). Whey processing with chitosan and isolation of lactose. *Process Biochemistry*, *39*(3), 381–385. doi:10.1016/S0032-9592(03)00126-2

Muller, D. M., Carrasco, M. S., Tonarelli, G. G., & Simonetta, A. C. (2009). Characterization and purification of a new bacteriocin with a broad inhibitory spectrum produced by *Lactobacillus plantarum* lp 31 strain isolated from dry-fermented sausage. *Journal of Applied Microbiology*, *106*(6), 2031–2040. doi:10.1111/j.1365-2672.2009.04173.x PMID:19302495

Muller, D. N., Kvakan, H., & Luft, F. C. (2011). Immune-related effects in hypertension and target-organ damage. *Current Opinion in Nephrology and Hypertension*, *20*(2), 113–117. doi:10.1097/MNH.0b013e3283436f88 PMID:21245763

Mulvihill, Erin E, & Huff, Murray W. (2012). Citrus flavonoids and the prevention of atherosclerosis. *Cardiovascular & Haematological Disorders-Drug Targets (Formerly Current Drug Targets-Cardiovascular & Hematological Disorders), 12*(2), 84-91.

Muncie, H. L. Jr, & Campbell, J. (2009). Alpha and beta thalassemia. *American Family Physician*, *80*(4), 339–344. PMID:19678601

Murakami, A., Ashida, H., & Terao, J. (2008). Multitargeted cancer prevention by quercetin. *Cancer Letters*, *269*(2), 315–325. doi:10.1016/j.canlet.2008.03.046 PMID:18467024

Murase, T., Yokoi, Y., Misawa, K., Ominami, H., Suzuki, Y., Shibuya, Y., & Hase, T. (2012). Coffee polyphenols modulate whole-body substrate oxidation and suppress postprandial hyperglycaemia, hyperinsulinaemia and hyperlipidaemia. *British Journal of Nutrition*, *107*(12), 1757–1765. doi:10.1017/S0007114511005083 PMID:22017960

Murphy, E. F., Cotter, P. D., Hogan, A., O'Sullivan, O., Joyce, A., Fouhy, F., ... Shanahan, F. (2013). Divergent metabolic outcomes arising from targeted manipulation of the gut microbiota in diet induced obesity. *Gut*, *62*(2), 220–226. doi:10.1136/gutjnl-2011-300705 PMID:22345653

Murray, C. J. L., & Lopez, A. D. (1996). T*he Global burden of disease : a comprehensive assessment of mortality and disability from diseases, injuries, and risk factors in 1990 and projected to 2020 : summary*. WHO. Retrieved from http://www.who.int/iris/handle/10665/41864

Mylonaki, M., Rayment, N. B., Rampton, D. S., Hudspith, B. N., & Brostoff, J. (2005). Molecular characterization of rectal mucosa-associated bacterial flora in inflammatory bowel disease. *Inflammatory Bowel Diseases*, *11*(5), 481–487. doi:10.1097/01.MIB.0000159663.62651.4f PMID:15867588

Nag, T., & Ghosh, A. (2015). Prevalence of cardiovascular disease risk factors in a rural community in West Bengal, India. *International Journal of Medicine and Public Health*, *5*(4), 259. doi:10.4103/2230-8598.165941

Nagy, L., Tontonoz, P., Alvarez, J. G. A., Chen, H., & Evans, R. M. (1998). Oxidized LDL Regulates Macrophage Gene Expression through Ligand Activation of PPAR[3]. *Cell*, *93*(2), 229–240. doi:10.1016/S0092-8674(00)81574-3 PMID:9568715

Nair, H. B., Sung, B., Yadav, V. R., Kannappan, R., Chaturvedi, M. M., & Aggarwal, B. B. (2010). Delivery of antiinflammatory nutraceuticals by nanoparticles for the prevention and treatment of cancer. *Biochemical Pharmacology*, *80*(12), 1833–1843. doi:10.1016/j.bcp.2010.07.021 PMID:20654584

Nakashima, Y., Fujii, H., Sumiyoshi, S., Wight, T. N., & Sueishi, K. (2007). Early human atherosclerosis: Accumulation of lipid and proteoglycans in intimal thickenings followed by macrophage infiltration. *Arteriosclerosis, Thrombosis, and Vascular Biology*, *27*(5), 1159–1165. doi:10.1161/ATVBAHA.106.134080 PMID:17303781

Nantitanon, W., Yotsawimonwat, S., & Okonogi, S. (2010). Factors influencing antioxidant activities and total phenolic content of guava leaf extract. *Lebensmittel-Wissenschaft + Technologie*, *43*(7), 1095–1103. doi:10.1016/j.lwt.2010.02.015

Napoli, F., Olivieri, G., Russo, M. E., Marzocchella, A., & Salatino, P. (2010). Butanol production by *Clostridium acetobutylicum* in a continuous packed bed reactor. *Journal of Industrial Microbiology & Biotechnology*, *37*(6), 603–608. doi:10.100710295-010-0707-8 PMID:20349108

Nash, K. M., & Shah, Z. A. (2015). Current Perspectives on the Beneficial Role of Ginkgo biloba in Neurological and Cerebrovascular Disorders. *Integrative Medicine Insights*, *10*, 1–9. doi:10.4137/IMI.S25054 PMID:26604665

Navarro, F., Liu, Y., & Rhoads, J. M. (2016). Can probiotics benefit children with autism spectrum disorders? *World Journal of Gastroenterology*, *22*(46), 10093–10102. doi:10.3748/wjg.v22.i46.10093 PMID:28028357

Nayak, D. U., Karmen, C., Frishman, W. H., & Vakili, B. A. (2001). Antioxidant vitamins and enzymatic and synthetic oxygen-derived free radical scavengers in the prevention and treatment of cardiovascular disease. *Heart Disease (Hagerstown, Md.)*, *3*(1), 28–45. doi:10.1097/00132580-200101000-00006 PMID:11975768

Nelson, B. M., Lichtenstein, A. H., Abrams, S., Adams-Campbell, L., & Anderson, C. J. (2015). 2015–2020 Dietary Guidelines for Americans (8th ed.). U.S. Department of Health and Human Services and the U.S. Department of Agriculture.

Nemetchek, M. D., Stierle, A. A., Stierle, D. B., & Lurie, D. I. (2017). The Ayurvedic plant Bacopa monnieri inhibits inflammatory pathways in the brain. *Journal of Ethnopharmacology*, *197*, 92–100. doi:10.1016/j.jep.2016.07.073 PMID:27473605

New York Health Department. (1932). *Practical Homeopathic Therapeutics*. New York: Oxford University Press.

Newman, D. J., & Cragg, G. M. (2007). Natural Products as Sources of New Drugs over the Last 25 Years. *Journal of Natural Products*, *70*, 461–477.

Ng, S. C., Plamondon, S., Al-Hassi, H. O., Kamm, M. A., Knight, S. C., & Stagg, A. J. (2008a). M1202 Effective probiotic treatment (VSL#3), but not placebo, in acute ulcerative colitis is associated with downregulation of inflammatory intestinal dendritic cells. *Gastroenterology*, *134*(4), A3610. doi:10.1016/S0016-5085(08)61677-7

Ng, S. C., Plamondon, S., Al-Hassi, H. O., Kamm, M. A., Knight, S. C., & Stagg, A. J. (2008b). Corticosteroids increase interleukin-10 and inhibit interleukin-12p40 production by intestinal dendritic cells in acute ulcerative colitis: Novel mechanisms of therapy. *Gastroenterology*, *134*(4), A646. doi:10.1016/S0016-5085(08)63015-2

Niccoli, T., & Partridge, L. (2012). Ageing as a risk factor for disease. *Current Biology*, *22*(17), R741–R752. doi:10.1016/j.cub.2012.07.024 PMID:22975005

Nieves, J. W. (2013). Skeletal effects of nutrients and nutraceuticals, beyond calcium and vitamin D. *Osteoporosis International*, *24*(3), 771–786. doi:10.100700198-012-2214-4 PMID:23152094

NIH. (2012). *Clinical Trials*. NIH.

Nishihara, M., Hirooka, Y., Matsukawa, R., Kishi, T., & Sunagawa, K. (2012). Oxidative stress in the rostral ventrolateral medulla modulates excitatory and inhibitory inputs in spontaneously hypertensive rats. *Journal of Hypertension*, *30*(1), 97–106. doi:10.1097/HJH.0b013e32834e1df4 PMID:22157590

Nishino, H., Murakoshi, M., Ii, T., Takemura, M., Kuchide, M., Kanazawa, M., ... Jinno, K. (2002). Carotenoids in cancer chemoprevention. *Cancer and Metastasis Reviews*, *21*(3/4), 257–264. doi:10.1023/A:1021206826750 PMID:12549764

Niu, Y.-G., & Evans, R. D. (2011). Very-Low-Density Lipoprotein: Complex Particles in Cardiac Energy Metabolism. *Journal of Lipids*, *9*. doi:10.1155/2011/189876 PMID:21773049

Nordestgaard, B. G., & Zacho, J. (2009). Lipids, atherosclerosis and CVD risk: Is CRP an innocent bystander? *Nutrition, Metabolism, and Cardiovascular Diseases*, *19*(8), 521–524. doi:10.1016/j.numecd.2009.07.005 PMID:19695857

Norshazila, S. Jr, Syed Zahir, I., Mustapha Suleiman, K., Aisyah, M. R., & Kamarul Rahim, K. (2010). Antioxidant levels and activities of selected seeds of malaysian tropical fruits. *Malaysian Journal of Nutrition*, *16*(1), 149–159. PMID:22691862

North, B. J., & Sinclair, D. A. (2012). The intersection between aging and cardiovascular disease. *Circulation Research*, *110*(8), 1097–1108. doi:10.1161/CIRCRESAHA.111.246876 PMID:22499900

Noviendri, D., Hasrini, R. F., & Octavianti, F. (2011). Carotenoids: Sources, medicinal properties and their application in food and nutraceutical industry. *Journal of Medicinal Plants Research*, *5*(33), 7119–7131.

Nutraceuticals - opportunities in an emerging market. (n.d.). Retrieved April 14, 2017, from http://www.fimdefelice.org/p2463.html

Nwofia, G. E., Ojimelukwe, P., & Eji, C. (2012). Chemical composition of leaves, fruit pulp and seeds in some Carica papaya (L) morphotypes. *International Journal of Medicinal and Aromatic Plants*, *2*(1), 200–206.

O'connor, T. (2017). Developing New Functional Food and Nutraceutical Products. *Journal of Nutrition Education and Behavior*, *49*(9), 793. doi:10.1016/j.jneb.2017.05.356

O'Hara, A. M., & Shanahan, F. (2006). The gut flora as a forgotten organ. *EMBO Reports*, *7*(7), 688–693. doi:10.1038j.embor.7400731 PMID:16819463

Obarzanek, E., Sacks, F. M., Vollmer, W. M., Bray, G. A., Miller, E. R. III, Lin, P. H., ... Proschan, M. A. (2001). Effects on blood lipids of a blood pressure-lowering diet: The Dietary Approaches to Stop Hypertension (DASH) Trial. *The American Journal of Clinical Nutrition*, *74*(1), 80–89. doi:10.1093/ajcn/74.1.80 PMID:11451721

Obodozie, O. O., Ameh, S. J., Afolabi, E. K., Oyedele, E. O., Ache, T. A., Onanuga, C. E., & Inyang, U. S. (2010). A normative study of the components of niprisan—an herbal medicine for sickle cell anemia. *Journal of Dietary Supplements*, *7*(1), 21–30. doi:10.3109/19390210903534988 PMID:22435571

Oboh, G., Bello, F. O., Ademosun, A. O., Akinyemi, A. J., & Adewuni, T. M. (2015). Antioxidant, hypolipidemic, and anti-angiotensin-1-converting enzyme properties of lemon (Citrus limon) and lime (Citrus aurantifolia) juices. *Comparative Clinical Pathology*, *24*(6), 1395–1406. doi:10.100700580-015-2088-x

Oduyebo, O. O., Anorlu, R. I., & Ogunsola, F. T. (2009). The effects of antimicrobial therapy on bacterial vaginosis in non-pregnant women. *Cochrane Database of Systematic Reviews*, *3*, CD006055. PMID:19588379

Oelschlaeger, T. A. (2010). Mechanisms of probiotic actions – a review. *International Journal of Medical Microbiology*, *300*(1), 57–62. doi:10.1016/j.ijmm.2009.08.005 PMID:19783474

Oh, D. Y., Talukdar, S., Bae, E. J., Imamura, T., Morinaga, H., Fan, W., ... Olefsky, J. M. (2010). GPR120 is an ω-3 fatty acid receptor mediating potent anti-inflammatory and insulin-sensitizing effects. *Cell*, *142*(5), 687–698. doi:10.1016/j.cell.2010.07.041 PMID:20813258

Ohland, C. L., & Macnaughton, W. K. (2010). Probiotic bacteria and intestinal epithelial barrier function. *AmericanJournal of Gastrointestinal and Liver Physiology*, *298*(6), G807–G819. doi:10.1152/ajpgi.00243.2009 PMID:20299599

Ohnishi, N., Kusuhara, M., Yoshioka, M., Kuroda, K., Soga, A., Nishikawa, F., ... Yokoyama, T. (2003). Studies on interactions between functional foods or dietary supplements and medicines. I. Effects of Ginkgo biloba leaf extract on the pharmacokinetics of diltiazem in rats. *Biological & Pharmaceutical Bulletin*, *26*(9), 1315–1320. doi:10.1248/bpb.26.1315 PMID:12951478

Oksanen, P. J., Salminen, S., Saxelin, M., Hämäläinen, P., Ihantola-Vormisto, A., Muurasniemi-Isoviita, L., ... Vapaatalo, H. (1990). Prevention of travel-lers' diarrhoea by *Lactobacillus* GG. *Annals of Medicine*, *22*(1), 53–93. doi:10.3109/07853899009147242 PMID:2184847

Olalla, M. T., Medrano, M. J., Sierra, M. J., & Almazán, J. (1999). Time trends, cohort effect and spatial distribution of cerebrovascular disease mortality in Spain. *European Journal of Epidemiology*, *15*(4), 331–339. doi:10.1023/A:1007555000016 PMID:10414373

Olesen, J., Gustavsson, A., Svensson, M., Wittchen, H. U., & Jönsson, B. (2012). The economic cost of brain disorders in Europe. *European Journal of Neurology*, *19*(1), 155–162. doi:10.1111/j.1468-1331.2011.03590.x PMID:22175760

Olveira, G., & González-Molero, I. (*In-press*). Actualización de probióticos, prebióticos y simbióticos en nutrición clínica. *Endocrinología y Nutrición*. doi:10.1016/j.endonu.2016.07.006

Omenn, G. S., Goodman, G. E., Thornquist, M. D., Balmes, J., Cullen, M. R., Glass, A., ... Hammar, S. (1996). Effects of a Combination of Beta Carotene and Vitamin A on Lung Cancer and Cardiovascular Disease. *The New England Journal of Medicine*, *334*(18), 1150–1155. doi:10.1056/NEJM199605023341802 PMID:8602180

Oncescu, V., Mancuso, M., & Erickson, D. (2014). Cholesterol testing on a smartphone. *Lab on a Chip*, *14*(4), 759–763. doi:10.1039/C3LC51194D PMID:24336861

Ong, L., Henriksson, A., & Shah, N. P. (2007). Angiotensin converting enzyme-inhibitory activity in Cheddar cheeses made with the addition of probiotic Lactobacillus casei sp. *Le Lait*, *87*(2), 149–165. doi:10.1051/lait:2007004

Ong, L., & Shah, N. P. (2009). Probiotic Cheddar cheese: Influence of ripening temperatures on survival of probiotic microorganisms, cheese composition and organic acid profiles. *Food Science and Technology (Campinas)*, *42*, 1260–1268.

Ono, K., Hasegawa, K., Naiki, H., & Yamada, M. (2004). Anti-amyloidogenic activity of tannic acid and its activity to destabilize Alzheimer's beta-amyloid fibrils in vitro. *Biochimica et Biophysica Acta*, *1690*(3), 193–202. doi:10.1016/j.bbadis.2004.06.008 PMID:15511626

Ooi, L. G., & Liong, M. T. (2010). Cholesterol-lowering effects of probiotics and prebiotics: A reviewof in vivo and in vitro findings. *International Journal of Molecular Sciences*, *11*(6), 2499–2522. doi:10.3390/ijms11062499 PMID:20640165

Oram, J. F., & Lawn, R. M. (2001). ABCA1: The gatekeeper for eliminating excess tissue cholesterol. *Journal of Lipid Research*, *42*(8), 1173–1179. PMID:11483617

Ostlund, R. E. Jr. (2007). Phytosterols, cholesterol absorption and healthy diets. *Lipids*, *42*(1), 41–45. doi:10.100711745-006-3001-9 PMID:17393209

Ostlund, R. E. Jr, Spilburg, C. A., & Stenson, W. F. (1999). Sitostanol administered in lecithin micelles potently reduces cholesterol absorption in humans. *The American Journal of Clinical Nutrition*, *70*(5), 826–831. doi:10.1093/ajcn/70.5.826 PMID:10539742

Ouwehand, A. C., Salminen, S., & Isolauri, E. (2002). Probiotics: An overview of beneficial effects. *Antonie van Leeuwenhoek*, *82*(1/4), 279–289. doi:10.1023/A:1020620607611 PMID:12369194

Over the Counter & Complementary Therapies. (2017). Parkinson's Foundation. Retrieved from www.parkinson.org/Understanding-Parkinsons/Treatment/Over-the-Counter-and-Complementary-Therapies

Overview of hypertension. (2015). Retrieved April 13, 2017, from http://www.uptodate.com/contents/overview-of-hypertension

Ovesen, L. F. (2005). Increased consumption of fruits and vegetables reduces the risk of ischemic heart disease. *Ugeskr Laeger, 167*(25-31), 2742-2747.

Oyagbemi, A., Saba, A., & Azeez, O. (2010). Capsaicin: A novel chemopreventive molecule and its underlying molecular mechanisms of action. *Indian Journal of Cancer*, *47*(1), 53. doi:10.4103/0019-509X.58860 PMID:20071791

Ozden, A. (2008). Other fermented dairy products: Bioyogurt-probioitc yogurt. *Guncel Gastroenteroloji*, *12*(3), 169–181.

Ozturk, S., & Cillier, A. E. (2006). Magnesium supplementation in the treatment of dementia patients. *Medical Hypotheses*, *67*(5), 1223–1225. doi:10.1016/j.mehy.2006.04.047 PMID:16790324

Packer, L. (1998). Alpha-Lipoic acid: A metabolic antioxidant which regulates NF-kappa B signal transduction and protects against oxidative injury. *Drug Metabolism Reviews*, *30*(2), 245–275. doi:10.3109/03602539808996311 PMID:9606603

Pala, V., Krogh, V., Muti, P., Chajès, V., Riboli, E., Micheli, A., ... Berrino, F. (2001). Erythrocyte membrane fatty acids and subsequent breast cancer: A prospective Italian study. *Journal of the National Cancer Institute*, *93*(14), 1088–1095. doi:10.1093/jnci/93.14.1088 PMID:11459870

Paliwal, S., Sundaram, J., & Mitragotri, S. (2005). Induction of cancer-specific cytotoxicity towards human prostate and skin cells using quercetin and ultrasound. *British Journal of Cancer*, *92*(3), 499–502. doi:10.1038j.bjc.6602364 PMID:15685239

Palloshi, A., Fragasso, G., Piatti, P., Monti, L. D., Setola, E., Valsecchi, G., ... Margonato, A. (2004). Effect of oral L-arginine on blood pressure and symptoms and endothelial function in patients with systemic hypertension, positive exercise tests, and normal coronary arteries. *The American Journal of Cardiology*, *93*(7), 933–935. doi:10.1016/j.amjcard.2003.12.040 PMID:15050504

Palozza, P., Simone, R., Catalano, A., Parrone, N., Monego, G., & Ranelletti, F. O. (2011). Lycopene regulation of cholesterol synthesis and efflux in human macrophages. *The Journal of Nutritional Biochemistry*, *22*(10), 971–978. doi:10.1016/j.jnutbio.2010.08.010 PMID:21208793

Palthur, P., Palthur, S., & Chitta, S. K. (2010). *Nutraceuticals: a conceptual definition*. Academic Press.

Pandey, K. R., Naik, S. R., & Vakil, B. V. (2015). Probiotics, prebiotics and synbiotics- a review. *Journal of Food Science and Technology*, *52*(12), 7577–7587. doi:10.100713197-015-1921-1 PMID:26604335

Pan, M.-H., Lin, C.-C., Lin, J.-K., & Chen, W.-J. (2007). Tea Polyphenol (−)-Epigallocatechin 3-Gallate Suppresses Heregulin-β1-Induced Fatty Acid Synthase Expression in Human Breast Cancer Cells by Inhibiting Phosphatidylinositol 3-Kinase/Akt and Mitogen-Activated Protein Kinase Cascade Signaling. *Journal of Agricultural and Food Chemistry*, *55*(13), 5030–5037. doi:10.1021/jf070316r PMID:17539658

Panossian, A., Wikman, G., & Wagner, H. (1999). Plant adaptogens III. Earlier and more recent aspects and concepts on their mode of action. *Phytomedicine*, *6*(4), 287–300. doi:10.1016/S0944-7113(99)80023-3 PMID:10589450

Pantoflikova, D. L., Theulaz, I. C., & Blum, A. L. (2007). *Helicobacter pylori* and probiotics. *The Journal of Nutrition, 137*(3), 812S–818S. doi:10.1093/jn/137.3.812S PMID:17311980

Panza, F., Frisardi, V., Capurso, C., D'Introno, A., Colacicco, A. M., Di Palo, A., & Solfrizzi, V. (2009). Polyunsaturated Fatty Acid and S-Adenosylmethionine Supplementation in Predementia Syndromes and Alzheimer's Disease: A Review. *The Scientific World Journal, 9*, 373–389. doi:10.1100/tsw.2009.48 PMID:19468660

Pardridge, W. M. (2002a). Targeting Neurotherapeutic Agents Through the Blood-Brain Barrier. *Archives of Neurology, 59*(1), 35. doi:10.1001/archneur.59.1.35 PMID:11790228

Pardridge, W. M. (2002b). Why is the global CNS pharmaceutical market so under-penetrated? *Drug Discovery Today, 7*(1), 5–7. doi:10.1016/S1359-6446(01)02082-7 PMID:11790589

Pardridge, W. M. (2007). Brain Drug Development and Brain Drug Targeting. *Pharmaceutical Research, 24*(9), 1729–1732. doi:10.100711095-007-9387-0 PMID:17629776

Park, D. Y., Ahn, Y. T., Park, S. H., Huh, C. S., Yoo, S. R., Yu, R., ... Choi, M. S. (2013). Supplementation of Lactobacillus curvatus HY7601 and Lactobacillus plantarum KY1032 in diet-induced obese mice is associated with gut microbial changes and reduction in obesity. *PLoS One, 8*(3), e59470. doi:10.1371/journal.pone.0059470 PMID:23555678

Parker-Athill, E., Luo, D., Bailey, A., Giunta, B., Tian, J., Shytle, R. D., & Tan, J. (2009). Flavonoids, a prenatal prophylaxis via targeting JAK2/STAT3 signaling to oppose IL-6/MIA associated autism. *Journal of Neuroimmunology, 217*(1–2), 20–27. doi:10.1016/j.jneuroim.2009.08.012 PMID:19766327

Parker, S. J., Koistinaho, J., White, A. R., & Kanninen, K. M. (2013). Biometals in rare neurodegenerative disorders of childhood. *Frontiers in Aging Neuroscience*, 5. PMID:23531702

Parracho, H. M., Gibson, G. R., Knott, F., Bosscher, D., Kleerebezem, M., & McCartney, A. L. (2010). A double-blind, placebo-controlled, crossover-designed probiotic feeding study in children diagnosed with autistic spectrum disorders. *International Journal of Probiotics & Prebiotics, 5*(2), 69–74.

Parrondo, J., Garcia, L. A., & Diaz, M. (2009). Whey Vinegars. In Vinegars of the World. Springer.

Pasternak, R. (2002). Adult Treatment Panel II vs Adult Treatment Panel III: What has changed and why? *The American Journal of Cardiology, 89*(5suppl), 3C–7C. doi:10.1016/S0002-9149(02)02221-X PMID:11900712

Patel, S., Celermajer, D. S., & Bao, S. (2008). Atherosclerosis-Underlying inflammatory mechanisms and clinical implications. *The International Journal of Biochemistry & Cell Biology, 40*(4), 576–580. doi:10.1016/j.biocel.2007.11.017 PMID:18203647

Pathak, Y. V. (Ed.). (2010). Handbook of Nutraceuticals: Vol. 1. Ingredients, Formulations, and Applications. CRC Press.

Pathak, A. K., Bhutani, M., Nair, A. S., Ahn, K. S., Chakraborty, A., Kadara, H., ... Aggarwal, B. B. (2007). Ursolic Acid Inhibits STAT3 Activation Pathway Leading to Suppression of Proliferation and Chemosensitization of Human Multiple Myeloma Cells. *Molecular Cancer Research*, *5*(9), 943–955. doi:10.1158/1541-7786.MCR-06-0348 PMID:17855663

Patil, S. P. D. (2011). Speech by her Excellency, the President of India, Shrimati Pratibha Devisingh Patil at the presentation of the National Florence Nightingale Awards for nursing personnel. *Nursing Journal of India*, *102*(7), 146–147. PMID:22482305

Patterson, G. W. (1991). Sterols of algae. In G. W. Patterson & D. W. Nes (Eds.), *Physiology and Biochemistry of Sterols* (pp. 118–156). Campaing, IL: American Oil's Chemists' Society.

Pecere, T., Gazzola, M. V., Mucignat, C., Parolin, C., Vecchia, F. D., Cavaggioni, A., ... Palù, G. (2000). Aloe-emodin Is a New Type of Anticancer Agent with Selective Activity against Neuroectodermal Tumors. *Cancer Research*, *60*(11). PMID:10850417

Pecorino, L. (2008). *Molecular biology of cancer : mechanisms, targets, and therapeutics*. Oxford University Press.

Pelikanova, T. (2009). Treatment of diabetes in metabolic syndrome]. *Vnitrni Lekarstvi*, *55*(7-8), 637–645. PMID:19731868

Pellegrino, L., Battelli, G., Resmini, P., Ferranti, P., Barone, F., & Addeo, F. (1997). Effects of heat load gradient occurring in moulding on characterization and ripening of Grana Padano. *Le Lait*, *77*(2), 217–228. doi:10.1051/lait:1997215

Penner, R. M., Madsen, K. L., & Fedorak, R. N. (2005). Postoperative Crohn's disease. *Inflammatory Bowel Diseases*, *11*(8), 765–777. doi:10.1097/01.MIB.0000171273.09757.f2 PMID:16043993

Penniston, K. L., & Tanumihardjo, S. A. (2006). The acute and chronic toxic effects of vitamin A. *The American Journal of Clinical Nutrition*, *83*(2), 191–201. doi:10.1093/ajcn/83.2.191 PMID:16469975

Pereira, D. I., Bruggraber, S. F., Faria, N., Poots, L. K., Tagmount, M. A., Aslam, M. F., & Powell, J. J. (2014). Nanoparticulate iron (III) oxo-hydroxide delivers safe iron that is well absorbed and utilised in humans. *Nanomedicine; Nanotechnology, Biology, and Medicine*, *10*(8), 1877–1886. doi:10.1016/j.nano.2014.06.012 PMID:24983890

Perera, T., & Thevathasan, W. (2014). *An Introduction to Parkinson's Disease*. Academic Press.

Pérez-Fons, L., Aranda, F. J., Guillén, J., Villalaín, J., & Micol, V. (2006). Rosemary (Rosmarinus officinalis) diterpenes affect lipid polymorphism and fluidity in phospholipid membranes. *Archives of Biochemistry and Biophysics*, *453*(2), 224–236. doi:10.1016/j.abb.2006.07.004 PMID:16949545

Pérez-Herrero, E., & Fernández-Medarde, A. (2015). Advanced targeted therapies in cancer: Drug nanocarriers, the future of chemotherapy. *European Journal of Pharmaceutics and Biopharmaceutics*, *93*, 52–79. doi:10.1016/j.ejpb.2015.03.018 PMID:25813885

Pérez-Jiménez, J., & Saura-Calixto, F. (2008). Grape products and cardiovascular disease risk factors. *Nutrition Research Reviews*, *21*(2), 158–173. doi:10.1017/S0954422408125124 PMID:19087369

Pericleous, M., Mandair, D., & Caplin, M. E. (2013). Diet and supplements and their impact on colorectal cancer. *Journal of Gastrointestinal Oncology*, *4*(4), 409–423. PMID:24294513

Perricone, N. V., Bagchi, D., Echard, B., & Preuss, H. G. (2010). Long-term metabolic effects of different doses of niacin-bound chromium on Sprague-Dawley rats. *Molecular and Cellular Biochemistry*, *338*(1-2), 91–103. doi:10.100711010-009-0342-8 PMID:20012467

Perticone, F., Ceravolo, R., Maio, R., Cloro, C., Candigliota, M., Scozzafava, A., ... Mattioli, P. L. (2000). Effects of atorvastatin and vitamin C on endothelial function of hypercholesterolemic patients. *Atherosclerosis*, *152*(2), 511–518. doi:10.1016/S0021-9150(00)00370-1 PMID:10998481

Peterson, A. L., Murchison, C., Zabetian, C., Leverenz, J. B., Watson, G. S., Montine, T., & Quinn, J. F. (2013). Memory, Mood, and Vitamin D in Persons with Parkinson's Disease. *Journal of Parkinson's Disease*, *3*(4), 547–555. PMID:24081441

Philip, M., Rowley, D. A., & Schreiber, H. (2004). Inflammation as a tumor promoter in cancer induction. *Seminars in Cancer Biology*, *14*(6), 433–439. doi:10.1016/j.semcancer.2004.06.006 PMID:15489136

Philippe, G. (2014). Metabolism of cholesterol and bile acids by the gut microbiota. *Pathogens (Basel, Switzerland)*, *3*, 14–24. PMID:25437605

Phillips, K. M., Ruggio, D. M., Toivo, J. I., Swank, M. A., & Simpkins, A. H. (2002). Free and esterified sterol composition of edible oils and fats. *Journal of Food Composition and Analysis*, *15*(2), 123–142. doi:10.1006/jfca.2001.1044

Piironen, V., Toivo, J., & Lampi, A. M. (2000). Natural sources of dietary plant sterols. *Journal of Food Composition and Analysis*, *13*(4), 619–624. doi:10.1006/jfca.2000.0898

Pillai, D. S., Prabhasankar, P., Jena, B. S., & Anandharamakrishnan, C. (2012). Microencapsulation of *Garcinia cowa* Fruit Extract and Effect of its use on Pasta Process and Quality. *International Journal of Food Properties*, *15*(3), 590–604. doi:10.1080/10942912.2010.494756

Piretti, M. V., Giampiero, P., Boni, L., Pistocchi, R., Diamante, M., & Gazzotti, T. (1997). Investigation of 4-methyl sterols from cultured dinoflagellate algal strains. *Journal of Phycology*, *33*(1), 61–67. doi:10.1111/j.0022-3646.1997.00061.x

Piwocka, K., Zabłocki, K., Wieckowski, M. R., Skierski, J., Feiga, I., Szopa, J., ... Sikora, E. (1999). A novel apoptosis-like pathway, independent of mitochondria and caspases, induced by curcumin in human lymphoblastoid T (Jurkat) cells. *Experimental Cell Research*, *249*(2), 299–307. doi:10.1006/excr.1999.4480 PMID:10366429

Pogodina, V. V. (1975). Elizaveta Nilolaevna Levkovich-75th birthday. *Acta Virologica. English Ed.*, *19*(6), 509. PMID:2002

Pohanka, M. (2014). Alzheimer s disease and oxidative stress: A review. *Current Medicinal Chemistry, 21*(3), 356–364. doi:10.2174/09298673113206660258 PMID:24059239

Position of the American Dietetic Association. (1999). Position of the American Dietetic Association. *Journal of the American Dietetic Association, 99*(10), 1278–1285. doi:10.1016/S0002-8223(99)00314-4 PMID:10524397

Powell, E. E., Jonsson, J. R., & Clouston, A. D. (2005). Steatosis: Co-factor in other liver diseases. *Hepatology (Baltimore, Md.), 42*(1), 5–13. doi:10.1002/hep.20750 PMID:15962320

Powolny, A. A., & Singh, S. V. (2008). Multitargeted prevention and therapy of cancer by diallyl trisulfide and related Allium vegetable-derived organosulfur compounds. *Cancer Letters, 269*(2), 305–314. doi:10.1016/j.canlet.2008.05.027 PMID:18579286

Premarajah, R. (2014). *The effects of drying conditions and carrier selection on the production of an antioxidant rich powder* (MPhil thesis). The University of Sydney.

Prieto, J. M., Iacopini, P., Cioni, P., & Chericoni, S. (2007). In vitro activity of the essential oils of Origanum vulgare, Satureja montana and their main constituents in peroxynitrite-induced oxidative processes. *Food Chemistry, 104*(3), 889–895. doi:10.1016/j.foodchem.2006.10.064

Prior, R. L., Wilkes, S. E., Rogers, T. R., Khanal, R. C., Wu, X., & Howard, L. R. (2010). Purified Blueberry Anthocyanins and Blueberry Juice Alter Development of Obesity in Mice Fed an Obesogenic High-Fat Diet. *Journal of Agricultural and Food Chemistry, 58*, 3970–3976. doi:10.1021/jf902852d PMID:20148514

Priyadarshani, W. M. D., & Rakshit, S. K. (2011). Screening selected strains of probiotic lactic acid bacteria for their ability to produce biogenic amines (histamine and tryamine). *International Journal of Food Science & Technology, 46*(10), 2062–2069. doi:10.1111/j.1365-2621.2011.02717.x

Puddu, P., Valenti, P., & Gessani, S. (2009). Immunomodulatory effects of lactoferrin on antigen presenting cells. *Biochimie, 91*(1), 11–18. doi:10.1016/j.biochi.2008.05.005 PMID:18539153

Qiang, X., Sang, Z., Yuan, W., Li, Y., Liu, Q., Bai, P., & Deng, Y. (2014). Design, synthesis and evaluation of genistein-O-alkylbenzylamines as potential multifunctional agents for the treatment of Alzheimer's disease. *European Journal of Medicinal Chemistry, 76*, 314–331. doi:10.1016/j.ejmech.2014.02.045 PMID:24589487

Qin, B., Polansky, M. M., Harry, D., & Anderson, R. A. (2010). Green tea polyphenols improve cardiac muscle mRNA and protein levels of signal pathways related to insulin and lipid metabolism and inflammation in insulin-resistant rats. *Molecular Nutrition & Food Research, 54*(1), S14–S23. doi:10.1002/mnfr.200900306 PMID:20112301

Queen, G. M., Surette, M., & Moayyedi, P. (2017). The gut microbiota and psychiatric illness. *Journal of Psychiatry & Neuroscience, 42*(2), 75–77. doi:10.1503/jpn.170028 PMID:28245172

Quideau, S. (2006). Flavonoids. Chemistry, Biochemistry and Applications. Edited by Øyvind M. Andersen and Kenneth R. Markham. *Angewandte Chemie, 45*(41), 6786–6787. doi:10.1002/anie.200685399

Quigley, E. M. M. (2016). Basic Definitions and Concepts: Organization of the Gut Microbiome. *Gastroenterology Clinics of North America*, 1–8. PMID:28164844

Quilez, J., Garcia-Lorda, P., & Salas-Salvado, J. (2003). Potential uses and benefits of phytosterols in diet: Present situation and future directions. *Clinical Nutrition (Edinburgh, Lothian)*, *22*(4), 343–351. doi:10.1016/S0261-5614(03)00060-8 PMID:12880600

Quirolo, K., & Vichinsky, E. (2016). Sickle cell anemia, thalassemia, and congenital hemolytic anemias. *Rossi's Principles of Transfusion Medicine*, 126-143.

Quiroz, Y., Johnson, R. J., & Rodríguez-Iturbe, B. (2012). The role of T cells in the pathogenesis of primary hypertension. *Nephrology, Dialysis, Transplantation*, *27*(Suppl 4), iv2–iv5. doi:10.1093/ndt/gfs421 PMID:23036901

Racette, S. B., Lin, X., Lefevre, M., Spearie, C. A., Most, M. M., Ma, L., & Ostlund, R. E. Jr. (2010). Dose effects of dietary phytosterols on cholesterol metabolism: A controlled feeding study. *The American Journal of Clinical Nutrition*, *91*(1), 32–38. doi:10.3945/ajcn.2009.28070 PMID:19889819

Rader, D. J. (2006). Molecular regulation of HDL metabolism and function: Implications for novel therapies. *The Journal of Clinical Investigation*, *116*(12), 3090–3100. doi:10.1172/JCI30163 PMID:17143322

Rains, T. M., Agarwal, S., & Maki, K. C. (2011). Antiobesity effects of green tea catechins: A mechanistic review. *The Journal of Nutritional Biochemistry*, *22*(1), 1–7. doi:10.1016/j.jnutbio.2010.06.006 PMID:21115335

Rajasekaran, A., Sivagnanam, G., & Xavier, R. (2008). Nutraceuticals as therapeutic agents: A Review. *Res J Pharm Tech*, *1*(4), 328–340.

Ramaa, C. S., Shirode, A. R., Mundada, A. S., & Kadam, V. J. (2006). Nutraceuticals--an emerging era in the treatment and prevention of cardiovascular diseases. *Current Pharmaceutical Biotechnology*, *7*(1), 15–23. doi:10.2174/138920106775789647 PMID:16472130

Ramachandran, C., & You, W. (1999). Differential sensitivity of human mammary epithelial and breast carcinoma cell lines to curcumin. *Breast Cancer Research and Treatment*, *54*(3), 269–278. doi:10.1023/A:1006170224414 PMID:10445426

Ramawat, K. G., & Merillon, J. M. (2007). *Biotechnology: Secondary metabolites : plants and microbes*. Science Publishers.

Rampen, S. W., Abbas, B. A., Schouten, S., & Sinninghe Damste, J. S. (2010). A comprehensive study of sterols in marine diatoms (Bacillariophyta): Implications for their use as tracers for diatom productivity. *Limnology and Oceanography*, *55*(1), 91–105. doi:10.4319/lo.2010.55.1.0091

Ranjan, D., Johnston, T. D., Reddy, K. S., Wu, G., Bondada, S., & Chen, C. (1999). Enhanced Apoptosis Mediates Inhibition of EBV-Transformed Lymphoblastoid Cell Line Proliferation by Curcumin. *The Journal of Surgical Research*, *87*(1), 1–5. doi:10.1006/jsre.1999.5719 PMID:10527697

Ravussin, E., & Swinburn, B. A. (1993). metabolic predictors of obesity cross-sectional versus longitudinal dataInt. *Journal of Obesity*, *17*, S28–S31. PMID:8124397

Ray, A., Joshi, J., & Gulati, K. (2016). Regulatory Aspects of Nutraceuticals. In Nutraceuticals (pp. 941–946). Elsevier. doi:10.1016/B978-0-12-802147-7.00066-8

Rayalam, S., Della-Fera, M. A., & Baile, C. A. (2008). Phytochemicals and regulation of the adipocyte life cycle. *The Journal of Nutritional Biochemistry*, *19*(11), 717–726. doi:10.1016/j.jnutbio.2007.12.007 PMID:18495457

Razzouk, L., Muntner, P., Bansilal, S., Kini, A. S., Aneja, A., Mozes, J., ... Farkouh, M. E. (2009). C-reactive protein predicts long-term mortality independently of low-density lipoprotein cholesterol in patients undergoing percutaneous coronary intervention. *American Heart Journal*, *158*(2), 277–283. doi:10.1016/j.ahj.2009.05.026 PMID:19619706

Reddy, K. R. (2012). *Kidwai memorial institute of oncology*. Retrieved from http://kidwai.kar.nic.in/statistics.html

Reddy, K. S. (1993). Cardiovascular diseases in India. *World Health Statistics Quarterly. Rapport Trimestriel De Statistiques Sanitaires Mondiales*, *46*(2), 101–107. PMID:8303903

Reedy, J., Wirfält, E., Flood, A., Mitrou, P. N., Krebs-Smith, S. M., Kipnis, V., ... Subar, A. F. (2010). Comparing 3 Dietary Pattern Methods—Cluster Analysis, Factor Analysis, and Index Analysis—With Colorectal Cancer Risk. *American Journal of Epidemiology*, *171*(4), 479–487. doi:10.1093/aje/kwp393 PMID:20026579

Reid, G., Beuerman, D., Heinemann, C., & Bruce, A. (2001). Probiotic Lactobacillus dose required to restore and maintain a normal vaginal flora. *FEMS Immunology and Medical Microbiology*, *32*(1), 37–41. doi:10.1111/j.1574-695X.2001.tb00531.x PMID:11750220

Rein, M. J., Renouf, M., Cruz-Hernandez, C., Actis-Goretta, L., Thakkar, S. K., & da Silva Pinto, M. (2013). Bioavailability of bioactive food compounds: A challenging journey to bioefficacy. *British Journal of Clinical Pharmacology*, *75*(3), 588–602. doi:10.1111/j.1365-2125.2012.04425.x PMID:22897361

Rembacken, B. J., Snelling, A. M., Hawkey, P. M., Chalmers, D. M., & Axon, A. T. R. (1999). Chalmers DM, Axon AT Non-pathogenic *Escherichia coli* versus mesalazine for the treatment of ulcerative colitis: A randomised trial. *Lancet*, *354*(9179), 635–639. doi:10.1016/S0140-6736(98)06343-0 PMID:10466665

Rengo, G., Pagano, G., Vitale, D. F., Formisano, R., Komici, K., Petraglia, L., ... Ferrara, N. (2016). Impact of aging on cardiac sympathetic innervation measured by (123) I-mIBG imaging in patients with systolic heart failure. *European Journal of Nuclear Medicine and Molecular Imaging*, *43*(13), 2392–2400. doi:10.100700259-016-3432-3 PMID:27287990

Riccardi, G., Capaldo, B., & Vaccaro, O. (2005). Functional foods in the management of obesity and type 2 diabetes. *Current Opinion in Clinical Nutrition and Metabolic Care*, *8*(6), 630–635. doi:10.1097/01.mco.0000171126.98783.0c PMID:16205464

Rice-Evans, C. A., & Miller, N. J. (1996). Antioxidant activities of flavonoids as bioactive components of food. *Biochemical Society Transactions*, *24*(3), 790–795. doi:10.1042/bst0240790 PMID:8878849

Rice, M. E. (2000). Ascorbate regulation and its neuroprotective role in the rat brain. *Trends in Neurosciences*, *23*(5), 209–216. doi:10.1016/S0166-2236(99)01543-X PMID:10782126

Richardson, G. H., Cheng, C. T., & Young, R. (1977). Lactic bulk culture system utilizing a whey-based bacteriophage inhibitory medium and pH control: Applicability to American style cheese. *Journal of Dairy Science*, *60*(3), 378–386. doi:10.3168/jds.S0022-0302(77)83876-9

Ricote, M., Li, A. C., Willson, T. M., Kelly, C. J., & Glass, C. K. (2009). The peroxisome proliferator-activated receptor-γ is a negative regulator of macrophage activation. *Nature*, *391*(6662), 79–82. doi:10.1038/34178 PMID:9422508

Ried, K., & Fakler, P. (2011). Protective effect of lycopene on serum cholesterol and blood pressure: Meta-analyses of intervention trials. *Maturitas*, *68*(4), 299–310. doi:10.1016/j.maturitas.2010.11.018 PMID:21163596

Riemersma, R. A., Rice-Evans, C. A., Tyrrell, R. M., Clifford, M. N., & Lean, M. E. (2001). Tea flavonoids and cardiovascular health. *QJM: Monthly Journal of the Association of Physicians*, *94*(5), 277–282. doi:10.1093/qjmed/94.5.277 PMID:11353103

Riggs, K. M., Spiro, A. I. I. I. III, Tucker, K., & Rush, D. (1996). Relations of vitamin B-12, vitamin B-6, folate, and homocysteine to cognitive performance in the Normative Aging Study. *The American Journal of Clinical Nutrition*, *63*(3), 306–314. doi:10.1093/ajcn/63.3.306 PMID:8602585

Rijkers, G. T., Bengmark, S., Enck, P., Haller, D., Herz, U., Kalliomaki, M., ... Antoine, J. M. (2010). Guidance for substantiating the evidence for beneficial effects of probiotics: Current status and recommendations for future research. *The Journal of Nutrition*, *140*(3), 671S–676S. doi:10.3945/jn.109.113779 PMID:20130080

Rimm, E. B., Willett, W. C., Hu, F. B., Sampson, L., Colditz, G. A., Manson, J. E., ... Stampfer, M. J. (1998). Folate and vitamin B6 from diet and supplements in relation to risk of coronary heart disease among women. *Journal of the American Medical Association*, *279*(5), 359–364. doi:10.1001/jama.279.5.359 PMID:9459468

Rincon, D., Vaquero, J., Hernando, A., Galindo, E., Ripoll, C., Puerto, M., ... Banares, R. (2014). Oral probiotic *VSL#3* attenuates the circulatory disturbances of patients with cirrhosis and ascites. *Liver International*, *34*(10), 1504–1512. doi:10.1111/liv.12539 PMID:24661740

Rinttilä, T., Lyra, A., Kurikka, L. K., & Palva, A. (2011). Real-time PCR analysis of enteric pathogens from faecal samples of irritable bowel syndrome subjects. *Gut Pathogens*, *3*(1), 1–9. doi:10.1186/1757-4749-3-6 PMID:21281494

Rissanen, T. H., Voutilainen, S., Virtanen, J. K., Venho, B., Vanharanta, M., Mursu, J., & Salonen, J. T. (2003). Low intake of fruits, berries and vegetables is associated with excess mortality in men: The Kuopio Ischaemic Heart Disease Risk Factor (KIHD) Study. *The Journal of Nutrition, 133*(1), 199–204. doi:10.1093/jn/133.1.199 PMID:12514290

Ritchie, M. L., & Romanuk, T. N. (2012). A Meta-Analysis of Probiotic Efficacy for Gastrointestinal Diseases. *PLoS One, 7*(4), e34938. doi:10.1371/journal.pone.0034938 PMID:22529959

Rivière, C., Richard, T., Quentin, L., Krisa, S., Mérillon, J.-M., & Monti, J.-P. (2007). Inhibitory activity of stilbenes on Alzheimer's beta-amyloid fibrils in vitro. *Bioorganic & Medicinal Chemistry, 15*(2), 1160–1167. doi:10.1016/j.bmc.2006.09.069 PMID:17049256

Rizvi, S. I., & Zaid, M. A. (2009). Effect of tea catechins on erythrocyte Ca $^{++}$ -pump in type 2 diabetes mellitus. *Pharmaceutical Biology, 47*(5), 440–443. doi:10.1080/13880200902822588

Roberfroid, M. B., & Delzenne, N. M. (1998). Dietary fructans. *Annual Review of Nutrition, 18*(1), 117–143. doi:10.1146/annurev.nutr.18.1.117 PMID:9706221

Roberts, S. B. (2003). Glycemic index and satiety. *Nutrition in Clinical Care, 6*, 20–26. PMID:12841427

Rockenstein, E., Crews, L., & Masliah, E. (2007). Transgenic animal models of neurodegenerative diseases and their application to treatment development. *Advanced Drug Delivery Reviews, 59*(11), 1093–1102. doi:10.1016/j.addr.2007.08.013 PMID:17869376

Rodríguez-Iturbe, B., Franco, M., Tapia, E., Quiroz, Y., & Johnson, R. J. (2012). Renal inflammation, autoimmunity and salt-sensitive hypertension. *Clinical and Experimental Pharmacology & Physiology, 39*(1), 96–103. doi:10.1111/j.1440-1681.2011.05482.x PMID:21251049

Rodriguez-Mateos, A., Heiss, C., Borges, G., & Crozier, A. (2014). Berry (Poly)phenols and Cardiovascular Health. *Journal of Agricultural and Food Chemistry, 62*(18), 3842–3851. doi:10.1021/jf403757g PMID:24059851

Rohdewald, P. (2002). A review of the French maritime pine bark extract (Pycnogenol®), a herbal medication with a diverse clinical pharmacology. *International Journal of Clinical Pharmacology and Therapeutics, 40*(04), 158–168. doi:10.5414/CPP40158 PMID:11996210

Rojas, P., Montes, P., Rojas, C., Serrano-García, N., & Rojas-Castañeda, J. C. (2012). Effect of a phytopharmaceutical medicine, Ginko biloba extract 761, in an animal model of Parkinson's disease: Therapeutic perspectives. *Nutrition (Burbank, Los Angeles County, Calif.), 28*(11–12), 1081–1088. doi:10.1016/j.nut.2012.03.007 PMID:22817828

Ros, E., Núñez, I., Pérez-Heras, A., Serra, M., Gilabert, R., Casals, E., & Deulofeu, R. (2004). A walnut diet improves endothelial function in hypercholesterolemic subjects: a randomized crossover trial. *Circulation, 109*(13), 1609–1614. .91474.FF10.1161/01.CIR.0000124477

Rosell, M., Appleby, P., Spencer, E., & Key, T. (2006). Weight gain over 5 years in 21 966 meat-eating, fish-eating, vegetarian, and vegan men and women in EPIC-Oxford. *International Journal of Obesity, 30*(9), 1389–1396. doi:10.1038j.ijo.0803305 PMID:16534521

Rossetti, L., Carminati, D., Zago, M., & Giraffa, G. (2009). A qualified presumption of safety approach for the safety assessment of Grana Padano whey starters. *International Journal of Food Microbiology, 130*(1), 70–73. doi:10.1016/j.ijfoodmicro.2009.01.003 PMID:19187995

Rossetti, L., Fornasari, M., Gatti, M., Lazzi, C., Neviani, E., & Giraffa, G. (2008). Grana Padano cheese whey starters: Microbial composition and strain distribution. *International Journal of Food Microbiology, 127*(1-2), 168–171. doi:10.1016/j.ijfoodmicro.2008.06.005 PMID:18620769

Ross, R. (1993). The pathogenesis of atherosclerosis: A perspective for the 1990s. *Nature, 362*(6423), 801–809. doi:10.1038/362801a0 PMID:8479518

Ross, R. (1999). Atherosclerosis - An Inflammatory Disease. *The New England Journal of Medicine, 340*(2), 115–126. doi:10.1056/NEJM199901143400207 PMID:9887164

Rouxinol-Dias, A. L., Pinto, A. R., Janeiro, C., Rodrigues, D., Moreira, M., Dias, J., & Pereira, P. (2016). Probiotics for the control of obesity – Its effect on weight change. *Porto Biomedical Journal, 1*(1), 12–24. doi:10.1016/j.pbj.2016.03.005

Roy, P., Madan, E., Kalra, N., Nigam, N., George, J., Ray, R. S., ... Shukla, Y. (2009). Resveratrol enhances ultraviolet B-induced cell death through nuclear factor-kappaB pathway in human epidermoid carcinoma A431 cells. *Biochemical and Biophysical Research Communications, 384*(2), 215–220. doi:10.1016/j.bbrc.2009.04.100 PMID:19397895

Rozner, S., & Garti, N. (2006). The activity and absorption relationship of cholesterol and phytosterols. *Colloids and Surfaces. A, Physicochemical and Engineering Aspects, 282*, 435–456. doi:10.1016/j.colsurfa.2005.12.032

Ruel, G., Pomerleau, S., Couture, P., Lamarche, B., & Couillard, C. (2005). Changes in plasma antioxidant capacity and oxidized low-density lipoprotein levels in men after short-term cranberry juice consumption. *Metabolism: Clinical and Experimental, 54*(7), 856–861. doi:10.1016/j.metabol.2005.01.031 PMID:15988692

Ruijschop, R. M., & Burgering, M. J. M. (2007). Aroma induced satiation possibilities to manage weight through aroma in food products. *Agro Food Industry Hi-Tech, 18*, 37–39.

Rund, D., & Rachmilewitz, E. (2001, October). Pathophysiology of α-and β-thalassemia: Therapeutic implications. *Seminars in Hematology, 38*(4), 343–349. doi:10.1016/S0037-1963(01)90028-9 PMID:11605169

Russell, R. M., & Mayer, J. (2002). Beta-carotene and lung cancer. *Pure and Applied Chemistry, 74*(8), 1461–1467. doi:10.1351/pac200274081461

Saavedra, J. M., Bauman, A., Oung, I., Perman, J. A., & Yolken, R. H. (1994). Feeding of *Bifidobacteriumbifidum*and *Streptococcus thermophilus*to infants in hospital for prevention of diarrhea and shedding of rotavirus. *Lancet, 344*(8929), 1046–1049. doi:10.1016/S0140-6736(94)91708-6 PMID:7934445

Sabate, J., & Ang, Y. (2009). Nuts and health outcomes: New epidemiologic evidence. *The American Journal of Clinical Nutrition*, *89*(5), 1643S–1648S. doi:10.3945/ajcn.2009.26736Q PMID:19321572

Sacks, F. M. (2015). The crucial roles of apolipoproteins E and C-III in apoB lipoprotein metabolism in normolipidemia and hypertriglyceridemia. *Current Opinion in Lipidology*, *26*(1), 56–63. doi:10.1097/MOL.0000000000000146 PMID:25551803

Saetan, S., Grove, K. A., & Lambert, J. D. (2011). Weight control and prevention of metabolic syndrome by green tea. *Pharmacological Research*, *64*(2), 146–154. doi:10.1016/j.phrs.2010.12.013 PMID:21193040

Sagara, M., Kanda, T., Jelekera, M. N., Teramoto, T., Armitage, L., Birt, N., ... Yamori, Y. (2004). Effects of Dietary Intake of Soy Protein and Isoflavones on Cardiovascular Disease Risk Factors in High Risk, Middle-Aged Men in Scotland. *Journal of the American College of Nutrition*, *23*(1), 85–91. doi:10.1080/07315724.2004.10719347 PMID:14963058

Sahib, P., Rakesh, P. K., Pal, S. S., Apoorva, S., & Nidhi, G. (2016). Awareness and knowledge of people towards probiotics products in punjab region Kaur. *International Journal of Applied Biology and Pharmaceutical Technology*, *7*(1), 154–160.

Salak-Johnson, J. L., & McGlone, J. J. (2007). Making sense of apparently conflicting data: Stress and immunity in swine and cattle. *Journal of Animal Science, 85*(13_suppl), E81-E88.

Salen, G., Shore, V., Tint, G. S., Forte, T., Shefer, S., Horak, I., ... Kwiterovich, P. O. Jr. (1989). Increased sitosterol absorption, decreased removal, and expanded body pools compensate for reduced cholesterol synthesis in sitosterolemia with xanthomatosis. *Journal of Lipid Research*, *30*, 1319–1330. PMID:2600539

Salminen, H., Herrmann, K., & Weiss, J. (2013). Oil-in-water emulsions as a delivery system for n-3 fatty acids in meat products. *Meat Science*, *93*(3), 659–667. doi:10.1016/j.meatsci.2012.11.035 PMID:23273478

Salminen, S., Bouley, C., Boutron-Ruault, M. C., Cummings, J. H., Franck, A., Gibson, G. R., ... Rowland, I. (1998). Functional food science and gastrointestinal physiology and function. *British Journal of Nutrition*, *80*(S1Suppl 1), S147–S171. doi:10.1079/BJN19980108 PMID:9849357

Salo, P. M. D., & Wester, I. M. S. (2005). Low fat formulations of plant stanols and sterols. *The American Journal of Cardiology*, *96*(1suppl.), 51D–54D. doi:10.1016/j.amjcard.2005.03.021 PMID:15992517

Salta, F. N., Kalogeropoulos, N., Karavanou, N., & Andrikopoulos, N. K. (2008). Distribution and retention of phytosterols in frying oils and fried potatoes during repeated deep and pan frying. *European Food Research and Technology*, *41*(2), 391–400. doi:10.100700217-007-0733-6

Sánchez, B., Urdaci, M. C., & Margolles, A. (2010). Extracellular proteins secreted by probiotic bacteriaas mediators of effects that promote mucosa- bacteria interactions. *Microbiology*, *156*(11), 3232–3242. doi:10.1099/mic.0.044057-0 PMID:20864471

Sanchez, M., Darimont, C., Drapeau, V., Emady-Azar, S., Lepage, M., Rezzonico, E., ... Tremblay, A. (2014). Effect of Lactobacillus rhamnosus CGMCC1.3724 supplementation on weight loss and maintenance in obese men and women. *British Journal of Nutrition*, *111*(08), 1507–1519. doi:10.1017/S0007114513003875 PMID:24299712

Sanders, M. E., Akkermans, L. M., Haller, D., Hammerman, C., Heimbach, J., Hörmannsperger, G., ... Vaughan, E. (2010). Safety assessment of probiotics for human use. *Gut Microbes*, *1*(3), 164–185. doi:10.4161/gmic.1.3.12127 PMID:21327023

Sanders, M. E., Guarner, F., Guerrant, R., Holt, P. R., Quigley, E. M. M., Sartor, R. B. E. A., & Mayer, P. M. S. (2013). An update on the use and investigation of probiotics in health and disease. *Gut*, *62*(5), 787–796. doi:10.1136/gutjnl-2012-302504 PMID:23474420

Sanfilippo, L., Li, C. K., Seth, R., Balwin, T. J., Menozzi, M. G., & Mahida, Y. R. (2000). *Bacteroidesfragilis*enterotoxin induces the expression of IL-8 and transforming growth factor-beta (TFG-_) by human colonic epithelial cells. *Clinical and Experimental Immunology*, *119*(3), 456–463. doi:10.1046/j.1365-2249.2000.01155.x PMID:10691917

Santhakumar, A. B., & Singh, I. (2016). Antioxidants as Functional Foods in Metabolic Syndrome. *Examining the Development, Regulation, and Consumption of Functional Foods*, 149.

Šaponjac, V. T., Cetkovic, G., Canadanovic-Brunet, J., Pajin, B., Djilas, S., Petrovic, J., ... Vulic, J. (2016). Sour cherry pomace extract encapsulated in whey and soy proteins: Incorporation in cookies. *Food Chemistry*, *207*, 27–33. doi:10.1016/j.foodchem.2016.03.082 PMID:27080876

Sarkar, F. H., & Li, Y. (2003). Soy isoflavones and cancer prevention. *Cancer Investigation*, *21*(5), 744–757. doi:10.1081/CNV-120023773 PMID:14628433

Sasayama, S. (2008). Heart Disease in Asia. *Circulation*, *118*(25), 2669–2671. doi:10.1161/CIRCULATIONAHA.108.837054 PMID:19106388

Savica, V., Bellinghieri, G., & Kopple, J. D. (2010). The effect of nutrition on blood pressure. *Annual Review of Nutrition*, *30*(1), 365–401. doi:10.1146/annurev-nutr-010510-103954 PMID:20645853

Scalbert, A., Manach, C., Morand, C., Rémésy, C., & Jiménez, L. (2005). Dietary polyphenols and the prevention of diseases. *Critical Reviews in Food Science and Nutrition*, *45*(4), 287–306. doi:10.1080/1040869059096 PMID:16047496

Schächinger, V., Britten, M. B., & Zeiher, A. M. (2000). Prognostic impact of coronary vasodilator dysfunction on adverse long-term outcome of coronary heart disease. *Circulation*, *101*(16), 1899–1906. doi:10.1161/01.CIR.101.16.1899 PMID:10779454

Scheiber, I. F., Mercer, J. F. B., & Dringen, R. (2014). Metabolism and functions of copper in brain. *Progress in Neurobiology*, *116*, 33–57. doi:10.1016/j.pneurobio.2014.01.002 PMID:24440710

Schenk, S., Saberi, M., & Olefsky, J. M. (2008). Insulin sensitivity: Modulation by nutrients and inflammation. *The Journal of Clinical Investigation*, *118*(9), 2992–3002. doi:10.1172/JCI34260 PMID:18769626

Schiffrin, E. J., & Blum, S. (2002). Interactions between the microbiota and the intestinal mucosa. *European Journal of Clinical Nutrition*, *56*(S3), S60–S64. doi:10.1038j.ejcn.1601489 PMID:12142966

Schloss, J. M., Colosimo, M., Airey, C., Masci, P. P., Linnane, A. W., & Vitetta, L. (2013). Nutraceuticals and chemotherapy induced peripheral neuropathy (CIPN): A systematic review. *Clinical Nutrition (Edinburgh, Lothian)*, *32*(6), 888–893. doi:10.1016/j.clnu.2013.04.007 PMID:23647723

Schloss, P. D. (2014). Microbiology: An integrated view of the skin microbiome. *Nature*, *514*(7520), 44–45. doi:10.1038/514044a PMID:25279916

Schmidt, J., Metselaar, J. M., Wauben, M. H. M., Toyka, K. V., Storm, G., & Gold, R. (2003). Drug targeting by long-circulating liposomal glucocorticosteroids increases therapeutic efficacy in a model of multiple sclerosis. *Brain*, *126*(Pt 8), 1895–1904. doi:10.1093/brain/awg176 PMID:12805101

Schmoldt, A., Benthe, H. F., & Haberland, G. (1975). Digitoxin metabolism by rat liver microsomes. *Biochemical Pharmacology*, *24*(17), 1639–1641. doi:10.1016/0006-2952(75)90094-5 PMID:10

Schrier, S. L. (1994). Thalassemia: Pathophysiology of red cell changes. *Annual Review of Medicine*, *45*(1), 211–218. doi:10.1146/annurev.med.45.1.211 PMID:8198378

Schroeter, H., Boyd, C., Spencer, J. P. E., Williams, R. J., Cadenas, E., & Rice-Evans, C. (n.d.). MAPK signaling in neurodegeneration: influences of flavonoids and of nitric oxide. *Neurobiology of Aging, 23*(5), 861–80.

Schuessler, W. H. (2013). *The Biochemic Handbook. An introduction to the cellular therapy and practical application of the twelve tissue cell salts in accordance with the Biochemic system of Medicine*. Retrieved from http://www.campbellmgold.com

Schultz, M., Timmer, A., Herfarth, H. H., Sartor, R. B., Vanderhoof, J. A., & Rath, H. C. (2004). *Lactobacillus GG* in inducing and maintaining remission of Crohn's disease. *BMC Gastroenterology*, *4*(1), 5. doi:10.1186/1471-230X-4-5 PMID:15113451

Schwartz, M. W., Peskind, E., Raskind, M., Boyko, E. J., & Porte, D. Jr. (1996). Cerebrospinal fluid leptin levels: Relationship to plasma levels and to adiposity in humans. *Nature Medicine*, *2*(5), 589–593. doi:10.1038/nm0596-589 PMID:8616722

Schwencke, J., & De Robichon-Szulmajster, H. (1976). The transport of S-adenosyl-L-methionine in isolated yeast vacuoles and spheroplasts. *European Journal of Biochemistry*, *65*(1), 49–60. doi:10.1111/j.1432-1033.1976.tb10388.x PMID:6283

Schwiertz, A., Taras, D., Schäfer, K., Beijer, S., Bos, N. A., Donus, C., & Hardt, P. D. (2010). Microbiota and SCFA in lean and overweight healthy subjects. *Obesity (Silver Spring, Md.)*, *18*(1), 190–195. doi:10.1038/oby.2009.167 PMID:19498350

Scicchitano, P., Cameli, M., Maiello, M., Modesti, P. A., Muiesan, M. L., Novo, S., ... di Studio Ipertensione, G. (2014). Nutraceuticals and dyslipidaemia: Beyond the common therapeutics. *Journal of Functional Foods*, *6*, 11–32. doi:10.1016/j.jff.2013.12.006

Sekirov, I., Russell, S. L., Antunes, L. C., & Finlay, B. B. (2010). Gut microbiota in health and disease. *Physiological Reviews*, *90*(3), 859–904. doi:10.1152/physrev.00045.2009 PMID:20664075

Semo, E., Kesselman, E., Danino, D., & Livney, Y. D. (2007). Casein micelle as a natural nano-capsular vehicle for nutraceuticals. *Food Hydrocolloids*, *21*(5), 936–942. doi:10.1016/j.foodhyd.2006.09.006

Semple, J. W., & Freedman, J. (2005, July). Autoimmune pathogenesis and autoimmune hemolytic anemia. *Seminars in Hematology*, *42*(3), 122–130. doi:10.1053/j.seminhematol.2005.04.002 PMID:16041661

Senftleber, F. C., Halline, A. G., Veening, H., & Dayton, D. A. (1976). Reversed-phase liquid-chromatographic analysis of hemodialysate from uremic patients. *Clinical Chemistry*, *22*(9), 1522–1527. PMID:8223

Serino, M., Baque, V. B., Nicolas, S., & Burcelin, R. (2014). Far from the eyes, close to the heart: Dysbiosis of gut microbiota and cardiovascular consequences. *Current Cardiology Reports*, *16*(11), 1–7. doi:10.100711886-014-0540-1 PMID:25303894

Serjeant, G. R., & Serjeant, B. E. (1992). *Sickle cell disease* (Vol. 3). New York: Oxford university press.

Serrano, J. C., Cassanyé, A., & Portero-Otin, M. (2012). Trends in functional food against obesity. In B. Valdez (Ed.), *Scientific, Health and Social Aspects of the Food Industry* (pp. 279–294). Intech Publishing.

Sesso, H. D., Buring, J. E., Christen, W. G., Kurth, T., Belanger, C., MacFadyen, J., ... Gaziano, J. M. (2008). Vitamins E and C in the prevention of cardiovascular disease in men: The Physicians' Health Study II randomized controlled trial. *Journal of the American Medical Association*, *300*(18), 2123–2133. doi:10.1001/jama.2008.600 PMID:18997197

Sgouras, M., Maragkoudakis, P., Petraki, K., Martinez-Gonzalez, B., Eriotou, E., Michopoulos, S., ... Mentis, A. (2004). *In vitro* and *in vivo* inhibition of *Helicobacter pylori* by Lactobacillus casei strain Shirota. *Applied and Environmental Microbiology*, *70*(1), 518–526. doi:10.1128/AEM.70.1.518-526.2004 PMID:14711683

Sharma, S., Arora, M., & Baldi, A. (2013). Probiotics in India: Current status and future prospects. *Pharm Aspire*, *4*(1), 1–11.

Shaw, J. E., Sicree, R. A., & Zimmet, P. Z. (2010). Global estimates of the prevalence of diabetes for 2010 and 2030. *Diabetes Research and Clinical Practice*, *87*(1), 4–14. doi:10.1016/j.diabres.2009.10.007 PMID:19896746

Shefa, U., Yeo, S. G., Kim, M.-S., Song, I. O., Jung, J., Jeong, N. Y., & Huh, Y. (2017). Role of Gasotransmitters in Oxidative Stresses, Neuroinflammation, and Neuronal Repair. *BioMed Research International*, *2017*, 1–15. doi:10.1155/2017/1689341 PMID:28386548

Shehzad, A., Khan, S., & Sup-Lee, Y. (2012). Curcumin molecular targets in obesity and obesity-related cancers. *Future Oncology (London, England)*, *8*(4), 179–190. doi:10.2217/fon.11.145 PMID:22335582

Shen, H., Zhang, J., Li Y., Xie, S., Jiang, Y., Wu, Y., Ye, Y., Yang, H., Mo, H., Situ, C., & Hu, Q. (2016). The 12 gastrointestinal pathogens spectrum of acute infectious diarrhea in a sentinel hospital, Shenzhen, China. *Frontiers in Microbiology, 7*(1926), 1-9.

Shenderov, B. A. (2012). Gut indigenous microbiota and epigenetics. *Microbial Ecology in Health and Disease*, *23*(0), 17195. doi:10.3402/mehd.v23i0.17195 PMID:23990811

Shen, L. (2015). Associations between B Vitamins and Parkinson's Disease. *Nutrients*, *7*(9), 7197–7208. doi:10.3390/nu7095333 PMID:26343714

Shi, H., Kokoeva, M. V., Inouye, K., Tzameli, I., Yin, H., & Flier, J. S. (2006). TLR4 links innate immunity and fatty acid-induced insulin resistance. *The Journal of Clinical Investigation*, *116*(11), 3015–3025. doi:10.1172/JCI28898 PMID:17053832

Shimakawa, Y., Matsubara, S., Yuki, N., Ikeda, M., & Ishikawa, F. (2003). Evaluation of Bifidobacterium breve strain Yakult-fermented soymilk as a probiotic food. *International Journal of Food Microbiology*, *81*(2), 131–136. doi:10.1016/S0168-1605(02)00224-6 PMID:12457587

Shimizu, M., Sakai, H., Shirakami, Y., Yasuda, Y., Kubota, M., Terakura, D., ... Moriwaki, H. (2011). Preventive Effects of (-)-Epigallocatechin gallate on diethylnitrosamine-induced liver tumorigenesis in obese and diabetic C57BL/KsJ-*db/db* mice. *Cancer Prevention Research (Philadelphia, Pa.)*, *4*(3), 396–403. doi:10.1158/1940-6207.CAPR-10-0331 PMID:21372039

Shimmyo, Y., Kihara, T., Akaike, A., Niidome, T., & Sugimoto, H. (2008). Multifunction of myricetin on A beta: Neuroprotection via a conformational change of A beta and reduction of A beta via the interference of secretases. *Journal of Neuroscience Research*, *86*(2), 368–377. doi:10.1002/jnr.21476 PMID:17722071

Shim, S. S., Hammonds, M. D., & Kee, B. S. (2008). Potentiation of the NMDA receptor in the treatment of schizophrenia: Focused on the glycine site. *European Archives of Psychiatry and Clinical Neuroscience*, *258*(1), 16–27. doi:10.100700406-007-0757-8 PMID:17901997

Shishodia, S., & Aggarwal, B. B. (2004). Guggulsterone Inhibits NF-κB and IκBα Kinase Activation, Suppresses Expression of Anti-apoptotic Gene Products, and Enhances Apoptosis. *The Journal of Biological Chemistry*, *279*(45), 47148–47158. doi:10.1074/jbc.M408093200 PMID:15322087

Shishodia, S., Potdar, P., Gairola, C. G., & Aggarwal, B. B. (2003). Curcumin (diferuloylmethane) down-regulates cigarette smoke-induced NF- B activation through inhibition of I B kinase in human lung epithelial cells: Correlation with suppression of COX-2, MMP-9 and cyclin D1. *Carcinogenesis*, *24*(7), 1269–1279. doi:10.1093/carcin/bgg078 PMID:12807725

Shofian, N. M., Hamid, A. A., Osman, A., Saari, N., Anwar, F., Dek, M. S., & Hairuddin, M. R. (2011). Effect of freeze-drying on the antioxidant compounds and antioxidant activity of selected tropical fruits. *International Journal of Molecular Sciences*, *12*(7), 4678–4692. doi:10.3390/ijms12074678 PMID:21845104

Shornikova, A. V., Casas, I. A., Isolauri, E., Mykkanen, H., & Vesikari, T. (1997). *Lactobacillus reuteri*as a therapeutic agent in acute diarrhea in young children. *Journal of Pediatric Gastroenterology and Nutrition*, *24*(4), 399–404. doi:10.1097/00005176-199704000-00008 PMID:9144122

Shrestha, S., Volek, J. S., Udani, J., Wood, R. J., Greene, C. M., Aggarwal, D., ... Fernandez, M. L. (2006). A combination therapy including psyllium and plant sterols lowers LDL cholesterol by modifying lipoprotein metabolism in hypercholesterolemic individuals. *The Journal of Nutrition*, *136*(10), 2492–2497. doi:10.1093/jn/136.10.2492 PMID:16988115

Shukitt-Hale, B., Lau, F. C., Carey, A. N., Galli, R. L., Spangler, E. L., Ingram, D. K., & Joseph, J. A. (2013). Blueberry polyphenols attenuate kainic acid-induced decrements in cognition and alter inflammatory gene expression in rat hippocampus. *Nutritional Neuroscience*. PMID:18681986

Shukla, S., & Gupta, S. (2005). Dietary Agents in the Chemoprevention of Prostate Cancer. *Nutrition and Cancer*, *53*(1), 18–32. doi:10.120715327914nc5301_3 PMID:16351503

Shukla, Y., & Singh, M. (2007). Cancer preventive properties of ginger: A brief review. *Food and Chemical Toxicology*, *45*(5), 683–690. doi:10.1016/j.fct.2006.11.002 PMID:17175086

Siddiqui, I. A., Shukla, Y., Adhami, V. M., Sarfaraz, S., Asim, M., Hafeez, B., & Mukhtar, H. (2008). Suppression of NFκB and its Regulated Gene Products by Oral Administration of Green Tea Polyphenols in an Autochthonous Mouse Prostate Cancer Model. *Pharmaceutical Research*, *25*(9), 2135–2142. doi:10.100711095-008-9553-z PMID:18317887

Siegel, A. B., & Zhu, A. X. (2009). Metabolic syndrome and hepatocellular carcinoma: Two growing epidemics with a potential link. *Cancer*, *115*(24), 5651–5661. doi:10.1002/cncr.24687 PMID:19834957

Sies, H., & Stahl, W. (1995). Vitamins E and C, beta carotene, and other carotenoids as antioxidants. *The American Journal of Clinical Nutrition*, *62*(6suppl), 1315S–1321S. doi:10.1093/ajcn/62.6.1315S PMID:7495226

Silva, G. A. (2007). Nanotechnology approaches for drug and small molecule delivery across the blood brain barrier. *Surgical Neurology*, *67*(2), 113–116. doi:10.1016/j.surneu.2006.08.033 PMID:17254859

Simon, A., Allais, D. P., Duroux, J. L., Basly, J. P., Durand-Fontanier, S., & Delage, C. (1998). Inhibitory effect of curcuminoids on MCF-7 cell proliferation and structure-activity relationships. *Cancer Letters*, *129*(1), 111–116.

Simpson, A., Tan, V. Y. F., Winn, J., Svensén, M., Bishop, C. M., Heckerman, D. E., ... Custovic, A. (2010). Beyond atopy: Multiple patterns of sensitization in relation to asthma in a birth cohort study. *American Journal of Respiratory and Critical Care Medicine*, *181*(11), 1200–1206. doi:10.1164/rccm.200907-1101OC PMID:20167852

Singh, P., Kesharwani, R. K., & Keservani, R. K. (2018). Antioxidants and Vitamins: Roles in Cellular Function and Metabolism. In Sustained Energy for Enhanced Human Functions and Activity (pp. 385-407). Academic Press.

Singh, R. B., Rastogi, S. S., Singh, N. K., Ghosh, S., Gupta, S., & Niaz, M. A. (1993). Can guava fruit intake decrease blood pressure and blood lipids? *Journal of Human Hypertension*, *7*(1), 33–38. PMID:8383769

Singh, S. V., Mohan, R. R., Agarwal, R., Benson, P. J., Hu, X., Rudy, M., ... Zaren, H. A. (1996). Novel anti-carcinogenic activity of an organosulfide from garlic: Inhibition of H-RAS oncogene transformed tumor growth in vivo by diallyl disulfide is associated with inhibition of p21H-ras processing. *Biochemical and Biophysical Research Communications*, *225*(2), 660–665.

Singh, T. K., Fox, P. F., & Healy, Á. (1997). Isolation and identification of further peptides in the diafiltrationretentate of the water-soluble fraction of Cheddar cheese. *The Journal of Dairy Research*, *64*(03), 433–443. doi:10.1017/S0022029997002227 PMID:9275258

Singh, U., Devaraj, S., & Jialal, I. (2005). Vitamin E, Oxidative Stress, and Inflammation. *Annual Review of Nutrition*, *25*(1), 151–174. doi:10.1146/annurev.nutr.24.012003.132446 PMID:16011463

Singh, U., & Jialal, I. (2008). Retracted: Alpha-lipoic acid supplementation and diabetes. *Nutrition Reviews*, *66*(11), 646–657. doi:10.1111/j.1753-4887.2008.00118.x PMID:19019027

Singleton, A. B., Farrer, M., Johnson, J., Singleton, A., Hague, S., Kachergus, J., ... Lincoln, S. (2003). α-Synuclein locus triplication causes Parkinson's disease. *Science*, *302*(5646), 841–841. doi:10.1126cience.1090278 PMID:14593171

Sissayb, Thierry, Regnier, & Lise. (2006). Citrus sinensisdisease survey: knowledge, attitude and management practices in Ethiopia. *Tropical Research Journal*, (4), 1-9.

Sivieri, K., Spinardi-Barbusan, A. L. T., Barbisan, L. F., Bedani, R., Pauly, N. D., Carlos, I. Z., ... Rossi, E. A. (2008). Probiotic Enterococcus faecium CRL 183 inhibit chemically induced colon cancer in male Wistar rats. *European Food Research and Technology*, *228*(2), 231–237. doi:10.100700217-008-0927-6

Skeggs, H. R., & Wright, L. D. (1944). The use of Lactobacillus arabinosus in the microbiological determination of pantothenic acid. *The Journal of Biological Chemistry*, *156*, 21–26.

Slavin, J. L. (2005). Dietary fiber and body weight. *Nutrition (Burbank, Los Angeles County, Calif.)*, *21*(3), 411–418. doi:10.1016/j.nut.2004.08.018 PMID:15797686

Smirnov, V. V., Reznik, S. R., V'iunitskaia, V. A., Sorokulova, I. B., Samgorodskaia, N. V., & Tofan, A. V. (1993). The current concepts of the mechanisms of the therapeutic-prophylactic action of probiotics from bacteria in the genus Bacillus. *Mikrobiolohichnyi Zhurnal (Kiev, Ukraine: 1993), 55*(4), 92–112.

Smith, J., & Charter, E. (Eds.). (2010). *Functional food product development*. Chichester, UK: Wiley-Blackwell. doi:10.1002/9781444323351

Smith, R. (2005). Medical Journals Are an Extension of the Marketing Arm of Pharmaceutical Companies. *PLoS Medicine*, *2*(5), e138. doi:10.1371/journal.pmed.0020138 PMID:15916457

Smith-Warner, S. A., Elmer, P. J., Tharp, T. M., Fosdick, L., Randall, B., Gross, M., ... Potter, J. D. (2000). Increasing vegetable and fruit intake: Randomized intervention and monitoring in an at-risk population. *Cancer Epidemiology, Biomarkers & Prevention*, *9*(3), 307–317. PMID:10750670

Sobenin, I. A., Pryanishnikov, V. V., Kunnova, L. M., Rabinovich, Y. A., Martirosyan, D. M., & Orekhov, A. N. (2010). The effects of time-released garlic powder tablets on multifunctional cardiovascular risk in patients with coronary artery disease. *Lipids in Health and Disease*, *9*(1), 119. doi:10.1186/1476-511X-9-119 PMID:20958974

Society, P. (2005). JBS 2: Joint British Societies' guidelines on prevention of cardiovascular disease in clinical practice. *Heart (British Cardiac Society)*, *91*(suppl 5), v1–v52. doi:10.1136/hrt.2005.079988 PMID:16365341

Somaye, F., Marzieh, M. N., & Lale, N. (2008). Single cell protein (SCP) production from UF cheese whey by *Kluyveromyces marxianus. 18th National Congress on Food Technology.*

Soobrattee, M. A., Bahorun, T., & Aruoma, O. I. (2006). Chemopreventive actions of polyphenolic compounds in cancer. *BioFactors (Oxford, England)*, *27*(1–4), 19–35. doi:10.1002/biof.5520270103 PMID:17012761

Sotiroudis, T. G., & Kyrtopoulos, S. A. (2008). Anticarcinogenic compounds of olive oil and related biomarkers. *European Journal of Nutrition*, *47*(S2), 69–72. doi:10.100700394-008-2008-9 PMID:18458836

Soupas, L. (2006). *Oxidative stability of phytosterols in food models and foods* (Academic dissertation). University of Helsinki, Helsinki, Finland.

Soupas, L., Huikko, L., Lampi, A. M., & Piironen, V. (2005). Esterification affects phytosterol oxidation. *European Journal of Lipid Science and Technology*, *107*(2), 107–118. doi:10.1002/ejlt.200401096

Spence, J. T. (2006). Challenges related to the composition of functional foods. *Journal of Food Composition and Analysis*, *19*(SUPPL.), 2005–2007. doi:10.1016/j.jfca.2005.11.007

Spencer, E. A., Appleby, P. N., Davey, G. K., & Key, T. J. (2003). Diet and body mass index in 38000 EPIC-Oxford meat-eaters, fish-eaters, vegetarians and vegans. *International Journal of Obesity and Related Metabolic Disorders: Journal of the International Association for the Study of Obesity*, *27*(6), 728–734. doi:10.1038j.ijo.0802300 PMID:12833118

Spielman, A., Pollack, R. J., Kiszewski, A. E., & Telford, S. R. III. (2001). Issues in public health entomology. *Vector Borne and Zoonotic Diseases (Larchmont, N.Y.)*, *1*(1), 3–19. doi:10.1089/153036601750137606 PMID:12653132

Sporn, M. B., & Suh, N. (2000). Chemoprevention of cancer. *Carcinogenesis*, *21*(3), 525–530. doi:10.1093/carcin/21.3.525 PMID:10688873

Srinivasan, M., Sudheer, A. R., & Menon, V. P. (2007). Recent Advances in Indian Herbal Drug Research Guest Editor: Thomas Paul Asir Devasagayam Ferulic Acid: Therapeutic Potential Through Its Antioxidant Property. Journal of Clinical Biochemistry and Nutrition, 40(2), 92–100.

Stahl, W., & Sies, H. (2003). Antioxidant activity of carotenoids. *Molecular Aspects of Medicine*, *24*(6), 345–351. doi:10.1016/S0098-2997(03)00030-X PMID:14585305

Stamatelatou, K., Georgia, A., Tremouli, A., & Lyberatos, G. (2011). Production of gaseous biofuels and electricity from cheese whey. *Industrial & Engineering Chemistry Research*, *50*(2), 639–644. doi:10.1021/ie1002262

Stampfer, M. J., Hu, F. B., Manson, J. E., Rimm, E. B., & Willett, W. C. (2000). Primary Prevention of Coronary Heart Disease in Women through Diet and Lifestyle. *The New England Journal of Medicine*, *343*(1), 16–22. doi:10.1056/NEJM200007063430103 PMID:10882764

Stankiewicz, J., Panter, S. S., Neema, M., Arora, A., Batt, C. E., & Bakshi, R. (2007). Iron in Chronic Brain Disorders: Imaging and Neurotherapeutic Implications. *Neurotherapeutics; the Journal of the American Society for Experimental NeuroTherapeutics*, *4*(3), 371–386. doi:10.1016/j.nurt.2007.05.006 PMID:17599703

Steinberg, D. (1997). Low Density Lipoprotein Oxidation and Its Pathobiological Significance. *The Journal of Biological Chemistry*, *272*(34), 20963–20966. doi:10.1074/jbc.272.34.20963 PMID:9261091

Steinberg, D., & Witztum, J. L. (1990). Lipoproteins and Atherogenesis: Current Concepts. *Journal of the American Medical Association*, *264*(23), 3047–3052. doi:10.1001/jama.1990.03450230083034 PMID:2243434

Stephen, W. J. (2008). Variable Isoflavone Contents of Red Clover Products Affect Intestinal Disposition of Biochanin A, Formononetin, Genistein and Daidzein. *Journal of Alternative and Complementary Medicine (New York, N.Y.)*, *14*(3), 287–297. doi:10.1089/acm.2007.0617 PMID:18370585

Stienstra, R., Tack, C. J., Kanneganti, T. D., Joosten, L. A., & Netea, M. G. (2012). The inflammasome puts obesity in the danger zone. *Cell Metabolism*, *15*(1), 10–18. doi:10.1016/j.cmet.2011.10.011 PMID:22225872

Stojanovic, M. R., Biagi, E., Heilig, H. G., Kajander, K., Kekkonen, R. A., Tims, S., & De Vos, W. M. (2011). Signatures in fecal samples from patients with irritable bowel syndrome. *Gastroenterology*, *141*(5), 1792–1801. doi:10.1053/j.gastro.2011.07.043 PMID:21820992

Stone, N. J., Bilek, S., & Rosenbaum, S. (2005). Recent National Cholesterol Education Program Adult Treatment Panel III Update: Adjustments and Options. *The American Journal of Cardiology*, *96*(4suppl), 53E–59E. doi:10.1016/j.amjcard.2005.06.006 PMID:16098845

Story, E. N., Kopec, R. E., Schwartz, S. J., & Harris, G. K. (2010). An update on the health effects of tomato lycopene. *Annual Review of Food Science and Technology*, *1*(1), 189–210. doi:10.1146/annurev.food.102308.124120 PMID:22129335

Strachan, P. (2000). Family size, infection and atopy: the first 416 decade of the "hygiene hypothesis". *Thorax, 417*(55-1), S2–S10.

Stulnig, T. M. (2003). Immunomodulation by polyunsaturated fatty acids: Mechanisms and effects. *International Archives of Allergy and Immunology*, *132*(4), 310–321. doi:10.1159/000074898 PMID:14707462

Suekawa, M., Ishige, A., Yuasa, K., Sudo, K., Aburada, M., & Hosoya, E. (1984). Pharmacological studies on ginger. I. Pharmacological actions of pungent constitutents, (6)-gingerol and (6)-shogaol. *Journal of Pharmacobio-Dynamics*, *7*(11), 836–848. doi:10.1248/bpb1978.7.836 PMID:6335723

Suganami, T., Nishida, J., & Ogawa, Y. (2005). A paracrine loop between adipocytes and macrophages aggravates inflammatory changes: Role of free fatty acids and tumor necrosis factor α. *Arteriosclerosis, Thrombosis, and Vascular Biology*, *25*(10), 2062–2068. doi:10.1161/01.ATV.0000183883.72263.13 PMID:16123319

Suganami, T., Tanimoto-Koyama, K., Nishida, J., Itoh, M., Yuan, X., Mizuarai, S., ... Ogawa, Y. (2007). Role of the toll-like receptor 4/NF-κB pathway in saturated fatty acid induced inflammatory changes in the interaction between adipocytes and macrophages. *Arteriosclerosis, Thrombosis, and Vascular Biology*, *27*(1), 84–91. doi:10.1161/01.ATV.0000251608.09329.9a PMID:17082484

Sumpio, B. E., Cordova, A. C., Berke-Schlessel, D. W., Qin, F., & Chen, Q. H. (2006). Green tea, the "Asian paradox," and cardiovascular disease. *Journal of the American College of Surgeons*, *202*(5), 813–825. doi:10.1016/j.jamcollsurg.2006.01.018 PMID:16648021

Sun, H.-X., Xie, Y., & Ye, Y.-P. (2009). Advances in saponin-based adjuvants. *Vaccine*, *27*(12), 1787–1796. doi:10.1016/j.vaccine.2009.01.091 PMID:19208455

Sunitha, Nandha Kishore Chary, & Hemalatha, & Unissa. (2016). A Review on Nutraceuticals. *International Journal of Pharmaceutical Research And Bio-Science.*, *5*(1), 123–135.

Sunkara, R., & Verghese, M. (2014). Functional foods for obesity management. *Food and Nutrition Sciences*, *5*(14), 1359–1369. doi:10.4236/fns.2014.514148

Surawicz, C. M., McFarland, L. V., Greenberg, R. N., Rubin, M., Fekety, R., Mulligan, M. E., ... Elmer, G. W. (2003). The search for a better treatment for recurrent Clostridium difficile disease: Use of high-dose vancomycin combined with *Saccharomyces boulardii. Clinical Infectious Diseases*, *31*(4), 1012–1017. doi:10.1086/318130 PMID:11049785

Surh, Y.-J. (2002). Anti-tumor promoting potential of selected spice ingredients with antioxidative and anti-inflammatory activities: A short review. *Food and Chemical Toxicology : An International Journal Published for the British Industrial Biological Research Association*, *40*(8), 1091–1097. doi:10.1016/S0278-6915(02)00037-6 PMID:12067569

Surh, Y.-J. (2003). Cancer Chemoprevention with Dietary Phytochemicals. *National Review*, *3*(10), 768–780. doi:10.1038/nrc1189 PMID:14570043

Suzuki, M., Yoshioka, M., Hashimoto, M., Murakami, M., Noya, M., Takahashi, D., & Urashima, M. (2013). Randomized, double-blind, placebo-controlled trial of vitamin D supplementation in Parkinson disease. *The American Journal of Clinical Nutrition*, *97*(5), 1004–1013. doi:10.3945/ajcn.112.051664 PMID:23485413

Switzer, C. H., Ridnour, L., Cheng, R. Y. S., Sparatore, A., Del Soldato, P., Moody, T. W., ... Wink, D. A. (2009). Dithiolethione compounds inhibit Akt signaling in human breast and lung cancer cells by increasing PP2A activity. *Oncogene*, *28*(43), 3837–3846. doi:10.1038/onc.2009.244 PMID:19701246

Sýkora, J., Valecková, K., Amlerová, J., & ... . (2005). Effects of a specially designed fermented milk product containing probiotic *Lactobacillus casei*dn-114 001 and the eradication of *H. pylori* in children: A prospective randomized double-blind study. *Journal of Clinical Gastroenterology*, *39*, 692–698. doi:10.1097/01.mcg.0000173855.77191.44 PMID:16082279

Szajewska, H., Horvath, A., & Piwowarczyk, A. (2010). Meta-analysis: The effects of *Saccharomyces boulardii* supplementation on *Helicobacter pylori* eradication rates and side effects during treatment. *Alimentary Pharmacology & Therapeutics*, *32*(9), 1069–1079. doi:10.1111/j.1365-2036.2010.04457.x PMID:21039671

Szajewska, H., Kotowska, M., Mrukowicz, J. Z., Armańska, M., & Mikołajczyk, W. (2001). Efficacy of *Lactobacillus* GG in prevention of nosocomial diarrhea in infants. *The Journal of Pediatrics*, *138*, 361–365. doi:10.1067/mpd.2001.111321 PMID:11241043

Szewczuk, L. M., Forti, L., Stivala, L. A., & Penning, T. M. (2004). Resveratrol is a peroxidase mediated inactivator of COX-1 but not COX-2: A mechanistic approach to the design of COX-1 selective agents. *The Journal of Biological Chemistry*, *279*(21), 22727–22737. doi:10.1074/jbc.M314302200 PMID:15020596

Szyman'ski, H., Pejcz, J., Jawien´, M., Chmielarczyk, A., Strus, M., & Heczko, P. B. (2006). Treatment of acute infectious diarrhoea in infants and children with a mixture of three *Lactobacillus rhamnosus*strains—a randomized, double-blind, placebo-controlled trial. *Alimentary Pharmacology & Therapeutics*, *23*(2), 247–253. doi:10.1111/j.1365-2036.2006.02740.x PMID:16393304

Taipale, S. J., Hiltunen, M., Vuorio, K., & Peltomaa, E. (2016). Suitability of Phytosterols alongside Fatty Acids as Chemotaxonomic Biomarkers for Phytoplankton. *Frontiers in Plant Science*, *7*, 212. doi:10.3389/fpls.2016.00212 PMID:26973664

Takahashi, Y., Otsuki, A., Mori, Y., Kawakami, Y., & Ito, H. (2015). Inhibition of leukocyte-type 12-lipoxygenase by guava tea leaves prevents development of atherosclerosis. *Food Chemistry*, *186*, 2–5. doi:10.1016/j.foodchem.2015.03.105 PMID:25976783

Tapas, A. R., Sakarkar, D. M., & Kakde, R. B. (2008). Flavonoids as nutraceuticals: A review. *Tropical Journal of Pharmaceutical Research*, *7*(3), 1089–1099. doi:10.4314/tjpr.v7i3.14693

Tarozzi, A., Angeloni, C., Malaguti, M., Morroni, F., Hrelia, S., & Hrelia, P. (2013). Sulforaphane as a Potential Protective Phytochemical against Neurodegenerative Diseases. *Oxidative Medicine and Cellular Longevity*, *2013*, e415078. doi:10.1155/2013/415078 PMID:23983898

Tarride, J.-E., Lim, M., DesMeules, M., Luo, W., Burke, N., O'Reilly, D., ... Goeree, R. (2009). A review of the cost of cardiovascular disease. *The Canadian Journal of Cardiology*, *25*(6), e195–e202. doi:10.1016/S0828-282X(09)70098-4 PMID:19536390

Tasan, B.M., Bilgin, U., & Gecgel, A.S., & Demirci. (2006). Phytosterols as functional food ingredients. *Tekirdag Ziraat Fakültesi Dergisi*, *3*(2), 153–159.

Tatli, I. I. (2015). Ginkgo biloba Extracts in Neurological Disorders Therapy: Clinical Trials. In R. R. Watson & V. R. Preedy (Eds.), *Bioactive Nutraceuticals and Dietary Supplements in Neurological and Brain Disease* (pp. 113–124). San Diego, CA: Academic Press. doi:10.1016/B978-0-12-411462-3.00012-6

Taylor, A. J., Burke, A. P., O'Malley, P. G., Farb, A., Malcolm, G. T., Smialek, J., & Virmani, R. (2000). A Comparison of The Framingham Risk Index, Coronary Artery Calcification, and Culprit Plaque Morphology in Sudden Cardiac Death. *Circulation*, *101*(11), 1243–1248. doi:10.1161/01.CIR.101.11.1243 PMID:10725282

Taylor, A. L., Hale, J., Wiltschut, J., Lehmann, H., Dunstan, J. A., & Prescott, S. L. (2006). Effects of probiotic supplementation for the first 6 months of life on allergen- and vaccine-specific immune responses. *Clinical and Experimental Allergy*, *36*(10), 1227–1235. doi:10.1111/j.1365-2222.2006.02553.x PMID:17014429

Taylor, S., Scuffham, P. A., McCollam, P. L., & Newby, D. E. (2007). Acute coronary syndromes in Europe: 1-year costs and outcomes. *Current Medical Research and Opinion*, *23*(3), 495–503. doi:10.1185/030079906X167462 PMID:17355731

Thaipisuttikul, P., & Galvin, J. E. (2012). Use of medical foods and nutritional approaches in the treatment of Alzheimer's disease. *Clinical Practice (London, England)*, *9*(2), 199–209. doi:10.2217/cpr.12.3 PMID:23362453

Thanh, T. T., Vergnes, M. F., Kaloustian, J., El-Moselhy, T. F., Amiot-Carlin, M. J., & Portugal, H. (2006). Effect of storage and heating on phytosterol concentrations in vegetable oils determined by GC/MS. *Journal of the Science of Food and Agriculture*, *86*(2), 220–225. doi:10.1002/jsfa.2322

Thannickal, V. J., & Fanburg, B. L. (2000). Reactive oxygen species in cell signaling. *American Journal of Physiology. Lung Cellular and Molecular Physiology*, *279*(6), L1005–L1028. doi:10.1152/ajplung.2000.279.6.L1005 PMID:11076791

The Nutritional Characteristics of a Contemporary Diet Based Upon Paleolithic Food Groups Abstract 4 I Diet (Nutrition). (n.d.). Retrieved April 13, 2017, from https://www.scribd.com/ document/94643426/The-Nutritional-Characteristics-of-a-Contemporary-Diet-Based-UponPaleolithic-Food-Groups-Abstract-4

Theuwissen, E., & Mensink, R. P. (2007). Simultaneous intake of beta-glucan and plant stanol esters affects lipid metabolism in slightly hyper-cholesterolemic subjects. *The Journal of Nutrition*, *137*(3), 583–588. doi:10.1093/jn/137.3.583 PMID:17311944

Thomä-Worringer, C., Sørensen, J., & López-Fandiño, R. (2006). Health effects and technological features of caseinomacropeptide. *International Dairy Journal*, *16*(11), 1324–1333. doi:10.1016/j.idairyj.2006.06.012

Thompson, G. A. Jr. (1996). Lipids and membrane function in green algae. *Biochimica et Biophysica Acta*, *1302*(1), 17–45. doi:10.1016/0005-2760(96)00045-8 PMID:8695653

Tian, N., Penman, A. D., Manning, R. D. Jr, Flessner, M. F., & Mawson, A. R. (2012). Association between Circulating Specific Leukocyte Types and Incident Chronic Kidney Disease: The Atherosclerosis Risk in Communities (ARIC) Study. *Journal of the American Society of Hypertension*, *6*(2), 100–108. doi:10.1016/j.jash.2011.10.001 PMID:22054781

Ting, Y., Jiang, Y., Ho, C. T., & Huang, Q. (2014). Common delivery systems for enhancing in vivo bioavailability and biological efficacy of nutraceuticals. *Journal of Functional Foods*, *7*, 112–128. doi:10.1016/j.jff.2013.12.010

Todoric, J., Löffler, M., Huber, J., Bilban, M., Reimers, M., Kadl, A., ... Stulnig, T. M. (2006). Adipose tissue inflammation induced by high-fat diet in obese diabetic mice is prevented by n-3 polyunsaturated fatty acids. *Diabetologia*, *49*(9), 2109–2119. doi:10.100700125-006-0300-x PMID:16783472

Tomkin, G. H., & Owens, D. (2011). The chylomicron: Relationship to atherosclerosis. *International Journal of Vascular Medicine*. PMID:22007304

Touyz, R. M. (2012). New insights into mechanisms of hypertension. *Current Opinion in Nephrology and Hypertension*, *21*(2), 119–121. doi:10.1097/MNH.0b013e328350a50f PMID:22257800

Traber, M. G., & Stevens, J. F. (2011). Vitamins C and E: Beneficial effects from a mechanistic perspective. *Free Radical Biology & Medicine*, *51*(5), 1000–1013. doi:10.1016/j.freeradbiomed.2011.05.017 PMID:21664268

Trachootham, D., Alexandre, J., & Huang, P. (2009). Targeting cancer cells by ROS-mediated mechanisms: A radical therapeutic approach? *Nature Reviews. Drug Discovery*, *8*(7), 579–591. doi:10.1038/nrd2803 PMID:19478820

Tranjan, B. C., Cruz, A. G., Walter, E. H. M., Faria, J. A. F., Bolini, H. M. A., Moura, M. R. L., & Carvalho, L. M. J. (2009). Development of goat cheese whey-flavoured beverages. *International Journal of Dairy Technology*, *62*(3), 438–443. doi:10.1111/j.1471-0307.2009.00491.x

Tran, T. T., Medline, A., & Bruce, W. R. (1996). Insulin promotion of colon tumors in rats. *Cancer Epidemiology, Biomarkers & Prevention*, *5*(12), 1013–1015. PMID:8959325

Tripathi, M. K., & Giri, K. (2014). Probiotic functional foods: Survival of probiotics during processing and storage. *Journal of Functional Foods*, *9*(1), 225–241. doi:10.1016/j.jff.2014.04.030

Tsao, A. S., Kim, E. S., & Hong, W. K. (2004). Chemoprevention of Cancer. *CA: a Cancer Journal for Clinicians*, *54*(3), 150–180. doi:10.3322/canjclin.54.3.150 PMID:15195789

Tse, W. Y., Maxwell, S. R., Thomason, H., Blann, A., Thorpe, G. H., Waite, M., & Holder, R. (1994). Antioxidant status in controlled and uncontrolled hypertension and its relationship to endothelial damage. *Journal of Human Hypertension*, *8*(11), 843–849. PMID:7853328

Tsuchida, A., Yamauchi, T., Takekawa, S., Hada, Y., Ito, Y., Maki, T., & Kadowaki, T. (2005). Peroxisome proliferator-activated receptor (PPAR) α activation increases adiponectin receptors and reduces obesity-related inflammation in adipose tissue: Comparison of activation of PPARα, PPARγ, and their combination. *Diabetes*, *54*(12), 3358–3370. doi:10.2337/diabetes.54.12.3358 PMID:16306350

Tsuda, T. (2008). Regulation of adipocyte function by anthocyanins; possibility of preventing the metabolic syndrome. *Journal of Agricultural and Food Chemistry*, *56*(3), 642–646. doi:10.1021/jf073113b PMID:18211021

Tuekpe, M. K.-N., Todoriki, H., Sasaki, S., Zheng, K.-C., & Ariizumi, M. (2006). Potassium excretion in healthy Japanese women was increased by a dietary intervention utilizing home-parcel delivery of Okinawan vegetables. *Hypertension Research: Official Journal of the Japanese Society of Hypertension*, *29*(6), 389–396. doi:10.1291/hypres.29.389 PMID:16940700

Tung, J. M., Dolovich, L. R., & Lee, C. H. (2009). Prevention of *Clostridium dif-ficile*infection with *Saccharomyces boulardii*: A systematicreview. *Canadian Journal of Gastroenterology*, *23*(12), 817–821. doi:10.1155/2009/915847 PMID:20011734

Turnbaugh, P. J., & Gordon, J. I. (2009). The core gut microbiome, energy balance and obesity. *The Journal of Physiology*, *587*(17), 4153–4158. doi:10.1113/jphysiol.2009.174136 PMID:19491241

Turnbaugh, P. J., Hamady, M., Yatsunenko, T., Cantarel, B. L., Duncan, A., Ley, R. E., ... Gordon, J. I. (2009). A core gutmicrobiome in obese and lean twins. *Nature*, *457*(7228), 480–484. doi:10.1038/nature07540 PMID:19043404

Turnbaugh, P. J., Ley, R. E., Mahowald, M. A., Magrini, V., Mardis, E. R., & Gordon, J. I. (2006). An obesity-associated gut microbiome with increased capacity for energy harvest. *Nature*, *444*(7122), 1027–1031. doi:10.1038/nature05414 PMID:17183312

Turroni, F., Ventura, M., Buttó, L. F., Duranti, S., O'Toole, P. W., Motherway, M. O., & Van Sinderen, D. (2014). Molecular dialogue between the human gut microbiota and the host: A *Lactobacillus* and *Bifidobacterium* perspective. *Cellular and Molecular Life Sciences*, *71*(2), 183–203. doi:10.100700018-013-1318-0 PMID:23516017

Tursi, A., Brandimarte, G., Giorgetti, G. M., Forti, G., Modeo, M. E., & Gigliobianco, A. (2004). Low-dose balsalazide plus a high-potency probiotic preparation is more effective than balsalazide alone or mesalazine in the treatment of acute mild-to-moderate ulcerative colitis. *Medical Science Monitor, 10*, PI126–PI131. PMID:15507864

Tu, S.-H., Ku, C.-Y., Ho, C.-T., Chen, C.-S., Huang, C.-S., Lee, C.-H., & Ho, Y.-S. (2011). Tea polyphenol (-)-epigallocatechin-3-gallate inhibits nicotine- and estrogen-induced α9-nicotinic acetylcholine receptor upregulation in human breast cancer cells. *Molecular Nutrition & Food Research, 55*(3), 455–466. doi:10.1002/mnfr.201000254 PMID:21370452

Uedo, N., Tatsuta, M., Iishi, H., Baba, M., Sakai, N., Yano, H., & Otani, T. (1999). Inhibition by D-limonene of gastric carcinogenesis induced by N-methyl-N'-nitro-N-nitrosoguanidine in Wistar rats. *Cancer Letters, 137*(2), 131–136.

Ueeda, M., Doumei, T., Takaya, Y., Shinohata, R., Katayama, Y., Ohnishi, N., ... Kusachi, S. (2008). Serum N-3 polyunsaturated fatty acid levels correlate with the extent of coronary plaques and calcifications in patients with acute myocardial infarction. *Circulation Journal, 72*(11), 1836–1843. doi:10.1253/circj.CJ-08-0249 PMID:18812674

Uicich, R., Pizarro, F., Almeida, C., Díaz, M., Boccio, J., Zubillaga, M., & O'Donnell, A. (1999). Bioavailability of microencapsulated ferrous sulfate in fluid cow's milk.Studies in human beings. *Nutrition Research (New York, N.Y.), 19*(6), 893–897. doi:10.1016/S0271-5317(99)00049-4

Ungvari, Z., Buffenstein, R., Austad, S. N., Podlutsky, A., Kaley, G., & Csiszar, A. (2008). Oxidative stress in vascular senescence: Lessons from successfully aging species. *Frontiers in Bioscience, 13*(13), 5056–5070. doi:10.2741/3064 PMID:18508570

Ungvari, Z., Kaley, G., de Cabo, R., Sonntag, W. E., & Csiszar, A. (2010). A. Mechanisms of vascular aging: New perspectives. *The Journals of Gerontology. Series A, Biological Sciences and Medical Sciences, 65*(10), 1028–1041. doi:10.1093/gerona/glq113 PMID:20576649

United Nations Food and Agriculture Organization of the United Nations/World Health Organization (UNFAO/WHO). (2001). *Health and Nutritional Properties of Probiotics in Food including Powder Milk with Live Lactic Acid Bacteria*. Retrieved from http://ftp.fao.org/es/esn/food/probio_report_en.pdf

United Nations Food and Agriculture Organization of the United Nations/World Health Organization (UNFAO/WHO). (2002). *Guidelines for the Evaluation of Probiotics in Food.* Retrieved from http://ftp.fao.org/es/esn/food/wgreport2.pdf

Upadhyay, J., Kesharwani, R. K., & Misra, K. (2009). Comparative study of antioxidants as cancer preventives through inhibition of HIF-1 alpha activity. *Bioinformation, 4*(6), 233–236. doi:10.6026/97320630004233 PMID:20975915

USFDA. (2015, July 25). *Consumer Updates - FDA 101: Dietary Supplements*. Retrieved April 14, 2017, from https://www.fda.gov/ForConsumers/ConsumerUpdates/ucm050803.htm

USFDA. (2016, July 26). *Dietary Supplement Products & Ingredients*. Retrieved March 17, 2017, from https://www.fda.gov/Food/DietarySupplements/ProductsIngredients/

Valko, M., Leibfritz, D., Moncol, J., Cronin, M. T., Mazur, M., & Telser, J. (2007). Free radicals and antioxidants in normal physiological functions and human disease. *The International Journal of Biochemistry & Cell Biology*, *39*(1), 44–84. doi:10.1016/j.biocel.2006.07.001 PMID:16978905

van den Broek, N. (1996). The aetiology of anemia in pregnancy in West Africa. *Tropical Doctor*, *26*(1), 5–7. doi:10.1177/004947559602600103 PMID:8693577

Vance, J. E. (2008). Thematic Review Series: Glycerolipids. Phosphatidylserine and phosphatidylethanolamine in mammalian cells: two metabolically related aminophospholipids. *Journal of Lipid Research*, *49*(7), 1377–1387. doi:10.1194/jlr.R700020-JLR200 PMID:18204094

Vandenplas, Y., Brunser, O., & Szajewska, H. (2009). *Saccharomyces boulardii*in childhood. *European Journal of Pediatrics*, *168*(3), 253–265. doi:10.100700431-008-0879-7 PMID:19096876

Vandenplas, Y., Huys, G., & Daube, G. (2015). Probiotics: An update. *Jornal de Pediatria*, *91*(1), 6–21. doi:10.1016/j.jped.2014.08.005 PMID:25458874

Vartiainen, E., Laatikainen, T., Peltonen, M., Juolevi, A., Männistö, S., Sundvall, J., ... Puska, P. (2010). Thirty-five-year trends in cardiovascular risk factors in Finland. *International Journal of Epidemiology*, *39*(2), 504–518. doi:10.1093/ije/dyp330 PMID:19959603

Veerappan, G. R., Betteridge, J., & Young, P. E. (2012). Probiotics for the treatment of inflammatory bowel disease. *Current Gastroenterology Reports*, *14*(4), 324–333. doi:10.100711894-012-0265-5 PMID:22581276

Velikov, K. P., & Pelan, E. (2008). Colloidal delivery systems for micronutrients and nutraceuticals. *Soft Matter*, *4*(10), 1964–1980. doi:10.1039/b804863k

Venkatachalam, H., Nayak, Y., & Jayashree, B. S. (2012). Synthesis, Characterization and Antioxidant Activities of Synthetic Chalcones and Flavones. *APCBEE Procedia*, *3*, 209–213.

Venkatramesh, M., Karunanandaa, B., Sun, B., Gunter, C. A., Boddupalli, S., & Kishore, G. M. (2003). Expression of a streptomyces 3-hydroxysteroid oxidase geve in oilseeds for converting phytosterols to phytostanols. *Phytochemistry*, *62*(1), 39–46. doi:10.1016/S0031-9422(02)00431-4 PMID:12475617

Ventura, M., Meylan, V., & Zink, R. (2003). Identification and tracing of *Bifidobacterium* species by use of enterobacterial repetitive intergenic consensus sequences. *Journal of Applied and Environmental Microbiology*, *69*(7), 4296–4301. doi:10.1128/AEM.69.7.4296-4301.2003 PMID:12839818

Viljanen, M., Savilahti, E., Haahtela, T., Juntunen-Backman, K., Korpela, R., Poussa, T., ... Kuitunen, M. (2005). Probiotics in the treatment of atopic eczema/dermatitis syndrome in infants: A double-blind placebo-controlled trial. *Allergy*, *60*(4), 494–500. doi:10.1111/j.1398-9995.2004.00514.x PMID:15727582

Vinson, J. A., Bose, P., Proch, J., Al Kharrat, H., & Samman, N. (2008). Cranberries and Cranberry Products: Powerful in Vitro, ex Vivo, and in Vivo Sources of Antioxidants. *Journal of Agricultural and Food Chemistry, 56*(14), 5884–5891. doi:10.1021/jf073309b PMID:18558697

Vitali, B., Ndagijimana, M., Maccaferri, S., Biagi, E., Guerzoni, M. E., & Brigidi, P. (2012). An *in vitro* evaluation of the effect of probiotics and prebiotics on the metabolic profile of human microbiota. *Anaerobe, 18*(4), 386–391. doi:10.1016/j.anaerobe.2012.04.014 PMID:22579985

Viteri, F. E., Álvarez, E., Batres, R., Torun, B., Pineda, O., Mejía, L. A., & Sylvi, J. (1995). Fortification of sugar with iron sodium ethylenediaminotetraacetate (FeNaEDTA) improves iron status in semirural Guatemalan populations. *The American Journal of Clinical Nutrition, 61*(5), 1153–1163. doi:10.1093/ajcn/61.5.1153 PMID:7733042

Vitolins, M. Z., Anderson, A. M., Delahanty, L., Raynor, H., Miller, G. D., Mobley, C., ... Mayer-Davis, E. (2009). Action for Health in Diabetes (Look AHEAD) Trial: Baseline evaluation of selected nutrients and food group intake. *Journal of the American Dietetic Association, 109*(8), 1367–1375. doi:10.1016/j.jada.2009.05.016 PMID:19631042

Vizoso Pinto, M. G., Rodríguez Gómez, M., Seifert, S., Waltz, B., Holzapfel, W. H., & Franz, C. M. (2009). Lactobacilli stimultates the innate immune response and modulate TLR expression of HT29 intestinal epithelial cells in vitro. *International Journal of Food Microbiology, 133*(1-2), 86–93. doi:10.1016/j.ijfoodmicro.2009.05.013 PMID:19523707

Volpi, E., Kobayashi, H., Sheffield-Moore, M., Mittendorfer, B., & Wolfe, R. R. (2003). Essential amino acids are primarily responsible for the amino acid stimulation of muscle protein anabolism in healthy elderly adults. *The American Journal of Clinical Nutrition, 78*(5), 250–258. doi:10.1093/ajcn/78.2.250 PMID:12885705

Vongpatanasin, W., Thomas, G. D., Schwartz, R., Cassis, L. A., Osborne-Lawrence, S., Hahner, L., ... Shaul, P. W. (2007). C-reactive protein causes downregulation of vascular angiotensin subtype 2 receptors and systolic hypertension in mice. *Circulation, 115*(8), 1020–1028. doi:10.1161/CIRCULATIONAHA.106.664854 PMID:17283257

Voutilainen, S., Nurmi, T., Mursu, J., & Rissanen, T. H. (2006). Carotenoids and cardiovascular health. *The American Journal of Clinical Nutrition, 83*(6), 1265–1271. doi:10.1093/ajcn/83.6.1265 PMID:16762935

Vural, H., Demirin, H., Kara, Y., Eren, I., & Delibas, N. (2010). Alterations of plasma magnesium, copper, zinc, iron and selenium concentrations and some related erythrocyte antioxidant enzyme activities in patients with Alzheimer's disease. *Journal of Trace Elements in Medicine and Biology, 24*(3), 169–173. doi:10.1016/j.jtemb.2010.02.002 PMID:20569929

Wade, W. G. (2013). The oral microbiome in health and disease. *Pharmacological Research, 69*(1), 137–143. doi:10.1016/j.phrs.2012.11.006 PMID:23201354

Walford, R. L., Mock, D., Verdery, R., & MacCallum, T. (2002). Calorie restriction in biosphere 2: Alterations in physiologic, hematologic, hormonal, and biochemical parameters in humans restricted for a 2-year period. *The Journals of Gerontology. Series A, Biological Sciences and Medical Sciences*, *57*(6), B211–B224. doi:10.1093/gerona/57.6.B211 PMID:12023257

Wall, M. M. (2006). Ascorbic acid, vitamin A, and mineral composition of banana (Musa sp.) and papaya (Carica papaya) cultivars grown in Hawaii. *Journal of Food Composition and Analysis*, *19*(5), 434–445. doi:10.1016/j.jfca.2006.01.002

Wang, G., & Hollingsworth, R. I. (1999). Synthetic routes to L-carnitine and L-gamma-amino-beta-hydroxybutyric acid from (S)-3-hydroxybutyrolactone by functional group priority switching. *Tetrahedron, Asymmetry*, *10*(10), 1895–1901. doi:10.1016/S0957-4166(99)00169-X

Wang, I. K., Wu, Y. Y., Yang, Y. F., Ting, I. W., Lin, C. C., Yen, T. H., ... Lin, H. C. (2015). The effect of probiotics on serum levels of cytokine and endotoxin in peritoneal dialysis patients: A randomised, double-blind, placebo-controlled trial. *Beneficial Microbes*, *6*(4), 423–430. doi:10.3920/BM2014.0088 PMID:25609654

Wang, J. Z., Du, W. T., Xu, Y. L., Cheng, S. Z., & Liu, Z. J. (2017). Gut microbiome-based medical methodologies for early-stage disease prevention. *Microbial Pathogenesis*, *105*, 122–130. doi:10.1016/j.micpath.2017.02.024 PMID:28219830

Wang, L.-S., & Stoner, G. D. (2008). Anthocyanins and their role in cancer prevention. *Cancer Letters*, *269*(2), 281–290. doi:10.1016/j.canlet.2008.05.020 PMID:18571839

Wang, S., Yang, D., & Lippman, M. E. (2003). Targeting Bcl-2 and Bcl-XL with nonpeptidic small-molecule antagonists. *Seminars in Oncology*, *30*(5Suppl 16), 133–142. doi:10.1053/j.seminoncol.2003.08.015 PMID:14613034

Wang, X., & Michaelis, E. K. (2010). Selective neuronal vulnerability to oxidative stress in the brain. *Frontiers in Aging Neuroscience*, *2*, 12. PMID:20552050

Wang, Y.-J., Thomas, P., Zhong, J.-H., Bi, F.-F., Kosaraju, S., Pollard, A., & Zhou, X.-F. (2009). Consumption of grape seed extract prevents amyloid-beta deposition and attenuates inflammation in brain of an Alzheimer's disease mouse. *Neurotoxicity Research*, *15*(1), 3–14. doi:10.100712640-009-9000-x PMID:19384583

Wang, Y., & Kasper, L. H. (2014). The role of microbiome in central nervous system disorders. *Brain, Behavior, and Immunity*, *38*(5), 1–12. doi:10.1016/j.bbi.2013.12.015 PMID:24370461

Ward, S., Chackalamannil, S., & Rotella, D. (2017). Comprehensive. *Medicinal Chemistry (Shariqah, United Arab Emirates)*, III. PMID:28724914

Watkinsa, M., & Nash, D. (2010). Dairy factory wastewaters, their use on land and possible environmental impacts – A mini review. *The Open Agriculture Journal*, *4*(1), 1–9. doi:10.2174/1874331501004010001

Watson, R. R., Gerald, J. K., & Preedy, V. R. (Eds.). (2011). *Nutrients, dietary supplements, and nutriceuticals: cost analysis versus clinical benefits*. New York: Humana Press.

Wei, W., Liu, Y.-H., Zhang, C.-E., Wang, Q., Wei, Z., Mousseau, D. D., & Liu, G.-P. (2011). Folate/vitamin-B12 prevents chronic hyperhomocysteinemia-induced tau hyperphosphorylation and memory deficits in aged rats. *Journal of Alzheimer's Disease. JAD, 27*(3), 639–650. PMID:21860088

Welberg, J. W., Monkelbaan, J. F., de Vries, E. G., Muskiet, F. A., Cats, A., Oremus, E. T., ... Kleibeuker, J. H. (1994). Effects of supplemental dietary calcium on quantitative and qualitative fecal fat excretion in man. *Annals of Nutrition & Metabolism, 38*(4), 185–191. doi:10.1159/000177810 PMID:7832578

Weltgesundheitsorganisation (Ed.). (2002). *Reducing risks, promoting healthy life*. Geneva: World Health Organization.

Westcott, N. R., & Muir, A. D. (2003). Flax seed lignan in disease prevention and health promotion. *Phytochemistry Reviews, 2*(3), 401–407. doi:10.1023/B:PHYT.0000046174.97809.b6

Westerterp-Plantenga, M. S. (2010). Green Tea Catechins, Caffeine and Body-Weight Regulation. *Physiology & Behavior, 100*(1), 42–46. doi:10.1016/j.physbeh.2010.02.005 PMID:20156466

Wetmur, J. G. (1976). Hybridization and renaturation kinetics of nucleic acids. *Annual Review of Biophysics and Bioengineering, 5*(1), 337–361. doi:10.1146/annurev.bb.05.060176.002005 PMID:7992

Whelton, S. P., Hyre, A. D., Pedersen, B., Yi, Y., Whelton, P. K., & He, J. (2005). Effect of dietary fiber intake on blood pressure: A meta-analysis of randomized, controlled clinical trials. *Journal of Hypertension, 23*(3), 475–481. doi:10.1097/01.hjh.0000160199.51158.cf PMID:15716684

WHO. (2007). *Prevention of cardiovascular disease*. World Health Organization.

Wildman, R. E. (Ed.). (2016). *Handbook of nutraceuticals and functional foods*. CRC press.

Williams, L. (2002). Third report of the National Cholesterol Education Program (NCEP) expert panel on detection, evaluation, and treatment of high blood cholesterol in adults (Adult Treatment Panel III) final report. *Circulation, 106*(25), 3143–3143. PMID:12485966

Wills, M. R., & Savory, J. (1989). Aluminum and chronic renal failure: Sources, absorption, transport, and toxicity. *Critical Reviews in Clinical Laboratory Sciences, 27*(1), 59–107. doi:10.3109/10408368909106590 PMID:2647415

Wilson, P. W., D'Agostino, R. B., Levy, D., Belanger, A. M., Silbershatz, H., & Kannel, W. B. (1998). Prediction of coronary heart disease using risk factor categories. *Circulation, 97*(18), 1837–1847. doi:10.1161/01.CIR.97.18.1837 PMID:9603539

Wilson, W. (1994). Established Risk Factors And Coronary Artery Disease. *American Journal of Hypertension, 7*(7_Pt_2), 7S–12S. doi:10.1093/ajh/7.7.7S PMID:7946184

Wine, E., Gareau, M. G., Henry, J. K., & Sherman, P. M. (2009). Strain-specific probiotic (*Lactobacillus helveticus*) inhibition of *Campylobacter jejuni* invasion of human intestinal epithelial cells. *FEMS Microbiology Letters*, *300*(1), 146–152. doi:10.1111/j.1574-6968.2009.01781.x PMID:19765084

Wiseman, H., O'Reilly, J. D., Adlercreutz, H., Mallet, A. I., Bowey, E. A., Rowland, I. R., & Sanders, T. A. (2000). Isoflavone phytoestrogens consumed in soy decrease F(2)-isoprostane concentrations and increase resistance of low-density lipoprotein to oxidation in humans. *The American Journal of Clinical Nutrition*, *72*(2), 395–400. doi:10.1093/ajcn/72.2.395 PMID:10919933

Wisnewsky, A. J., & Clément, K. (2016). The gut microbiome, diet, and links to cardiometabolic and chronic disorders. *Nature Reviews. Nephrology*, *12*(3), 169–181. doi:10.1038/nrneph.2015.191 PMID:26616538

Woodgate, D. E., & Conquer, J. A. (2003). Prevalence of self-treatment with complementary products and therapies for weight loss: A randomized, cross-sectional Study in Overweight and Obese Patients in Colombia. *Curr Thera Res*, *64*, 248–262. doi:10.1016/S0011-393X(03)00058-4

World Health Organization Fact Sheet: Obesity and Overweight. (n.d.). Retrieved from http://www.who.int/mediacentre/factsheets/fs311/en/

World Health Organization. (2009). *Cardiovascular disease; Fact sheet N°317. Geneva,473.* World Health Organization.

World Health Organization. (2010). *Global strategy on diet, physical activity and health.* Retrieved from http://www.who.int/dietphysicalactivity/publications/facts/obesity/en/

World Health Organization. (2015). *The global prevalence of anemia in 2011.* WHO.

Woyengo, T. A., Ramprasath, V. R., & Jones, P. J. H. (2009). Anti-cancer effects of phytosterols. *European Journal of Clinical Nutrition*, *63*(7), 813–820. doi:10.1038/ejcn.2009.29 PMID:19491917

Wullt, M., Hagslätt, M. L., & Odenholt, I. (2003). Lactobacillus plantarum 299v forthe treatment of recurrent Clostridium difficile-associated diarrhoea: A doubleblind,placebo-controlled trial. *Scandinavian Journal of Infectious Diseases*, *35*(6-7), 365–367. doi:10.1080/00365540310010985 PMID:12953945

Wynne, K., Stanley, S., McGowan, B., & Bloom, S. (2005). Appetite control. *The Journal of Endocrinology*, *184*(2), 291–318. doi:10.1677/joe.1.05866 PMID:15684339

Xia, S., & Xu, S. (2005). Ferrous sulfate liposomes: Preparation, stability and application in fluid milk. *Food Research International*, *38*(3), 289–296. doi:10.1016/j.foodres.2004.04.010

Xing, T., Wang, F., Li, J., & Wang, N. (2012). Hypertension: An immunologic disease? *Journal of Hypertension*, *30*(12), 2440–2441. doi:10.1097/HJH.0b013e32835953f9 PMID:23151885

Xu, H., Barnes, G. T., Yang, Q., Tan, G., Yang, D., Chou, C. J., ... Chen, H. (2003). Chronic inflammation in fat plays a crucial role in the development of obesity-related insulin resistance. *The Journal of Clinical Investigation*, *112*(12), 1821–1830. doi:10.1172/JCI200319451 PMID:14679177

Xu, J., Kochanek, K., Murphy, S., & Tejada-Vera, B. (2010). Deaths: Final data for 2007. *National Vital Statistics Reports*, *58*, 1–136. PMID:25075874

Yadav, H., Lee, J. H., Lloyd, J., Walter, P., & Rane, S. G. (2013). Beneficial metabolic effects of a probiotic via butyrate induced GLP-1 secretion. *The Journal of Biological Chemistry*, *288*(35), 25088–25097. doi:10.1074/jbc.M113.452516 PMID:23836895

Yamada, T., Hayasaka, S., Shibata, Y., Ojima, T., Saegusa, T., Gotoh, T., ... Kayaba, K. (2011). Frequency of Citrus Fruit Intake Is Associated With the Incidence of Cardiovascular Disease: The Jichi Medical School Cohort Study. *Journal of Epidemiology*, *21*(3), 169–175. doi:10.2188/jea.JE20100084 PMID:21389640

Yang, F., Wolk, A., Håkansson, N., Pedersen, N. L., & Wirdefeldt, K. (2017). Dietary antioxidants and risk of Parkinson's disease in two population-based cohorts. *Movement Disorders*, *32*(11), 1631–1636. doi:10.1002/mds.27120 PMID:28881039

Yang, H., & Irudayaraj, J. (2001). Comparison of near-infrared, fourier transform-infrared, and fourier transform-raman methods for determining olive pomace oil adulteration in extra virgin olive oil. *Journal of the American Oil Chemists' Society*, *78*(9), 889. doi:10.100711746-001-0360-6

Yang, S.-F., Yang, W.-E., Kuo, W.-H., Chang, H.-R., Chu, S.-C., & Hsieh, Y.-S. (2008). Antimetastatic potentials of flavones on oral cancer cell via an inhibition of matrix-degrading proteases. *Archives of Oral Biology*, *53*(3), 287–294. doi:10.1016/j.archoralbio.2007.09.001 PMID:17936716

Yarandi, S. S., Peterson, D. A., Treisman, G. J., Moran, T. H., & Pasricha, P. J. (2016). Modulatory effects of gut microbiota on the central nervous system: How gut could play a role in neuropsychiatric health and diseases. *Journal of Neurogastroenterology and Motility*, *22*(2), 201–212. doi:10.5056/jnm15146 PMID:27032544

Yasmin, A., Butt, M. S., Afzaal, M., van Baak, M., Nadeem, M. T., & Shahid, M. Z. (2015). Prebiotics, gut microbiota and metabolic risks: Unveiling the relationship. *Journal of Functional Foods*, *17*, 189–201. doi:10.1016/j.jff.2015.05.004

Yasuda, Y., Shimizu, M., Sakai, H., Iwasa, J., Kubota, M., Adachi, S., ... Moriwaki, H. (2009). (-)-Epigallocatechin gallate prevents carbon tetrachloride-induced rat hepatic fibrosis by inhibiting the expression of the PDGFR beta and IGF-1R. *Chemico-Biological Interactions*, *182*(2-3), 159–164. doi:10.1016/j.cbi.2009.07.015 PMID:19646978

Yehuda, S. (2003). Omega-6/omega-3 ratio and brain-related functions. *World Review of Nutrition and Dietetics*, *92*, 37–56. doi:10.1159/000073791 PMID:14579682

Yen, C. C., Lin, C. Y., Chong, K. Y., Tsai, T. C., Shen, C. J., Lin, M. F., ... Chen, C. M. (2009). Lactoferrin as a natural regimen for selective decontamination of the digestive tract: Recombinant porcine lactoferrin expressed in the milk of transgenic mice protects neonates from pathogenic challenge in the gastrointestinal tract. *The Journal of Infectious Diseases*, *199*(4), 590–598. doi:10.1086/596212 PMID:19125673

Yetukuri, L., Söderlund, S., Koivuniemi, A., Seppänen-Laakso, T., Niemelä, P. S., Hyvönen, M., ... Orešič, M. (2010). Composition and lipid spatial distribution of HDL particles in subjects with low and high HDL-cholesterol. *Journal of Lipid Research*, *51*(8), 2341–2351. doi:10.1194/jlr.M006494 PMID:20431113

Yoshida, H., & Kisugi, R. (2010). Mechanisms of LDL oxidation. *Clinica Chimica Acta*, *411*(23–24), 1875–1882. doi:10.1016/j.cca.2010.08.038 PMID:20816951

Young, N. S., Bacigalupo, A., & Marsh, J. C. (2010). Aplastic anemia: Pathophysiology and treatment. *Biology of Blood and Marrow Transplantation*, *16*(1), S119–S125.

Younis, K., Ahmad, S., & Jahan, K. (2015). Health benefits and application of prebiotics in foods. *Journal of Food Processing & Technology*, *6*, 433. doi:10.4172/2157-7110.1000433

Yu, R., Kim, C. S., Kwon, B. S., & Kawada, T. (2006). Mesenteric adipose tissue-derived monocyte chemo-attractant protein-1 plays a crucial role in adipose tissue macrophage migration and activation in obese mice. *Obesity (Silver Spring, Md.)*, *14*(8), 1353–1362. doi:10.1038/oby.2006.153 PMID:16988077

Yussif, N. M., Abdul Aziz, M. A., & Abdel Rahman, A. R. (2016). Evaluation of the Anti-Inflammatory Effect of Locally Delivered Vitamin C in the Treatment of Persistent Gingival Inflammation: Clinical and Histopathological Study. *Journal of Nutrition and Metabolism*, *2016*, e2978741. doi:10.1155/2016/2978741 PMID:28050280

Yusuf, S., Islam, S., Chow, C. K., Rangarajan, S., Dagenais, G., Diaz, R., ... Avezum, A. (2011). Use of secondary prevention drugs for cardiovascular disease in the community in high-income, middle-income, and low-income countries (the PURE Study): A prospective epidemiological survey. *Lancet*, *378*(9798), 1231–1243. doi:10.1016/S0140-6736(11)61215-4 PMID:21872920

Zafar, S., & Owais, M. (2005). Ethanol production from crude whey by *Kluyveromyces marxianus*. *Biochemical Engineering Journal*, *27*(3), 295–298. doi:10.1016/j.bej.2005.05.009

Zaied, K.A., Kawther, S., & Kash, E.A., & Aliaa, A.D. (2009). Enhancement the Fermentation of Lactose–Whey Using Recombinants between *Lactobacillus* and *Tetragenococcus*. *Australian Journal of Basic and Applied Sciences*, *3*(2), 761–775.

Zecca, L., Youdim, M. B. H., Riederer, P., Connor, J. R., & Crichton, R. R. (2004). Iron, brain ageing and neurodegenerative disorders. *Nature Reviews. Neuroscience*, *5*(11), 863–873. doi:10.1038/nrn1537 PMID:15496864

Zee, J., Carmichael, L., Codère, D., Poirier, D., & Fournier, M. (1991). Effect of storage conditions on the stability of vitamin C in various fruits and vegetables produced and consumed in Quebec. *Journal of Food Composition and Analysis*, *4*(1), 77–86. doi:10.1016/0889-1575(91)90050-G

Zemel, M. B., & Miller, S. L. (2004). Dietary calcium and dairy modulation of adiposity and obesity risk. *Nutrition Reviews*, *62*(4), 125–131. doi:10.1111/j.1753-4887.2004.tb00034.x PMID:15141427

Zhang, L., Cao, H., Wen, J., & Xu, M. (2009). Green tea polyphenol (-)-epigallocatechin-3-gallate enhances the inhibitory effect of huperzine A on acetylcholinesterase by increasing the affinity with serum albumin. *Nutritional Neuroscience*, *12*(4), 142–148. doi:10.1179/147683009X423283 PMID:19622237

Zhang, M., Xuan, S., Bouxsein, M. L., von Stechow, D., Akeno, N., Faugere, M. C., ... Clemens, T. L. (2002). Osteoblast-specific knockout of the insulin-like growth factor (IGF) receptor gene reveals an essential role of IGF signaling in bone matrix mineralization. *The Journal of Biological Chemistry*, *277*(46), 44005–44012. doi:10.1074/jbc.M208265200 PMID:12215457

Zhao, C., Giusti, M. M., Malik, M., Moyer, M. P., & Magnuson, B. A. (2004). Effects of Commercial Anthocyanin-Rich Extracts on Colonic Cancer and Nontumorigenic Colonic Cell Growth. *Journal of Agricultural and Food Chemistry*, *52*(20), 6122–6128. doi:10.1021/jf049517a PMID:15453676

Zhao, L., Lee, J. Y., & Hwang, D. H. (2011). Inhibition of pattern recognition receptor-mediated inflammation by bioactive phytochemicals: A review of recent research. *Nutrition Reviews*, *69*(6), 310–320. doi:10.1111/j.1753-4887.2011.00394.x PMID:21631512

Zhao, S. P., Smelt, A. H., Van den Maagdenberg, A. M., Van Tol, A., Vroom, T. F., Gevers Leuven, J. A., ... Van 't Hooft, F. M. (1994). Plasma lipoprotein profiles of normocholesterolemic and hypercholesterolemic homozygotes for apolipoprotein E2(Arg158-->Cys) compared. *Clinical Chemistry*, *40*(8), 1559–1566. PMID:8044997

Zhou, C., Lin, H., Ge, X., Niu, J., Wang, J., Wang, Y., ... Tan, X. (2015). The Effects of dietary soybean isoflavones on growth, innate immune responses, hepatic antioxidant abilities and disease resistance of juvenile golden pompano Trachinotus ovatus. *Fish & Shellfish Immunology*, *43*(1), 158–166. doi:10.1016/j.fsi.2014.12.014 PMID:25541076

Zhu, Y., Huang, X., Zhang, Y., Wang, Y., Liu, Y., Sun, R., & Xia, M. (2014). Anthocyanin Supplementation Improves HDL-Associated Paraoxonase 1 Activity and Enhances Cholesterol Efflux Capacity in Subjects With Hypercholesterolemia. *The Journal of Clinical Endocrinology and Metabolism*, *99*(2), 561–569. doi:10.1210/jc.2013-2845 PMID:24285687

Zierler-Brown, S. (2007). Nutraceuticals: A Guide for Healthcare Professionals. *American Journal of Pharmaceutical Education, 71*(5). Retrieved from http://www.ncbi.nlm.nih.gov/pmc/articles/ PMC2064899/

Zilberman, D., Yarkin, C., & Heiman, A. (1997, August). *Agricultural biotechnology: economic and international implications.* Invited paper presented at the International Agricultural Economics Association meeting, Sacramento, CA.

Zimmet, P., Alberti, K. G., & Shaw, J. (2001). Global and societal implications of the diabetes epidemic. *Nature, 414*(6865), 782–787. doi:10.1038/414782a PMID:11742409

Zuidam, N., & Shimoni, E. (Eds.). (2010). Encapsulation Technologies for Active Food Ingredients and Food Processing. Springer Science Plus Business Media.

Zunjar, V., Dash, R. P., Jivrajani, M., Trivedi, B., & Nivsarkar, M. (2016). Antithrombocytopenic activity of carpaine and alkaloidal extract of Carica papaya Linn. leaves in busulfan induced thrombocytopenic Wistar rats. *Journal of Ethnopharmacology, 181*, 20–25. doi:10.1016/j.jep.2016.01.035 PMID:26812680

About the Contributors

Raj K. Keservani, M.Pharm, working as Associate Professor, Chhatrapati Shahu Ji Maharaj Group of Institutions, Allahabad Uttar Pradesh, India. He has more than 10 years of academic (teaching) experience from various institutes of India in pharmaceutical education. He has published 35 peer-reviewed papers in the field of pharmaceutical sciences in national and international journals, sixteen book chapters, and nine books as co-author. He is also active as a reviewer for several international scientific journals. His research interests include Nutraceutical and Functional Foods, Novel Drug Delivery Systems (NDDS), Transdermal Drug Delivery/ Drug Delivery, Health Science/Life Science, and Biology/Cancer Biology/Neurobiology. Mr. Keservani graduated with a pharmacy degree from the Department of Pharmacy at Kumaun University, Nainital (UA), India. He received a Master of Pharmacy (MPharm) degree from the School of Pharmaceutical Sciences, Rajiv Gandhi Proudyogiki Vishwavidyalaya (Technical University) Bhopal, India, with a specialization in pharmaceutics.

Anil K. Sharma, MPharm, PhD, is a lecturer at the Delhi Institute of Pharmaceutical Sciences & Research, New Delhi, India. He has published 27 peer-reviewed papers in the field of pharmaceutical sciences in national and international reputed journals as well as fifteen book chapters. In addition he has edited 10 books with publishers of repute. His research interests include nutraceutical and functional foods, novel drug delivery systems (NDDs), drug delivery, nanotechnology, health science/life science, and biology/cancer biology/neurobiology. He graduated with a degree in pharmacy from the University of Rajasthan, Jaipur, India, and received a Master of Pharmacy (MPharm) from the School of Pharmaceutical Sciences, Rajiv Gandhi Proudyogiki Vishwavidyalaya, Bhopal, India, with specialization in pharmaceutics. He has earned his Ph.D. in pharmacy from the University of Delhi.

Rajesh K. Kesharwani, M.Tech, PhD, has more than 8 years of teaching & research experience in various institutes of India, imparting bioinformatics and biotechnology education. He has received several awards, including the NASI-Swarna Jayanti Puruskar-2013 by The National Academy of Sciences of India. He has authored over 34 peer-reviewed articles, sixteen book chapters and six books as co-editor with publishers of repute. He has been a member of many scientific communities as well as a reviewer for many international journals. His research fields of interest are medical informatics, protein structure and function prediction, computer aided drug designing, structural biology, drug delivery, cancer biology and next generation sequence analysis. Dr. Kesharwani received a BSc in biology from Ewing Christian College, Allahabad, India, an autonomous college of University of Allahabad; his MSc (Biochemistry)from Awadesh Pratap Singh University, Rewa, Madhya Pradesh, India; and MTech-IT (Specialization in Bioinformatics) from the Indian Institute of Information Technology, Allahabad, India. He earned his Doctorate (Ph.D.) from the Indian Institute of Information Technology, Allahabad and received a Ministry of Human Resource Development, India, fellowship and Senior Research Fellowship from the Indian Council of Medical Research, India.

* * *

Auni Fatin Abdul Hamid received her BSc in Biochemistry, Iowa State University, Iowa, USA in 2012. She then pursued MSc (Molecular Biology) in 2013 at the Advanced Medical and Dental Institute, Universiti Sains Malaysia. She is currently a PhD candidate in the field of Molecular Pathology. Her work is related to oxidized low-density lipoprotein and its role in cancer biology. She has presented her findings in scientific conferences and postgraduate colloquium.

Sakshi Bajaj is currently working as Assistant Professor, Department of Pharmacognosy, at Delhi Institute of Pharmaceutical Sciences & Research (now known as Delhi Pharmaceutical & Research University), New Delhi, India. Her area of specialization & interest is Isolation & separation of phytoconstituents, standardization of herbal drugs, HPTLC method development & validation etc.

Manisha Choudhary working as Assistant Professor, Nims University Rajasthan Jaipur since June 2014. Her research expertise in metal ion neurotoxicity. She is exploring neurochemical and behavioral changes during neurotoxicity. She has received Best PhD Scholar Award during her PhD and also recipient of prestigious

ELSEVIER London fellowship Award to attend 12th Biennial conference of International Society of Developmental Neuroscience 2012. She has guided many graduate and postgraduate thesis. She has published more than 25 research publications in national and International Journal of repute. She is also member of various International and National Societies (IAN, ISN, ACBI, SFRR, IABS and SOPI).

Shrikant Dhage is Ph.D. (Tech.) Research scholar studying at Department of Pharmaceutical Sciences and Technology, Institute of chemical Technology, Mumbai. He has been awarded research fellowship by University Grant Commission – Special Assistance program (UGC-SAP), Government of India. He has participated in a number of national & international conferences and symposia. He has several technical posters in his credit. He is working on the development of novel excipients for the solubility enhancement of the natural bioactive. He has a keen interest in pharmaceutical innovations specifically related to the novel drug delivery strategies for challenging drug molecules.

John I. Disouza, PhD, is a professor in pharmaceutics and principal at Tatyasaheb Kore College of Pharmacy in Warananagar, India. He has over 17 years of teaching and research experience. He also has an executive MBA (Higher education) degree. Dr. Disouza has written two books and published over 100 research papers in peer reviewed journals. He has worked in diverse research areas including herbal formulations, micro/nanoparticulate, self-emulsifying, liposomal, fast and modified release drug delivery systems. His areas of interest include probiotics, novel diagnostic tools and therapies in cancer, and structural modifications of natural polymers for their pharmaceutical potential. He is an active consultant to pharmaceutical industry.

Srijan Goswami is currently associated as a Assistant Professor at Department of Molecular Biology at Institute of Genetic Engineering, Kolkata, India. He is also an Honorary Professor at Department of Biochemistry of Shree Krishna Biochemic College, Kolkata, India. He is one of the co-founder and Director of Indian School of Complementary Therapy& Allied Sciences, India, (autonomous nonprofit organization for development, promotion and training of complementary medicine and associated sciences). His area of specialization is human genetics, biochemistry and medicine. He completed his Masters in Medical Biotechnology from Institute of Genetic Medicine and Genomic Sciences, Kolkata, India in 2012 and received his B.Sc. (Honours) in Biotechnology from Institute of Genetic Engineering, Kolkata, India in 2010. He is trained in Medical Microbiology from Department of Microbiology, R.G.Kar Medical College Kolkata, India and in Medical Biochemistry from Department of Biochemistry, Calcutta National Medical College, Kolkata, India. He have research and teaching experience of around four years. He has several research publications in various national and international journals and conferences. He is also Editorial Review Member of International Journal of Public Health Management and Ethics, IGI Global, USA.

Charu Gupta (Gold Medal; ICAR-NET, GATE qualified), Assistant Professor, Amity Institute of Herbal Research & Studies, Amity University Uttar Pradesh carries with over 8 years of experience in teaching and research at University level. She has published around 30 research and review papers in SCI journals, authored 4 books and 70 abstracts in both national and international conferences. During her tenure at Amity, she has filed several patents and related to the medicinal plants and microbiology. Her research interests are in probiotics & utilization of agro-industrial wastes for production of value added products.

Sneh Gupta, Principal, RG(PG) college has over 40 years of vast teaching experience in Zoology. She has published around 15 research & review papers, contributed 5 book chapters & has attended several national conferences.

Shahrul Bariyah Sahul Hamid received her PhD in Chemical Pathology from Universiti Sains Malaysia in 2003. In 2004, she was employed as a lecturer at the School of Medical Sciences, Universiti Sains Malaysia. Later in 2010, she joined as a senior lecturer at the Advanced Medical and Dental Institute, Universiti Sains Malaysia. Her expertise is in lipid research and cancer molecular biology. She has published in journals and presented her work in scientific conferences and authored a lipid book for the blind and visually impaired elementary school children.

Amita Joshi has been working as SERB-DST Young Scientist at the Department of Pharmaceutics, B. V. Patel PERD Centre and has more than 10 years of research experience. Dr. Joshi is a post-graduate from Panjab University, Chandigarh and has a doctoral degree from Nirma University, Ahmedabad. Her doctoral work was focused on novel formulation for the treatment of tuberculosis. This novel anti-Tb formulation was later evaluated at AIIMS, New Delhi. Prior to Ph.D., she was associated with Ranbaxy Research Laboratory, Gurgaon, and Cadila Pharmaceuticals, Ahmedabad in formulation development department. Her research areas of interest include lipid-based formulations, lymphatic delivery, and infectious diseases. She has more than 17 international publications, 3 book chapter and 1 patent application to her credit. She has been awarded Gandhian Young Technology Innovation

(GYTI) award in 2015, for her work on lymphatic targeting. She has been awarded best paper presentation award at APTICON 2014. She is the reviewer for projects submitted to Science and Engineering Research Board (SERB), Department of Science and Technology, Govt. of India, New Delhi and also on the reviewing board of the peer-reviewed journals like AAPS Pharm SciTech, International Journal of Nanomedicine, Nanotechnology, ChronoPhysiology and Therapy etc.

Namrata A. Kadwadkar is currently pursuing PhD. (Tech) in Pharmaceutics at Department of Pharmaceutical Sciences and Technology, Institute of Chemical Technology, Mumbai. She has completed Masters in Pharmacognosy and Phytochemistry. She has been awarded research fellowship by University Grant Commission – Special Assistance program (UGC-SAP), Government of India. Her area of research includes Application of Nanophytomedicine using traditional knowledge for treatment of hemoglobinopathies. She has participated and presented in a of national & international conferences and symposia and banked in a few awards as an additional feather in the cap. Her keen interest includes development of nanophytomedicine.

Pratik S. Kakade is senior research fellow perusing Ph.D. (Tech) degree in Department of Pharmaceutical Sciences and Technology at Institute of Chemical Technology, Mumbai, India. He has 3 International publications to his credit. He has participated in various National and International forums as an Oral/Poster presenter and won awards. He has successfully completed industrial M. Pharm and a project on Herbal solid oral dosage form sponsored by an Industry. He was bestowed 'Best outgoing student award' by his alma mater.

Satish Manchanda is occupied at the position of Assistant Professor, Department of Pharmaceutics at Delhi Institute of Pharmaceutical Sciences & Research (now known as Delhi Pharmaceutical & Research University), New Delhi, India. As an academician, he is involved with the postgraduate students in research projects in the area of Pharmaceutics & Quality Assurance along with the regular academic activities of undergraduate students. He is also associated with some professional associations like IPGA etc. His area of interest involves solubility enhancement, drug delivery, particulate drug delivery, HPLC method development & validation etc.

Shivraj Vasantrao Naik is currently pursuing PhD (Tech.) in Pharmaceutics at Department of Pharmaceutical Sciences and Technology, Institute of Chemical Technology, Mumbai. He has completed Master of Technology in Pharmaceutical Technology and secured the first rank in the university. His area of research is 'Development of novel formulations for the treatment of neurodegenerative disease.' He has participated in many national and international conferences and presented his work there. He has a number of technical poster presentations to his credit. He has been awarded research fellowship by University Grant Commission (UGC-SAP), Government of India.

Consuelo Pacheco is a Researcher and Assistant Professor specialized in Food Engineering. She has conducted three research stays at Université de Technologie de Compiègne (FRANCE), Universitat Politècnica de València (SPAIN), and Instituto Politécnico de Veracruz (MEXICO). She has published 7 research papers in SCI journals, 17 works in both national and international conferences and she has collaborated in 2 technological consultancies. She currently works on the microencapsulation of bioactive compounds.

Kiran Shivaji Patil is an assistant professor in quality assurance department at Tatyasaheb Kore College of pharmacy, Warananagar. He has over 06 years of teaching and research experience. He is perusing Ph.D. (Tech) degree in Shivaji University, Kolhapur. He also has an MBA degree in Marketing and Finance. Mr. Kiran Patil has published over 10 research papers and review articles in various national and international journals. He has participated in various National and International conferences, workshops, symposiums and won numerous awards.

Shalaka Ramakant Patki is serving as Assistant Professor in Pharmaceutics at Tatyasaheb Kore College of Pharmacy Warananagar. She has 7 years of teaching & research experience. She has done her M.Pharm in Pharmaceutics and has a Diploma in Drug Regulatory Affairs.She has 8 national and international presentations in various conferences. She has guided a number of degree & postgraduate students. Her research areas include novel drug delivery systems, community pharmacy & regulatory affairs. She has worked as organizing comittee member for various conferences, seminars, FDP's held nationally and internationally. She is a life member of various professional organizations like IPA, APTI, ISTE.

Vandana B. Patravale is currently Professor of Pharmaceutics at the Institute of Chemical technology (previously, UDCT). Her areas of expertise encompass lipid and colloidal drug delivery systems for enhanced solubilisation, bioavailability, and targeting. Her interests additionally include the use of indigenous excipients and development of cosmeceuticals, nutraceuticals, and medical devices. Prof. Patravale owns 8 granted patents, 3 trademark registries and 1 industrial design with 23 additional filed patents in the pipeline that include European as well as US patents. She has over 100 publications in peer reviewed journals and has delivered over 100 invited talks. Prof. Patravale receives and elucidates multifarious projects from the pharmaceutical industry at ICT. She is a recipient of many Government (BRNS, DBT, ICMR, DST, AICTE, UGC) and private grants including Bill and Melinda Gates Foundation grant. She is recipient of VASVIK award, OPPI Pharmaceutical scientist award, P. D. Patil best pharmaceutical scientist award, APTI best teacher award to name a few. She is a reviewer for many international journals. She has been actively collaborating with various Government and private institutes in India and abroad including UK, Japan, Germany, and Switzerland.

Piyasee Paul is currently associated as Assistant Professor at the Department of Genetics of Institute of Genetic Engineering, India. Her area of specialization are Clinical Cytogenetics and Human Genetics. She has teaching and research experience of about 2 years.

Amrita Poonia, PhD, is Assistant Professor in Centre of Food Science and Technology, Institute of Agricultural Sciences, Banaras Hindu University, Varanasi (U.P), India where she teaches various postgraduate and PhD level courses and guides research projects at PhD and masters levels. Her research interest includes development of functional foods; value added dairy products and shelf-stable foods. She has published various research papers in peer –reviewed international and national journals and book chapters. She has attended, chaired and presented various papers at international and national conferences. She is a member of various professional bodies, including the Association of Food Scientists and Technologists (India), the Indian Dairy Association (IDA).

Dhan Prakash has 39 years of research experience in life sciences, worked as guest scientist at GSF-Munich, (GERMANY), Freiburg University, (GERMANY) and Ecole Normale Superieur, Lyon (FRANCE); guided more than 25 Ph. D. thesis, published 152 research papers in SCI journals, 32 book chapters, 177 abstracts in conferences, filed 39 patents and edited 6 books.

Kirti Rani is working as Assistant Professor (III) in Amity Institute of Biotechnology, Amity University Uttar Pradesh, Noida, INDIA (2008-till date). She has done M.Sc in 2000 and Ph.D. in 2004 Biochemistry from Maharashi Dayanand University, Rohtak (INDIA) in the collaboration with Post Graduate Institute of Medical Sciences, Rohtak (INDIA) and in the collaborative research training followed CSIR-Institute of Genomics and Integrative Biology (CSIR-IGIB) New Delhi (2000). She has also worked as Ex-senior resident in Deptt. of Biochemistry, Post Graduate Institute of Medical Education & Research, Chandigarh, INDIA (2004-2007). She is expertise in Enzyme Technology, Clinical Biochemistry & Nanotechnology. She has more than 100 international/ national publications including research articles/ books/ patents/ abstracts in various reputed and peer reviewed journals including RSC, elesvier and Scopus indexed journals and 12 complete filed patents. She is also member, reviewer and editor of various recognized international/ national scientific societies and journals.

Syed Ibrahim Rizvi, Professor since 2006. Working in the area of metabolic syndrome, aging, longevity and natural products. Have published more than 150 research papers. Received research grants from International Foundation for Science, Sweden, Department of Science and Technology, Government of India.

Sandeep Tripathi is associated with the developmental activities of the department since last six years. He is involved in post graduate and doctorate research projects. He has an expertise in neuroscience research (Neurobehavioral and Neurotoxicity), Biomedical Science. He has received Best PhD thesis Award (Gold Medal) from King George's Medical University Lucknow. Received International award "Niloufer Chinoy Award" for the research on fluoride. Received Best paper presentation Award by Association of Clinical Biochemist of India and Nizam Institute of Medical Science, Hyderabad. Many meritorious and appreciation awards received during service period at Nims University. Four PhD students completed their thesis under the supervision of Dr. Tripathi and Four PhDs are under process. He has published 83 national and International papers index journals. He has contributed many chapters in the national and International Books. Dr. Tripathi is the member of editorial board of many journals. He is the member of various International and National Societies (IBRO, ISNR, SOT, IAN, ACBI, SFRR, SOPI, SPGHTN and InSLAR).

Index

O

P

S

T

V

www.ingramcontent.com/pod-product-compliance
Lightning Source LLC
LaVergne TN
LVHW080354011026
849161LV00009B/2297